FRCEM Intermediate SAQ

Volume 2

Moussa Issa

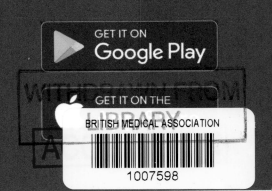

Disclaimer

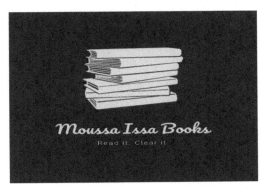

First Edition 2017 by Moussa Issa Bookstore Limited.
Second edition 2018
Third edition 2019
Reprinted with Revisions 2020
Distributed by Moussa Issa Bookstore

ISBN-13: **978-1999957582**
8.5" x 11" (21.59 x 27.94 cm)
BISAC: Medical / Emergency Medicine
Authored by Moussa Issa
Published by: Moussa Issa Bookstore Ltd

Website: www.moussaissabooks.com
Email: info@moussaissabooks.com
eBook subscription: www.moussaissabooks.com/read-ebook-online

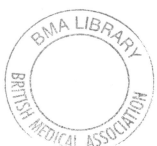

Preface

The Royal College Emergency exams are no mean feat. Anyone who has gone through the process knows the extensive amount of knowledge one needs to amass for these examinations. The new edition of the SAQ intermediate comes at a crucial time in one's preparation for these exams.

This is a constant & fast evolving branch of medicine. As Emergency Medicine Doctors in practice we are required to be quick and efficient decision makers, taking carefully calculated risks but this can be done only on a strong knowledge base. It is exactly this that the College evaluates on, if as Emergency doctors we can make the right decision when the time comes. The new edition of this book endeavours to do just that, prepare you on this journey towards the examination by giving concise and specific points on all topics covered by the syllabus of the Royal college. As new guidelines keep getting published, as changes in treatment and drug therapy keep evolving, it has been my constant endeavour to keep up with these changes.

There are new topics added to this edition:
- ➢ Short and concise Chapters
- ➢ Major changes to resuscitation guidelines.
- ➢ Complete rewriting of Palpitation section.
- ➢ Changes to drug overdose sections in toxicology
- ➢ Acute coronary syndrome management
- ➢ Significant updating of following newly tested topics:
  - ○ Headache Section
  - ○ Dental Emergency
  - ○ Traumatic ocular Injuries
  - ○ Traveller's Fever and Diarrhoea
  - ○ Penile Conditions
  - ○ BRUE, The New ALTE
  - ○ Sepsis, what is Really New?
  - ○ Wound Management
  - ○ Ultrasound in the ED

Relevant guidelines from NICE & from the college have been added on all repeatedly tested topics. To make learning easier, images have been added with details. The format of each topic is covered in bullet points to make learning and retention easy.

The organization of this book is divided according to the curriculum on the RCEM website and follows the pattern of acute and major presentations, Trauma Emergencies, Paediatrics, Anaesthesia, Procedures and Common competencies.

This book was one I first made from my extensive collection of notes which I personally made to study for the MRCEM and FRCEM. And now after successful completion of these exams not just for me but for countless others, I hope this book helps you successfully bridge the gap to success in these daunting but not impossible exams.

Dr Moussa Issa
MBChB MRCEM FRCEM

Acknowledgments

To my wife and children: Marlene, Tatiana, Kevin, Ryan and Brandon. I thank you for your love and support. You've always been by my side and never complained watching me working on my books when you needed me the most.

To my co-Editors: Tina Cardoza, Muhammad Amjad, Faizan Alam and Nasir Mahmood. Thank you for taking the time to lay this out and providing me the inspiration to do this. **Muhammad Amjad** you are an amazing colleague, a kind brother and a great friend; thank you and I appreciate you more than you'll ever know.

To some other important people: Sayed Ramadan, Zain Ul Abadin, Russel Hall, Robyn Pretorius, Rana Tanweer, Moez Ibrahim, Mohanad Ibrahim, Yasser Mohamad, Awwad El Mahdi, Luke Joseph Chirayil, Donna Edano, Abubakar Bin Omer Badam, Pintu Syed, and all the others who took the time to help me find some needed corrections to my books that only made this workbook and latest printing even better. I would like to thank you for your interest in my work and I encourage you to continue to send me your invaluable feedback and ideas for further improvement of the FRCEM Exam book series. I am grateful to you.

To all my clients and Colleagues: Your continued patronage has helped me keep this book running. For this, I never mind the arthritis on my writing hand. We have ventured many roads together, some new and some well-travelled, but we have continued to sharpen each other with patience, perception and perseverance. The pain cannot overcome the happiness that I am feeling right now, thanks to you.

To you: The only thing that can stop you from showing the best results is you being so extremely nervous. There's no need to be scared, buddy. You are ready to show everyone that you are the smartest fella in the world! Good luck!

I feel blessed that social media have given me the chance to reconnect or stay connected with many colleagues all over the world. I am grateful to you all and wish you success throughout your exams. Remember, few years ago, I was also at the beginning like you, with little effort and perseverance, I managed to clear all FRCEM Exams.

An exam is not a game. It's a background for your future.
Wish you to pass all exams.

Dr Moussa Issa
MBChB MRCEM FRCEM

My sources:

Disclaimer: Information and images included in these notes originate from multiples sources such as academic journals, textbooks, published articles, Emergency Medicine websites and Blogs etc.

The Editor and the Publisher have gone to every effort to seek permission from and acknowledge the sources of clinical guidelines and images which appear in this compilation that is public on the internet. Nevertheless, should there be any cases where Copyright holders have not been identified or suitably acknowledged, the author welcome advice from such Copyright holders and will endeavor to amend the text accordingly on future prints.

Many guidelines presented in this book originated from:
- Royal College of Emergency Medicine (www.rcem.ac.uk),
- National Institute for Health and Care Excellence (www.nice.org.uk),
- British Thoracic Society (www.brit-thoracic.org.uk),
- Resuscitation Council UK (www.resus.org.uk),
- American Heart Association (www.heart.org),
- Advanced cardiovascular Life Support (ACLS),
- Advanced Trauma Life Support (ATLS),
- Advanced Paediatric Life Support (APLS),
- Toxbase (www.toxbase.org),
- Life in the fast lane (www.lifeinthefastlane.com)

I owe my dedicated work to the above organizations.

Ebook for only £3/month!

Get our Reading App for your Android smartphone or tablet to start enjoying the Moussa Issa eBookstore discovery and digital reading experience.

Download our APP on your Smart device Now.

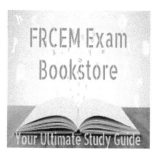

FRCEM Exam eBookstore

FRCEM Exam Bookstore   Books & Reference

▣ PEGI 3

Offers in-app purchases
ⓘ This app is compatible with all of your devices.

Installed

A static eBook with little interactivity cannot draw your attention any more. Thus it is essential to engage readers with interactive reading experience.
Moussa Issa eBookstore proves to be on top of the interactive eBook game, enabling readers to watch integrated videos related to the subject directly on the page.
The additional flipping effect makes the eBook fully interactive and dynamic.

Customize your experience with multiple font and page styles and social sharing tools.

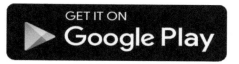
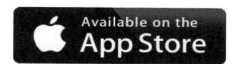

Distributed by Moussa Issa Bookstore Ltd
Website: www.moussaissabooks.com
Email: info@moussaissabooks.com
eBook subscription: www.moussaissabooks.com/read-ebook-online

Table of Contents

Section III: Trauma

Section 3: Trauma

6 Questions

By Moussa Issa

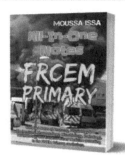 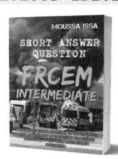 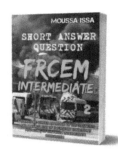
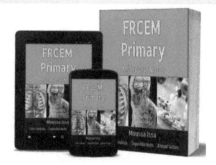 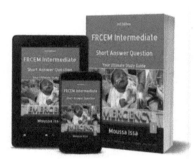 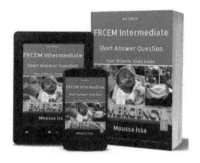
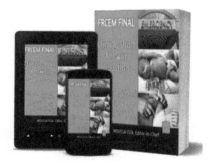 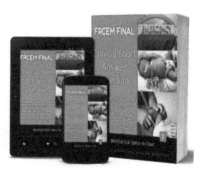 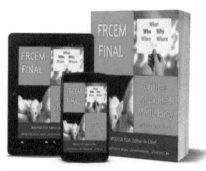
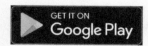
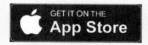

1.ED Approach to Major Trauma
1. INITIAL APPROACH TO TRAUMA

What is major trauma?

- According to the World Health Organization (WHO), road traffic injuries accounted for 1.25 million deaths in 2014, and trauma is expected to rise to the third leading cause of disability worldwide by 2030[1].
- Major trauma is any traumatic injury which involves multiple body areas. The management of major trauma patients involves a systematic approach which starts with a primary survey to identify immediate life threats, and then proceeds to a secondary survey looking for additional injuries which are not life threatening.
- The final tertiary survey is a complete examination of the patient and a review of all the ordered investigations. It occurs in a delayed fashion generally 24 hours after the initial admission to hospital.

What are the criteria for activation of a trauma team?

- Care by specialized trauma teams at designated trauma centers has been shown to improve survival, especially in critically injured patients[2].
- The criteria for activation of a trauma team varies between institutions.
- Generally, the activation is based on three major criteria: **mechanism**, **specific injuries** and **physiological signs**.

1. Mechanism

- Falls > 5 m height.
- High speed motor vehicle accident.
- Ejection from vehicle.
- MBA > 30 kph.
- Pedestrian vs vehicle > 30 kph.
- Fatality in same vehicle.

2. Specific Injuries

- Injury to two or more body regions.
- Spinal Cord Injury.

- Penetrating Injury to Head, Neck, Torso or Proximal Limb.
- Limb amputations (Proximal to wrist and ankle).
- Burns > 15% BSA in adult and > 10% in children, or airway burns.
- Airway Obstruction.
- Multiple Long Bone Fractures.

3. Physiological Derangement

- Systolic BP < 90 mmHg or Pulse > 130 bpm.
- RR < 10 or > 30 per minute.
- GCS < 14/15, or seizures.
- Deterioration in the ED.
- Age > 70 years with chest injury.
- Pregnancy > 24 weeks with torso injury.

Who are the members of a trauma team?

The Trauma Team consists of:

- Trauma Team Leader (usually an Emergency Physician, but can also be a Surgeon)
- Airway Doctor / Nurse
- Procedure or Circulation Doctor
- Nurse (depending on the case, there can be two of these)
- Scribe Nurse
- Trauma Fellow / Surgeon
- Orthopaedic Registrar
- Wardsperson
- Radiographer
- Social Worker
- Blood Bank (required for activation of the massive transfusion protocol)

What are the key steps in assessment and management of a major trauma patient?

The key steps, according to ATLS principles (with a few additions and clarifications) are:

- **Preparation,**
- **Triage**
- **Activation of the trauma resuscitation team.**

- Transfer the patient from the ambulance stretcher to the ED resuscitation bed using spinal injury precautions if indicated.

---

[1] World Health Organization. Global burden of disease. www.who.int/healthinfo/global_burden_disease/en/ (Accessed on May 01, 2010).

[2] MacKenzie EJ, Rivara FP, Jurkovich GJ, Nathens AB, Frey KP, Egleston BL, et al. A national evaluation of the effect of trauma-center care on mortality. N Engl J Med. 2006;354:366–78.

- Obtain a handover from prehospital care providers including history, the mechanism of injury, field treatment, and response to treatment. Obtain vital signs while the patient is being undressed.
- **Primary survey (ABCDE) and resuscitation** as needed, while obtaining large bore IV access. Take blood tests for group and hold/ cross-match, and baseline laboratory testing (e.g. blood gas, Hb, coagulation studies)
- **Adjuncts to primary survey and resuscitation** (IDC, NGT, ECG, monitoring, trauma X-ray series and bedside ultrasound)
- **Consider need for patient transfer** (initiate as soon as adequate information is available)
- **Secondary survey**
- **Adjuncts to the secondary survey** (further imaging and investigations)
- **Continued post-resuscitation monitoring and reevaluation**
- **Definitive care** and disposition

PREPARATION

ATLS describes 2 phases of preparation for major trauma: **prehospital and hospital phases.** Here, we are interested in the latter. This simple set of headings is worth remembering when preparing for the 'hospital phase' management of any critically ill patient: **"PPE"**

- *People*
- *Place*
- *Equipment and drugs*

1. People

- Consider trauma team activation
- Ensure continued safe running of the rest of the emergency department
- Patient and family may need social support.
- Security (especially if gunshot wound... someone might come to finish off the job)
- Notify other hospital areas as required (e.g. radiology, operating theatres, ICU, laboratory)

2. Place

- Ideally a designated trauma bay with facilites for resuscitation

3. Equipment and drugs

- Anticipate what you might need, thinking through systems in an ABCDE approach
- For example: universal precautions, advanced airway equipment, analgesia and rapid sequence intubation drugs, chest tubes, rapid transfusers, activate massive transfusion protocol, pelvic binders, femoral splints, warming equipment, emergency thoracotomy tray.

TRAUMA TEAM AND WHAT ARE THEIR ROLES

- Team structures vary between systems and hospitals. In small centres the team may consist of only a doctor and a nurse. In trauma centres there are defined roles, and the team members assemble when activated by a trauma call.
- More important than the composition of the trauma team is that the team members are trained in the emergency care of trauma patients and work effectively as a team with:
  - *Clear roles and organization*
  - *Effective communication*
  - *Support from other hospital areas, transfer services and trauma centres*

TEAM ROLES INCLUDE:

- **Team Leader** — usually a senior emergency medicine doctor who coordinates assessment and management.
- **Airway doctor** — doctor with advanced airway skills (ED, anaesthetics or ICU)
- **Procedures doctor** — emergency doctor
- **Assessment doctor** — emergency doctor or surgical doctor
- **Airway nurse** — nurse trained to assist with advanced airway management
- **Drugs/ procedures nurse(s)** — nurse(s)s assist with
- **Scribe** — nurse who keeps a real time written record of events and interventions
- **Runners** — healthcare assistants who relay messages, source equipment and assist in transfers

In addition to the trauma/ general surgical doctor, other surgical specialties may be alerted to the trauma call as the scenario demands.
These specialties may include orthopedics, neurosurgery, cardiothoracics, plastics, ENT and ophthalmology. Early notification of operating theatre staff and ICU is also crucial for critically ill trauma patients. Notification of radiography and radiology staff is also a key part of trauma team activation.

What is the standard handover received from the paramedics?

- This is based on 2 acronyms: **MIST & AMPLE:**
  - **M** - Mechanism of Injury
  - **I** - Injuries Sustained
  - **S** - Signs
  - **T** - Treatment and Trends in the Vital Signs
  - **A** – Allergies
  - **M** – Medications
  - **P** - Past Medical History
  - **L** - Last Ate / LMP (in females)
  - **E** - Events (This is usually the MIST)

2. PRIMARY SURVEY

- This is the initial assessment of a major trauma patient, and is designed to identify immediate life-threatening problems[3].
- This used to be an ABCDE approach, but recently C (circulation) has become the number one priority in recognition of hypovolaemic shock being a major cause to mortality: "C-ABCDE"
  - **C**irculation (including haemorrhage control)
  - **A**irway Maintenance (cervical spine control)
  - **B**reathing and Ventilation
  - **C**irculation (reassess again - this is **IMPORTANT**)
  - **D**isability (check neurological status)
  - **E**xposure (undress patient completely - strip and flip, examining both sides of the patient) - cover as soon as practical to prevent hypothermia.

Using a team-based approach, life threatening conditions are identified and management is begun simultaneously.

A. AIRWAY WITH CERVICAL SPINE CONTROL
ASSESSMENT
- **Look** for signs of airway obstruction, examine for airway foreign bodies and injuries to face & neck.
- **Listen** for stridor.
- Always assume a cervical spine injury in any patient with multi-trauma (especially if they have an altered LOC or evidence of injury above the clavicle).
- In general, patients with a GCS < 8/15 are unable to protect their airway.
- Patients with evidence of an airway burn should be intubated early. With severe burns, there can be delayed onset of swelling and airway compromise.

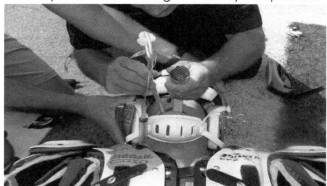

MANAGEMENT
- To relieve obstruction in a trauma patient, the **jaw thrust** technique should only be used as it maintains a neutral alignment of the cervical spine.

- Following a jaw thrust to open the airway, **simple oral airway devices** can be placed as a temporising measure (guerdal and nasopharyngeal).
- Patients requiring airway manouevres to maintain patency should have a **definitive airway** placed (intubation).
- Assume any intubation in a trauma patient will be a difficult airway, and prepare for that (have plan A, B & C ready, and then a few more)
- The usual method of securing the airway in trauma would be via an RSI and endotracheal tube placement.

Indications for advanced airway management (Intubation):
- **A** – e.g.: impending airway obstruction (burns, penetrating or blunt neck injury) or injury that may distort airway anatomy (e.g. neck hematoma)
- **B** – e.g.: Respiratory insufficiency due to a large pulmonary contusion, flail chest, or other thoracic injury.
- **C** – e.g.: multisystem trauma with shock
- **D** – e.g.: Reduced GCS (especially <8), penetrating cranial vault injury

EXAMINATION OF THE NECK OF A TRAUMA PATIENT
Look for **TWELVE things** (OK, there's only six, so check them twice...):
- **T**racheal deviation
- **W**ounds
- **E**xternal markings
- **L**aryngeal disruption
- **V**enous distention
- **E**mphysema (surgical)

These findings suggest life-threatening injuries to the neck or thorax (e.g. tension pneumothorax, cardiac tamponade). I like to look for these when I'm the airway doctor as part of an assessment of A and B. I've specifically stressed the importance of examining the neck because it is easily forgotten when hidden by a hard collar...

B. BREATHING & VENTILATION
ASSESSMENT[4]
- Respiratory rate and SpO2
- **Inspection:** Exposure and inspection essential: external signs of trauma, asymmetrical chest movements
- **Palpation:** over entire chest wall may reveal unsuspected injury e.g. crepitus / surgical emphysema.

---

[3] *Advanced Trauma Life Support® (ATLS) Student Course Manual 10th edition*

[4] *Advanced Trauma Life Support® (ATLS) Student Course Manual 10th edition*

- **Percussion:** often difficult in a noisy trauma bay
- **Auscultation:** listening for air entry bilaterally, gauge adequacy and assess for added sounds
- **Trachea:** palpate to see if deviated, although true tracheal deviation due to a tension pneumothorax is pre-terminal and it is unlikely to be the only sign
- May be appropriate to log roll at this stage if concerned about a posterior chest injury
- **Investigations** should include a chest x-ray and lung ultrasound.

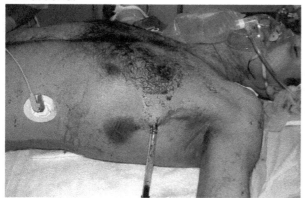

MANAGEMENT

- High flow oxygen 15L/min via non-rebreather mask on arrival. Non-invasive ventilation is rarely indicated in trauma patients.
- Patients requiring respiratory support are usually intubated and mechanically ventilated.
- Needle thoracotomy, finger thoracotomy or intercostal catheter insertion may be required urgently
- **Tension Pneumothorax** - the initial treatment is needle thoracocentesis (this procedure is only effective 50% of the time - if there is a failure, then you should proceed to an open finger thoracostomy).
- Decompression should be immediately followed by a formal intercostal catheter insertion.
- **Massive haemothorax** is defined as greater than 1500 ml blood loss on insertion of an intercostal catheter or persistent blood loss of 200 ml per hour over 2-3 hours.
- In this setting, the patient may need to go to the OT for urgent thoracotomy to control the bleeding.
- Most bleeding will start to settle as the lung re-expands causing a tamponade effect against the chest wall.

C. CIRCULATION & HAEMORRHAGE CONTROL

ASSESSMENT

- Pulse rate, blood pressure, capillary refill and the warmth of peripheries
- Systematically look for evidence of bleeding.

- In a haemodynamically unstable trauma patient there are five potential sites of major blood loss: **"On the floor and the four more"** [5]:
  1. External (Floor),
  2. Thoracic cavity,
  3. Abdominal cavity,
  4. Pelvis and retroperitoneum
  5. The long bones.
- Removal of all prehospital bandaging is vital – a poorly applied 'turban' can mask major scalp haemorrhage.
- Each of these areas needs to be assessed in the setting of major trauma.
- Standard imaging on arrival will include a **CXR, PXR and an eFAST.**

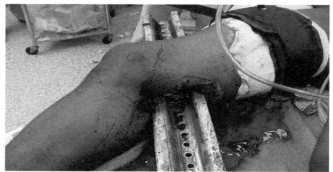

MANAGEMENT

- Insert 2 large bore (at least 16 gauge) intravenous cannulae, ideally in the antecubital fossae.
- If this cannot be rapidly achieved obtain intraosseous access. Send off 'trauma bloods' emergently, most importantly crossmatch blood.
- Venous blood gas is useful for rapid determination of lactate and initial hemoglobin.
- Others tests include full blood count, urea and electrolytes, creatinine, glucose, coagulation profile and lipase. These rarely alter initial management.
- Traditional ATLS teaching is to commence IV fluids - usually Normal Saline or Hartman's Solution (1-2 L STAT). Change to blood if remains haemodynamically unstable after 2 L of crystalloid, or earlier if obvious signs of major bleeding.
- This approach is being superseded by the concept of **damage control resuscitation.**
- **Haemorrhage control:**
  - Most external bleeding can be at least temporarily controlled with direct pressure, tourniquets or by tying off vessels.
  - Other measures are considered in 'major haemorrhage', and ultimately damage control surgery may be needed

---

[5] *Management of Hypovolaemic Shock in the Trauma Patient.pdf*

D. DISABILITY & NEURO EVALUATION

ASSESSMENT

- Assess GCS and document it's components (e.g. E4, V5, M6 = GCS 15)
- Assess pupillary size and responsiveness (if you can open the eyelids due to swelling, consider using ocular ultrasound)
- Assess gross motor and sensory function in all 4 limbs
- If you suspect a spinal injury is present a full neurological assessment is vital at the earliest opportunity — check for priapism, loss of anal sphincter tone and the bulbocavernosus reflex
- Check glucose

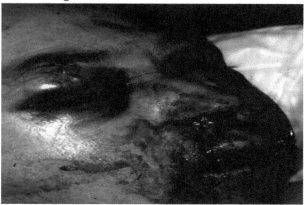

MANAGEMENT

- Airway maintenance (see above)
- Seizure control — midazolam 5-10mg IV, followed by phenytoin 18mg/kg IV over 30 minutes
- Treat hypoglycaemia (glucose <3 mmol/L) with 50 mL 50% glucose
- Anxiety or agitation — treat pain, shock and search for underlying cause
- Treat raised intracranial pressure — 30 degree head up positioning, analgesia and sedation, neuromuscular blockade, mannitol or hypertonic saline, arrange for urgent surgical decompression

E. EXPOSURE AND ENVIRONMENTAL CONTROL

- While maintaining thermostasis, completely expose the patient[6]
- If not yet done, consider log-rolling the patient now
- Areas where potentially life-threating injuries can be missed are:
  - o Back of head
  - o Back
  - o Buttocks
  - o Perineum
  - o Axillae
  - o Skin folds

---

[6] *Advanced Trauma Life Support® (ATLS) Student Course Manual 10th edition*

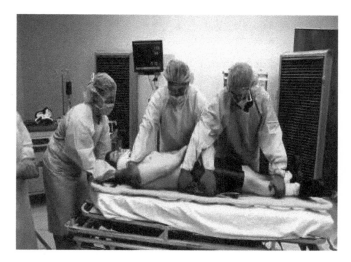

LABORATORY INVESTIGATIONS

In a major trauma patient, a full panel of investigations should be ordered.

- FBC - Hb, Hct, Platelets
- ABG with Lactate - check for ventilatory failure and marker of shock (lactate)
- Coag's - evidence of early trauma associated coagulopathy.
- Blood alcohol
- U&E
- Group and Hold +/- X-Match as indicated.
- ECG
- CXR, PXR
- eFAST (extended FAST ultrasound scan)
- CT scans as indicated (generally in the obtunded major trauma patient a panscan is performed if the patient is haemodynamically stable)
- Urinalysis

3. SECONDARY SURVEY

This is a head to toe examination of the patient looking for other injuries, which are not life threatening.

1. FOCUSED HISTORY AND PHYSICAL EXAM

- The focused history and physical exam include a physical examination that focuses on a specific injury or medical complaint, or it may be a rapid examination of the entire body.
- It also includes obtaining a patient history and vital signs.
- **Patient History**
  - o **S** - Signs/symptoms
  - o **A** - Allergies
  - o **M** - Medications
  - o **P** - Past medical history
  - o **L** - Last oral intake/ **L**MP
  - o **E** - Events leading to the illness or injury

- **Rapid assessment:** This a quick, less detailed head - to toe assessment of the most critical patients

- **Focused assessment:** This is an exam conducted on stable patients. It focuses on a specific injury or medical complaint.

- **Vital signs**
  - This include: BP, HR, RR, SpO2, skin signs, pupils.
  - **Pulse** - Assess for rate, rhythm, and strength
  - **Respiration** - Assess for rate, depth, sound, and ease of breathing
  - **Skin signs** - Assess for color, temperature, and moisture
  - **Pupils** - Check pupils for size, equality, and reaction to light. Constricted pupils in a mass casualty event are highly suggestive of nerve agent/organophosphate toxicity.

2. HEAD TO TOE EXAMINATION OF A TRAUMA PATIENT

- The physical examination of the patient should take no more than two to three minutes
- **Head**
  - Check the scalp for cuts, bruises, swellings, and other signs of injury.
  - Examine the skull for deformities, depressions, and other signs of injury.
  - Inspect the eyelids/eyes for impaled objects or other injury.
  - Determine pupil size, equality, and reactions to light.
  - Note the color of the inner surface of the eyelids.
  - Look for blood, clear fluids, or bloody fluids in the nose and ears.
  - Examine the mouth for airway obstructions, blood, and any odd odours.

- **Neck**
  - Examine the patient for point tenderness or deformity of the cervical spine.
  - Any tenderness or deformity should be an indication of a possible spine injury.
  - If the patient's C-spine has not been immobilized immobilize now prior to moving on with the rest of the exam.
  - Check to see if the patient is a neck breather, check for tracheal deviation.

- **Chest**
  - Examine the chest for cuts, bruises, penetrations, and impaled objects.

  - Check for fractures and Note chest movements a look for equal expansion.
- **Abdomen**
  - Examine the abdomen for cuts bruises, penetrations, and impaled objects.
  - Feel the abdomen for tenderness.
  - Gently press on the abdomen with the palm side of the fingers, noting any areas that are rigid, swollen, or painful.
  - Note if the pain is in one spot or generalized and Check by quadrants and document any problems in a specific quadrant.

- **Lower Back**
  - Feel for point tenderness, deformity, and other signs of injury.

- **Pelvis**
  - Feel the pelvis for injuries and possible fractures.
  - After checking the lower back, slide your hands from the small of the back to the lateral wings of the pelvis.
  - Press in and down at the same time noting the presence of pain and/ or deformity

- **Genital Region**
  - Look for wetness caused by incontinence or bleeding or impaled objects.
  - In male patients check for priapism (persistent erection of the penis). This is an important indication of spinal injury.

- **Lower Extremities**
  - Examine for deformities, swellings, bleedings, discolorations, bone protrusions and obvious fractures.
  - Check for a distal pulse. The most useful is **the posterior tibial pulse** which is felt behind the medial ankle.
  - If a patient is wearing boots and has indications of a crush injury do not remove them.
  - Check the feet for motor function and sensation.

- **Upper Extremities**
  - Examine for deformities, swellings, bleedings, discolorations, bone protrusions and obvious fractures and Check for the **radial pulse** (wrist).
  - In children check for capillary refill. Check for motor function and strength.

2. Shock in Trauma

INITIAL PATIENT ASSESSMENT

- Shock refers to inadequate tissue perfusion, which manifests clinically as hemodynamic disturbances and organ dysfunction. At the cellular level, shock results from insufficient delivery of required metabolic substrates, principally oxygen, to sustain aerobic metabolism. In the setting of trauma, loss of circulating blood volume from hemorrhage is the most common cause of shock.

- Inadequate oxygenation, mechanical obstruction (eg, cardiac tamponade, tension pneumothorax), neurologic dysfunction (eg, high-spinal cord injury), and cardiac dysfunction represent other potential causes or contributing factors[7]. Shock is a common and frequently treatable cause of death in injured patients and is second only to brain injury as the leading cause of death from trauma[8].

- Specific attention should be directed to **pulse rate**, **pulse character**, **respiratory rate**, **skin circulation**, and **pulse pressure** (i.e., the difference between systolic and diastolic pressure).

- To rely solely on systolic blood pressure as an indicator of shock may result in delayed recognition of the shock state. Compensatory mechanisms can preclude a measurable fall in systolic pressure until up to 30% of the patient's blood volume is lost.

- Tachycardia and cutaneous vasoconstriction are the typical early physiologic responses to volume loss in most adults. Any injured patient who is cool and has tachycardia is considered to be in shock until proven otherwise. Occasionally, a normal heart rate or even bradycardia is associated with an acute reduction of blood volume; other indices of perfusion must be monitored in these situations.

- The normal heart rate varies with age. Elderly patients may not exhibit tachycardia because of their limited cardiac response to catecholamine stimulation or the concurrent use of medications, such as ß-adrenergic blocking agents. The ability of the body to increase the heart rate also may be limited by the presence of a pacemaker.

- **A narrowed pulse pressure** suggests significant blood loss and involvement of compensatory mechanisms.

- **Laboratory values for haematocrit or haemoglobin concentration** may be unreliable for estimating acute blood loss and should not be used to exclude the presence of shock.

- Massive blood loss may produce only a minimal acute decrease in the haematocrit or haemoglobin concentration. Thus, a very low haematocrit value obtained shortly after injury suggests either massive blood loss or a preexisting anaemia, whereas a normal haematocrit does not exclude significant blood loss.

- **Base deficit and/or lactate levels** can be useful in determining the presence and severity of shock. Serial measurement of these parameters may be used to monitor a patient's response to therapy.

CAUSE OF SHOCK

- Shock in a trauma patient is classified as haemorrhagic or nonhemorrhagic[9]:

HEMORRHAGIC SHOCK

- Hemorrhagic shock is a condition of reduced tissue perfusion, resulting in the inadequate delivery of oxygen and nutrients that are necessary for cellular function. Whenever cellular oxygen demand outweighs supply, both the cell and the organism are in a state of shock.

- If signs of shock are present, treatment usually is instituted as if the patient is hypovolemic. However, as treatment is instituted, it is important to identify the small number of patients whose shock has a different cause (e.g., a secondary condition such as cardiac tamponade, tension pneumothorax, spinal cord injury, or blunt cardiac injury, which complicates hypovolemic or haemorrhagic shock). Specific information about the treatment of haemorrhagic shock is provided in the next section of this chapter.

- Management priorities in the bleeding patient include controlling blood loss, replenishing intravascular volume and sustaining tissue perfusion.

- In a haemodynamically unstable trauma patient there are five potential sites of major blood loss: externally, long bones, the chest, the abdomen and the retroperitoneum[10].

[7] Britt LD, Weireter LJ Jr, Riblet JL, et al. Priorities in the management of profound shock. Surg Clin North Am 1996; 76:645.

[8] Advanced Trauma Life Support® (ATLS) Student Course Manual 10th edition

[9] Management of Hypovolaemic Shock in the Trauma Patient.pdf

[10] Management of Hypovolaemic Shock in the Trauma Patient.pdf

- Chest x-ray, pelvic x-ray, abdominal assessment with either focused assessment sonography in trauma (FAST) or diagnostic peritoneal lavage (DPL), and bladder catheterization may all be necessary to determine the source of blood loss.

NONHEMORRHAGIC SHOCK

- Nonhemorrhagic shock includes cardiogenic shock, cardiac tamponade, tension pneumothorax, neurogenic shock, and septic shock.

I. HEMORRHAGIC SHOCK

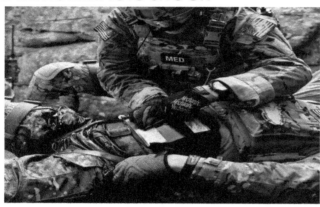

- Hemorrhage is the most common cause of shock in trauma patients.
- Acute blood loss or the redistribution of blood, plasma, or other body fluid predisposes the injured patient to hypovolaemic shock.
- Absolute hypovolaemia refers to the actual loss of volume that occurs in the presence of haemorrhage.
- Relative hypovolaemia refers to the inappropriate redistribution of body fluids such as that that occurs following major burn trauma[11].
- Acute blood loss is a very common problem following traumatic injury.
- Rapid recognition and restoration of homeostasis is the cornerstone of the initial care of any seriously injured patient.
- Delay in recognising and quickly treating a state of shock results in a progression from compensated reversible shock to widespread multiple system organ failure to death.
- Morbidity may be widespread and can include renal failure, brain damage, gut ischaemia, hepatic failure, metabolic derangements, disseminated intravascular coagulation (DIC), systemic inflammatory response syndrome (SIRS), cardiac failure, and death.

- The average adult blood volume represents 7% of body weight (or 70 ml/kg of body weight)[12]. Estimated blood volume (EBV) for a 70 kg person is approximately 5 l.
- Blood volume varies with age and physiologic state.
- When indexed to body weight, older individuals have a smaller blood volume. Children have EBVs of 8–9% of body weight, with infants having an EBV as high as 9–10% of their total body weight[13].
- The blood volume for a child is calculated as 8% to 9% of body weight (80–90 mL/kg).

CLASSIFICATION OF HEMORRHAGE

- The Advanced Trauma Life Support (ATLS) manual produced by the American College of Surgeons describes four classes of hemorrhage to emphasize the early signs of the shock state[14].
- Clinicians should note that significant drops in blood pressure are generally not manifested until Class III hemorrhage develops, and up to 30 percent of a patient's blood volume can be lost before this occurs.
- Class I is a nonshock state, such as occurs when donating a unit of blood, whereas class IV is a preterminal event requiring immediate therapy[15].
- Massive hemorrhage may be defined as loss of total EBV within a 24-hour period, or loss of half of the EBV in a 3-hour period.
  o **Class I hemorrhage:** is exemplified by the condition of an individual who has donated a unit of blood.
  o **Class II hemorrhage:** is uncomplicated haemorrhage for which crystalloid fluid resuscitation is required.
  o **Class III hemorrhage:** is a complicated haemorrhagic state in which at least crystalloid infusion is required and perhaps also blood replacement.
  o **Class IV haemorrhage:** is considered a preterminal event; unless very aggressive measures are taken, the patient will die within minutes.
- Below table outlines the estimated blood loss and other critical measures for patients in each classification of shock.

[11] Jordan KS 2000, Fluid resuscitation in acutely injured patients, Journal of Intravenous Nursing 23(2):81-7, 2000 Mar;-Apr

[12] Kasuya H, Onda H, Yoneyama T, Sasaki T, Hori T. Bedside monitoring of circulating blood volume after subarachnoid hemorrhage. Stroke. 2003;34:956–960.

[13] Changes in blood and plasma volumes during growth. Cropp GJJ Pediatr. 1971 Feb; 78(2):220-9.

[14] Advanced Trauma Life Support® (ATLS) Student Course Manual 10th edition

[15] Committee on Trauma . Advanced Trauma Life Support Manual. Chicago: American College of Surgeons; 1997. pp. 103–112.

- Several confounding factors profoundly alter the classic hemodynamic response to an acute loss of circulating blood volume, and these must be promptly recognized. These factors include:
  o Patient's age
  o Severity of injury, with special attention to type and anatomic location of injury
  o Time lapse between injury and initiation of treatment
  o Prehospital fluid therapy
  o Medications used for chronic conditions
- It is dangerous to wait until a trauma patient fits a precise physiologic classification of shock before initiating appropriate volume restoration.
- Hemorrhage control and balanced fluid resuscitation must be initiated when early signs and symptoms of blood loss are apparent or suspected — not when the blood pressure is falling or absent.
- Bleeding patients need blood!

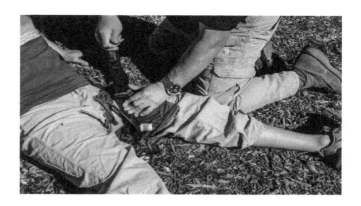

Class of shock	Class I	Class II	Class III	Class IV
Volume Blood loss (ml)	Up to 750	750-1500	1500-2000	>2000
Volume of blood loss (%)	0-15%	15-30%	30-40%	>40%
Heart Rate	<100	>100	>120	>140
Blood Pressure	Normal	Normal	Decrease	Decrease
Pulse Pressure	Normal or increase	Decrease	Decrease	Decrease
Respiratory Rate	14-20	20-30	30-40	>35
Urine output (ml/h)	>30	20-30	5-15	Negligible
Mental State	Slightly anxious	Mildly anxious	Anxious, confused	Confused, lethargic
Initial fluid replacement	Crystalloid	Crystalloid	Crystalloid & blood	Crystalloid & blood

1. CLASS I HEMORRHAGE
- **Up to 15% Blood Volume Loss.**
- The heart rate is minimally elevated or normal, and there is no change in blood pressure, pulse pressure, or respiratory rate.
- For otherwise healthy patients, this amount of blood loss does not require replacement, because transcapillary refill and other compensatory mechanisms will restore blood volume within 24 hours, usually without the need for blood transfusion.

2. CLASS II HEMORRHAGE
- **15% to 30% Blood Volume Loss.**
- In a 70-kg male, volume loss with class II haemorrhage represents 750 to 1500 mL of blood.
- It is manifested clinically as tachycardia (heart rate of 100 to 120), tachypnea (respiratory rate of 20 to 24), and a decreased pulse pressure, although systolic blood pressure (SBP) changes minimally if at all. The skin may be cool and clammy, and capillary refill may be delayed.
- Despite the significant blood loss and cardiovascular changes, urinary output is only mildly affected. The measured urine flow is usually 20-30mL/hour in an adult.
- Accompanying fluid losses can exaggerate the clinical manifestations of class II hemorrhage. Some patients in this category may eventually require blood transfusion, but most are stabilized initially with crystalloid solutions.

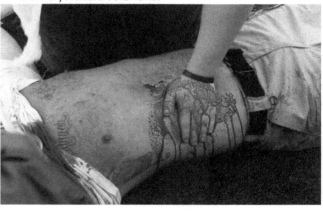

3. CLASS III HEMORRHAGE
- **30% to 40% Blood Volume Loss.**
- The blood loss with class III hemorrhage (approximately **1500–2000 mL in an adult**) can be devastating.
- It results in a significant drop in blood pressure and changes in mental status. Any hypotension (SBP less than 90 mmHg) or drop in blood pressure greater than 20 to 30 percent of the measurement at presentation is cause for concern.

- While diminished anxiety or pain may contribute to such a drop, the clinician must assume it is due to hemorrhage until proven otherwise.
- Heart rate (≥120 and thready) and respiratory rate are markedly elevated, while urine output is diminished.
- Capillary refill is delayed.
- Patients with this degree of blood loss almost always require transfusion. However, the priority of initial management is to stop the hemorrhage, by emergency operation or embolization if necessary.
- Most patients in this category will require packed red blood cells (pRBCs) and blood product resuscitation in order to reverse the shock state.
- The decision to transfuse blood is based on the patient's response to initial fluid resuscitation.

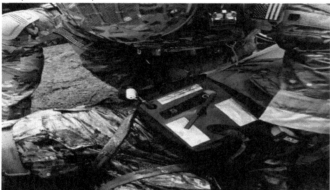

4. CLASS IV HEMORRHAGE

- **More than 40% Blood Volume Loss** leading to significant depression in blood pressure and mental status. Most patients in Class IV shock are hypotensive (SBP less than 90 mmHg).
- Pulse pressure is narrowed (≤25 mmHg), and tachycardia is marked (>120 beats per minute). Urine output is minimal or absent.
- The skin is cold and pale, and capillary refill is delayed.

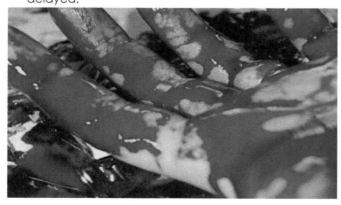

- Patients with class IV hemorrhage frequently require rapid transfusion and immediate surgical intervention.

- Loss of more than 50% of blood volume results in loss of consciousness and decreased pulse and blood pressure.

ED MANAGEMENT OF HEMORRHAGIC SHOCK

- Management priorities in the bleeding patient include controlling blood loss, replenishing intravascular volume and sustaining tissue perfusion[16]. When services are needed that exceed available resources, it is of critical importance that early consultation with a trauma specialist and rapid transportation to definitive care occurs.

PHYSICAL EXAMINATION

- The physical examination is directed toward the immediate diagnosis of life-threatening injuries and includes assessment of the ABCDEs.
- Baseline recordings are important to monitor the patient's response to therapy, and measurements of vital signs, urinary output, and level of consciousness are essential.
- A more detailed examination of the patient follows as the situation permits.

AIRWAY AND BREATHING

- Establishing a patent airway with adequate ventilation and oxygenation is the first priority.
- Supplementary oxygen is provided to maintain oxygen saturation at greater than 95%.

CIRCULATION—HEMORRHAGE CONTROL

- Priorities for managing circulation include controlling obvious hemorrhage, obtaining adequate intravenous access, and assessing tissue perfusion. Bleeding from external wounds usually can be controlled by direct pressure to the bleeding site, although massive blood loss from an extremity may require a tourniquet.
- A sheet or pelvic binder from an extremity may be used to control bleeding from pelvic fractures.
- The adequacy of tissue perfusion dictates the amount of fluid resuscitation required.
- Surgical or angiographic control may be required to control internal hemorrhage. The priority is to stop the bleeding, not to calculate the volume of fluid lost.

DISABILITY—NEUROLOGIC EXAMINATION

- A brief neurologic examination will determine the patient's level of consciousness, eye motion and pupillary response, best motor function, and degree of sensation.

[16] Nolan J 2001, Fluid resuscitation for the trauma patient, Resuscitation, 48(1):57-69.

- This information is useful in assessing cerebral perfusion, following the evolution of neurologic disability, and predicting future recovery.
- Alterations in CNS function in patients who have hypotension as a result of hypovolemic shock do not necessarily imply direct intracranial injury and may reflect inadequate brain perfusion.
- Restoration of cerebral perfusion and oxygenation must be achieved before ascribing these findings to intracranial injury.

EXPOSURE—COMPLETE EXAMINATION

- After lifesaving priorities are addressed, the patient must be completely undressed and carefully examined from head to toe to search for associated injuries.
- When undressing the patient, it is essential to prevent hypothermia. The use of fluid warmers and external passive and active warming techniques are essential to prevent hypothermia.

GASTRIC DILATION—DECOMPRESSION

- Gastric dilation often occurs in trauma patients, especially in children, which can cause unexplained hypotension or cardiac dysrhythmia, usually bradycardia from excessive vagal stimulation.
- In unconscious patients, gastric distention increases the risk of aspiration of gastric contents, which is a potentially fatal complication.
- Proper positioning of the tube does not completely obviate the risk of aspiration.

URINARY CATHETERIZATION

- Bladder catheterization allows for assessment of the urine for hematuria (indicating the retroperitoneum may be a significant source of blood loss) and continuous evaluation of renal perfusion by monitoring urinary output.
- **Blood at the urethral meatus** or a **high-riding, mobile, or nonpalpable prostate** in males is an absolute contraindication to the insertion of a transurethral catheter prior to radiographic confirmation of an intact urethra.

INITIAL FLUID THERAPY

- If blood products are not immediately available, we suggest that initial fluid resuscitation for trauma patients in hemorrhagic shock consist of **500 mL boluses of isotonic crystalloid** given as rapidly as possible through short, large gauge (16 or larger) peripheral IVs.
- Fluid resuscitation using such boluses continues until blood products are available or a systolic blood pressure (SBP) of 90 mmHg is achieved.

- Central venous catheters are used when peripheral IVs are not available. Many hospitals have blood products immediately available in the emergency department (ED). In such hospitals, immediate transfusion of blood products, rather than fluid resuscitation, can be performed for patients with severe hemorrhage in obvious need of transfusion.
- Absolute volumes of resuscitation fluids should be based on patient response.
- The patient's response is observed during this initial fluid administration, and further therapeutic and diagnostic decisions are based on this response.
- It is most important to assess the patient's response to fluid resuscitation and identify evidence of adequate end-organ perfusion and oxygenation (i.e., via urinary output, level of consciousness, and peripheral perfusion).
- If blood pressure is raised rapidly before the hemorrhage has been definitively controlled, increased bleeding can occur. Persistent infusion of large volumes of fluid and blood in an attempt to achieve a normal blood pressure is not a substitute for definitive control of bleeding. Excessive fluid administration can exacerbate the lethal triad of **coagulopathy, acidosis, and hypothermia** with activation of the inflammatory cascade.
- Fluid resuscitation and avoidance of hypotension are important principles in the initial management of blunt trauma patients, particularly those with traumatic brain injury (TBI).
- In penetrating trauma with hemorrhage, delaying aggressive fluid resuscitation until definitive control may prevent additional bleeding.
- Although complications associated with resuscitation injury are undesirable, the alternative of exsanguination is even less so. A careful, balanced approach with frequent re-evaluation is required.
- Balancing the goal of organ perfusion with the risks of rebleeding by accepting a lower-than-normal blood pressure has been termed **"controlled resuscitation," "balanced resuscitation," "hypotensive resuscitation," and "permissive hypotension."**
- The goal is the balance, not the hypotension.
- Such a resuscitation strategy may be a bridge to, but is not a substitute for, definitive surgical control of bleeding.
- Challenges in the diagnosis and treatment of shock include equating blood pressure with cardiac output, extremes of age, athletes, pregnancy, medications, hypothermia, and pacemakers.

Management according to clinical scenario

1. SEVERE ONGOING HEMORRHAGE

- For trauma patients with severe, ongoing hemorrhage that is unlikely to be controlled quickly or adequately, we suggest immediate transfusion of blood products in a **1:1:1 ratio of PRBCs, fresh frozen plasma (FFP), and platelets.** The hospital's massive transfusion protocol (MTP) should be activated immediately in such circumstances.
- In other words, as soon as the treating clinician recognizes that the patient will require 4 or more units of PRBCs over one hour (or 10 or more units over 6 hours), he or she should begin transfusing 6 units of PRBCs, 6 units of FFP, and 6 units of random donor platelets (or 1 unit of apheresis platelets). Note that 1 unit of apheresis platelets is equivalent to 6 units of non-apheresis (ie, random donor or whole-blood derived) platelets. Evidence to support this approach of transfusing components in a 1:1:1 ratio is presented separately.
- **Tranexamic acid (TXA)** may be given to trauma patients with signs of significant hemorrhage who present within three hours of injury.
- **Hypothermia** must be controlled during transfusions.
- Excessive infusion of crystalloid (ie, ratio of crystalloid to PRBCs >1.5:1) has been associated with worse outcomes in patients with severe hemorrhage and should be avoided.

2. MASSIVE TRANSFUSION PROTOCOL

- A massive transfusion protocol (MTP) should be in place for any hospital that manages trauma.
- This protocol should be activated in anticipation of the need for large-scale transfusion or as soon as the clinician treating the patient recognizes the presence or likelihood of severe, ongoing hemorrhage. Traditionally, a massive transfusion was considered 10 units of PRBCs or more transfused over a 24-hour period, but many experts now advocate a revised definition of 10 units or more transfused over 6 hours. We prefer the revised definition.
- Determining when to initiate an MTP has been the subject of considerable research. As early implementation of massive transfusion in the appropriate patient improves outcomes, identifying those trauma patients early in their ED course is important[17]. While a number of scores have been developed for this purpose, the Assessment of Blood Consumption (ABC) score has been validated and is easy to use.

- The ABC score relies on 4 parameters that can be determined upon arrival to the ED:
  - Penetrating mechanism of injury
  - Positive FAST (Focused Assessment with Sonography in Trauma) examination (ie, evidence of hemorrhage)
  - SBP of 90 mmHg or less
  - Heart rate of 120 beats per minute (bpm) or greater
  - Each positive parameter receives a score of one. A score of 2 or more predicts the need for massive transfusion with a sensitivity of 75 percent and a specificity of 86 percent.

3. MODERATE ONGOING HEMORRHAGE

- For patients with bleeding that is not massive but is ongoing and significant (eg, more than 4 units of PRBCs are transfused in the first few hours, or chest tube continues to drain >200 mL of blood per hour), we suggest using the same transfusion ratios used for patients with severe hemorrhage: a **1:1:1 ratio of PRBCs, FFP, and random donor platelets**.
- Hypothermia must be controlled during transfusions.

4. BLEEDING READILY CONTROLLED IN ED

- Severe bleeding can sometimes be controlled effectively in the ED or trauma bay. Closure of scalp lacerations and compression of venous extremity wounds reduce the threat of further bleeding, even though significant hemorrhage may have occurred. Application of a tourniquet can prevent further bleeding from what would otherwise be a life-threatening extremity wound.
- Whether to transfuse after bleeding has been controlled depends on the clinical situation and the patient's underlying comorbidities. Patients that are experiencing symptoms due to anemia from blood loss may require transfusion even after bleeding is well controlled. As an example, a patient with coronary artery disease who is experiencing chest pain suggestive of an acute coronary syndrome should be given blood.
- There is no evidence of benefit from transfusing patients in whom bleeding has been controlled and who are not experiencing any symptoms related to anemia. Therefore, we do not recommend transfusion in this situation.

5. FLUID RESUSCITATION AND BLOOD TRANSFUSION IN THE PATIENT TO BE TRANSFERRED

- Clinicians transferring trauma patients for definitive care must determine what fluids or blood products to send with the patient. The answer depends on the clinical scenario, including the extent of known or suspected injuries, the blood products available, and the capabilities of the transport team.

[17] *Cantle PM, Cotton BA. Prediction of Massive Transfusion in Trauma. Crit Care Clin 2017; 33:71.*

- Radiology studies in patients to be transferred should be kept to a minimum and focus only on identifying pathology that the transferring center is capable of addressing. Transfer must not be delayed to perform radiology or laboratory studies that cannot be acted on prior to transfer.
- Sometimes it is necessary to transfer a patient being actively resuscitated for as yet unknown injuries.
- In these situations, we recommend limiting the administration of crystalloid prior to transfer (in part to prevent infusions of large volumes during transfer), and emphasizing transfusion of blood products in a 1:1:1 ratio whenever possible.
- We exceed two liters of crystalloid only if blood products are not available. If only one blood product can accompany the patient during transfer, PRBCs should be taken, bearing in mind the ultimate goal of giving a **1:1:1 ratio** of blood products[18].
- Prior to arrival at a trauma center where definitive management of the bleeding can take place, a goal of SBP >90 with a MAP of 65 mmHg for penetrating trauma, and a MAP of 85 mmHg for blunt trauma with possible head injury is appropriate.

6. SPINAL CORD INJURY IN THE SETTING OF HEMORRHAGIC SHOCK

- Patients with a spinal cord injury (SCI) who are in hemorrhagic shock pose a special challenge.
- While controlled hypotension may be appropriate for many trauma patients, those with SCI, like those with traumatic brain injury, are at greater risk for complications from hypotension. Thus, a higher blood pressure is needed to ensure adequate perfusion of the spinal cord.
- Guidelines from 2013 recommend **maintaining a MAP of at least 85 to 90 mmHg for patients with SCI**, and subsequent studies support this goal[19]. Acute SCI and the management of TBI are discussed separately.
- In the uncommon circumstance when hemorrhagic shock and SCI coexist, the most immediate life threat is blood loss. Therefore, transfusion of blood products is prioritized. However, long-term morbidity in such patients depends largely upon the ability to maintain MAP in the goal range.

- Thus, vasopressor therapy should be added expeditiously if an appropriate MAP cannot be achieved with blood products alone.
- For patients with SCI and hemorrhagic shock, we recommend transfusing blood as described above for patients with severe ongoing bleeding, with the goal of maintaining a MAP of 85 to 90 mmHg.
- Vasopressor therapy is needed for patients with SCI when blood products alone have failed to raise or maintain the MAP in the 85 to 90 mmHg range.
- While there is no clearly defined combination of blood products and vasopressor treatment for these patients, **norepinephrine** is recommended over dopamine or phenylephrine by some authorities when vasopressors are required for patients with SCI, and we concur with this approach[20].
- Patients with SCI and hemorrhagic shock who are being transferred should be sent with both blood products and norepinephrine, assuming each is available, and managed using the same approach: give blood products first and add the vasopressor if MAP goals are not achieved.

7. PREGNANT PATIENT WITH HEMORRHAGE

- The indications for and general approach to fluid resuscitation and blood transfusion do not differ in the pregnant trauma patient.
- Evaluation and management of the pregnant trauma patient are reviewed in detail separately.
- Important considerations related to hemorrhage in the pregnant patient include:
  o Rapid obstetrical consultation should be obtained in case cesarean delivery is needed.
  o Displacing the uterus to the patient's left side may significantly improve cardiac output.
  o Substantial changes in vital signs may not occur until more than 20 percent of total blood volume has been lost due to the hypervolemia and normal physiology of pregnancy.
  o Fetal heart rate monitoring, when appropriate based on viability (>20 weeks gestation), is essential for determining the condition of the fetus.
  o Treatment with **anti-D immune globulin** may be needed. Rh(D)-negative women with abdominal or pelvic trauma or with vaginal bleeding (who are not already alloimmunized, if this is known) should receive anti-D immune globulin, per standard protocols.

---

[18] Cannon JW, Khan MA, Raja AS, et al. Damage control resuscitation in patients with severe traumatic hemorrhage: A practice management guideline from the Eastern Association for the Surgery of Trauma. J Trauma Acute Care Surg 2017; 82:605.

[19] Hawryluk G, Whetstone W, Saigal R, et al. Mean Arterial Blood Pressure Correlates with Neurological Recovery after Human Spinal Cord Injury: Analysis of High Frequency Physiologic Data. J Neurotrauma 2015; 32:1958.

[20] Inoue T, Manley GT, Patel N, Whetstone WD. Medical and surgical management after spinal cord injury: vasopressor usage, early surgerys, and complications. J Neurotrauma 2014; 31:284.

INITIAL ASSESSMENT & SHOCK MANAGEMENT

Condition	Assessment (physical examination)	Management
Tension pneumothorax	• Tracheal deviation • Distended neck veins • Tympany • Absent breath sounds	• Needle decompression • Tube thoracostomy
Massive hemothorax	• Tracheal deviation • Flat neck veins • Percussion dullness • Absent breath sounds	• Venous access • Volume replacement • Surgical consultation • Thoracotomy • Tube thoracostomy
Cardiac tamponade	• Distended neck veins • Muffled heart tones • Ultrasound	• Venous access • Volume replacement • Thoracotomy • Pericardiocentesis
Intraabdominal hemorrhage	• Distended abdomen • Uterine lift, if pregnant • DPL • Ultrasonography • Vaginal examination	• Venous access • Volume replacement • Surgical consultation • Displace uterus from vena cava
Obvious external bleeding	• Identify source of obvious external bleeding	• Direct pressure • Splints • Closure of actively bleeding scalp wounds

PELVIC FRACTURES

Condition	Image findings	Significance	Intervention
	Pelvic x-ray		
Pelvic fracture	• Pubic ramus fracture	• Less blood loss than other types • Lateral compression mechanism	• Volume replacement • Probable transfusion • Decreased pelvic volume • Pelvic binder • External fixator • Angiography • Skeletal traction • Orthopaedic consultation
	• Open book	• Pelvic volume increased • Major source of blood loss	
	• Vertical shear	• Major source of blood loss	
Visceral organ injury	• CT scan		
	• Intra-abdominal hemorrhage	• Potential for continuing blood loss • Performed only in hemodynamically normal patients	• Volume replacement • Possible transfusion • Surgical consultation

3. Burns and Scalds

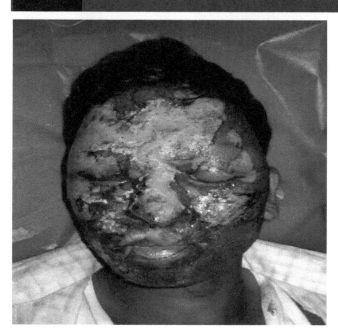

DEFINITION

- Burns are commonly thought of as injury to the skin caused by excessive heat.
- More broadly, burns result from traumatic injuries to the skin or other tissues primarily caused by thermal or other acute exposures.
- Burns occur when some or all of the cells in the skin or other tissues are destroyed by heat, electrical discharge, friction, chemicals, or radiation.
- Burns are acute wounds caused by an isolated, non-recurring insult, and healing ideally progresses rapidly through an orderly series of steps[21].

TYPES OF BURN

- **Thermal:**
  o The depth of the thermal injury is related to contact temperature, duration of contact of the external heat source, and the thickness of the skin.
  o Because the thermal conductivity of skin is low, most thermal burns involve the epidermis and part of the dermis[22].
  o The most common thermal burns are associated with flames, hot liquids, hot solid objects, and steam.

- **Chemical:**
  o Injury is caused by a wide range of caustic reactions, including alteration of pH, disruption of cellular membranes, and direct toxic effects on metabolic processes.
  o In addition to the duration of exposure, the nature of the agent will determine injury severity.
  o Contact with acid causes coagulation necrosis of the tissue, while alkaline burns generate liquefaction necrosis.
  o Systemic absorption of some chemicals is life-threatening, and local damage can include the full thickness of skin and underlying tissues.

- **Electrical:**
  o Electrical energy is transformed into heat as the current passes through poorly conducting body tissues. Electroporation (injury to cell membranes) disrupts membrane potential and function. The magnitude of the injury depends on the pathway of the current, the resistance to the current flow through the tissues, and the strength and duration of the current flow. It is still very important that domestic electrical burns are taken seriously and an ECG is performed as the alternating nature of domestic current can cause arrhythmias.

- **Cold exposure (frostbite):**
  o These burns are caused by ice crystals which can form both intra and extracellularly. The subsequent fluid and electrical fluxes cause cell membrane lysis and cell death and a damaging inflammatory process is set up.

- **Radiation:**
  o Radio frequency energy or ionizing radiation can cause damage to skin and tissues. The most common type of radiation burn is the sunburn.
  o Radiation burns are most commonly seen today following therapeutic radiation therapy and are also seen in patients who receive excessive radiation from diagnostic procedures. Radiation burns can be seen in individuals who work in the nuclear industry.
  o Radiation burns are often associated with cancer due to the ability of ionizing radiation to interact with and damage DNA.

---

[21] *Surgical management of the burn wound and use of skin substitutes.*

[22] *Orgill DP, Solari MG, Barlow MS, O'Connor NE. A finite-element model predicts thermal damage in cutaneous contact burns. J Burn Care Rehabil 1998; 19:203.*

o The clinical results of ionizing radiation depend on the dose, time of exposure, and type of particle that determines the depth of exposure. Depending on the photon energy, radiation can cause very deep internal burns.

- **Higher risk groups include:**
  o Children
  o Older adults
  o Alcoholics,
  o Epileptics,
  o Those with chronic psychiatric or medical conditions
  o Those who have a low socio-economic status.

INITIAL ASSESSMENT & RESUSCITATION

A. AIRWAY
- Despite advances in ventilatory management, inhalation injury remains a leading cause of death in adult burn victims[23]. It is critical to maintain the airway and provide supplemental oxygen in patients with major burns[24].

The airway is at risk by three major mechanisms:
- **Generalized oedema:** can cause swelling of the airway and compromise airflow.
- **Localized oedema:** can obstruct airflow.
- **Inhalation injury:** can cause damage to the airway.

ASSESSMENT
Factors that increase the suspicion of airway obstruction or inhalation injury include:

1. Hoarse voice
2. Carbonaceous sputum
3. Raised carbon monoxide (CO)
4. Deep facial burns
5. A history of burns in an enclosed space
6. Respiratory distress
7. Stridor
8. Depressed mental status, including evidence of drug or alcohol use
9. Nares with inflammation or singed hair
10. Blistering or edema of the oropharynx

Airway compromise can develop over a matter of hours and may only come to light when the patient is in crisis. Figure below shows airway change over a period of 1 hour.

---

[23] *Bloemsma GC, Dokter J, Boxma H, Oen IM. Mortality and causes of death in a burn centre. Burns 2008; 34:1103.*

[24] *Cancio LC. Airway management and smoke inhalation injury in the burn patient. Clin Plast Surg 2009; 36:555.*

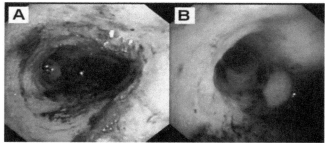
Smoke Inhalation Lung Injury

MANAGEMENT
1. Sit patient upright
2. Senior anaesthetic review if any suspected airway injury to identify and predict deterioration.
3. If indicated, **early intubation** with an uncut tube prevents the tube moving in the event of further swelling.

B. BREATHING
Gas exchange can be compromised for a number of reasons:
- Direct lower airway and gas exchange surface **damage** from inhalation injury
- **Carbon monoxide (CO)** can quickly build up impairing oxygen carrying capacity.
- **Eschar:** Burnt tissues with significant loss of the elasticity in superficial fibres are known as an **eschar.** This creates a constricting effect and inhibits expansion. When circumferential around the chest/torso/neck this can lead to impaired chest expansion and subsequent ventilation.

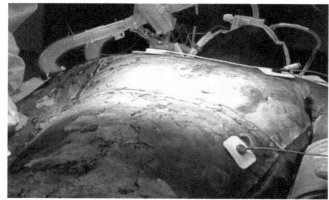

ASSESSMENT:
- Exposure of the chest to perform comprehensive assessment of ventilation and any injury to the chest. Prompt assessment of oxygenation with saturation probe
- Baseline ABG/VBG (if there is a reliable saturation trace) to assess oxygenation, ventilation and CO.

MANAGEMENT

1. **Supplementary oxygen** to target appropriate saturations of 94-98%
2. Immediate discussion with burns center if any restriction of movement of chest
3. Suspected inhalation injury may warrant **intubation.**

- *Escharotomy can be a lifesaving procedure that relieves restriction of movement and allows chest expansion.*
- *Cyanide poisoning is common in patients that have been exposed to inhalation of burnt household items. In profound hypoxia consider early administration of* **cyanokit.**

C. CIRCULATION

- Burns **>15% BSA in Adults and >10% in children** can cause profound circulatory shock that can occur from both large fluid losses through tissue damage and from a systemic inflammatory response.
- Haemodynamic instability is rarely due to the burn alone and should prompt us to look for other causes
- Circumferential limb burns can compromise blood supply distally

ASSESSMENT

- Burns <15% in adults and <10% in children do not require immediate fluid resuscitation
- Capillary refill time (CRT), blood pressure and mucous membrane assessment are important indicators of hydration status but may be hard to measure due to location of the burn.
- Though rarely immediately helpful in the Emergency Department setting, **early catheterization** is important as urine output is a reliable sign that can demonstrate poor perfusion and serve as a guide to ongoing resuscitation. In a significant burn there can be an increased metabolic demand on the patient which can cause organ dysfunction.
- Therefore, important baseline tests to consider are FBC, U&E, LFT, coagulation profile, amylase, CRP and capillary blood glucose. This also helps to identify any other issues impacting on the patient. If the patient is likely to go to theatre a serum group and save is warranted.
- In circumferential limb burns, blood supply to the extremities should be checked regularly. If unable to do this clinically, a Doppler ultrasound can be used.

MANAGEMENT

1. Immediate intravenous (IV) access and, if required, fluid resuscitation are critical steps in initial care.
2. Blood tests
3. Evaluate any areas of circumferential burns in limbs and regularly reassess perfusion
4. Any deterioration in the circulation to a limb could indicate ischemia or a compartment syndrome. This warrants immediate discussion with a burns center and may require urgent intervention such as escharotomy or fasciotomy.

FLUIDS

- Adequate volume replacement decreases the morbidity and mortality associated with severe burn injury. The goal of initial fluid resuscitation is to restore and maintain vital organ perfusion.
- In adults, IV fluid resuscitation is usually necessary in second- or third-degree burns involving greater than 20% TBSA[25].
- There are a number of methods to calculate appropriate fluid replacement. One of the most used is the **Parkland equation:**

2-4mls x % BSA of Burn x weight in kg

- This estimates the recommended total fluid administration **over 24 hours.** Half of this volume should be administered over the first **8 hours from the time of the burn.** This fluid, ideally a warmed physiological crystalloid e.g. Hartmann's should be administered **in addition to the maintenance fluids.**
- Careful monitoring is paramount as adjustments may be needed to achieve an appropriate urine output of 0.5ml/kg/hr.

D. DISABILITY AND EXPOSURE

- Like any trauma patient disability and exposure cannot be ignored.
- Appropriate exposure is fundamental for the assessment of patients with burns.
- A thorough assessment of size and depth of burns is impossible without **full exposure** and a good secondary survey. However, patients with burns are physiologically vulnerable to getting cold so it is critical to keep them warm and minimize fluid loss.

---

[25] *Morehouse JD, Finkelstein JL, Marano MA, et al. Resuscitation of the thermally injured patient. Crit Care Clin 1992;8:355-365.*

MANAGEMENT

1. Consideration should be made to **maintain body temperature** by both **active and passive warming.**
2. This is balanced with the need to adequately expose the burn in order to assess, photograph and clean.
3. Clean the burn with normal saline and cover with strips of cling film. Do not use cling film on the face.
4. Consider imaging e.g. X-ray, CT etc. based on findings of the secondary survey
5. Consider Analagesia

ASSESSING THE EXTENT OF A BURN

In order to guide management goals, it is important to assess both **extent** and **depth** of the burn.

In order to assess the extent of a burn it is vital to expose all areas to accurately estimate correct % BSA affected.

This can help:

- Predict the physiological response the body will have to the burn
- Calculate the fluid requirement during the initial resuscitation period
- Burns are graded into **Severe** and **Non-Severe** according to the physiological effect exerted on the body.
- **Severe burns** are defined as a **>10% BSA in a child and >15% BSA in an Adult**

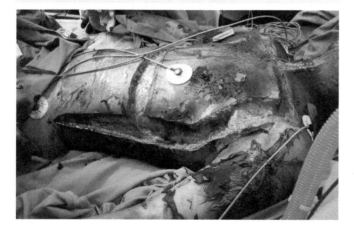

COMMON TOOLS OF ESTIMATING % BURN OF BSA ARE:

- **Palmar surface** -The surface area of a patient's palm (including fingers) is roughly 0.8% of total body surface area. Palmar surface are can be used to estimate relatively small burns (< 15% of total surface area) or very large burns (> 85%, when unburnt skin is counted). For medium sized burns, it is inaccurate.

- **Wallace rule of nines** - This is a good, quick way of estimating medium to large burns in adults. The body is divided into areas of 9%, and the total burn area can be calculated. It is not accurate in children.
- **Lund and Browder chart** - This chart, if used correctly, is the most accurate method. It compensates for the variation in body shape with age and therefore can give an accurate assessment of burns area in children.
- It is important that all of the burn is exposed and assessed. During assessment, the environment should be kept warm, and small segments of skin exposed sequentially to reduce heat loss. Pigmented skin can be difficult to assess, and in such cases it may be necessary to remove all the loose epidermal layers to calculate burn size.

Burn Percentage in Adults: Rule of Nines

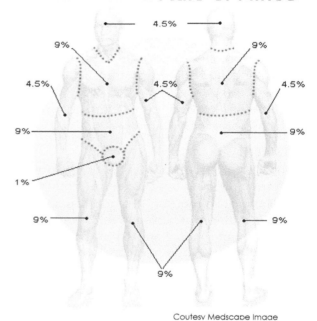

Coutesy Medscape Image

✦ *Epidermal burns are not included when calculating the size of the burn*

ASSESSING THE DEPTH OF A BURN

- Severe burns can be life changing.
- They can cause excruciating physical pain and suffering leaving victims with permanent scars.
- The course of treatment and prognosis vary greatly depending on the degree and type of the burn.
- Burns can be categorized into degrees based on the severity of the injury and by type, which describes the source of the heat that caused the injury.

Depht of Burn	Layer of skin affected	Clinical features	
Epidermal Burn	Epidermal only	Skin is red and painful, but not blistered. This is typical of SUN BURN	
Superficial partial Thickness Burn	The epidermis & Upper layer of dermis	The skin is pale pink and painful with blistering. **Capillary refill:** blanches and rapidly returns	
Deep partial thickness Burn	The epidermis , Upper and deeper layers of dermis	The skin appears dry or moist, blotchy and cherry red, or may be painful or painless. There may be blisters. **Capillary refill:** blanches with a sluggish return or does not blanch.	
Full thickness Burn	The burn extends through all the layers of skin to subcutaneous tissues.	The skin is dry and white, brown, or black in color, with no blisters. It may be described as leathery or waxy. It is painless. **Capillary refill:** does not blanch	

DEFINITIVE TREATMENT MEASURES

- After completion of the primary and secondary survey, priority should be given to pain management.
- Partial-thickness burns are intensely painful and patients may require IV narcotics. Because intramuscular narcotics may have erratic and unpredictable absorption in patients with capillary leak syndrome, repeated boluses of IV narcotics are safer and more effective. If the wound requires debridement, the patient must be given adequate analgesia and sedation.
- Complications associated with eschar formation may occur in any patient with circumferential, deep partial- or full-thickness burns.
- **Emergent escharotomy** can relieve life- or limb-threatening constrictions caused by circumferential burns. When these burns involve the chest, they can cause ventilatory restriction; neck burns also can lead to airway compromise. Circumferential extremity burns may impair distal circulation.
- When life or limb is threatened, the physician should incise the eschar through the dermis into the level of the subcutaneous fat.
- The wound should open significantly and bleed if the incision is made to the proper depth.

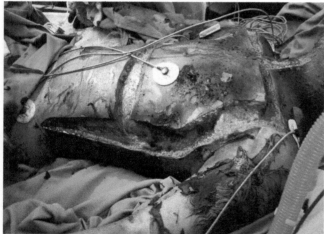

- If a chest escharotomy is required, cut the skin from the clavicles to the costal margin along the anterior axillary line. This incision may be joined by a transverse incision along the superior, anterior abdominal wall. If a neck escharotomy is required, place the incisions posterio-laterally to avoid vascular structures. On the extremities, incisions are made on the medial and lateral surfaces, paying careful attention when crossing the joints so as not to injure neuro-vascular structures.
- Tetanus status needs to be determined and adequate cover given

SPECIAL CIRCUMSTANCES

- In certain circumstances it is recommended patients are discussed with and referred to the local burns centre.
- An important one not to miss is **non-accidental injury (NAI)**. It should always be considered in paediatric presentations and particular attention given to whether the history is consistent with the pattern, location, and type of burn seen.
- Elderly patients are also at risk of NAI.
- **Toxic shock syndrome (TSS)** is another key situation to discuss with the local burns service.
- Any patient, with any size burn, with any of the symptoms below are at risk:
  - *Temperature > 38⁰C*
  - *Rash*
  - *Diarrhoea & vomiting*
  - *General malaise*
  - *Not eating or drinking*
  - *Tachycardia/tachypnoea*
  - *Hypotension*
  - *Reduced urine output*

BURNS REFERRAL CRITERIA

Causes	• Inhalation injury • Deep partial thickness • Full thickness • Electrical, Chemical • Burns with trauma
Affected area	• Face, Hands, Feet, • Genitals, • Joints, Scalp, Ears • Circumferential
Size	• >1% BSA in children • >3% BSA in adults
Ages	• Any neonatal burn • Consider in older people (60+)
Wound	• Not healed within 2 weeks • Infected site
Discuss	• Suspected NAI • Suspected Toxic Shock Syndrome • Progressive non-burn skin loss (TENS, Necrotising Fasciitis) • Significant co-morbidities (e.g. diabetes) or immunocompromised patients • Cold burns with full thickness skin loss • Any other cases that cause concerns

4. Compartment Syndrome

BACKGROUND

- Musculoskeletal compartment syndrome is a limb threatening condition resulting from increased pressure within a muscular compartment, which causes compression of the nerves, muscles and vessels within the compartment.
- Acute compartment syndrome occurs when the tissue pressure within a closed muscle compartment exceeds the perfusion pressure and results in muscle and nerve ischemia. It typically occurs subsequent to a traumatic event, most commonly a fracture[26].
- The incidence of compartment syndrome depends on the patient population studied and the etiology of the syndrome. In a study by Qvarfordt and colleagues, 14% of patients with leg pain were noted to have anterior compartment syndrome[27]; compartment syndrome was seen in 1-9% of leg fractures.

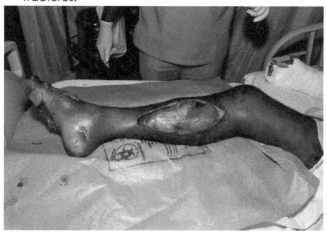

CAUSES

- **Fractures** (about 75% of cases):
  o Tibia,
  o Humeral shaft,
  o Combined radius and ulna fractures,
  o Supracondylar fractures in children.
  o May be open or closed

- **Soft tissue injuries** due to:
  o Crush injury
  o Snake bite
  o Excessive exertion

[26] Torlincasi AM, Waseem M. Compartment Syndrome, Extremity. 2018 Jan

[27] Qvarfordt P, Christenson JT, Eklof B, et al. Intramuscular pressure, muscle blood flow, and skeletal muscle metabolism in chronic anterior tibial compartment syndrome. Clin Orthop. 1983 Oct. (179):284-90.

  o Prolonged immobilisation
  o Constrictive dressings and plaster casts
  o Soft tissue infection
  o Seizures
  o Extravasation of intravenous fluids and medications
  o Burns
  o Tourniquets

- Patients with a **coagulopathy** are at particular risk of compartment syndrome.

COMPLICATIONS INCLUDE:

- **Gangrene** or loss of limb viability requiring amputation
- **Volkmann's ischemic contracture** and loss of function
- **Rhabdomyolysis**
- **Renal failure**

ASSESSMENT

- **History**
  o Suspect if:
    ▪ One of the fractures listed above is present
    ▪ One of the soft tissue injuries listed above is present (e.g. Crush injury)
    ▪ Patient has a coexistent bleeding disorder or coagulopathy

  o Remember the **6Ps**
    ▪ **Pain:**
      • Out of proportion to the injury
      • Increased with passive stretch of compartment muscles (most specific)
      • Not relieved by analgesia
    ▪ **Pallor**
    ▪ **Paraesthesia**
    ▪ **Polar:** cold limb (late finding)
    ▪ **Paralysis** (late finding)
    ▪ **Pulselessness** (late finding)

  o **Pain is the key symptom.** It occurs early, is persistent, tends to be disproportionate compared with the original injury and is not relieved by immobilisation.
  o Increase pain with passive stretch is the most sensitive clinical exam finding for compartment syndrome.

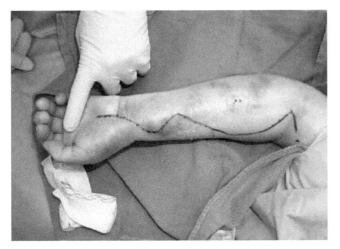

- **Examination**
  - Pain is exacerbated by passive stretching, which is the most sensitive sign.
  - The extremity may be swollen and affected compartments may feel tense and tender on palpation.
  - Assess loss of sensation by light touch and two-point discrimination, rather than just pinprick, which is less sensitive.
  - Refer to a surgeon if compartment syndrome is suspected — do not rely on clinical signs — **have a high index of suspicion!**
  - Palpable distal pulses and normal capillary refill **does not exclude** compartment syndrome.
  - Pulse oximetry is insensitive and is not recommended in the detection of compartment syndrome.

IMAGING
- Imaging has no role in the diagnosis of compartment syndrome, but may show the presence of fractures and soft tissue injuries that are associated with the condition.

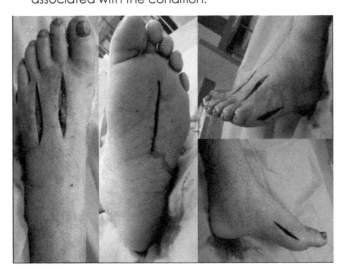

MANAGEMENT
- **RESUSCITATION**
  - Attend to any coexistent life threats
  - Ensure adequate oxygenation and systemic circulation if compartment syndrome is potentially present

- **SPECIFIC TREATMENT**
  - Arrange immediate **FASCIOTOMY**
  - Remove all constrictive dressings (casts, splints)
  - Elevate the limb.
  - Reassess in 20 minutes
  - Consider measurement of compartment pressures.
  - BUT the diagnosis is primarily clinical and if a compartment syndrome is suspected definitive treatment is SURGERY.

  - **Consider injury specific measures:**
    - Relieve flexion of the elbow if the forearm is involved
    - Apply traction for a partially reduced supracondylar fracture
  - If there is no relief within 30 minutes, go straight to the operating theatre

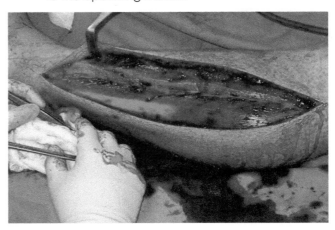

- **SUPPORTIVE CARE AND MONITORING**
  - Provide adequate analgesia
  - Provide IV hydration to maintain an adequate urine output in case of rhabdomyolysis
  - Frequent monitoring of compartments and neurovascular status of the affected limb

- **DISPOSITION**
  - **Urgent surgical referral** (usually an orthopaedic surgeon) and transfer to the operating theatre
  - Patients require admission for ongoing monitoring.

5. Traumatic Brain Injury

INTRODUCTION

- Traumatic brain injury (TBI) is a major cause of mortality and morbidity. In England and Wales, ~1.4 million patients per year attend hospital following head injury and it is the most common cause of death under the age of 40 years[28].
- Over the past 30 years, advances in management including the introduction of Advanced Trauma Life Support National Institute for Health and Care Excellence (NICE) guidelines[29] and protocol-driven therapy have improved outcomeand reduced mortality[30].
- Recently, Regional Trauma Networks have been implemented in England and Wales.

TYPES OF BRAIN INJURY

1. PRIMARY AND SECONDARY INJURIES

- **Primary injury:** Induced by mechanical force and occurs at the moment of injury; the 2 main mechanisms that cause primary injury are contact (eg, an object striking the head or the brain striking the inside of the skull) and acceleration-deceleration. [31]
- **Secondary injury:** Not mechanically induced; it may be delayed from the moment of impact, and it may superimpose injury on a brain already affected by a mechanical injury.

2. FOCAL AND DIFFUSE INJURIES

- These injuries are commonly found together; they are defined as follows:
  - **Focal injury:** Includes scalp injury, skull fracture, and surface contusions; generally caused by contact
  - **Diffuse injury:** Includes diffuse axonal injury (DAI), hypoxic-ischemic damage, meningitis, and vascular injury; usually caused by acceleration-deceleration forces

MEASURES OF SEVERITY

- **Glasgow Coma Scale (GCS):** A 3- to 15-point scale used to assess a patient's level of consciousness and neurologic functioning[32]; scoring is based on best motor response, best verbal response, and eye opening (eg, eyes open to pain, open to command)
- **Duration of loss of consciousness:** Classified as mild (mental status change or loss of consciousness [LOC] < 30 min), moderate (mental status change or LOC 30 min to 6 hr), or severe (mental status change or LOC >6 hr)
- **Posttraumatic amnesia (PTA):** The time elapsed from injury to the moment when patients can demonstrate continuous memory of what is happening around them·

CLINICAL FEATURES OF INCREASING ICP

o Vomiting,
o Headache,
o Irritability,
o Reducing GCS
o Seizures,
o **Cushing's triad**—hypertension, bradycardia, irregular respirations.
o Focal neurology.
o Dilated pupil and contralateral hemiparesis—uncal herniation causes compression of the 3rd cranial nerve against the tentorium cerebelli, resulting in loss of parasympathetic supply to the ipsilateral eye and unopposed sympathetic activity dilating the pupil; in addition, compression of the corticospinal tract in the midbrain results in contralateral weakness.

INDICATIONS FOR IMAGING

- CT scanning is the recommended imaging in head injured patients. NICE[33] have produced guidance on when CT scanning is indicated.
- Plain X-rays of the skull are not recommended unless as part of a skeletal survey in children presenting with suspected non-accidental injury.
- Consideration should always be made about possible associated neck injuries.

---

[28] Head injury: triage, assessment, investigation and early management of head injury in children, young people and adults (NICE guideline CG 176).

[29] Advanced trauma life support (ATLS®): the ninth edition. ATLS Subcommittee., American College of Surgeons' Committee on Trauma., International ATLS working group. J Trauma Acute Care Surg. 2013 May; 74(5):1363-6.

[30] Relationship of aggressive monitoring and treatment to improved outcomes in severe traumatic brain injury. Stein SC, Georgoff P, Meghan S, Mirza KL, El Falaky OM.J Neurosurg. 2010 May; 112(5):1105-12.

[31] Silver JM, McAllister TW, Yodofsky SC, eds. Textbook of Traumatic Brain Injury. Arlington, Va: American Psychiatric Publishing; 2005. Arlington, VA: 27-39.

[32] Teasdale G, Jennett B. Assessment of coma and impaired consciousness. A practical scale. Lancet. 1974 Jul 13. 2(7872):81-4.

[33] Head injury: triage, assessment, investigation and early management of head injury in children, young people and adults (NICE guideline CG 176).

NICE CRITERIA FOR CT HEAD SCAN

1. ADULTS

- For adults who have sustained a head injury and have any of the following risk factors, **perform a CT head scan within 1 hour of the risk factor being identified:**
  - GCS less than 13 on initial assessment in the ED.
  - GCS less than 15 at 2 hours after the injury on assessment in the ED.
  - Suspected open or depressed skull fracture.
  - Any sign of basal skull fracture (haemotympanum, 'panda' eyes, cerebrospinal fluid leakage from the ear or nose, Battle's sign).
  - Post-traumatic seizure.
  - Focal neurological deficit.
  - More than 1 episode of vomiting
- A provisional written radiology report should be made available within 1 hour of the scan being performed. **[new 2014]**

- For adults with any of the following risk factors **who have experienced some loss of consciousness or amnesia since the injury**, perform a **CT head scan within 8 hours of the head injury:**
  - Age 65 years or older.
  - Any history of bleeding or clotting disorders.
  - Dangerous mechanism of injury (a pedestrian or cyclist struck by a motor vehicle, an occupant ejected from a motor vehicle or a fall from a height of greater than 1 metre or 5 stairs).
  - More than 30 minutes' retrograde amnesia of events immediately before the head injury
- A provisional written radiology report should be made available within 1 hour of the scan being performed. **[new 2014]**

2. CHILDREN

- For children who have sustained a head injury and have any of the following risk factors, perform a **CT head scan within 1 hour of the risk factor being identified:**
  - Suspicion of non-accidental injury
  - Post-traumatic seizure but no history of epilepsy.
  - On initial ED assessment, GCS less than 14, or for children under 1-year GCS (Paeds) less than 15.
  - At 2 hours after the injury, GCS less than 15.
  - Suspected open or depressed skull fracture or tense fontanelle.
  - Any sign of basal skull fracture (haemotympanum, 'panda' eyes, CSF leakage from the ear or nose, Battle's sign).
  - Focal neurological deficit.

  - For children under 1 year, presence of bruise, swelling or laceration of more than 5 cm on the head
- A provisional written radiology report should be made available within 1 hour of the scan being performed. **[new 2014]**

- For children who have sustained a head injury and have more than 1 of the following risk factors (and none of those in recommendation above), **perform a CT head scan within 1 hour of the risk factors being identified:**
  - Loss of consciousness lasting more than 5 minutes (witnessed).
  - Abnormal drowsiness.
  - Three or more discrete episodes of vomiting.
  - Dangerous mechanism of injury (high-speed road traffic accident either as pedestrian, cyclist or vehicle occupant, fall from a height of greater than 3 metres, high-speed injury from a projectile or other object).
  - Amnesia (antegrade or retrograde) lasting more than 5 minutes.
- A provisional written radiology report should be made available within 1 hour of the scan being performed. **[new 2014]**

- Children who have sustained a head injury and have **only 1 of the risk factors** in recommendation above should be observed for **a minimum of 4 hours** after the head injury.
- If during observation any of the risk factors below are identified, **perform a CT head scan within 1 hour:**
  - GCS less than 15.
  - Further vomiting.
  - A further episode of abnormal drowsiness.
- A provisional written radiology report should be made available within 1 hour of the scan being performed. If none of these risk factors occur during observation, use clinical judgement to determine whether a longer period of observation is needed.

PATIENTS HAVING WARFARIN TREATMENT[34]

- For patients (adults and children) who have sustained a head injury with no other indications for a CT head scan and who are having warfarin treatment, **perform a CT head scan within 8 hours of the injury**.
- A provisional written radiology report should be made available within 1 hour of the scan being performed.

---

[34] *Head injury: triage, assessment, investigation and early management of head injury in children, young people and adults (NICE guideline CG 176).*

CT HEAD APPEARANCES

EXTRADURAL OR EPIDURAL HAEMORRHAGE (EDH)

Biconvex.
Cannot cross skull suture lines.
Commonly temporo-parietal
Usually middle meningeal artery.
Good prognosis with early treatment.
"Lucid' interval" in one third of patients—can be minutes or hours.

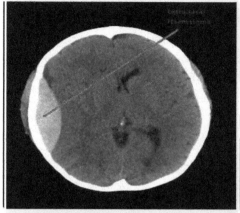

INTRACEREBRAL HAEMATOMA

Looks white when acute.
Size will often cause midline shift (mass effect).
Location and size determine neurological signs and treatment.
If in posterior fossa, then evacuation more likely to be required.

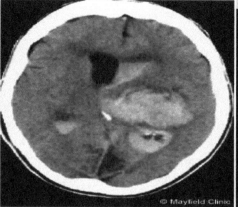

SUBARACHNOID HAEMORRHAGE (SAH)

Blood in subarachnoid space, i.e. around the brain (blood conforms to sulci and gyri), and in ventricles (wherever CSF goes). Due to tearing of small leptomeningeal arteries and veins. Prognosis better in traumatic rather than spontaneous SAH.

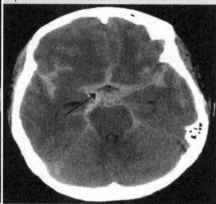

SUBDURAL HAEMORRHAGE

Uniconvex.
Most common focal lesion.
Venous bleed (from bridging dural veins). Can be:
Acute: RTA, NAI
Chronic: elderly, alcoholics, warfarin, i.e. frequent falls with cerebral atrophy and/ or increased bleeding potential.
Acute-on-chronic: acute is whiter; chronic is nearly the same shade of grey as brain tissue. Often able to visualise a line demarcating the two ages of blood.

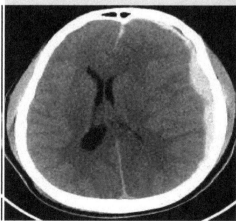

CEREBRAL CONTUSION

Small bleeds = white spots on CT Scan be subtle. Often frontal/temporal due to impact of brain tissue with orbital plates or Sphenoid ridge.
Often associated with SDH.

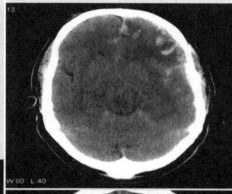

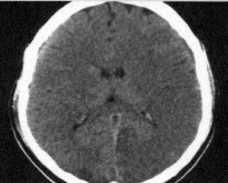

DIFFUSE AXONAL INJURY

Often very little to see on scans initially.
May be pinpoint haemorrhages in corpus callosum and lateral brainstem due to capillary rupture.
Widespread, severe white matter injury.
Shear strains in acceleration/deceleration injury causes severing of neuronal axons.
Commonest cause of a persistent vegetative state.

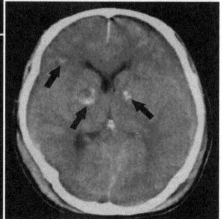

PREVENTING SECONDARY BRAIN INJURY

- **Primary brain injury** occurs during the initial trauma and results from the displacement of physical structures of the brain. The only way to significantly reduce such injuries is **with accident prevention.**
- **Secondary brain injury** occurs after the initial insult. Many factors are involved in secondary brain injury and are potentially preventable or treatable.

CAUSES OF SECONDARY BRAIN INJURY:

o Hypoxia and hypercapnea
o Hypovolaemia and cerebral hypoperfusion
o Intracranial haematoma with localized pressure effects
o Increased ICP and cerebral oedema
o Hyperthermia and seizures
o Infection.
- The focus of ED management in head-injured patients is the prevention and treatment of secondary brain injury:
  o **Ensure adequate oxygenation** (PaO_2>13 kPa).
  o **Aim for $PaCO_2$ in normal range** (NICE recommend $PaCO_2$ 4.5–5 kPa). Intubate and ventilate as required to achieve these aims.
  o **Avoids increases in ICP:**
    ▪ Consider 30° head-up tilt,
    ▪ Avoid cervical collars/ compressions;
    ▪ Tape the ET Tube in place rather than tie it
    ▪ Avoid excessive intra-thoracic pressures.
    ▪ Consider mannitol on specialist advice.
  o **Maintain end organ perfusion** (NICE recommend MAP≥80 mmHg). Use urine output as indicator of adequate renal perfusion.
  o **Maintain normoglycaemia.**
  o **Treat seizures**: benzodiazepines, prophylactic phenytoin.
  o **Monitor for signs** of neurological deterioration.
  o **Pain management** to avoid increases in ICP.
  o **Temperature control**: aim for normothermia.
  o **Infection control**: wound management; tetanus booster/immunoglobulin and antibiotics.

- **INDICATIONS FOR REFERRAL TO/DISCUSSION WITH NEUROSURGERY**
  o 'New, surgically significant abnormalities on imaging'.
  o Persisting coma (GCS≤8) after initial resuscitation.
  o Unexplained confusion >4 hours.
  o Deterioration in GCS after admission.
  o Progressive focal neurology.
  o Seizure without full recovery.
  o Penetrating injury (definite or suspected).
  o CSF leak.

ADMISSION CRITERIA FOR HEAD INJURIES

o CT with clinically significant abnormalities.
o GCS not returned to normal.
o Awaiting scan.
o Continued clinical concern (e.g. vomiting).
o Other ongoing concerns (e.g. intoxication, other injuries, suspected NAI, etc.)

RECOMMENDED OBSERVATIONS OF HEAD INJURED PATIENTS

- The following observation should be recorded:
  o GCS &Pupil size and reactivity.
  o Limb movements.
  o RR, HR, BP, T°, SPO2

NICE RECOMMEND THE FOLLOWING FREQUENCY OF OBSERVATIONS:

o Half-hourly until GCS 15.
o Then half-hourly for 2 hours.
o Then hourly for 4 hours.
o Then 2-hourly.

DISCHARGE ADVICE POST HEAD INJURY[35]

o Verbal and written advice should be given to all patients discharged following a head injury.
o Advice should be appropriate to the age and language of the patient/carer.
o If patients have had a CT scan, they should have follow-up arranged with their GP **within 1 week.**
o Discharge advice should include symptoms that the patient/carer should observe for and return to the ED if they develop.
o There should also be a section describing symptoms of post-concussional syndrome and where to get help if these are persistent.
o Return to the ED if any of the following develop:
  ▪ Unconsciousness or lack of full consciousness.
  ▪ Any confusion.
  ▪ Any drowsiness that goes on for longer than 1 h when you would normally be wide awake.
  ▪ Any problems understanding or speaking.
  ▪ Any loss of balance or problems walking.
  ▪ Any weakness in one or both arms or legs.
  ▪ Any problems with your eyesight.
  ▪ Very painful headache that won't go away.
  ▪ Any vomiting.
  ▪ Any fits (collapsing or passing out suddenly).
  ▪ Clear fluid coming out of your ear or nose.
  ▪ Bleeding from one or both ears and New deafness in one or both ears.

---

[35] Head injury: triage, assessment, investigation and early management of head injury in children, young people and adults (NICE guideline CG 176).

6. Spinal Trauma

I. NEUROGENIC SHOCK & SPINAL SHOCK

INTRODUCTION

- Although there haven't been any significant studies on the incidence of spinal cord injuries over the last 10 years, the annual incidence is about 12,000 new cases per year (not including the patients who die at the scene)[36]. Nearly half of all the injuries occur in patients between the ages of 16 and 30 and the majority (80%) of them are men.
- Motor vehicle crashes account for the majority of causes at ~36%, followed by falls, acts of violence and sports. There's a tremendous financial cost associated with these injuries both in hospital charges and in wages and productivity lost.

DEFINITIONS

- **Neuorgenic shock:** A form of distributive shock that results from unopposed parasympathetic response after a disruption of the spinal cord at mid-thoracic levels (T6) and above.
- **Parasympathetic nervous system:** A division of the autonomic nervous system that performs many functions, including increased intestinal activity during digestion and slowed heart rates.
- **Spinal cord:** Long, round structure found in the spinal canal and reaching from the base of the skull to the lumbar spine. The cord carries sensory and motor signals to and from the brain and controls many reflexes.
- **Spinal shock:** Characterized by similar cardiovascular signs of neurogenic shock (bradycardic, hypotensive and hypothermic) but more often includes a marked reduction or loss of somatic and/or reflex functions of the spinal cord beyond the level of the injury.
- **Sympathetic nervous system:** A division of the autonomic nervous system that functions during strenuous muscular work and other stresses. Functions include dilating blood vessels in the skeletal muscle; increasing adrenal secretion, heart rate and pupillary size, and decreases digestive functions in preparation for fight-or-flight reactions.

NEUROGENIC SHOCK/SPINAL SHOCK

- Although frequently used interchangeably, true definitions of neurogenic and spinal shock are hard to identify. Multiple definitions have been used, but, from a practical standpoint, **neurogenic shock** is a form of distributive shock that results from unopposed parasympathetic response after a disruption of the spinal cord at mid-thoracic levels (T6) and above.
- There's some indication that a transient hypertension exists immediately after injury, but, most commonly, because of the loss of sympathetic activity, these patients can present bradycardic, hypotensive and hypothermic.
- Because of the profound vasodilation that occurs, the patient's extremities will be warm as opposed to the cool, clamped down feeling one normally finds in hemorrhagic shock.
- **Spinal shock** is an entity that can encompass the earlier noted cardiovascular findings but is more often characterized by a marked reduction or loss of somatic and/or reflex functions of the spinal cord beyond the level of the injury. This has the potential to last for days or weeks post injury.
- It should be noted that the patient with spinal cord injury and neurogenic shock as a result of trauma often has other injuries that could result in hemorrhagic shock.
- This could cloud the presentation and make diagnosis difficult. It's therefore imperative to exclude other causes of hypotension before attributing the cause to neurogenic shock, as their treatments may be different.

CLASSIFICATIONS OF SPINAL CORD INJURIES

- Spinal cord injuries can be classified according to:
  o Level,
  o Severity of neurologic deficit,
  o Spinal cord syndromes, and
  o Morphology.

1. LEVEL

- The neurologic level is the most caudal segment of the spinal cord that has normal sensory and motor function on both sides of the body.

---

[36] *Spinal Cord Injury (SCI) Fact Sheet. (Nov. 10, 2010.) Centers for Disease Control and Prevention. Retrieved Sept. 10, 2014,*

- When the term **sensory level** is used, it refers to the most caudal segment of the spinal cord with normal sensory function.
- **The motor level** is defined similarly with respect to motor function as the lowest key muscle that has a **grade of at least 3/5.**
- In complete injuries, when some impaired sensory and/or motor function is found just below the lowest normal segment, this is referred to as **the zone of partial preservation**.
- As described above, the determination of the level of injury on both sides is important. A broad distinction may be made between lesions above and below T1. Injuries of the first eight cervical segments of the spinal cord result in quadriplegia, and lesions below the T1 level result in paraplegia.
- The bony level of injury is the vertebra at which the bones are damaged, causing injury to the spinal cord. The neurologic level of injury is determined primarily by clinical examination.
- Frequently, there is a discrepancy between the bony and neurologic levels because the spinal nerves enter the spinal canal through the foramina and ascend or descend inside the spinal canal before actually entering the spinal cord.
- The further caudal the injury is, the more pronounced this discrepancy becomes.

2. SEVERITY OF NEUROLOGIC DEFICIT

- Spinal cord injury may be categorized as:
  o Incomplete paraplegia (incomplete thoracic injury)
  o Complete paraplegia (complete thoracic injury)
  o Incomplete quadriplegia (incomplete cervical injury)
  o Complete quadriplegia (complete cervical injury)
- It is important to assess for any sign of preservation of function of the long tracts of the spinal cord.
- Any motor or sensory function below the level of the injury constitutes an incomplete injury.
- Signs of an incomplete injury include any sensation (including position sense) or voluntary movement in the lower extremities, sacral sparing, voluntary anal sphincter contraction, and voluntary toe flexion.
- Sacral reflexes, such as the bulbocavernosus reflex or anal wink, do not qualify as sacral sparing.

3. SPINAL CORD SYNDROMES

- Motor and sensory function loss from an injury can be classified as complete or incomplete.
- A complete cord injury will present with motor paralysis and sensory loss below the level of the cord that's involved.

- These are the injuries that most often result in spinal or neurogenic shock.
- An incomplete injury will present in multiple different ways depending on what part of the cord is injured.

CENTRAL CORD SYNDROME
o This is a type of incomplete lesion to the cord that results in dysfunction in the upper extremities as opposed to the lower extremities.
o The patient will present with upper extremity weakness or paralysis and minimal if any dysfunction of the lower extremities.

ANTERIOR CORD SYNDROME
o This is found when the mechanism results in an injury to the anterior portion of the spinal cord. Because of the specific nerve fibers that run through this region, the patient will present with absence of motor function, pain and sensation below the level of the injury.
o The patient will retain the ability to feel light touch, proprioception and vibration.

BROWN-SEQUARD SYNDROME
o These lesions result from injury to half the cord, which results in paralysis on the side of the injury and loss of pain and temperature sensation on the opposite side.

4. MORPHOLOGY
- Spinal injuries can be described as fractures, fracture dislocations, spinal cord injury without radiographic abnormalities (SCIWORA), and penetrating injuries.
- Each of these categories may be further described as stable or unstable. However, determining the stability of a particular type of injury is not always simple and, indeed, even experts may disagree.
- Therefore, especially in the initial treatment, all patients with radiographic evidence of injury and all those with neurologic deficits should be considered to have an unstable spinal injury.
- These patients should be immobilized until after consultation with an appropriately qualified doctor, usually a neurosurgeon or orthopaedic surgeon.

SUSPECTED CERVICAL SPINE INJURY
- The presence of paraplegia or quadriplegia is presumptive evidence of spinal instability.
- Patients who are awake, alert, sober, and neurologically normal, and have no neck pain or midline tenderness, or a distracting injury: These patients are extremely unlikely to have an acute c-spine fracture or instability.
- With the patient in a supine position, remove the c-collar and palpate the spine.

- If there is no significant tenderness, ask the patient to voluntarily move his or her neck from side to side.
- Never force the patient's neck. When performed voluntarily by the patient, these manoeuvers are generally safe.
- If there is no pain, have the patient voluntarily flex and extend his or her neck. Again, if there is no pain, c-spine films are not necessary. Patients who are awake and alert, neurologically normal, cooperative, and do not have a distracting injury and are able to concentrate on their spine, but do have neck pain or midline tenderness: The burden of proof is on the clinician to exclude a spinal injury.
- Where available, all such patients should undergo multi-detector axial CT from the occiput to T1 with sagittal and coronal reconstructions.
- Where not available, patients should undergo lateral, AP, and open mouth odontoid x-ray examinations of the c-spine with axial CT images of suspicious areas or of the lower cervical spine if not adequately visualized on the plain films.

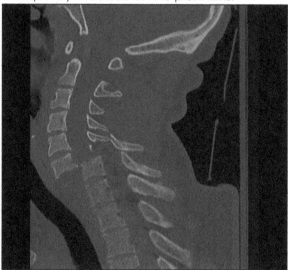

- **Assess the c-spine films for:**
  - o Bony deformity
  - o Fracture of the vertebral body or processes
  - o Loss of alignment of the posterior aspect of the vertebral bodies (anterior extent of the vertebral canal)
  - o Increased distance between the spinous processes at one level
  - o Narrowing of the vertebral canal
  - o Increased prevertebral soft tissue space
- If these films are normal, remove the c-collar.
- Under the care of a knowledgeable clinician, obtain flexion and extension, and lateral cervical spine films with the patient voluntarily flexing and extending his or her neck.

- If the films show no subluxation, the patient's c-spine can be cleared and the c-collar removed. However, if any of these films are suspicious or unclear, replace the collar and obtain consultation from a spine specialist.
- Patients who have an altered level of consciousness or are too young to describe their symptoms: Where available, all such patients should undergo multi-detector axial CT from the occiput to T1 with sagittal and coronal reconstructions.
- Where not available, all such patients should undergo lateral, AP, and open-mouth odontoid films with CT supplementation through suspicious areas (e.g., C1 and C2, and through the lower cervical spine if areas are not adequately visualized on the plain films).
- In children, CT supplementation is optional.
- If the entire c-spine can be visualized and is found to be normal, the collar can be removed after appropriate evaluation by a doctor/consultant skilled in the evaluation/ management of patients with spine injuries.
- Clearance of the c-spine is particularly important if pulmonary or other care of the patient is compromised by the inability to mobilize the patient. When in doubt, leave the collar on.

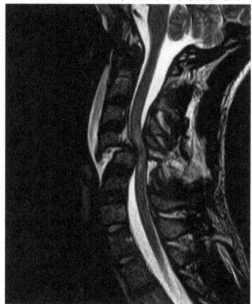

SUSPECTED THORACOLUMBAR SPINE INJURY

- The presence of paraplegia or a level of sensory loss on the chest or abdomen is presumptive evidence of spinal instability.
- Patients who are awake, alert, sober, neurologically normal, and have no midline thoracic or lumbar back pain or tenderness: The entire extent of the spine should be palpated and inspected.

- If there is no tenderness on palpation or ecchymosis over the spinous processes, an unstable spine fracture is unlikely, and thoracolumbar radiographs may not be necessary.
- Patients who have spine pain or tenderness on palpation, neurologic deficits, an altered level of consciousness, or in whom intoxication is suspected: AP and lateral radiographs of the entire thoracic and lumbar spine should be obtained.
- Thin-cut axial CT should be obtained through suspicious areas identified on the plain films.
- All images must be of good quality and interpreted as normal by an experienced doctor before discontinuing spine precautions. Consult a doctor skilled in the evaluation and management of spine injuries if a spine injury is detected or suspected.

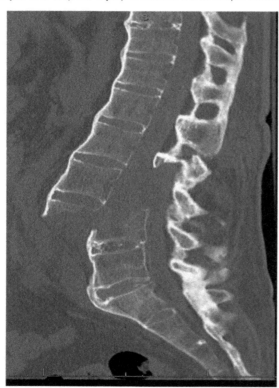

TRANSFER

- Patients with spine fractures or neurologic deficit should be transferred to a definitive-care facility.
- The safest procedure is to transfer the patient after telephone consultation with a spine specialist.
- Avoid unnecessary delay.
- Stabilize the patient and apply the necessary splints, backboard, and/or semirigid cervical collar.
- Remember, cervical spine injuries above C6 can result in partial or total loss of respiratory function.
- If there is any concern about the adequacy of ventilation, the patient should be intubated prior to transfer.

NICE CRITERIA FOR CERVICAL SPINE IMAGING[37]
1. ADULTS

- For adults who have sustained a head injury and have any of the following risk factors, perform a CT cervical spine scan **within 1 hour** of the risk factor being identified:
  - o GCS less than 13 on initial assessment.
  - o The patient has been intubated.
  - o Plain X-rays are technically inadequate (for example, the desired view is unavailable).
  - o Plain X-rays are suspicious or definitely abnormal.
  - o A definitive diagnosis of cervical spine injury is needed urgently (for example, before surgery).
  - o The patient is having other body areas scanned for head injury or multi-region trauma.
  - o The patient is alert and stable, there is clinical suspicion of cervical spine injury and any of the following apply:
    - Age 65 years or older
    - Dangerous mechanism of injury (fall from a height of greater than 1 metre or 5 stairs; axial load to the head, for example, diving; high-speed motor vehicle collision; rollover motor accident; ejection from a motor vehicle; accident involving motorised recreational vehicles; bicycle collision)
    - Focal peripheral neurological deficit
    - Paraesthesia in the upper or lower limbs.
- A provisional written radiology report should be made available within 1 hour of the scan being performed. **[new 2014]**

- For adults who have sustained a head injury and have neck pain or tenderness but no indications for a CT cervical spine scan (see recommendation above), **perform 3-view cervical spine x-rays within 1 hour** if either of these risk factors are identified:
  - o It is not considered safe to assess the range of movement in the neck (see recommendation below).
  - o Safe assessment of range of neck movement shows that the patient cannot actively rotate their neck to 45 degrees to the left and right.
  - o The X-rays should be reviewed by a clinician trained in their interpretation within 1 hour of being performed.

---

[37] *Head injury: triage, assessment, investigation and early management of head injury in children, young people and adults (NICE guideline CG 176).*

ASSESSING RANGE OF MOVEMENT IN THE NECK[38]

- Be aware that in adults and children who have sustained a head injury and in whom there is clinical suspicion of cervical spine injury, **range** of movement in the neck can be assessed safely before imaging only if no above high-risk factors present and at least 1 of the following low-risk features apply.
- The patient:
  - Was involved in a simple rear-end motor vehicle collision
  - Is comfortable in a sitting position in the emergency department
  - Has been ambulatory at any time since injury
  - Has no midline cervical spine tenderness
  - Presents with delayed onset of neck pain. **[new 2014]**

2. CHILDREN

- For children who have sustained a head injury, perform a CT cervical spine scan only if any of the following apply (because of the increased risk to the thyroid gland from ionising radiation and the generally lower risk of significant spinal injury):
  - GCS less than 13 on initial assessment.
  - The patient has been intubated.
  - Focal peripheral neurological signs.
  - Paraesthesia in the upper or lower limbs.
  - A definitive diagnosis of cervical spine injury is needed urgently (for example, before surgery).
  - The patient is having other body areas scanned for head injury or multi-region trauma.
  - There is strong clinical suspicion of injury despite normal X-rays.
  - Plain X-rays are technically difficult or inadequate.
  - Plain X-rays identify a significant bony injury.
- The scan should be performed within 1 hour of the risk factor being identified.
- A provisional written radiology report should be made available within 1 hour of the scan being performed. **[new 2014]**
- For children who have sustained a head injury and have neck pain or tenderness but no indications for a CT cervical spine scan (see recommendation above), **perform 3-view cervical spine x-rays before assessing range of movement in the neck** if either of these risk factors are identified:

  - Dangerous mechanism of injury (that is, fall from a height of greater than 1 metre or 5 stairs; axial load to the head, for example, diving; high-speed motor vehicle collision; rollover motor accident; ejection from a motor vehicle; accident involving motorised recreational vehicles; bicycle collision).
  - Safe assessment of range of movement in the neck is not possible.
- The X-rays should be carried out within 1 hour of the risk factor being identified and reviewed by a clinician trained in their interpretation within 1 hour of being performed. **[new 2014]**
- If range of neck movement can be assessed safely in a child who has sustained a head injury and has neck pain or tenderness but no indications for a CT cervical spine scan, **perform 3-view cervical spine X-rays if the child cannot actively rotate their neck 45 degrees to the left and right**.
- The X-rays should be carried out within 1 hour of this being identified and reviewed by a clinician trained in their interpretation within 1 hour of being performed. **[new 2014]**
- In children who can obey commands and open their mouths, **attempt an odontoid peg view. [2003, amended 2014]**

---

[38] Head injury: triage, assessment, investigation and early management of head injury in children, young people and adults (NICE guideline CG 176).

7. Thoracic Trauma
I. TENSION PNEUMOTHORAX

DEFINITION AND CONTEXT

- A tension pneumothorax is a life-threatening condition that develops when air is trapped in the pleural cavity under positive pressure, displacing mediastinal structures and compromising cardiopulmonary function.
- Tension pneumothorax arises from numerous causes and rapidly progresses to respiratory insufficiency, cardiovascular collapse, and, ultimately, death if not recognized and treated. Therefore, if the clinical picture fits a tension pneumothorax, it must be emergently treated before it results in hemodynamic instability and death.
- Given that the expansion is dynamic, be vigilant in patients with a chest x-ray proven small pneumothorax in whom you elect not to insert a chest drain.

CLINICAL ASSESSMENT AND IDENTIFICATION

- Symptoms and signs depend on where your patient is on the expanding pneumothorax continuum – clinical features become more obvious with expansion.

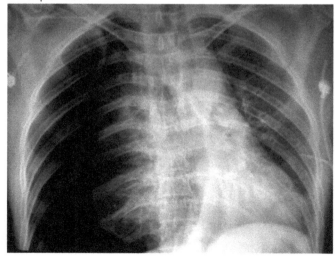

A. FOR AWAKE PATIENTS:

- Universal features of tension pneumothorax are **chest pain** and **respiratory compromise**, neither of which are discriminatory of course.
- **Low oxygen saturations** may be an early feature; **hypotension** tends to be late. Both may have other causes.
- Lateralising the pneumothorax may not be straightforward – listen for **decreased breath sounds on the affected side**.
- Listen in the axillae rather than over the anterior chest wall. Note the classical signs of **hyper-resonance** and **tracheal deviation** are soft and difficult to elicit.

B. FOR VENTILATED PATIENTS:

- Early reliable signs are: ↓**SPO2**, ↓**BP**, ↑**HR**, ↑**VP**
  - Decrease in oxygen saturations – this is likely to be prompt
  - Decrease in BP, Tachycardia
  - Look too for raised ventilation pressure (VP>40) – ensure that the ventilator pressure alarm settings are set appropriately.
  - **Lateralising signs** are the same as for awake patients.
- A portable CXR is recommended for tension pneumothorax, unless the patient is critical
- Radiological evidence of tensioning does not necessarily correlate clinically

ED MANAGEMENT[39]

- **Emergent Needle Thoracentesis**
  - Do not wait for Chest XRay
  - Use 14 gauge (5 cm long) angiocatheter in children and 10 gauge (7.5 cm long) angiocatheter in adults
  - Insert angiocatheter over the top of the third rib in the mid-clavicular line
- **Chest Tube**
  - Perform immediately after needle decompression
  - Insert over the top of the 5th rib in the mid-axillary line

Needle thoracocentesis is advocated for tension pneumothorax in the first instance in the ATLS manual.

- Potential drawbacks to this strategy are:
  - **It tends to get over used**, particularly in stable resus room patients in whom portable CXR is readily available and chest drain is the preferred treatment.

---

[39] *2012 ATLS 9th ed, American College of Surgeons, Committee on Trauma, p. 96-9*

o **A lack of hiss** (or bubbling, if you have put some saline in a syringe attached to the needle) might be considered as evidence of no tension pneumothorax – the procedure doesn't have 100% sensitivity.

Three potential drawbacks to the recommendation of using needle thoracocentesis:

o A (4.5 cm) 14-gauge cannula may not reach the pleural space via the second intercostal space.
o The cannula can kink and cease to function.
o A pneumothorax may be caused if the diagnosis is incorrect.

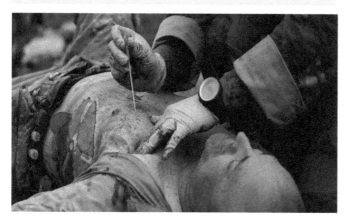

2. Thoracostomy (Finger)

o Avoid needle thoracocentesis in peri-arrest patients with suspected tension pneumothorax – thoracostomy is the better option.

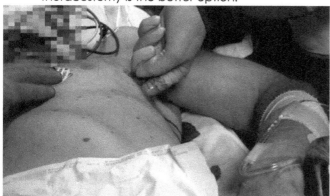

3. Chest drain insertion

o The most common cause of serious injury (and death) as a result of chest drain insertion, is insertion at the incorrect site, usually too low
o Confirm that the drain lies within the chest wall cavity by looking for fogging of the tube and swinging of the chest drain with respiration.
o Do not clamp the chest drain or apply suction
o The underwater seal needs to remain below the insertion site at all times

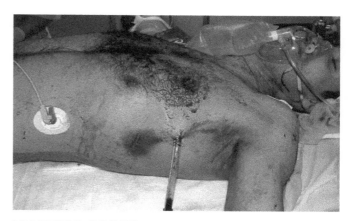

LEARNING POINTS

- If you do perform needle thoracocentesis, have some saline in the syringe to demonstrate bubbling when the tension is hit. Gross surgical emphysema with pneumomediastinum (as per CXR) and a chest drain that continues to bubble, suggests **tracheobronchial injury.**
- If there is good clinical and radiological evidence of significant lateral chest wall injury, consider the second intercostal space anteriorly for the chest drain insertion – it's safer for the operator and less painful for the awake patient.
- One third of initial CXRs in trauma will not detect pneumothorax; anaesthetic colleagues need to be aware of this if your patient leaves for theatre.
- Cardiac tamponade may give similar signs clinically shock, with distended neck veins.
- A combination of your FAST skills, urgent CXR and consideration of the mechanism of injury should help you distinguish the two.

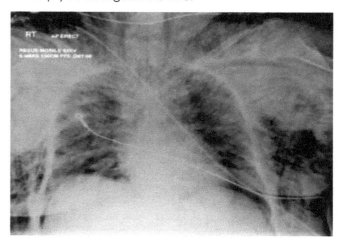

- Beware other pathology masquerading as large (possibly tensioning?) pneumothorax on the CXR, for example an emphysematous bulla or gastrothorax.
- Reconsider the clinical presentation and consider CT where the CXR diagnosis remains in doubt.

II. OPEN PNEUMOTHORAX

DEFINITION AND CONTEXT

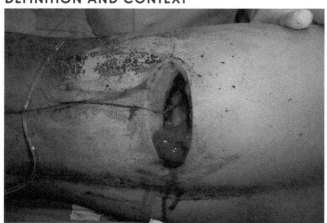

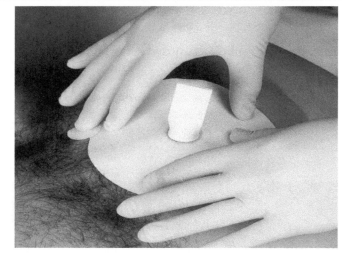

- Think hole in the chest. It is also known as a **communicating pneumothorax** or **sucking chest wound**.
- A hole of only 1 or 2 cm in radius may cause serious respiratory compromise, particularly in patients with comorbidities, and/or other injuries
- Rarely, it is caused by ballistic (shot gun) injury.
- Clearly, this unlikely to be missed clinically.
- As the patient takes a breath in, the hole in the chest competes with the normal airway (mouth/nose to trachea) for delivery of air.

CLINICAL ASSESSMENT AND IDENTIFICATION

- Prompt clinical inspection front and back; a small sucking chest wound is usually audible.

ED MANAGEMENT[40]

- **Apply a sterile Occlusive Dressing to wound**
  - Tape dressing on 3 of the 4 sides (Valve effect)
  - Offers only temporary stabilization until Chest Tube can be placed
  - Chest Tube is the primary management for an open chest wound
  - Do not completely occlude the wound until Chest Tube is in place (Tension Pneumothorax risk)
- **Place Chest Tube remote from open wound**
  - Typical Chest Tube placement is over the 5th rib in the mid-axillary line
  - Do not use the wound site for insertion of Chest Tube (contamination risk)
- **Surgical Consultation**
  - Provides definitive chest wound closure

- **Early intubation:** IPPV solves the respiratory embarrassment created by the hole in the chest
- For small open pneumothoraces, insert a **chest drain** remote from the wound on that side; this is practically easier once the patient is anaesthetised.
- Do not insert a chest drain in patients with a large open pneumothorax since muscle flaps may be needed for closure and can be damaged in the procedure. Definitive treatment is surgical repair.

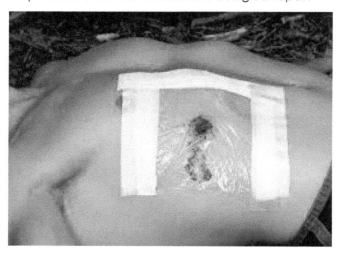

---

[40] *2012 ATLS 9th ed, American College of Surgeons, Committee on Trauma, p. 96-9*

III. MASSIVE HAEMOTHORAX

DEFINITION AND CONTEXT

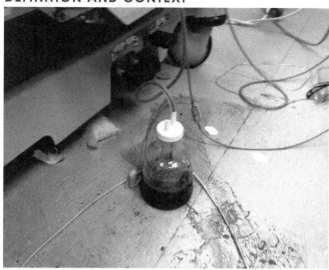

- Massive Haemothorax is a haemothorax with a **volume greater than 1500 ml**, or greater than **one third of the patient's blood volume**.
- This is an uncommon injury which can be caused by blunt or penetrating trauma, and is unlikely to be missed radiologically.
- It creates a problem because of shock (haemorrhagic and impaired venous return from the vena cava) and decreased ventilation (the lung on that side gets compressed).

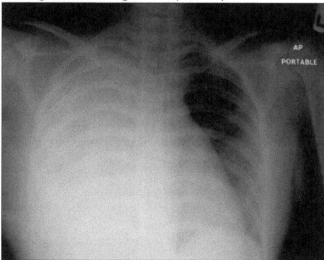

CLINICAL ASSESSMENT AND IDENTIFICATION

- Think of the concept of expanding haemothorax (another continuum!): the signs will be less reliable in moderate haemothorax.
- Listen at the lung bases (Figure above).

- There should be clear signs of shock prompting you to rule out the diagnosis.
- Use CXR and FAST to guide you.
- You may underestimate the size of the haemothorax on a supine CXR.

- **FAST SIGNS:**
  - o **The absence of a mirror image of liver/ lung or spleen/lung** across the diaphragm suggests a haemothorax;
  - o Alternatively, free fluid in the abdomen alone should prompt you to reconsider the source of haemorrhage.

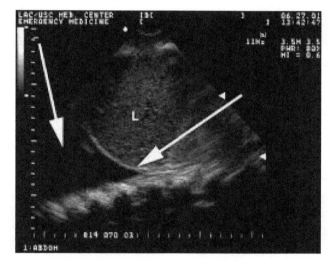

TREATMENT[41]

- **ABCD approach.**
- **Intravenous fluid** resuscitation
- Consider autotransfusion device (e.g. hemovac, cell saver)
- Large bore Chest Tube (36-40 french) at the 5th intercostal space in the midaxillary line
- Operative management as below

ATLS indications for Thoracotomy

- ❖ Chest Tube output >1500-2000 cc total or
- ❖ Chest Tube output 150-200 cc/hour for several hours or
- ❖ Refractory hemodynamic instability or
- ❖ Penetrating anterior Chest Trauma medial to the nipple line

---

[41] *2012 ATLS 9th ed, American College of Surgeons, Committee on Trauma, p. 96-9*

IV. CARDIAC TAMPONADE

DEFINITION AND CONTEXT

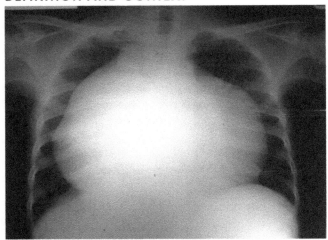

- Cardiac tamponade is a collection of fluid (blood in the context of trauma) in the pericardial sack causing haemodynamic compromise.
- When faced with a penetrating injury to chest, back or upper abdomen, **think tension pneumothorax, think massive haemothorax, and think cardiac tamponade.**
- Exclude or confirm tamponade with a FAST scan.

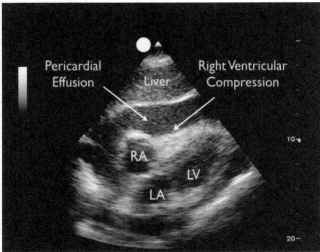

Subxiphoid view of the heart demonstrating a moderate sized pericardial effusion.

- Cardiac tamponade is not an on/off phenomenon (yet another continuum), though the progression to PEA cardiac arrest may be rapid.
- **50 to 200 ml** of blood in the pericardial sac may be enough.
- Cardiac tamponade as a result of blunt injury is exceptionally rare in those patients reaching hospital alive.

CLINICAL ASSESSMENT AND IDENTIFICATION

- FAST has particularly high sensitivity (about 95% according to ATLS).
- Do note that there are drawbacks in detecting and interpreting the classical clinical signs **(Beck's Triad):**
  o **Neck veins** may not be distended if the patient has haemorrhagic shock
  o **Hypotension** (and a raised respiratory rate) may have other causes
  o **Muffled heart sounds** unlikely to be heard in the ED!

TREATMENT[42]

- **ABCD approach** with **Fluid resuscitation** to increase pre-load
- **Immediate Pericardiocentesis under Ultrasound gui dance (ATLS)**
  o Emergency Pericardiocentesis
  o Sub-xiphoid approach
  o Needle angled toward left Shoulder
  o Constant suction applied to syringe on entry
  o Send fluid for cytology if not Traumatic in origin
- **Emergency Thoracotomy**
  o Indicated in Cardiac Tamponade due to Trauma (especially penetrating), refractory to Pericardiocentesis
- **Emergent Cardiothoracic surgery**
  o Pericardial window placement and other definitive management
- **Intravenous Fluids**
  o Transient stabilization to increase venous pressure
- **Precautions**
  o Avoid Positive Pressure Ventilation until after decompression with Pericardiocentesis
    ▪ Negative intrathoracic pressure is the last safeguard maintaining venous return in Pericardial Tamponade
    ▪ Positive Pressure Ventilation eliminates negative intrathoracic pressure
    ▪ Pulseless Electrical Activity arrest (PEA arrest) results
  o Avoid measures that reduce cardiac filling
    ▪
    ▪ Avoid inotropes (increased Heart Rate decreases filling time)

---

[42] *Mallemat and Swadron in Herbert (2013) EM:Rap 13(12): 10-11*

V. FLAIL CHEST

DEFINITION AND CONTEXT

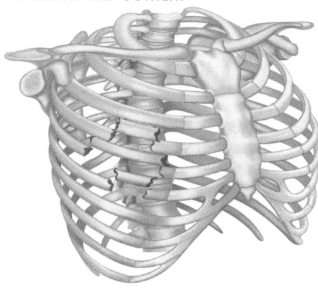

- Chest Trauma resulting in 2 or more contiguous Rib Fractures at 2 or more sites along each rib resulting in paradoxical chest wall movement and associated with other lung injury (Lung Contusion, pain with Splinting and Atelectasis)and Results in hypoventilation and Hypoxia
- This injury is relatively common – small flails may be missed clinically.
- Beware **underlying pulmonary contusions** which are inevitable, and may cause significant morbidity and mortality in any age group
- Considerable force is required to create a flail chest in young people look carefully for other injuries, both intra and extra-thoracic.
- Multiple rib fractures are a potential source of significant haemorrhage.

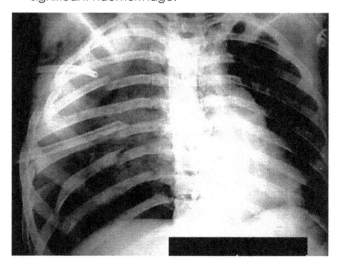

CLINICAL ASSESSMENT AND IDENTIFICATION

- By palpation as well as inspection.
- A CXR might identify associated pneumothorax, haemothorax and pulmonary contusions.
- The appearance of early pulmonary contusions is particularly worrying; evidence of further and perhaps extensive contusion (with physiological effect) may evolve.

TREATMENT

- Treatment options depend largely on the respiratory embarrassment caused: consider your patient's clinical condition, the size of the flail chest, associated injuries, age, co-morbidities and destination from resus (theatre, CT scan, ITU or ward)

If no life-threatening injuries[43]:
- Stabilize flail segment
- Supplemental Oxygen
- Pain management
    o Narcotic Analgesics (e.g. Dilaudid or Morphine Sulfate)
    o Consider intercostal Nerve Block
    o Consider intrapleural or extrapleural anesthesia
    o Consider Epidural Anesthesia
- Consider intubation
    o Indicated for Respiratory Failure

- **For patients with major trauma (Life-threatening):**
    o **Intubation and ventilation (IPPV):** This enables you to take better control of respiratory compromise,
    o **Pain management** (remember to give **adequate morphine post RSI**) and facilitates clinical procedures e.g. chest drain insertion and CT scan.
    o Insert a **chest drain** for associated pneumothorax and haemothorax
    o **CT** is likely to pick up occult pneumothoraces; whilst usually small, chest drain insertion is recommended if the treatment option is ventilation
    o Judicious **fluid resuscitation** since excessive fluid floods injured lung tissue
    o **Definitive surgery** (internal fixation of ribs) at the discretion of cardiothoracic surgeons.
    o Discuss treatment options with **ICU and thoracic surgical** colleagues.

---

43 2012 ATLS, ACOS, Chicago, p. 99

VI. PULMONARY CONTUSION

DEFINITION AND CONTEXT

- Bruised lung; unlikely to be missed radiologically unless the CXR is early.
- Potentially life threatening since:
  - o The patient is at **risk of hypoxaemia**
  - o Because of the force involved to cause the injury, **associated injuries are common**
  - o Injured lung is **vulnerable to flooding** from aggressive fluid resuscitation
  - o Patients with co-morbidities and/or advanced age are particularly at risk from this injury.

CLINICAL ASSESSMENT AND IDENTIFICATION

- Look for patchy white areas progressing to frank consolidation on the CXR (aspiration and haemorrhage are differential diagnoses)
- Contusions visible on the initial CXR suggests significant injury, with further radiological changes and blood gas derangement likely to follow.
- Look for associated rib fractures and haemo/pneumothorax
- Rib fractures do not always co-exist, particularly in the young (where their existence indicates that significant force created the injury)

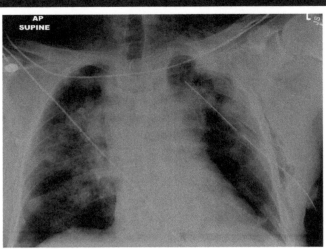

TREATMENT

- **A&B: IPPV with Positive End Expiratory Pressure** (PEEP) for the sicker patients
- **C: Judicious use of fluids**
  - o Consider insertion of a central line and arterial line
  - o **Avoid colloids** since these will breach injured lung tissue and worsen hypoxia
- **D:** No evidence for steroids or prophylactics antibiotics
- Discuss disposition of each patient with **ITU and thoracic surgical colleague**

VII. MYOCARDIAL CONTUSION

DEFINITION AND CONTEXT

- Myocardial bruising caused by blunt injury, including deceleration and ballistic mechanisms.
- The key problem with interpreting the literature is the lack of a diagnostic gold standard (apart from post mortem).

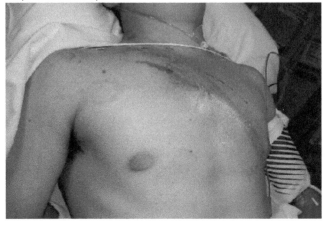

CLINICAL ASSESSMENT AND IDENTIFICATION

- A normal ECG effectively rules out the condition.
- Unexplained tachycardia may be a clue.
- Look too for atrial and ventricular ectopics.
- Consider bedside echocardiogram.
- Consider troponin.
- Beware labelling ST changes as myocardial contusion; there may have been a primary cardiac event that precipitated the accident.

TREATMENT

- There is no direct ED-based intervention to treat the myocardial contusion itself; treat the following if identified:
  - o Hypoxaemia
  - o Acidaemia
  - o Fluid status
  - o Low haemoglobin
- Monitor ECG.
- Consider a central and arterial line.

VIII. DIAPHRAGMATIC INJURY

DEFINITION AND CONTEXT

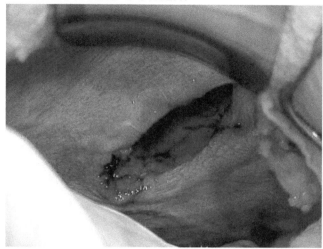

- Diaphragmatic injury is usually caused by penetrating rather than blunt injury.
- It is easily missed both clinically and radiologically.
- In blunt injury it is three times more common on the left (the right hemi-diaphragm being protected by the liver) and nearly always at the weakest point, posterolaterally.
- A diaphragmatic breach will not heal spontaneously because of the differential pressure gradients between chest and abdomen.
- Abdominal content herniation is a possibility and may be picked up years later.

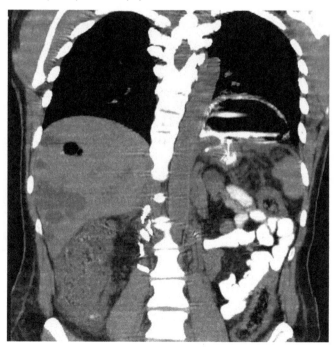

CLINICAL ASSESSMENT AND IDENTIFICATION

- Symptoms are likely to be masked by associated injuries.
- Diaphragm injuries resulting from knives or bullets are more likely to be detected on surgical exploration.
- In blunt injuries, particularly those causing an abrupt rise in intra-abdominal pressure, be careful not to interpret a gastrothorax for a large pneumothorax; both will cause respiratory embarrassment.

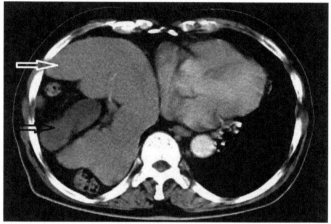

Right diaphragmatic hernia

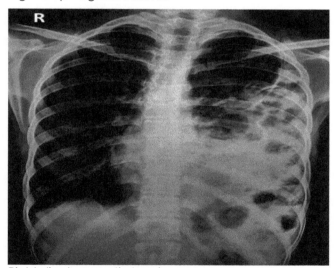

Right diaphragmatic hernia

TREATMENT

- **Insert a nasogastric tube** gently to drain stomach content.
- A cautiously placed **chest drain** using the traditional open technique, not Seldinger, is indicated.
- **Surgical repair** needs to be considered in the context of associated injuries.

IX. OESOPHAGEAL INJURY

- This rare injury is often initially missed both clinically and radiologically.
- Other associated injuries will normally predominate the clinical presentation e.g. a neck stabbing with tracheal and vascular disruption.

TREATMENT

- Operative repair or endoluminal stenting should be considered in the context of other associated injuries.

X. TRACHEAL/BRONCHIAL INJURYDEFINITION AND CONTEXT

- This rare injury is typically caused by significant deceleration injuries; most patients die at the scene of the accident.
- It is unlikely to be missed clinically or radiologically in survivors, since clinical effects are usually dramatic.

CLINICAL ASSESSMENT AND IDENTIFICATION

- **A massive air leak** is suggested by **gross surgical emphysema**, **pneumomediastinum** and **a vigorously bubbling chest drain** that has failed to alleviate respiratory compromise.
- **Haemoptysis** is an additional clue.

TREATMENT

- Discuss **intubation strategy** with senior anaesthetic colleagues (consider single or double cuffed tubes, use of fibre optics, etc).
- Consider **additional large bore chest drain** on the affected side (one intercostal space further up).
- Do not attach suction to the chest drain.
- Other significant patient injuries may influence your resuscitation strategy.

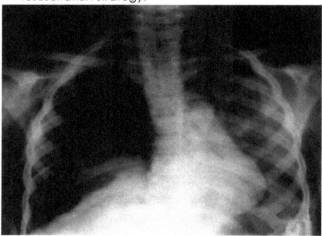

XI. SIMPLE PNEUMOTHORAX

DEFINITION AND CONTEXT

- This is a common injury which is readily missed on CXR and subsequently discovered on CT.
- Small, asymptomatic/occult pneumothoraces may be observed, even if the patient is ventilated.
- About a third may deteriorate clinically, necessitating a drain.
- No guideline regarding the safe timing for flying following a simple traumatic pneumothorax exists.
- A pragmatic approach may be to adopt British Thoracic Society guidelines for spontaneous pneumothorax: **flying is permissible, once chest x-ray confirms resolution of the pneumothorax**

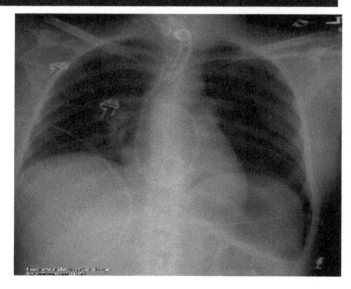

XII. RIB FRACTURES

DEFINITION AND CONTEXT

- Significant force is required to break ribs in the young; underlying injury is typical, especially lung contusions.
- Whilst less force is required in the elderly, even an isolated rib fracture can result in significant morbidity (e.g. secondary pneumonia) particularly in those with pre-existing comorbidities.

TREATMENT

- In addition to standard therapy consider the role of patient-controlled **analgesia**, **thoracic epidural** and **physiotherapy** for vulnerable patients.

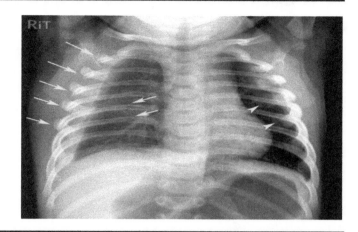

XIII. STERNAL FRACTURES

DEFINITION AND CONTEXT

- These are relatively benign injuries but may be associated with underlying myocardial or pulmonary contusion.

TREATMENT

- Consider the role of patient-controlled **analgesia** or **local anaesthetic** via a sternal catheter in vulnerable patients.

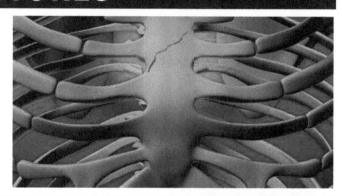

XIV. POSTERIOR STERNOCLAVICULAR JOINT DISLOCATION

- This an exceptionally rare injury.
- It is clinically important since the medial clavicular head may compromise the airway or major vessels.
- If there is evidence of compromise, reduction of the dislocation should be attempted.

- Abduct the arm to 90° and extend 10-15° and apply traction (with counter attraction to the torso from another colleague); maintain traction and pull the medial end of the clavicle forward with your fingers and thumb.
- If this fails, prepare the skin with iodine and local anaesthetic and repeat with a towel clip.

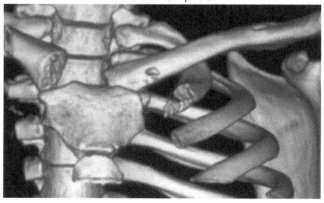

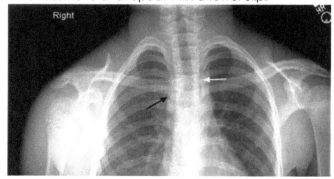

8. Acute Aortic Dissection

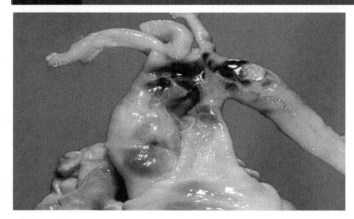

1. DEFINITION

- **Aortic dissection** occurs following a tear in the aortic intima with subsequent separation of the tissue within the weakened media by the propagation of blood.
- **A ruptured or leaking abdominal aneurysm** is a different disease, requires immediate surgery with only occasional need for any imaging, can be performed in most hospitals by a vascular surgeon and does not require the use of cardiopulmonary bypass. An acute aortic dissection is considered chronic at 2 weeks. The dissection usually stops at an aortic branch vessel or at the level of an atherosclerotic plaque[44].

2. CLASSIFICATION[45]

STANFORD CLASSIFICATION

o There are 4 different classifications of aortic dissection and the commonest one used is the **Stanford classification** dividing them into **Type A** and **Type B**.
- **Type A** dissection involves the Ascending Aorta
- **Type B** dissections involve only the Descending Aorta and occur distal to the origin of the left subclavian artery.

DEBAKEY'S CLASSIFICATION

o **Type I** dissections involve the entire aorta whilst
o **Type II** only involves the ascending aorta and, or the arch of the aorta.
o **Type III** involves only the descending aorta.

REUL AND COOLEY

- Further subdivided **DeBakey's** classification into subtypes **IIIa** and **IIIb**.

---

44 *Siegal EM. Acute aortic dissection.* J Hosp Med. *2006 Mar. 1(2):94-105.*

45 *https://teachmesurgery.com/vascular/arterial/aortic-dissection/*

o **In IIIa** the dissection involves the aorta just distal to the left subclavian artery but extends proximal or distal to this but is largely above the diaphragm.
o **In IIIb** the dissection occurs only distal to the left subclavian artery and may extend below the diaphragm.

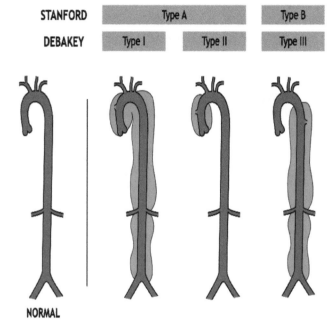

3. PATHOPHYSIOLOGY

- There are 3 possibilities as to how the blood gets into the media:
  o Atherosclerotic ulcer leading to intimal tear
  o Disruption of vasa vasorum causing intramural haematoma
  o De novo intimal tear
- Following dissection, blood flow into the media may cause:
  o Extension up or down
  o Rupture
  o Vessel branch occlusion
  o Aortic regurgitation
  o Pericardial effusion / tamponade
- 80% of aortic dissections are in non-aneurysmal vessels

4. RISK FACTORS

o Hypertension
o Coarctation of the aorta
o Giant cell arteritis

- o Cocaine abuse
- o Iatrogenic
- o Pregnancy
- o Ehlers-Danlos Syndrome
- o Marfan's syndrome
- o Turners Syndrome
- o Bicuspid aortic valve
- o Annulaortic ectasia and familial aortic dissection

5. HISTORY

- Chest pain (ripping, tearing in nature, sudden onset, maximal @ onset) – not always present!
  - o Retrosternal chest pain – anterior dissection
  - o Interscapular pain – descending aorta
  - o Severe pain ('worst ever-pain') (90%)
  - o Sudden onset (90%)
  - o Sharp (64%) or tearing (50%)
  - o Migrating pain (16%)
  - o Down the back (46%)
  - o Maximal at onset (not crescendo build up, as in an AMI)
- **Other**
  - o End-organ symptoms: neurological, syncope, seizure, limb paraesthesias, pain or weakness, flank pain, SOB + haemoptysis
  - o Aortic regurgitation
  - o Hypertension
  - o Most have ischaemic heart disease

6. EXAMINATION

- Aortic regurgitation is common
- Hypertension (if hypotensive ensure it is not due to limb discrepancy caused by an occluded vessel – check BP in the arm with best radial pulse)
- Shock – ominous signs: tamponade, hypovolaemia, vagal tone
- Heart failure
- Neurological deficits: limb weakness, paraesthesia, Horner's syndrome
- SVC syndrome – compression of SVC by aorta
- Asymetrical pulses (carotid, brachial, femoral)
- Haemothorax

7. COMPLICATIONS

- Suspect if hypotensive (check for limb discrepancy!)
  - o Aortic rupture
  - o Aortic regurgitation
  - o Acute Myocardial Infarction
  - o Cardiac Tamponade
  - o End-organ ischaemia – brain, limbs, spine, renal, gut, liver
  - o Death

8. INVESTIGATIONS

- **Bedside**
  - o **ECG**
    - ▪ Normal
    - ▪ Inferior ST elevation (right coronary dissection) but can be any STEMI (0.1% of STEMIs are dissections)
    - ▪ Pericarditis changes, electrical alternans (tamponade)

- **Laboratory**
  - o Leukocytosis/ Creatinine elevation with renal artery involvement
  - o Troponin elevated if dissection causes myocardial ischaemia
  - o D-dimer – if negative dissection is very unlikely, but not sufficient to rule out
  - o X-match
  - o Various biomarkers being investigated (e.g. elastin fragments, d-dimer, smooth muscle myosin heavy-chain protein)

- **Imaging**
  - o **CXR**
    - ▪ Widened mediastinum (56-63%), **the most reliable sign**
    - ▪ Abnormal aortic contour (48%),
    - ▪ Aortic knuckle: Double calcium sign >5mm (14%),
    - ▪ Pleural effusion (L>R),
    - ▪ Left apical cap,
    - ▪ Depressed left main stem bronchus
    - ▪ Fractures of the first and second ribs
    - ▪ Tracheal shift to the right,
    - ▪ Deviation of the nasogastric tube to the right
    - ▪ Normal in 11-16%.

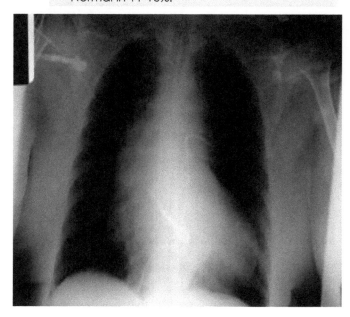

- o **ECHOCARDIOGRAPHY**
  - **Transthoracic (TTE)** 75% diagnostic Type A (ascending), 40% descending (Type B). Good for Aortic Regurgitation.
  - **Transoesophageal (TOE).** Much higher sensitivity/specificity, though operator-dependent, need sedation, and is less available. Useful in ICU / perioperative. Upper ascending aorta and arch not well visualised.

- o **HELICAL CT (CT MEDIASTINUM)**
  - Useful screen for widened mediastinum.
  - Newer multiplane/slice scanners may now negate additional need for TOE or aortography to plan operative management.

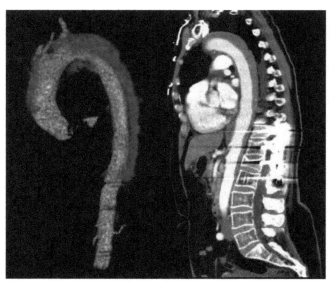

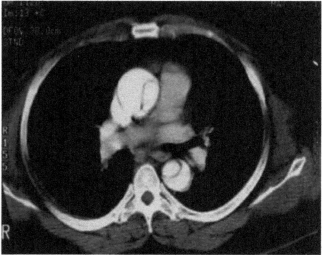

Contrast-enhanced axial CT image demonstrates an intimal flap that separates the 2 channels in the ascending and descending aorta diagnostic of a Stanford type A dissection.

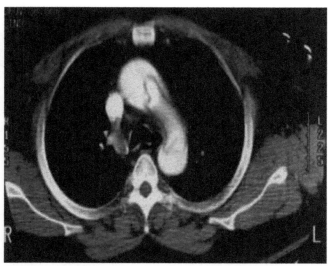

Contrast-enhanced CT scan obtained at the level of the aortic arch demonstrates an aortic dissection with almost complete separation of the aortic intima. The slight prolapse may be the beginning of a configuration at risk for intimo-intimo intussusception, a potentially fatal event.

- o **AORTOGRAPHY**
  - Was the traditional gold standard, delineating aortic incompetence and associated branch vessel involvement as well.

- o **MRI / MRA**
  - Excellent sensitivity and specificity limited by availability

9. ED MANAGEMENT OF AORTIC DISSECTION

- **Emergent priorities**
  - o Control BP
  - o Control bleeding
  - o Fluid resuscitation
- Supplemental Oxygen
- Wide bore IV access (Swan sheath)
- Invasive monitoring
- Warn blood bank (**X-match 6U** + need for other products)
- Correct coagulopathy
- Control HR and BP (**aim for P 60-80 & BP 100-120 SBP**)
- IV beta blocker (propranolol, Esmolol or labetalol) combined with vasodilators (e.g. GTN, labetalol, SNP)
- Start β-blocker first to avoid increased aortic wall stress from reflex tachycardia
- Refer to cardiothoracic surgeon

10. INDICATIONS FOR SURGERY

- Persistent pain
- Type A
- Branch Occlusion
- Leak
- Continued extension despite optimal medical management

10. Abdominal Trauma
I. PENETRATING ABDOMINAL TRAUMA

INTRODUCTION

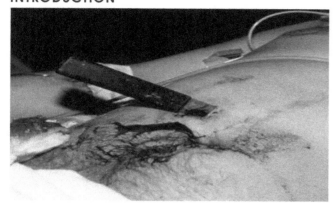

- Penetrating abdominal trauma is seen in many countries. The most common cause is a stab or gunshot. The most common organs injured are the small bowel (50%), large bowel (40%), liver (30%), and intra-abdominal vascular (25%).
- When the injury is close range, there is more kinetic energy than those injuries sustained from a distance. Even though most gunshot wounds typically have a linear projection, the high-energy wounds are associated with unpredictable injuries.
- There may also be secondary missile injuries from bone or bullet fragments. Stab wounds that penetrate the abdominal wall are difficult to assess.
- Occult injuries can be missed, resulting in delayed complications that can add to the morbidity[46].

ETIOLOGY

- Penetrating trauma occurs when a foreign object pierces the skin and enter the body creating a wound. In blunt or non-penetrating trauma the skin is not necessarily broken. In penetrating trauma, the object remains in the tissue or passes through the tissues and exits the body.
- An injury in which an object enters the body and passes through is called a perforating injury.
- Perforating trauma is associated with an entrance wound and an exit wound[47].

---

[46] Taghavi S, Askari R. StatPearls [Internet]. StatPearls Publishing; Treasure Island (FL): Jan 13, 2019. Liver Trauma.

[47] Revell MA, Pugh MA, McGhee M. Gastrointestinal Traumatic Injuries: Gastrointestinal Perforation. Crit Care Nurs Clin North Am. 2018 Mar;30(1):157-166.

- Penetrating trauma suggests the object does not pass through. Penetrating trauma can be caused by violence and may result from:
  o Fragments of a broken bone
  o Gunshots
  o Knife wounds
- Penetrating trauma often causes damage to internal organs resulting in shock and infection. The severity depends on the body organs involved, the characteristics of the object, and the amount of energy transmitted. Assessment includes x-rays, CT scans, and MRI. Treatment involves surgery to repair damaged structures and remove foreign objects.
- Puncture and penetration are similar.
  o A puncture is different from a penetration wound in that there is no exit wound in a puncture.
  o This type of trauma is seen in a stabbing or a gunshot wound in which a low-velocity pistol bullet was used.

HISTORY AND PHYSICAL

- Penetrating abdominal trauma is due to stabbings, ballistic injuries, and industrial accidents.
- These injuries may be life-threatening because abdominal organs bleed profusely.
- If the pancreas is injured, further injury occurs from autodigestion.
- Injuries of the liver often present in shock because the liver tissue has a large blood supply.
- The intestines are at risk of perforation with concomitant fecal matter complicating penetration. Penetrating abdominal trauma may cause hypovolemic shock and peritonitis.
- Penetration may diminish bowel sounds due to bleeding, infection, and irritation, and injuries to arteries may cause bruits.
- Percussion reveals hyperresonance or dullness suggesting blood. The abdomen may be distended or tender indicating surgery is needed.
- The standard management of penetrating abdominal trauma is a **laparotomy.**
- A greater understanding of mechanisms of injury and improved imaging has resulted in conservative operative strategies in some cases.

EVALUATION

- Gross assessment may be difficult as damage is often internal.
- The patient should be examined physically followed by **ultrasound, x-ray, and/or CT scanning**.
- Sometimes before an x-ray is performed a paper clip is taped over entry and exit wounds[48].
- The patient is treated with intravenous fluids and/or blood.
- Surgery is often required; impaled objects are secured in place so that they do not move and they should only be removed in an operating room.
- Foreign bodies such as bullets may be removed, but if there is a possibility that they may cause more damage, they should be left in place.
- Wounds are debrided to remove tissue that cannot survive and will lead to infection.

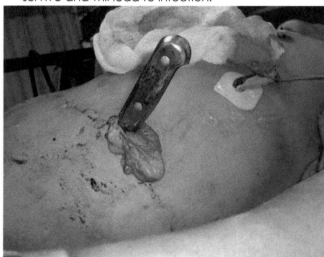

MANAGEMENT

- The presentation of a patient with penetrating abdominal injury may reveal shock, hypotension, narrow pulse pressure, tachypnea, oliguria, and an apparent trajectory or open wound.
- Examination in awake patients may reveal signs of peritonitis such as guarding or rebound tenderness.
- The approach to patients with penetrating abdominal trauma depends on the type of instrument that caused the injury and hemodynamic status.
- In general, gunshots to the abdomen are usually associated with hollow viscus injury and usually require exploration.
- Knife wounds are associated with lower incidence of intra-abdominal injury, and hence, their work-up requires clinical judgment and experience.

- Many protocols exist for evaluating patients with a stab wound to the abdomen.
- Blood work is always done but is nonspecific.
- The use of DPL and FAST can be performed to assess the stable patient with a knife or gunshot wound, but both these modalities have a high rate of false negatives.
- **CT scan** is used in patients with wounds of the flank and back and can help assess solid organ injury.
- The diagnostic test of choice is a **triple contrast CT scan** in hemodynamically stable patients.
- Other imaging tests may be done to assess for any associated head or skeletal injury.
- In most hospitals, penetrating trauma is handled by a trauma team. After the ABCs are completed, most gunshot patients require an exploratory laparotomy. This view is now changing, and stable patients with gunshot wound with no signs of peritonitis who have been evaluated by a triple contrast CT scan may be observed if there is no evidence of intra-abdominal injury.
- The indications for surgical intervention include:
  - Patient with hemodynamic instability,
  - Development of peritoneal findings such as involuntary guarding, point tenderness or rebound tenderness, and
  - Diffuse abdominal pain that does not resolve[49].
- Patients with a stab wound with clear signs of peritonitis similarly require a laparotomy.
- Stable patients with stab wounds may be locally explored or undergo a triple contrast CT scan.
- The prognosis of patients with penetrating abdominal trauma is variable and depends on the extent of injury and time of presentation to the emergency department.

DIFFERENTIAL DIAGNOSIS

- Abdominal compartment syndrome
- Hemorrhagic shock
- Trauma to pelvis, diaphragm or genitourinary system
- Sepsis

COMPLICATIONS

- Open wounds
- Sepsis
- Fistulas
- Wound dehiscence
- Colostomy/ileostomy
  Short bowel syndrome

---

48 Wortman JR, Uyeda JW, Fulwadhva UP, Sodickson AD. Dual-Energy CT for Abdominal and Pelvic Trauma. Radiographics. 2018 Mar-Apr;38(2):586-602.

49 Tarchouli M, Elabsi M, Njoumi N, Essarghini M, Echarrab M, Chkoff MR. Liver trauma: What current management? HBPD INT. 2018 Feb;17(1):39-44.

II. BLUNT ABDOMINAL TRAUMA

INTRODUCTION

- In civilian practice approximately 20% of trauma injuries requiring surgery involve the abdomen[50].
- Abdominal trauma may be blunt or penetrating, but generally in civilian practice, blunt trauma is more common than penetrating and usually follows a road traffic crash. However, in the American urban civilian practice penetrating trauma is more common than blunt trauma, gunshot wounds being more frequent than stab wounds[51].
- In the UK stab wounds predominate[52]. In military practice, penetrating abdominal wounds are greater than blunt with a high mortality from the high velocity missile/bullet/fragment wounds.
- The diagnosis of abdominal injury by clinical examination is unreliable and, thus in the initial management of abdominal trauma in adults following rapid assessment and resuscitation selection of appropriate investigations is of key importance[53].

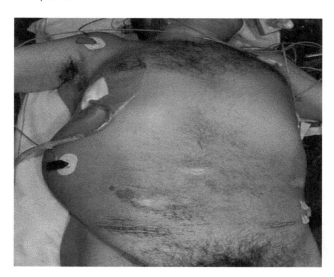

PATTERNS OF INJURIES

- Particular pattern of injuries occur with blunt abdominal trauma.
- Steering wheel injuries commonly involve the sternum (with the risk of myocardial contusion), liver and spleen.

---

[50] Gilroy D (2005) Deaths from blunt trauma, after arrival at hospital: What goes around comes around. Injury 36: 47-50.

[51] Buckman RF, Scalea TM (1999) International approaches to trauma care. Trauma Quarterly, USA.

[52] Greaves I, Porter KM, Ryan JM (2001) Trauma London: Arnold, UK

[53] National Confidential Enquiry into Perioperative Deaths (NCEPOD) (2007) Trauma: who cares?, UK.

- Pelvic fractures are associated with urethral and urinary bladder injuries and with rupture of the diaphragm.
- Different types of lumbar vertebral fractures from acceleration or deceleration injuries, are associated with various abdominal injuries.
- Transverse spinous process fractures may occur with renal trauma and horizontal fractures of the vertebrae through the body are associated with pancreatic, duodenal or small bowel mesentery injuries.
- It is important to understand the concept of the trimodal distribution of death (%) during a road traffic crash:
  - The first phase is death within seconds to minutes (40%) from the impact of the crash (energy being converted from one form to the other according to the first law of thermodynamics) causing instant damage to the brain, heart and great vessels and cervical cord.
  - The second phase is the 'golden hour' as death occurs within minutes to hours (30%) and thus can clinically be acted upon, influenced and death prevented. **This 'golden hour' phase** forms the basis of the primary survey (ABCDE) of the Advanced Trauma Life Support (ATLS) system of management in which immediately life-threatening injuries are identified and treated in the correct order[54].
  - The third phase is death within days to weeks (30%) from infection, multiple organ failure, abdomen (haemorrhage) and injury to the skeleton (pelvis and long bones).

ABDOMINAL ANATOMY

Region	Organs potentially injured
Lower chest	• Liver, Spleen, Diaphragm, Stomach
Anterior abdomen	• Liver, Spleen, Colon, Bladder, • Stomach, Pancreas, • Transverse colon, Ileum, Jejunum
Flank	• Kidneys, Ureters, • Ascending and Descending colon
Posterior abdomen	• Great vessels, Duodenum, • Pancreas, Spinal Cord

---

[54] Committee on Trauma (1981) Field Surgery Pocket Book. London, UK.

ASSESSMENT

- The initial assessment and resuscitation of the injured patient should follow the ATLS sequence of airway, breathing and circulation as airway compromise causes death within seconds, breathing derangement causes death within minutes and circulatory impairment causes death within hours[55].
- Shock, in the presence of obvious abdominal injuries, should prompt a laparotomy for haemorrhage control (resuscitation laparotomy) during the circulation stage of the primary survey.
- The assessment of the trauma patient following resuscitation includes obtaining a detailed history of the event from pre-hospital personnel. Knowledge of accident details (e.g. use of seat belts, estimated speeds, injuries to other passengers or any deaths) may enable the clinician to build a picture of likely injury patterns[56]. A thorough examination of the abdomen is part of the secondary survey and must include rectal, penile and vaginal examination.
- Physical examination of the abdomen in the trauma patient is unreliable and a single negative examination does not exclude serious injury.
- Regular review and documentation of findings are therefore essential as physical findings may undergo subtle changes with time[57].
- Many injuries are not an immediate threat to life but will become fatal if not diagnosed and treated expeditiously. Thus, the role of the secondary survey. The decision on which injuries mandate an urgent operation apart from obvious and exsanguinating bleeding is frequently difficult and best made by an experienced surgeon.

INVESTIGATIONS

- If patient's primary survey is intact, the adjuncts to the primary survey and resuscitation begins. The adjuncts to the primary survey include any of the following as necessary: EKcG, ABG, chest Xray, pelvis xray, urinary catheter, eFAST exam, and/or DPL and computed tomography.
- Bedside sonography should be used to perform an eFAST exam. The sole purpose of FAST **is to detect free fluid**. In the setting of hypotension, free fluid on the eFAST exam suggests hemoperitoneum, necessitating emergent surgical intervention.

- The sensitivity of FAST in abdominal trauma is 88% and it is therefore an ideal screening investigation for all trauma patients who do not need to go directly to theatre and patients who are unstable because of its rapid assessment[58].
- A normal FAST does not exclude injury as signs of blood loss and hollow viscus injury may initially be subtle. If the patient remains cardiovascularly stable, this can be augmented by computed tomography (CT) scan either to confirm the negative FAST or determine organ injury for non-operative management[59].
- As it will also miss injuries not associated with intra-abdominal fluid, FAST may not be very useful in haemodynamically stable patients.
- It is therefore the investigation of choice in the haemodynamically unstable patient whereas CT is the investigation of choice in the haemodynamically stable patient.

1. LIVER

- Liver injuries account for 15-20% of intra-abdominal organ injuries but up to 50% of mortality, and 45% have associated splenic injury. **Conservative management** is appropriate in 80% of cases, with surgical intervention reserved for ongoing and uncontrolled bleeding.
- If hepatic or splenic injuries are detected on CT, the source of any ongoing bleeding can be detected through angiography.
- Through interventional radiology it can be possible to embolise the bleeding vessel and remove the need for surgical intervention.

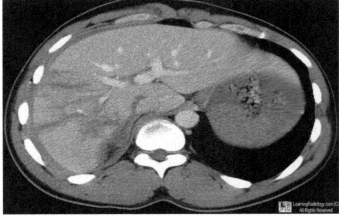

CT scan showing laceration to the liver (Courtesy Learning Radiology)

[55] American College of Surgeons (1997) ATLS for Doctors: Student Course manual. 6th edn, Chicago, USA.

[56] Doersch KB, Dozier WE (1968) The seat belt syndrome: the seat belt sign, intestinal and mesenteric injuries. Am J Surg 116: 831-833.

[57] Janson JO, Yule SR, Loudon MA (2008) Investigation of blunt abdominal trauma. BMJ 336: 938-942.

[58] Myers J (2007) Focused assessment with sonography for trauma (FAST): The truth about ultrasound in blunt trauma. J Trauma 62: S28

[59] Rodriguez C, Barone JE, Wilbanks TO, Rha CK, Miller K (2002) Isolated free fluid on computed tomographic scan in blunt abdominal trauma: a systematic review of incidence and management. J Trauma 53: 79-85

2. SPLEEN

- **Splenic injury is graded according to CT findings and treatment is guided by grade:**

Grade 1	Minor subcapsular tear or haematoma
Grade 2	Parenchymal injury not extending to the hilum
Grade 3	Major parenchymal injury involving vessels and hilum
Grade 4	Shattered spleen

- The spleen contains approximately one unit of blood at any time.
- Grade 1 or 2 injuries can usually be managed conservatively.

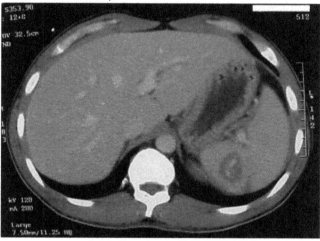

CT scan showing ruptured spleen

3. PANCREAS

- Injury to the pancreas may cause pancreatitis, which may develop over days.
- Blunt pancreatic injury may not be immediately recognised. It is relatively uncommon, occurring in around 10% of blunt abdominal injuries but it is rarely an isolated injury due to the position of the pancreas.
- Amylase elevation will often not occur until 3-4 hours after injnury, if at all, and lipase is no more specific for pancreatic trauma.

4. HOLLOW VISCUS

- Peritoneal contamination with bowel contents will produce peritonism.
- There may be accompanying blood loss but the degree of hypovolaemia is generally less significant than in solid organ injury.
- Damage to the retroperitoneal portion of the bowel will not produce classical signs of peritonism as the leak will be contained.

5. VASCULAR STRUCTURES

- Catastrophic blood loss may occur with injury to any of the large vessels in the abdomen.
- **Aortic injury** is usually fatal, but may be tamponaded if it occurs retroperitoneally.
- Injury to the **inferior vena cava** is likely to be associated with more insidious blood loss unless there is a large tear.

6. GU TRACT

- Bruising, haematuria or meatal blood are often the only signs of a GU injury.
- Injury to the intraperitoneal portion of the bladder may result in chemical peritonitis.

ED MANAGEMENT

All trauma patients must be managed in accordance with Advanced Trauma Life Support (ATLS) algorithms[60]:

- **A (Airway with c-spine protection):** Is the patient speaking in full sentences?
- **B (Breathing and Ventilation):** Is the breathing labored? Bilateral symmetric breath sounds and chest rise?
  - o O2 – Nasal cannula, Face Mask
- **C (Circulation with hemorrhage control):** Pulses present and symmetric? Skin appearance (cold clammy, warm well perfused)
  - o IV – 2 large bore (minimum 18 Gauge) Antecubital IV
  - o Monitor: Place patient on monitor.
- **D (Disability):** GCS scale? Moving all extremities?
- **E (Exposure/Environmental Control):** Completely expose the patient. Rectal tone? Gross blood per rectum?

- Early consultation by relevant speciality teams (surgeons, radiologists, anaesthetists, theatre staff, critical care) and transfer teams if definitive care is not available in your hospital. In a trauma centre, early trauma CT should be carried out, ideally once the patient has been haemodynamically stabilised through fluid resuscitation.

  If a patient remains unstable despite resuscitation then senior members of the trauma team (emergency, surgical and anaesthetics) should make a team decision weighing up the merits of CT versus immediate theatre.

---

[60] ATLS: Advanced Trauma Life Support for Doctors (Student Course Manual). Ninth ed. American College of Surgeons; 2013.

11. Fractures
I. CERVICAL SPINES FRACTURES

INTRODUCTION

- Approximately 3 % of patients who present to the emergency department as the result of a motor vehicle accident or fall have a major injury to the cervical spine[61]. 10-20% patients with head injury also have a cervical spine injury. Up to 17% of patients have a missed or delayed diagnosis of cervical spine injury, with a risk of permanent neurologic deficit after missed injury of 29%.
- Most cervical spine fractures occur predominantly at two levels. One third of injuries occur at the level of C2, and one half of injuries occur at the level of C6 or C7.

1. HYPERFLEXION

- **Chance fractures:** The combination of flexion and distraction forces can cause a *Chance* (or **seatbelt**) fracture. This is a type of thoracolumbar injury in which the posterior column is involved with injury to ligamentous components, bony components, or both. Chance fractures are often associated with intra abdominal injuries[62].
- **Tear drop fractures:** fracture of the anteroinferior vertebral body (**teardrop sign**)
- **Rupture of posterior ligament.**
- **The odontoid peg may also be fractured:** by sudden severe flexion.
- **Unstable wedge fracture** is an unstable flexion injury due to damage to both the anterior column (anterior wedge fracture) as the posterior column (interspinous ligament).

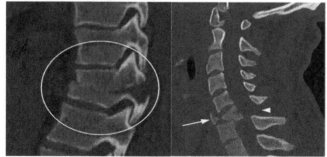

Chance fracture (healthline.com) & Tear drop fracture (cambridge.org)

---

[61] *Adam Flanders and adapted for the Radiology Assistant by Robin Smithuis*

[62] *Bernstein MP, Mirvis SE, Shanmuganathan K AJR Am J Roentgenol. 2006 Oct; 187(4):859-68.*

2. FLEXION & ROTATION

Clay Shoveller Fracture
- Stable fracture of one or more of the spinous processes of the C6-T3 vertebra
- Avulsion fracture by the supraspinous ligament of the spinous process caused hyperflexion
- All **intervertebral ligaments may tear** and the upper vertebral body can be displaced relative to the one below

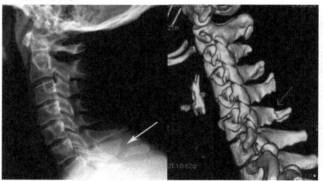

3. HYPEREXTENSION

- **Hangman's fracture:** Unstable fracture through pedicles of C2 following hyperextension with distraction or compression.
- Bilateral fracture of the posterior arch of C2 and disruption of the C2-3 junction
- Neurological injury may result from damage to the posterior longitudinal ligament allowing significant anterior displacement of C2 on C3
- Typical history: car accident with patient striking head on dashboard

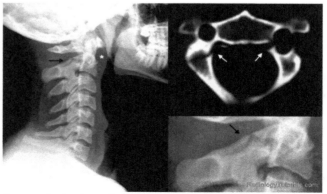

Hangman's fracture: fracture through pedicles of C2 following hyperextension with distraction or compression.

---

4. ROTATION

o   May result in **facet joint dislocation.**
o   Rarely occurs in isolation and it is often unstable
o   Unilateral interfacet dislocation is due to a hyperflexion injury with rotation.
o   The superior facet on one side slides over the inferior facet and becomes locked.

5. COMPRESSION

o   This mechanism is common in thoracic and lumbar spine injuries and results in wedge fractures.
o   **Jefferson fracture** is a burst fracture of the ring of C1 with lateral displacement of both articular masses . it is an unstable fracture.
o   Combined anterior and posterior arch fractures
o   Can result from hyperextension causing a posterior arch fracture.
o   Typical history: diving head first into water, thrown against roof of car

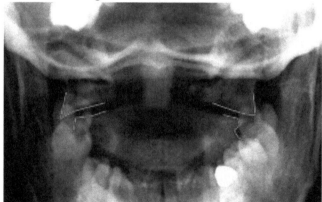

In the above odontoid view, the lateral displacement of C1 indicates a Jefferson fracture.

Unstable fractures	
Flexion	o Bilateral interfacetal dislocation o Flexion teardrop fracture o Wedge fracture with posterior ligamentous rupture
Extension	o Odontoid fracture type II o Hangman's fracture o Extension teardrop fracture
Vertical compression	o Burst fracture, e.g. Jefferson fracture

DIFFERENCES BETWEEN ADULTS & CHILDREN

•   The anatomy and relationships of the child's cervical spine is different to that in adults:
    o   Children have relatively larger heads
    o   Their ligaments and joint capsules are more lax
    o   Their facet joints are more horizontal
    o   Their vertebral bodies are wedge shaped

•   The pattern of injuries is determined by these progressive changes. Most spine injuries in children occur in the cervical region; in younger patients, these are more often subluxations or dislocations, more often in the upper cervical spine, and more often associated with neurological injury[63].
•   **Pseudosubluxation**: refers to the appearance of forward slippage of one vertebral body on another;
•   Pseudosubluxation of C2 on C3 occurs in 24% of under 8-year olds and of C3 on C4 in 14% of under 8-year olds.
•   In pediatric spinal injury, four patterns tend to predominate: fracture with subluxation, fracture without subluxation, subluxation without fracture [purely ligamentous injury and spinal cord injury without radiographic abnormality (SCIWORA)][64].
•   **SCIWORA** (**S**pinal **C**ord **I**njury **with**out **r**adiological **a**bnormality) which is defined as objective signs of myelopathy as a result of trauma with no evidence of fracture or ligamentous instability on plain radiographs or tomography.

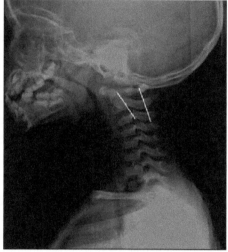

Pseudosubluxation of C2 on C3 in 2-year-old girl who fell.

CLINICAL ASSESSMENT

•   For the purposes of clearing the cervical spine, patients can be divided into two groups:
    o   Conscious and cooperative
    o   Unconscious and/or uncooperative

1. CONSCIOUS COOPERATIVE PATIENTS

•   This is the most commonly encountered group of patients who present to the ED or pre-hospital practitioner.

[63] *A prospective multicenter study of cervical spine injury in children. Viccellio P, Simon H, Pressman BD, Shah MN, Mower WR, Hoffman JR, NEXUS Group. Pediatrics. 2001 Aug; 108(2):E20.*

[64] *Hickman ZL, McDowell M, Anderson RCE. Principles of pediatric spinal column trauma. 3rd ed In: Albright AL, Pollack IF, Adelson PD, editors. , editors. Principles and Practice of Pediatric Neurosurgery. New York, NY: Thieme; (2015):789–805.*

- They have a low incidence (less than 3%) of cervical spine injury and are able to cooperate with clinical assessment. Therefore, a focussed history and examination can be used to clinically clear their necks – various clinical decision rules have been developed to be used in these patients:
  o **Nexus Low Risk Criteria**
  o **Canadian Cervical Spine Rules**

A. NEXUS LOW RISK CRITERIA (NLC)[65]

- This was developed from a prospective study of patients undergoing cervical spine radiography in 21 centres in the USA. The study looked at 5 criteria; if all were negative the patient was classified as having a low risk of injury:

NEXUS LOW PROBABILITY CRITERIA (NSAID)
o No focal **N**eurological deficit
o No midline **S**pinal (cervical) tenderness
o Normal **A**lertness
o No **I**ntoxication
o No painful **D**istracting injury

B. CANADIAN C-SPINE RULE (CCR)[66]

- The Canadian C-Spine Rules are designed for alert and stable trauma patients; it is a validated tool that is said to be 100% sensitive in identifying clinically important injuries.
- It includes assessment for all GCS 15 patients age> 65 with a dangerous mechanism or parenthesis in the extremities requires some radiology. The remainder of the indications include low risk criteria and a physical examination to assess 45 degree rotation of the neck.
- Unlike the NEXUS rule, this study excluded children <16 years of age, and all patients with a Glasgow Coma Scale (GCS) score of <15.
- There is no robust evidence base for a clinical rule-out for cervical spine injury in children less than 10 years of age.

- The decision rule resulting from this study asks 3 questions:
  o Is there any high-risk factor present which mandates radiography? Age ≥65 or dangerous mechanism of injury or parasthaesia of extremities?
  Yes>>> Radiography
  o Is there any low-risk factor present that allows safe assessment of the range of neck motion?

Simple rear MVC or sitting position in ED or ambulatory anytime or Delayed onset of pain or Absence of midline tenderness?
  No>>> Radiography
  o Is the patient able to actively rotate their neck 45° to the left, and right?
  Unable>>> Radiography

2. UNCONSCIOUS / UNCOOPERATIVE PATIENTS

- These patients are not able to have their cervical spines cleared clinically as a reliable clinical assessment cannot be made.
- These patients require imaging to clear their spines.

INVESTIGATION STRATEGIES

a. PLAIN CERVICAL SPINE SERIES
- Plain X-ray films are a 'quick & dirty' way to assess the spine, and are readily available in most hospitals and trauma centers. Normal imaging of the cervical spine consists of three views: **The Lateral, Antero-posterior (AP) and odontoid peg views.** In children under 5, the PEG view is considered unnecessary.

b. SWIMMERS VIEW
- In the case of an inadequate lateral view:

c. FLEXION / EXTENSION VIEWS
- There is no role for flexion/extension views in the acutely injured neck.

d. COMPUTERISED TOMOGRAPHY (CT)
- Computed tomography (CT), and in particular MDCT, plays a critical role in the rapid assessment of the (poly-)traumatized patient[67].
- CT screening has a higher sensitivity and specificity for evaluating cervical spine injury compared with plain film radiographs[68].
- In the cervical spine, CT detects 97–100% of fractures, but its accuracy in detection of purely ligamentous injuries has not been documented.

e. MAGNETIC RESONANCE IMAGING (MRI)
- MRI scanning is very sensitive for soft tissue injuries including ligament injuries, disc herniation and haemorrhage, which are less well visualised on CT[69].
- It has been recommended that cervical spine trauma patients with negative standard radiographs and suspected occult cervical injury should be investigated by MR imaging to detect ligamentous injuries that were not seen on plain X-ray studies.

[65] Hoffman J, Mower W, Wolfson A, Todd K, Zucker M, Group NEX-RUS. Validity of a set of clinical criteria to rule out injury to the cervical spine in patients with blunt trauma. The New England Journal of Medicine. 2000; 343:94-99.

[66] Stiell I, Wells G, McKnight R, et al. Canadian C-Spine Rule study for alert and stable trauma patients: II. Study objectives and methodology. Canadian Journal of Emergency Medicine. May 2002;4(3):185-193

[67] Linsenmaier U, Krötz M, Häuser H, Rock C, Rieger J, Bohndorf K, Pfeifer KJ, Reiser M Eur Radiol. 2002 Jul; 12(7):1728-40.

[68] Antevil JL, Sise MJ, Sack DI, Kidder B, Hopper A, Brown CV J Trauma. 2006 Aug; 61(2):382-7.

[69] Wilmink JT Eur Radiol. 1999; 9(7):1259-66.

II. FACIAL BONES INJURY

INTRODUCTION

- Facial injuries occur in a significant proportion of trauma patients requiring prompt diagnosis of fractures and soft tissue injuries, with possible emergency interventions[70].

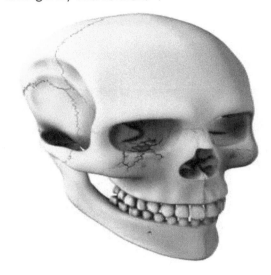

CLINICAL ASSESSMENT

Initial assessment

- Injuries to the head and neck frequently involve the airway or major vessels. The initial assessment, therefore, should begin with airway, breathing, and circulation (ABCs). In facial injuries, associated head and neck injury must also be considered.
- First, protect the airway by removing any foreign bodies and by placing the patient in a sitting position or on the side to facilitate expectoration of blood.
- If severe maxillofacial trauma is present, the athlete is at risk for airway obstruction because of a lack of tongue support from the mandibular structures.

History

- Following initial stabilization of the ABCs, the EP should proceed with the history and physical examination. In addition to obtaining a basic history of the injury and past medical problems, the clinician should seek to answer the following questions[71]:
  - o Can you breathe out of both sides of your nose?
  - o Are you having any trouble speaking?

---

[70] Erol B, Tanrikulu R, Görgün B. Maxillofacial fractures: Analysis of demographic distribution and treatment in 2901 patients (25-year experience) J Craniomaxillofac Surg. 2004;32:308–13.

[71] Mayersak RJ. Facial trauma in adults. Up To Date. Available at http://www.uptodate.com/contents/facial-trauma-in-adults

- o Do you have double vision or any other trouble with your vision?
- o Is your hearing normal?
- o Are you experiencing any numbness of your face?
- o Have you had any previous facial injuries or surgeries, including procedures to correct vision (eg, LASIK [laser-assisted in situ keratomileusis])?
- o Do your teeth come together the way they normally would?
- o Are any of your teeth painful or loose?
- o The patient should be questioned regarding the mechanism of the injury, the presence of numbness or pain over any parts of the face, and visual disturbances.

- For injuries of the **ZMC** and **zygomatic arch**, the history must also include:
  - o **Visual disturbance** indicating possible orbital or globe injury
  - o **Alteration in bite or difficulty moving the jaw** suggests mandible, maxilla or zygomatic arch injury
  - o **Sensory disturbance to the cheek and upper gum** a sign of infraorbital nerve injury

- **For nasal injury**, the history must include:
  - o **Previous nasal injury / deformity** often a perceived nasal deformity is pre-existing.
  - o **Epistaxis** this may be extensive with nasal trauma but a history of epistaxis alone is not predictive of a new nasal deformity.
  - o **Anticoagulant medication** may complicate the management of post-traumatic epistaxis
  - o **Any persistent nasal discharge** since the injury this symptom may indicate a nasoethmoid injury with CSF leak.

Physical Examination

- A general examination is important to identify any potential threat to the airway and the systemic effects of bleeding. If airway compromise is identified or threatened, senior EM and anaesthetic support should be called urgently.
- **Face**: Using a look, feel and move approach:
  - o **Look**: Look for the following, remembering to use a head light, nasal speculum and suction when examining the nose:
    - **Areas of swelling, bruising and bleeding**: persisting bleeding and / or discharge from the nose may indicate a nasoethmoidal fracture.

- **Deformity of the nose and zygomatic arch depression** of the zygomatic arch (flattened face) is best identified by looking from above or below.
- **Septal haematoma of the nose:** a haematoma on the side of the nasal septum which needs draining urgently to prevent a **"Saddle Nose Deformity"** from ischaemic necrosis.
- **Evidence of injury to the eye(s):** the position of the eye and visual acuity should be checked.
- **Enophthalmos and proptosis** both indicate a significant orbital injury.
- **Subconjunctival haemorrhage:** if the posterior limit of the haemorrhage cannot be seen, it is likely that blood has tracked round the eye from a fracture of the orbital wall. A clear posterior border suggests a direct blunt injury to the globe.

o **Feel:** palpation of facial bony landmarks and an assessment of neurological function should be undertaken, specifically identifying:

- **Zygomatic arch:** check for a step or flattening caused by a depressed fracture.
- **Periorbital region:** for the crepitus of surgical emphysema this indicates a fracture involving a sinus, usually the maxillary.
- **Intraorally:** to assess the maxilla in the upper buccal sulcus for tenderness or a step.
- Assessing **sensation to the skin** supplied by the infraorbital nerve

o **Move:** Movement of the eye and jaw must be assessed;

- **Eye movement:** particularly upward gaze, may be restricted in orbital blow-out fracture **due to trapping of the herniated inferior rectus muscle.**
- **Limited jaw movement:** caused by restricted movement of the coronoid process of the mandible under the zygomatic arch may be found in depressed fractures of the zygomatic arch.

INVESTIGATION STRATEGIES
Imaging Studies

- Plain radiograph has poor sensitivity for detection of facial fractures. It should not play a role in the diagnosis of head trauma, except in limited circumstances such as detection of a radiodense foreign body[72].

- Generally, **computed tomography (CT) scanning** is the study of choice when evaluating facial fractures because visualization of fractures among the complex curves of facial bones is best achieved using this modality. Its use in the ED is restricted to either a second line investigation, usually initiated by the maxillofacial team, or when other injuries (e.g. cervical spine injury) prevent routine facial x-rays being performed.
- The diagnosis of **orbital blow-out fracture** may be made on routine facial x rays (e.g. a **teardrop sign**) but CT scan remains the gold standard if this injury is suspected or identified.

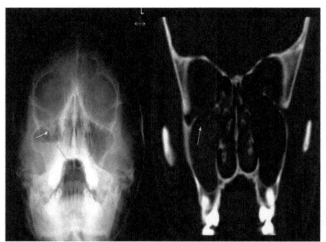

TEAR DROP SIGN: There is a **fracture of the inferior floor of the right orbit**, and there is evidence of orbital contents (such as the inferior rectus muscle) bulging into the right maxillary sinus (yellow arrow). There is **an air-fluid level in the sinus** in this example (orange arrow), which is due to haemorrhage and is a very helpful radiographic sign when the fracture itself is less obvious. CT is usually performed in these cases; in this example, it confirms the **displacement of some orbital fat** through the fracture (arrow).

- **Focused Ocular Ultrasound** (FOUS) has been evaluated in the ED and found to be highly accurate in both diagnosing and excluding both orbital and ocular trauma.
- Radiographic evaluation, however, should not be substituted for a complete external and internal examination[73]. See the following:
  o **Frontal sinus fractures:** Plain posteroanterior, lateral, and Waters radiographic projections demonstrate the fracture, whereas a **CT scan** with a thin 2-mm cut through the sinuses demonstrates the anatomy, the integrity of the posterior wall, and any pneumocephali that are pathognomonic for a posterior wall fracture.

[72] Shetty VS, Reis MN, Aulino JM, Berger KL, et al. ACR Appropriateness Criteria® Head Trauma.

[73] Reyes Mendez D, Lapointe A. Nasal trauma and fractures in children. Up To Date.

o **Orbital fractures**: **Facial CT scanning** in the axial and coronal planes with thin cuts through the orbits is the study of choice. Herniation of the orbital contents into the maxillary sinus, observed as clouding of the maxillary sinuses on plain radiographs, suggests an orbital floor fracture.

o **Nasal fractures**: Radiographs are not usually necessary to diagnose this injury. There can be no justification for ordering x-rays of the nasal bones for a patient with suspected nasal fracture. If a nasoorbitoethmoid fracture is suspected, **facial CT scanning** confirms the diagnosis. In patients with nasal injury and persisting discharge form the nose, it can be difficult to differentiate between nasal secretion and CSF arising from a **nasoethmoidal fracture.** Although often advocated:

  - **Testing for the Presence of glucose**, which is present in CSF but not normally in nasal secretion, may be falsely positive due to contamination of nasal secretions by blood or tears.

  - **Halo sign or Ring sign:** Dab some of the blood on a tissue. If there is CSF mixed with the blood, it will move by capillary action further away from the centre than the blood will.

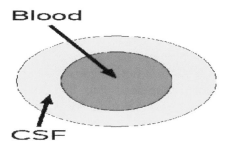

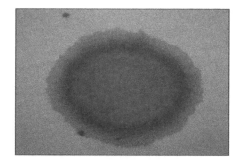

❖ **Beta-2 transferrin** (also known as the **Tau protein**) is almost exclusively found in the CSF and is a highly sensitive and specific test for the presence of CSF. The presence of beta-2 transferrin in nasal discharge is the most accurate diagnostic test to confirm CSF rhinorrhoea.

o **Zygomatic/zygomaticomaxillary fractures**: If a fracture is suspected, a **facial CT scan** with coronal and axial cuts elucidates the injury. A plain Waters view may be used as a scout radiograph.

o **Maxillary (Le Fort) fractures**: These fractures are very difficult to assess with plain radiography. If the clinical examination findings are equivocal, then a plain Waters image may provide additional information; otherwise, **facial CT scanning** with coronal and axial cuts is the criterion standard. Radiographically, Le Fort I fracture is the only one of the 3 Le Fort fractures to involve the nasal fossa; Le Fort II fracture is the only one of the 3 Le Fort fractures to involve the inferior orbital rim; and Le Fort III fracture is the only one of the 3 Le Fort fractures to involve the zygomatic arch[74].

o **Mandibular fractures**: The study of choice is panoramic radiography. Simple radiographs of the mandible are less sensitive for detecting fractures when compared to panoramic radiographs and can miss condylar fractures. If this study is not available, then a mandibular series consisting of a right and left lateral oblique, posteroanterior, and Towne view may be obtained. Fractures of the condyle may require coronal plane CT scanning.

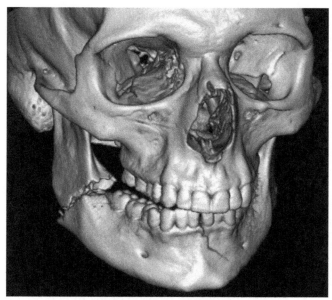

CT reconstruction of Mandibular fracture – Courtesy Wikipedia

---

[74] *Reehal P. Facial injury in sport. Curr Sports Med Rep. 2010 Jan-Feb. 9(1):27-34.*

1. ZMC FRACTURE

o Zygomaticomaxillary Complex (ZMC) fractures result from blunt trauma to the periorbital area.

o They are also referred to as **tripod, tetrapod, quadripod, malar or trimalar fractures**, are seen in the setting of traumatic injury to the face.

o They comprise fractures of the:
   ▪ Zygomatic arch
   ▪ Inferior orbital rim, and anterior and posterior maxillary sinus walls
   ▪ Lateral orbital rim

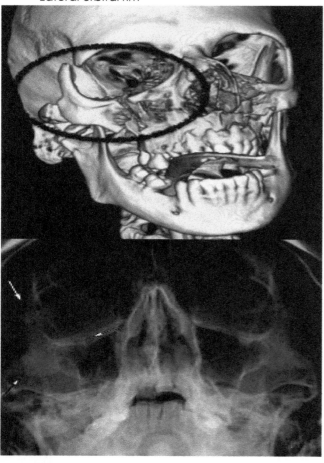

o **If eye involvement** (e.g. reduced visual acuity or diplopia): urgent referral to a maxillofacial surgeon and / or an ophthalmologist.

o **If infraorbital nerve involvement:** is not an indication for urgent referral.

o Patients should be given **general advice** regarding their injury including:
   ▪ Avoidance of nose blowing as this **may produce surgical emphysema.**
   ▪ Not to occlude the nose when sneezing.
   ▪ Application of ice packs to the area to reduce swelling.
   ▪ Take regular analgesia.
   ▪ General head injury advice.

2. ZYGOMATIC ARCH FRACTURE

o Fracture of the zygomatic bone is a common fracture of the facial skeleton; the zygomatic bone forms the most anterolateral projection one on each side of the middle face.

o If there is restriction of mouth opening due to **trapping of the temporalis muscle or mandibular condyle**, is an indication for urgent referral to a maxillofacial surgeon.

o Follow-up and advice should follow that of ZMC fracture.

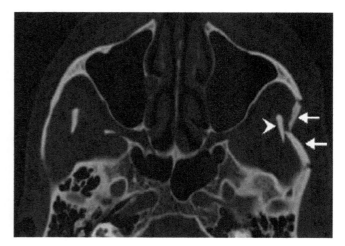

3. ORBITAL BLOW-OUT FRACTURE

• Orbital blow-out fractures generally occur with blunt trauma to the orbit with an object larger in diameter than the orbital entrance (eg, baseball, fist). A blow-in fracture results when a fracture fragment is displaced into the orbit, resulting in decreased orbital volume and impingement on orbital soft tissues, such as from high-velocity trauma (eg, falls from a height, severe blows to the orbit with a weapon).

• Patients may report diplopia.

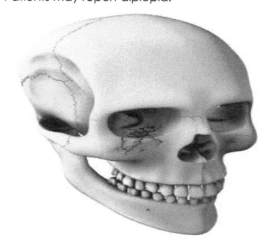

o **Visual disturbance, limitation of eye movements** and a **teardrop sign** on facial x ray are all signs of an orbital blow-out fracture: **Immediate referral to an ophthalmologist or maxillofacial surgeon is essential.**

o Facial CT will be needed to visualise the fracture in detail and plan surgical repair.

o There is no evidence to support routine antibiotic prophylaxis in orbital floor fracture.

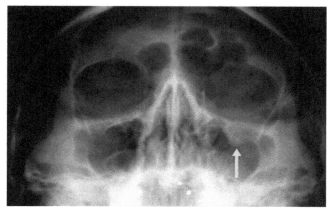

Left Orbital Blow-out Fracture with **Tear Drop Sign**

• Associated clinical findings of facial bones injuries may include:

❖ **Enophthalmos and proptosis:** *due to* **increased orbital volume**

❖ **Diplopia:** *due to trapping of the herniated* **inferior rectus muscle**

❖ **Orbital emphysema:** *especially when fracture is into an adjacent* **paranasal sinus**

❖ **Sensory disturbance to the cheek and upper gum:** *a sign of* **infraorbital nerve injury**

❖ **Restriction of mouth opening in ZMC Fracture:** *due to trapping of the* **temporalis muscle** *or* **mandibular condyle.**

4. LE FORT FRACTURES (MIDDLE THIRD)

• The Maxilla is a complex bone made up of strong buttresses but with areas of weakness around the maxillary sinus.

• **Le Fort I**
  o Transverse fracture through floor of maxillary sinuses (only palate moves)

• **Le Fort II**
  o Through nose, lower orbits and maxillary sinuses (pyramidal shaped fracture)

• **Le Fort III**
  o Through orbits (craniofacial dysjunction) (separates the entire midface from the base of the skull)
  o Combinations occur and fractures are often comminuted

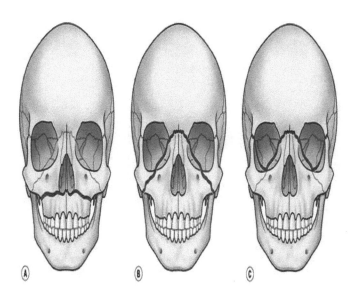

EXAMINATION

• **Inspection**
  o Displacement: lengthening of the midface, bruising, lacerations
  o Subconjunctival haemorrhage,
  o Enophthalmos, diplopia
  o Bleeding/CSF from nostrils, or post-nasally
  o Disruption of occlusion or dental arch
  o Missing or loose teeth- bruising in centre of palate or buccal sulcus

• **Palpation**
  o Rock maxilla against stable point e.g. upper basal skeleton
  o Check orbital margins for palpable steps
  o Check infra-orbital nerve

IMAGING

• **Plain radiographs**
  o Plain films are limited by their ability to penetrate through extensive soft tissue oedema and to help distinguish between multiple planes of complex bony framework.
  o OM15 and OM30 views
  o Lateral view facial bones

• **CT scans**
  o CT scan images are the imaging modality of choice for facial fractures.
  o CT imaging is superior to plain films for delineating multiple fractures, evaluating associated cartilaginous or soft tissue injury, and assessing for the presence of impingement into the optic canal.
  o Three-dimensional CT scans are highly recommended for the treatment planning of fractures of moderate or greater complexity.

5. MANDIBULAR FRACTURE

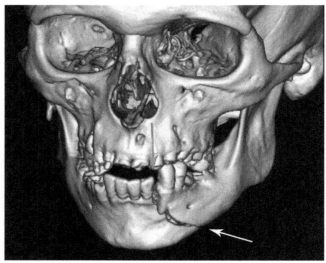

CT of Mandibular fracture (courtesy www.wikem.org)

- Mandible fractures are a frequent injury because of the mandible's prominence and relative lack of support. As with any facial fracture, consideration must be given for the need of emergency treatment to secure the airway or to obtain hemostasis if necessary before initiating definitive treatment of the fracture.
- Condylar fractures are classified as extracapsular, subcondylar, or intracapsular.

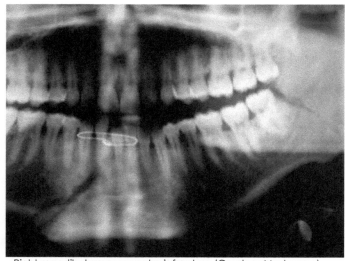

Right mandibular parasymphysis fracture (Courtesy Medscape)

- Treatment can be conservative or may involve formal reduction (which can be open or closed).
- Closed reduction may be supported with intermaxillary fixation or splints.
- **Possible complications of mandibular fracture include:**
  o Osteomyelitis
  o Permanent malocclusion
  o Permanent paraesthesia

6. NASAL FRACTURE

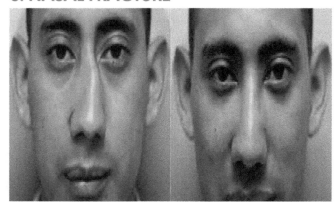

Nasal fracture (courtesy www.ohniww.com)

o Nasal fractures occur as a result of direct blows in contact sports and many other different causes, including traffic accidents, assault, external trauma from other objects, and falls.

o The nasal bones are the most commonly fractured bony structures of the maxillofacial complex[75] as they have an exposed, prominent position and little structural support.

o X-rays have little value in confirming or ruling out this condition due to the difficult imaging of these bones (plain films miss approximately 50% of fractures). Therefore, the management of nasal injuries is guided only by the clinical findings.

o **Septal haematoma** occur as a significant complication of nasal trauma in 2% of nasal injuries[76]. Blood vessels in the overlying mucoperichondrium supply the septal cartilage, which can be injured resulting in formation of septal haematoma. If left undrained, a septal haematoma can develop into a septal abscess or lead to ischaemic necrosis of the septal cartilage in a delayed manner and subsequent saddle nose deformity. Septal abscesses can result in meningitis, intracranial abscesses and cavernous sinus thrombosis because of the valveless venous drainage pathways creating an intracranial entry point[77].

o **Traumatic epistaxis** is common with nasal injuries caused by trauma to the nasal mucosa and vessels. Nasal packing may be required to stabilise a patient for transfer.

[75] Erdmann D, Follmar KE, Debruijn M, et al. A retrospective analysis of facial fracture etiologies. Ann Plast Surg. 2008 Apr. 60(4):398-403.

[76] Elcock M. Nasal septal haematomas: A case series and literature review. Emerg Med 1999;11(1):41–44.

[77] Alshaikh N, Lo S. Nasal septal abscess in children: From diagnosis to management and prevention. Int J Pediatr Otorhinolaryngol 2011;75(6):737–44.

o All patients with nasal packing should be placed on oral antibiotics (eg amoxicillin, cephalexin) to prevent toxic shock syndrome[78]. These patients should be referred promptly to ENT services for admission as there is a risk of inadvertently dislodging the nasal pack into the oropharynx.

ED MANAGEMENT OF EPISTAXIS

- **If CSF rhinorrhoea** is confirmed, the patient should be **referred immediately** to an otolaryngologist for further assessment.
- **Uncontrolled epistaxis, CSF rhinorrhoea** and **septal haematoma** are all indications for urgent ENT referral in nasal injury.
- The management of nasal injuries varies greatly across the United Kingdom and therefore a suggested flow chart is as follows[79]:

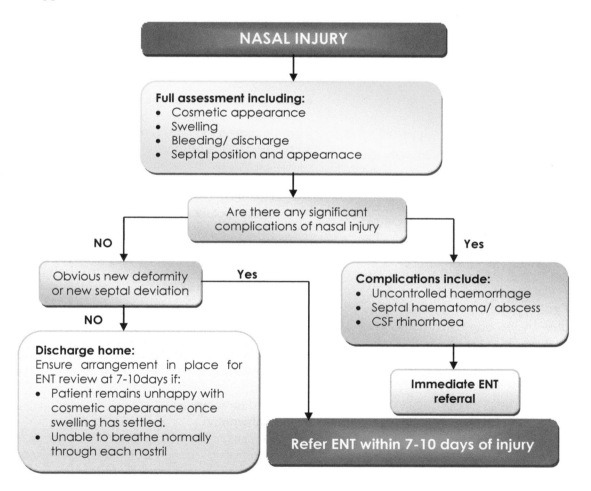

---

[78] Kasperek Z, Pollock G. Epistaxis: An overview. Emerg Med Clin North Am 2013;31(2):443–54.

[79] Management Algorithm adapted from RCEM Learning: https://www.rcemlearning.co.uk/reference/zygomatic-and-nasal-injury/#1571913781415-37b97970-6700

III. SHOULDER & BRACHIAL PLEXUS INJURY

ANATOMY

THE ROTATOR CUFF

o Stability is mostly conferred by robust neuromuscular control of the rotator cuff group of muscles.

o These arise from the scapula and insert on the tuberosities of the humerus, giving them the mechanical capacity to stabilise the ball in the socket against the pull of the powerful muscles that move the arm.

- **Supraspinatus:** abduction
- **Subscapularis:** internal rotation
- **Infraspinatus and Teres minor:** external rotation

STERNOCLAVICULAR JOINT

o The clavicle acts as a strut, keeping the upper limb away from the chest.

o The sternoclavicular joint relies on powerful ligaments to prevent displacement, which is therefore relatively unusual.

ACROMIOCLAVICULAR JOINT

o The clavicle has a complex relationship with the scapula. This allows scapular rotation in full abduction, while assisting in maintaining the position of the upper limb.

o It achieves this by the strong conoid and trapezoid ligaments which anchor the clavicle to the coracoid process of the scapula.

SCAPULO-THORACIC JOINT

o In full abduction, the glenohumeral joint can only achieve around 90° of abduction at which point the scapula rotates on the chest wall to achieve the remainder of the arc.

BRACHIAL PLEXUS

o The upper limb is supplied from the C4 to T1 nerve roots.

o Occasionally T2 is also involved.

o The myotomes are as follows:

- **Shoulder Joint**
  - C4-5: Abduction
  - C7: Adduction
- **Elbow Joint**
  - C5-6: Flexion
  - C7-8: Extension
  - C6: Pronation/Supination
  - C6-7: Flexion
- **Wrist Joint and Fingers**

- C6-7: Extension
- T1: Abduction/Adduction (small muscles of the hand)

CLINICAL ASSESSMENT

- Generally, be reluctant to diagnose a sprain.
- A minor sprain may be the diagnosis, but often there is something more significant to find.
- Always examine the rotator cuff.
- If it is intact and there is no bony tenderness or neurological impairment, most will resolve.
- Examination should take the form of the traditional sequence of: look, feel, move and image:
  o **Look:** for deformity, swelling, congestion etc.
  o **Feel:** for site and nature of tenderness (e.g. bony, diffuse, subacromial space.). Check for sensory loss.
  o **Move:** passively, then look for the active range of movement. Bear in mind the myotomes if there appears to be any motor loss.
  o Next assess the rotator cuff.
  o Active resisted movements are tested as follows;
  - **Supraspinatus** abduction 20-40° in extreme internal rotation with palms outwards
  - **Subscapularis** extending hand away from back
  - **Infraspinatus** and **Teres minor** external rotation

INVESTIGATION STRATEGIES

- **Plain Radiographs**
  o Always ask for 2 views, i.e. AP, and a modified axial.
  o The modified axial is preferable to the often-used Y view as it is less likely to be misinterpreted.
- **Ultrasound**
- **Computed Tomography (CT)**
- **Bone scintigraphy**
  o Bone scintigraphy is a highly sensitive method for demonstrating bone pathology, particularly covert fractures and bone metastases.
- **Magnetic resonance (MRI)**
  o MRI has the advantage of high contract resolution, making it particularly useful for the assessment of soft tissue injuries.

1. ACROMIO-CLAVICULAR DISRUPTION

MECHANISM OF INJURY:

o Injury to the acromioclavicular (AC) joint with disruption of the AC ligaments with or without coracoclavicular (CC) ligament disruption

o Usually being caused by direct blow to the shoulder or sustained while falling onto the shoulder[80].

SIGNS AND SYMPTOMS

o Pain at the end of the collar bone.

o Pain may feel widespread throughout the shoulder until the initial pain resolves; following this it is more likely to be a very specific site of pain over the joint itself.

o Swelling often occurs.

o Depending on the extent of the injury a step-deformity may be visible. This is an obvious lump where the joint has been disrupted and is visible on more severe injuries.

o Pain on moving the shoulder, especially when trying to raise the arms above shoulder height.

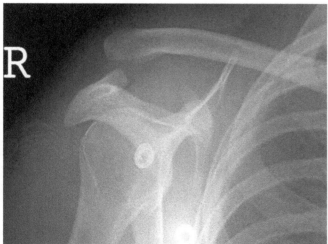

Acromioclavicular joint disruption (Courtesy Orthobullets.com)

MANAGEMENT:

o The immediate treatment of any soft tissue injury consists of the **RICER** protocol – **rest, ice, compression, elevation and referral.**

o RICE protocol should be followed for 48–72 hours.

o The aim is to reduce the bleeding and damage within the joint. The shoulder should be rested in an elevated position with an ice pack applied for 20 minutes every two hours (never apply ice directly to the skin).

o The arm should also be immobilised in a sling. This may be for as little as two days in a mild injury or up to six weeks in a more severe case.

---

[80] *https://www.orthobullets.com/shoulder-and-elbow/3047/acromio-clavicular-injuries-ac-separation*

o The No HARM protocol should also be applied – no heat, no alcohol, no running or activity, and no massage. This will ensure decreased swelling and bleeding in the injured area.

o A sports medicine professional should be seen as soon as possible to determine the extent of the injury and to provide advice on treatment required. A sports medicine professional may perform a physical examination and take x-rays of the shoulder.

2. STERNO-CLAVICULAR DISRUPTION

MECHANISM OF INJURY:

o Dislocations of the SCJ generally occur following a fall on the outstretched hand or a direct blow to the shoulder. Sporting injuries and motor vehicle accidents account for the most causes of SCJ dysfunction. However, they can also occur without any history of injury.

o Sternoclavicular dislocations account for 3% of all shoulder girdle injuries. 95% of SCJ dislocations are unilateral and anterior dislocations are far more common than posterior dislocations due to the weaker anterior sternoclavicular ligament (ratio 9:1). Bilateral superior dislocations, as in the case above, are rarely described.

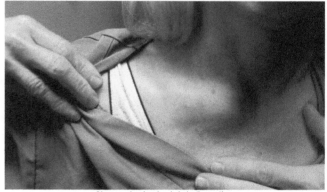

Sternoclavicular joint disruption
(Courtesy northlandscycling.wordpress.com)

CLINICAL:

o Patients commonly present with pain and swelling in the proximal sternum and sternoclavicular region. The pain will be exacerbated by lateral shoulder compression, arm movements, deep breathing or coughing.

o Patients often laterally flex their neck towards the affected side to relieving pressure on the SCJ. Asymmetry is best appreciated when viewed from above the patient's head.

o Additional symptoms include dysphonia, dysphagia or dyspnoea, Cough, Hoarseness, Pneumothorax and Tracheal compression.

o There may be venous congestion due to compression of the **internal jugular vein**, along with ipsilateral arm venous congestion.

IMAGING:

- Plain X-ray: standard views may not provide a definitive diagnosis. Alternate views such as 'serendipity view' (40-degree cephalic tilt) may provide more information.
- CTA or MRA to determine direction of dislocation and potential for vascular compromise. A contrast study is required for definitive evaluation of surrounding structures.

COMPLICATIONS

- Subclavian compression and laceration
- Mediastinal compression
- Pneumothorax
- Oesophageal rupture
- Myocardial conduction abnormalities
- Brachial plexopathy
- Tracheal tear
- Thoracic outlet syndrome

MANAGEMENT

o **Analgesia**
o An attempt can be made at **closed reduction**.
o Traction is applied to the arm and it is sometimes possible to grasp the clavicle through the skin and pull it forwards, hopefully resulting in a pop as reduction occurs.
o In extremis, the traditional method of bringing the clavicle away from the trachea is to grasp it with a towel clip through the skin and pull forwards.

3. ANTERIOR/ INFERIOR SHOULDER DISLOCATION

MECHANISM OF INJURY:

o Anterior dislocations account for 95% of all presented cases of shoulder dislocation, making them the most common type[81].
o They may be caused by a fall on an outstretched arm, trauma to the posterior humerus, or—more frequently—trauma to the arm while it is extended, externally rotated, and abducted (eg, blocking a shot in basketball).

CLINICAL:

o A patient with an anterior dislocation will enter the ED with a slightly abducted and externally rotated arm (see illustration) and will resist any movement by the examiner.

o Typically, the shoulder loses its rounded appearance, and in thin individuals, the acromion may be prominent. A detailed neurovascular examination of the arm must be performed.
o Dislocation of the humerus in any direction may compromise the axillary nerve, artery, or both. The axillary nerve and artery run parallel to each other, beneath and in close proximity to the humeral head.
o Any patient presenting with an anterior shoulder dislocation should also be screened for two other potential abnormalities.
o **Hill-Sachs lesion**, which occurs in up to 40% of anterior dislocations and 90% of all dislocations, is a cortical depression occurring in the humeral head.
o **Bankart lesions**, which occur in less than 5% of all dislocations, are avulsed bone fragments that occur when there is a glenoid labrum disruption[82]. Both can be seen on plain films, although Bankart lesions are best seen on CT.

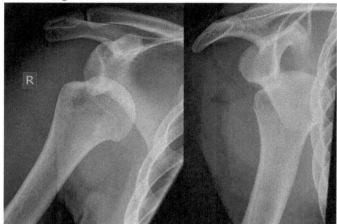

Anterior Shoulder dislocation with Hill-Sachs deformity (Source- Wikipaedia)

IMAGING:

o The x-ray is typical-Anterior and inferior dislocations are simply diagnosed with the humeral head and outline of the glenoid being incongruent, the humeral head is medially displaced and overlies the glenoid.
o In the axial view, a **Hill-Sachs deformity** always occurs in recurrent dislocations, and tells the treating physician that at least one previous dislocation has occurred.
o Another lesion can occur as the shoulder dislocates because it **tears the anterior labrum**, especially in younger patients. The tear is usually to lower part of the labrum, and this is called a **Bankart lesion.**

---

[81] Sachit M, Shekhar A, Shekhar S, Joban SH. Acute spontaneous atraumatic bilateral anterior dislocation of the shoulder joint with Hill-Sach's lesions: a rare case. J Orthop Case Rep. 2015;5(1):55-57.

[82] Greenspan A. Orthopedic Imaging: A Practical Approach. 5th ed. Philadelphia, PA: Lippincott Williams & Wilkins; 2011.

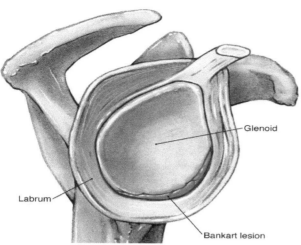

Bankart lesion (Source pathologies.lexmedicus.com)

- Sometimes a tear develops in the upper labrum, often referred to as a **S**uperior **L**abral **A**ntero-**P**osterior tear (or **SLAP lesion**), though this is often due to sports injuries and not dislocation.

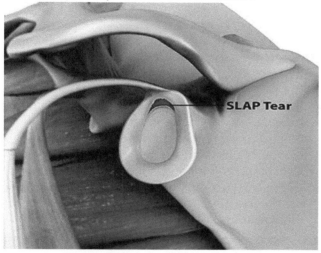

SLAP tear (Source drjeffreywitty.com)

MANAGEMENT

o **Reduction** is the only treatment option for a dislocated shoulder. The sooner these injuries are diagnosed the easier they are to **reduce**.
o Reduction is usually performed in the Emergency Department following sedation and appropriate analgesia. This can often be achieved under **entonox alone**.
o A number of techniques can be used to reduce the shoulder (**See** Procedure Competences section, Chapter 16).
    - **The Hippocratic method**
    - **The Spaso manoeuvre**
    - **The classic Kochers manoeuvre**.
o Discharge the patient with an arm sling for 3 weeks

4. POSTERIOR SHOULDER DISLOCATION

- **Mechanism of injury:**
    o Posterior shoulder dislocations occur far less frequently than anterior dislocations, representing 2% to 5% of all shoulder dislocations[83].
    o They often result from blows to the anterior portion of the shoulder (ie, motor vehicle accidents or sports-related collisions) or violent muscle contractions (eg, electrocution, electroconvulsive therapy, or seizures).
    o They occur with forced **internal rotation and adduction of the shoulder** and characteristically the patient **loses the ability to externally rotate.**
    o **The light bulb sign** seen on an AP view of the shoulder is characteristic.

IMAGING:

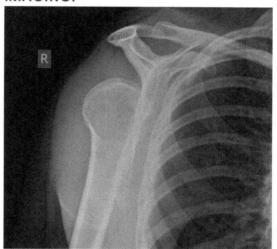

Posterior Shoulder dislocation (Source lifeinthefastlane)

Radiographic findings include:

o Internal rotation of the humerus - absence of external rotation on a standard shoulder series
o **Trough line sign:** dense vertical line in the medial humeral head due to impaction of the humeral head
o **Lightbulb sign:** The head of the humerus in the same axis as the shaft producing a lightbulb shape
o **Rim sign:** Widening of the glenohumeral space >6 mm
o The '**vacant glenoid sign**' – Where the anterior glenoid fossa looks empty

MANAGEMENT

o **Reduction** is the only treatment option for a dislocated shoulder.

---

[83] *Rouleau DM, Hebert-Davies J. Incidence of associated injury in posterior shoulder dislocation: systematic review of the literature. J Orthop Trauma. 2012;26(4):246-251.*

5. CLAVICLE FRACTURE

- **MECHANISM OF INJURY:**
  - o Clavicle fractures are most common in children and young adults, typically occurring in persons younger than 25 years.
  - o Its superficial location, its thin midshaft, and the forces transmitted across it make the clavicle a common site for injury.
  - o The usual mechanism of a clavicle fracture is a fall directly on the shoulder with the arm at the side. Rarely, clavicle fractures can occur from a direct blow or from a fall on an outstretched hand[84].

CLINICAL:

- o Patients who have sustained clavicle fractures typically hold the affected arm adducted close to the body, often supporting the affected side with the opposite hand.
- o Physical examination may reveal ecchymosis, edema, focal tenderness, and crepitation on palpation over the clavicle.
- o The defect in the bone may be seen by visual inspection or localized by palpation.

IMAGING:

- o Most fractures can be seen on a standard anteroposterior view of the clavicle; however, an anteroposterior view with 45-degree cephalic tilt minimizes the overlap of the ribs and scapula and allows for better assessment of displacement in the anterior and posterior plane[85].

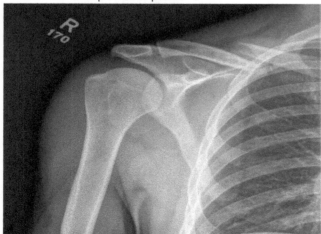

Right Clavicle fracture (Source Coreem.net)

MANAGEMENT

- o **Uncomplicated fracture:**
  - ▪ Immobilization in a sling or figure-of-eight dressing
  - ▪ Analgesia
  - ▪ Monitoring progress with X-rays every week or few weeks.
- o **Indications of surgical repair**
  - ▪ Skin penetration
  - ▪ Significant shortening of the clavicle
  - ▪ Comminution with separation
  - ▪ Associated neurological or vascular injury
  - ▪ Non-Union after 3-6 months

6. SCAPULAR FRACTURE

- Scapular fractures are uncommon, accounting for approximately 3-5% of all fractures of the shoulder girdle and less than 1% of total fractures.
- This is thought to be because they typically required high-energy trauma which also results in multi-system injuries[86].
- As high as 80-90% of all scapular fractures occurred during high-energy trauma such as motor vehicle collisions, falls, and other high impact trauma such as being thrown from a horse.
- The injury may not be noticed because it may be accompanied by other, more severe injuries.
- Diagnosis may require a **skyline view**
- Most scapular fractures are managed effectively with closed treatment and medical management.
- Treatment involves **pain control** and **immobilizing** the affected area, and, subsequently **physiotherapy.**

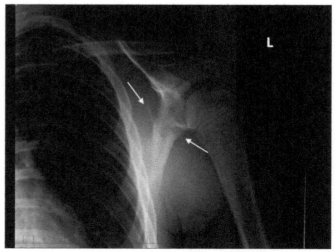

Left Scapular fracture (Source FIFA Medical Network)

[84] Nowak J, Mallmin H, Larsson S. The aetiology and epidemiology of clavicular fractures. A prospective study during a two-year period in Uppsala, Sweden. Injury. 2000;31:353–8.

[85] Johnson TR, Steinbach LS. Fracture of the clavicle. In: Essentials of Musculoskeletal Imaging. Rosemont, Ill.: American Academy of Orthopaedic Surgeons, 2003:180–1.

[86] Ideberg R, Grevsten S, Larsson S. Epidemiology of scapular fractures. Incidence and classification of 338 fractures. Acta Orthop Scand. 1995 Oct;66(5):395-7.

7. WINGING SCAPULA

OVERVIEW

o The **scapula (shoulder blade)** is the largest bone of the shoulder complex and has the greatest number of **muscles** attached to it.

o These muscles both stabilise the arm to the body and move the arm around in space.

o All these muscles act at the same time sometimes and oppose each other at other times, but work together like a well-trained team to allow the arm to move in space.

o If any of these muscles are not working in the right way at the right time this leads to a break in the rhythmic motion of the scapula.

o This is known as a scapula ' **dysrhythmia** '.

o This leads to apparent **'winging' of the scapula.**

o **Winging of the scapula** is a surprisingly common physical sign, but because it is often asymptomatic it receives little attention.

o Diagnosis is essentially clinical and should be considered in any patient presenting with **shoulder pain or weakness**, as delay in recognition may cause permanent disability

o Winging may be caused by injury or dysfunction of the muscles themselves or the nerves that supply the muscles.

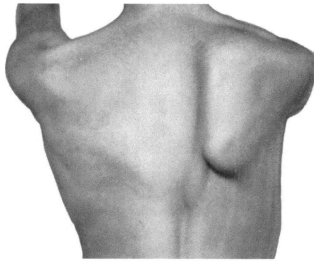

Winging of the left scapula (Source medbullets.com)

CAUSES

o **Serratus anterior muscle dysfunction**: traumatic injury to the nerve supplying the serratus anterior muscle, **the long thoracic nerve;** or due to damage to the nerve from pressure lesions or a neuritis (inflammation of the nerve).

o **Lesion of the accessory nerve** or **the dorsal nerve of the scapula**, affecting the trapezius or rhomboids, respectively.

o Important etiologies causing nerve palsy include compression injury, trauma, vigorous exercise causing traction, or viral illnesses. At times the cause may be idiopathic.

• **Guillain–Barré syndrome** can rarely present with winging of the scapula as the first symptom/sign.

• The test for identifying a long thoracic nerve injury is the **'serratus wall test':** The patient is asked to face a wall, standing about two feet from the wall and then push against the wall with flat palms at waist level.

• A majority of patients respond to conservative treatments involving **physical therapy and range of motion exercises.**

• If conservative treatment fails over the course of 6 months to 1-year, surgical intervention may be considered:

o **Exploration and decompression of the nerve** can be performed, where it gets trapped or damaged at the scalene muscles in the neck.

o For more advanced cases, **pectoralis muscle transfer** can be performed.

8. HUMERAL NECK FRACTURE

• Proximal humeral fractures are common, particularly in the elderly. Along with proximal femoral, distal radial, and vertebral-body fractures, they are a common type of osteoporotic fracture. Women are affected two to three times as often as men[87].

• **The surgical neck of the humerus** is so called because it is the area of the neck where fractures occur, rather than the anatomical neck.

• A fracture in this area may cause **damage to the axillary nerve.**

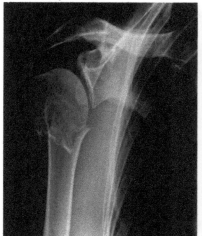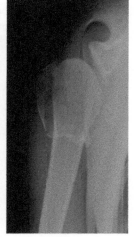

Surgical neck of the humerus fracture (Source imageinterpretation.co.uk)

[87] *The epidemiology of proximal humeral fractures. Court-Brown CM, Garg A, McQueen MM Acta Orthop Scand. 2001 Aug; 72(4):365-71*

9. SLIPPED UPPER HUMERAL EPIPHYSIS

- Proximal humeral fractures represent <5% of all paediatric fractures. This is a child/adolescent injury, seen most often between ages of 11 and 15 years.
- These fractures may occur either through the physis (growth plate) or in the metaphysis. They are usually the result of a fall on an outstretched hand, with the humeral head locked against the glenoid and the force transmitted to the physeal or metaphyseal region. The majority are, in fact, **Salter I or II fractures**. Occasionally an associated brachial plexus injury occurs.
- They may give the clinical appearance of anterior dislocation, but have a typical x-ray appearance.

MANAGEMENT:

- The proximal physis contributes 80% of the length of the humerus. Due to the enormous remodelling potential, most of these injuries do not require reduction. There is no role for attempted reduction in the ED.
- The older child with greater deformity may be treated with closed reduction. This is controversial and there are no agreed figures to guide closed operative reduction.
- Approximate indications are:
  - **5-12 years** - accept 60 degree angulation and 50% displacement
  - **>12 years** - accept 30 degrees angulation and 30% displacement
- Isolated greater tuberosity fractures with displacement in the adolescent are an exception group in which surgical reduction and fixation is usually required.
- Operative treatment is rarely indicated.
- An injury associated with a neurovascular complication is an indication for surgical treatment.

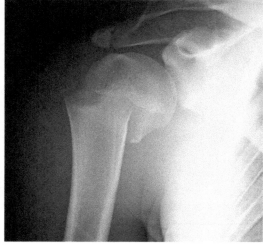

Slipped Upper Humeral Epiphysis (Source orthobullets.com)

10. BICEPS TENDON RUPTURES

- The biceps tendon consists of 2 heads originating from the coracoid process (short head) and supraglenoid tubercle of the superior labrum (long head). The tendon attaches to the radial tuberosity of the humerus. The biceps tendon is a strong supinator of the forearm and serves as a weak elbow flexor.
- Rupture of the long head of the biceps tendon leads to bunching of the muscle lower in the arm the so-called **Popeye sign.**
- It occurs through a degenerate tendon in the upper part of the bicipital groove.
- The etiology of biceps tendon rupture is mainly attributed to a sudden eccentric load on the flexed and supinated forearm, which can result in rupture of the tendon proximal and distal attachments.
- Risk factors include age, smoking, use of corticosteroids, and overuse.
- Rare causes include the use of quinolones, diabetes, lupus, and chronic kidney disease.
- In weight lifters, excessive loading and sudden stress can also lead to biceps tendon rupture.
- Rupture of the biceps tendon affects the strength of elbow flexion and supination. There is no absolute indication of surgical intervention. However, an operation is recommended for patients who want to have a faster recovery and to return to sports[88].

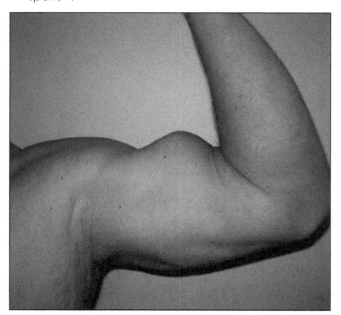

Popeye sign (Source doctorfrisella.com)

[88] Lang NW, Bukaty A, Sturz GD, Platzer P, Joestl J. Treatment of primary total distal biceps tendon rupture using cortical button, transosseus fixation and suture anchor: A single center experience. Orthop Traumatol Surg Res. 2018 Oct;104(6):859-863.

11. BRACHIAL PLEXUS INJURIES

- The brachial plexus may be injured in severe distracting injuries to the shoulder, particularly when the shoulder is forced caudally.
- This is typically seen in rugby injuries, falls from horses and falls from motorcycles.
- Success in the repair of proximal brachial plexus injuries is well documented.
- More distal, the axillary nerve is particularly vulnerable as it winds around the neck of the humerus.

A. AXILLARY NERVE INJURY

o Associated with **humeral neck fracture** and **Dislocated shoulder.** It can result in paralysis of the teres minor muscle and deltoid muscle; so that abduction of the shoulder is impaired and loss of sensation over a small part of the lateral upper arm.

o **Motor functions**: Paralysis of the deltoid and teres minor muscles. This renders the patient unable to abduct the affected limb.

o **Sensory functions**: The upper lateral cutaneous nerve of arm will be affected, resulting in loss of sensation over the regimental badge area.

o **Characteristic clinical signs**: In long standing cases, the paralysed deltoid muscle rapidly atrophies, and the greater tuberosity can be palpated in that area.

B. INJURY TO THE BRACHIAL PLEXUS

- There are two major types of injuries that can affect the brachial plexus.
- An upper brachial plexus injury affects the superior roots, and a lower brachial plexus injury affects the inferior roots.

1. UPPER BRACHIAL PLEXUS INJURY (ERB'S PALSY)

- Erb's palsy commonly occurs where there is excessive increase in the angle between the neck and shoulder, this stretches (or can even tear) the nerve roots, causing damage.
- It can occur as a result of a difficult birth or shoulder trauma.
- **Nerves affected:** Nerves derived from solely **C5-C6 roots**; **M**usculocutaneous, **A**xillary, **S**uprascapular and Nerve to **S**ubclavius. (**MASS nerves**)
- **Muscles paralysed:** Supraspinatus, infraspinatus, subclavius, biceps brachii, brachialis, coracobrachialis, deltoid and Teres minor.
- **Motor functions:** The following movements are lost or greatly weakened (**FALS**):
  o *Flexion at shoulder.*
  o *Abduction at shoulder,*
  o *Lateral rotation of arm,*
  o *Supination of forearm,*

- **Sensory functions:** Loss of sensation down lateral side of arm, which covers the sensory innervation of the axillary and musculocutaneous nerves.
- The affected limb hangs limply, **medially rotated** by the unapposed action of pectoralis major.
- The forearm is pronated due to the loss of biceps brachii. This is position is known as **'waiter's tip'**, and is characteristic of **Erb's palsy**.

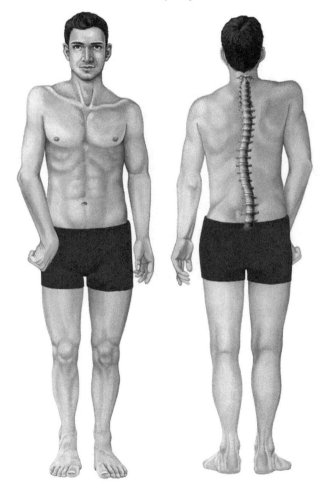

Erb's Palsy (Source agara.magdalene-project.org/erb-palsy/)

2. LOWER BRACHIAL PLEXUS INJURY (KLUMPKE'S PALSY)

- A lower brachial plexus injury results from excessive abduction of the arm (e.g. person catching a branch as they fall from a tree).
- It has a much lower incidence than Erb's palsy.
- **Nerves affected:** Nerves derived from the **C8-T1 root: Ulna and Median Nerves.**

- **Muscles paralysed:** All the small muscles of the hand.
- **Sensory functions:** Loss of sensation along medial side of arm.
- The classic presentation of KLUMPKE'S palsy is the **"claw hand" deformity.**
- There is associated **Horner syndrome** if there is involvement of the cervical sympathetic chain.

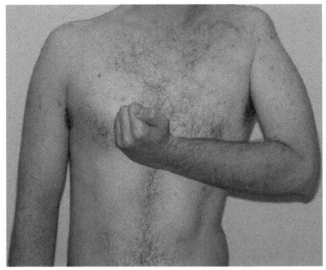

Klumpke's Palsy (Source medscape)

There is usually also a disparity in the length of the limbs; the affected limb is usually shorter than the unaffected.

- **Prognosis:** Less than 50% of those affected with Klumpke's palsy will spontaneously recover; the prognosis is worse if there is associated Horner syndrome.
- **Horner syndrome** results from an interruption of the sympathetic nerve supply to the eye and is characterized by the classic triad of **Miosis** (i.e., constricted pupil), **Partial Ptosis**, and Loss of Hemifacial Sweating (i.e., **Anhidrosis**) and **Enophthalmos**.
- **Pancoast syndrome** is characterized by a malignant neoplasm of the superior sulcus of the lung (lung cancer) with destructive lesions of the thoracic inlet and involvement of the brachial plexus and cervical sympathetic nerves (stellate ganglion).

↳ *Note that the flexors muscles in the forearm are supplied by the Ulnar and Median Nerves, but are innervated by different roots.*

12. PATHOLOGICAL FRACTURE

- **The commonest causes are:**
  o Simple bone cysts,
  o Fragility fractures
  o Metastatic lesions,
  o Fibrous dysplasia,
  o Giant cell tumor of bone
  o Multiple myeloma
- **Bone scintigraphy** may reveal other bone lesions which are not evident from radiographs, (but multiple myeloma is not usually hot).
- Sometimes it is clear that a fracture is pathological, but the cause is not immediately clear.

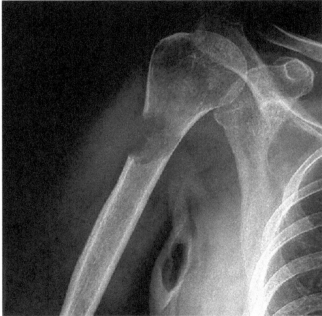

Pathologic Fracture (Source semanticscholar.org)

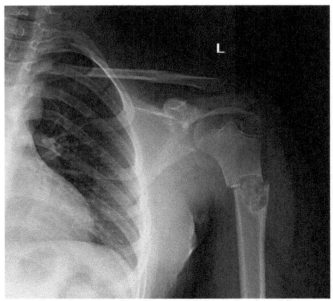

Pathologic Fracture (Source http://wuterpic.pw/)

IV. ELBOW INJURIES

IMPORTANT RADIOLOGICAL LINES

1. ANTERIOR HUMERAL LINE

o   The anterior humeral line is a line drawn down the anterior part of the distal humerus.

o   Normally this line should pass through the middle or middle third of the capitellum on the true lateral view of the elbow. When a fracture occurs in children, it is usually a supracondylar fracture through the weakest part of the humerus (note the wine glass shape) and this results in posterior displacement, moving the capitellum backwards.

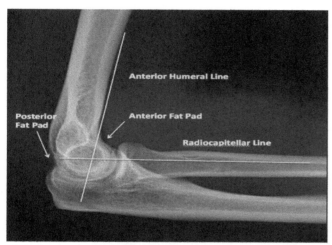

Anterior Humeral & radiocapitellar lines (Source Coreem.net)

2. THE RADIO-CAPITELLAR LINE

•   The radiocapitellar line is a line drawn along the longitudinal axis of the proximal radius.

•   Normally the line passes through the capitellum.

•   If it does not, there is radiocapitellar dislocation.

•   This should occur in every direction, no matter which x-ray view is taken.

3. FAT PADS

Anterior Fat Pad

•   Radiographically, the anterior fat pad is a superimposition of the radial and coronoid fat pads when viewing a lateral radiograph. Their location is anterior to the coronoid and radial fossae located on the distal anterior humerus.

•   The anterior fat pad can be elevated in a patient with an occult fracture. This is known as the **"sail sign"** due to the triangular sail-like appearance of the anterior fat pad[89].

---

[89] *Anatomy for medical students. University of Newfoundland Web site. Available at: www.med.mun.ca/anatomyts/ radioanat/radiology/ken/elbowbreak2.htm*

Posterior Fat Pad

•   In contrast, the posterior fat pad is located deep within the concavity of the olecranon fossa and is not normally visualized on a properly positioned lateral radiograph.

•   It is important to understand that a fat pad sign may demonstrate a false positive if the lateral has been improperly positioned. Proper positioning requires 90° flexion of the elbow joint. Other angles may tempt the posterior fat pad to emerge from the olecranon fossa, mimicking the fat pad sign.

•   In the setting of acute trauma, it represents **blood in the joint.**

•   In the non-trauma setting effusion may be due to an inflammatory cause.

•   Note that if the fracture is extra-articular, then there may not be a joint effusion and therefore the fad pad sign will be absent.

•   Examine the radial head closely in these injuries as there is often a subtle fracture.

•   Presence of a **posterior fat** pad has been associated with a **75% rate of occult fracture.**

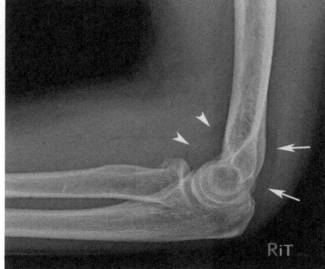

Anterior & Posterior fat pad signs (by Rathachai Kaewlai)

4. OSSIFICATION CENTRES

•   The order of the appearance of the osiification centres on radiographs of the elbow can be remembered using **CRITOL or CRITOE.**

•   The ages at when the ossification centres first appear is variable but the sequence remains constant. In general, the pattern of ossification occurs earlier in girls than boys.

- The capitellum and trochlea fuse between 10-12 years of age leaving the medial epicondyle separate until 14-17 years of age.
- It is the presence of these centres that make paediatric elbow x-rays notoriously difficult to interpret.
- Knowledge of these ossification centres and the age at which they appear will assist the observer in identifying whether a fracture is present or not.

Capitellum	1 year
Radial head	3 years
Internal (medial) epicondyle	5 years
Trochlear	7 years
Olecranon	9 years
Lateral (External) epicondyle	11 years

Note that these ages vary but a broad guide of 1, 3, 5, 7, 9 and 11 years is easy to remember.

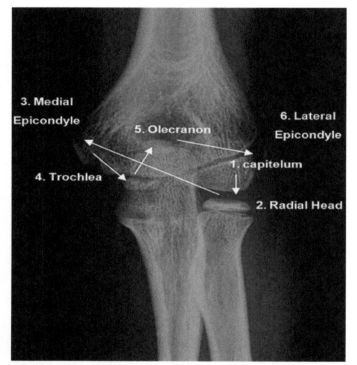

Elbow ossification centres (source wikiradiography.net)

5. CONTOURS

- It is important to analyse all 3 bones of the elbow joint and follow the contours looking for irregularities and steps that may indicate subtle disruptions and fractures in the cortex.
- Common subtle injuries that may be difficult to identify include **undisplaced radial head fractures in adults** and **undisplaced supracondylar fractures in children**.

1. ELBOW DISLOCATION

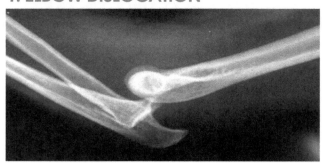

Posterior Elbow dislocation (source clinic-hq.co.uk)

MECHANISM OF INJURY

o Seen in both children and adults. More common in children than dislocation of the shoulder.

o Elbow dislocations are not common. Elbow dislocations typically occur when a person falls onto an outstretched hand.

CLINICAL

o Examination may reveal obvious deformity of the elbow. The triangular relationship of the epicondyles and olecranon will be disrupted.

o Neurovascular injury is uncommon, but should always be sought. Clinical evaluation should include median and ulna nerve function.

o Damage to the brachial artery can be assessed by palpating for a radial pulse. The dislocation is most commonly in a posterior or posterolateral direction and will be confirmed on x-ray, along with the presence of any associated fractures.

o Associated epicondylar fractures and fractures of the lateral condyle are known to occur in children.

MANAGEMENT

o **Analgesia** should be provided prior to attempts to reduce the dislocation.

o Reduction can usually be carried out in the emergency department. It requires adequate muscular relaxation and appropriate analgesia.

o **Procedural sedation** (with full monitoring) is likely to be required. In some cases, **reduction under general anaesthetic** may be necessary.

o Reduction should be immediately followed by a **further assessment of limb neurovascular status**.

o Successful reduction is then confirmed by **repeat x-ray**. This will also enable assessment of the new position of any associated fractures.

o The reduced elbow can be immobilised in a **backslab in 90° of flexion**. Admit for observation where there are concerns over neurovascular impairment or significant elbow swelling.

o **Outpatient orthopaedic** review should subsequently be arranged.

2. RADIAL HEAD FRACTURES

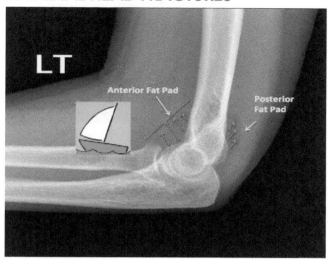

Radial head fracture with sail sign (Source Coreem.net)

MECHANISM IOF INJURY:

o Fractures of the radial head are common[90], constituting approximately one-third of all elbow fractures.

o These fractures typically follow a fall onto an outstretched wrist or direct trauma.

o Usually occur in adults and account for 30% of all adult elbow fractures.

CLINICAL

o Radial head fractures have been classified according to the **Mason classification**[91], of which there are three types: nondisplaced; displaced but without comminution, and comminuted. (A fourth type has been added to denote a radial head fracture with concomitant elbow dislocation.)

o Injuries associated with radial head fractures include the **Essex-Lopresti lesion** (tear of the interosseous membrane, distal radioulnar joint disruption) and the so-called terrible triad of the elbow (elbow dislocation, coronoid fracture, and radial head fracture).

o The physical examination of elbow injuries always must include the wrist, because injury to the radial head also may involve the distal radioulnar joint.

o If the wrist is unstable, this instability may not only need direct treatment, but also affect the choice of treatment at the elbow; when there is a risk of proximal migration in association with a distal radioulnar joint injury, excision of the radial head (without replacement) may be contraindicated.

MASON JOHNSTON CLASSIFICATION OF RADIAL HEAD FRACTURE

o *I - Nondisplaced*

o *II - Minimally displaced with depression, angulation and impaction*

o *III - Comminuted and displaced*

o *IV - Radial head fracture with dislocation of the elbow*

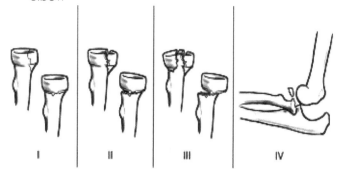

Radial Head Fractures classification | From SpringerLink

IMAGING:

• Standard radiographic evaluation of radial head fractures includes AP and lateral views of the elbow.

MANAGEMENT:

o **Undisplaced fractures:**

 ▪ Can be treated with a sling or splint for a few days followed by early ROM[92].

 ▪ Early mobilization to prevent loss of elbow extension.

o **Comminuted or displaced fractures:**

 ▪ Manipulation under anaesthetic or internal fixation.

 ▪ Occasionally the radial head may need to be excised and replaced.

o **Radial neck fractures:**

 ▪ Seen more commonly in children and are managed similar to radial head fractures.

 ▪ Greater than 20º of angulation in the adult requires reduction.

3. OLECRANON FRACTURES

MECHANISM OF INJURY:

o Olecranon fractures are most often caused by:

 ▪ Falling directly on the elbow

 ▪ Receiving a direct blow to the elbow from something hard, like a baseball bat or a dashboard or car door during a vehicle collision.

 ▪ Falling on an outstretched arm with the elbow held tightly to brace against the fall.

---

90 Pike JM, Athwal GS, Faber KJ, King GJ. Radial head fractures: an update. J Hand Surg Am. 2009;34:557–565. doi: 10.1016/j.jhsa.2008.12.024.

91 MASON ML Br J Surg. 1954 Sep; 42(172):123-32.

92 Rosenblatt Y, Athwal GS, Faber KJ Orthop Clin North Am. 2008 Apr; 39(2):173-85, vi.

CLINICAL:

Symptoms

o   Pain well localized to posterior elbow

Physical exam

o   Palpable defect
o   Indicates displaced fracture or severe comminution
o   Inability to extend elbow
o   Indicates discontinuity of triceps (extensor) mechanism

IMAGING:

o   Radiography will confirm the diagnosis and also reveal any displacement due to the pull of the triceps tendon.
o   Identification of paediatric olecranon fractures may be complicated by the appearance of the olecranon ossification centre, which may be bifid.

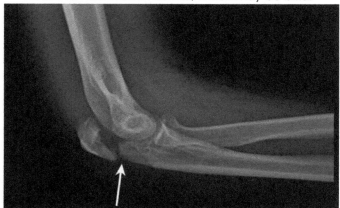

Elbow (Olecranon) Fractures - From OrthoInfo - AAOS

MANAGEMENT

o   **Undisplaced fractures**: backslab in 90° of elbow flexion and orthopaedic clinic follow-up.
o   **Displaced fractures (> 2mm)** and **those with comminution**: are more likely to require operative fixation and therefore warrant orthopaedic referral.

4. MONTEGGIA FRACTURE-DISLOCATION

MECHANISM OF INJURY:

o   A fracture of the shaft of the ulna associated with an anterior dislocation of the radial head was described by an Italian surgeon, Giovanni Battista Monteggia, in 1814[93].
o   This injury comprises **dislocation of the radial head with an ulna fracture (GRUM)**
o   It may result from a direct blow to the ulna or forced pronation.

---

[93] *Monteggia GB. Lussazioni delle ossa delle estremita superiori. In: Monteggia GB, editor. Instituzioni Chirurgiches. 2nd Vol. 5. Maspero; Milan, Italy: 1814. pp. 131–133.*

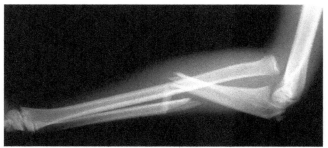

Monteggia Fractures - From Orthobullets

IMAGING:

•   The radiographic appearance of a dislocated radial head (suspect if a line bisecting the radius longitudinally does not pass through the center of the capitellum) should prompt further imaging of the forearm to exclude an ulna fracture.

MANAGEMENT:

o   Refer for reduction and internal fixation.

5. GALEAZZI FRACTURE-DISLOCATION

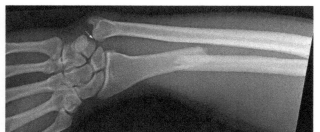

Galeazzi fractures - From Wikiradiography.net

MECHANISM OF INJURY:

o   The Galeazzi fracture is a fracture of the middle to distal one-third of the radius associated with dislocation or subluxation of the distal radioulnar joint **(GRUM)**.
o   Fall on an outstretched hand (FOOSH) with a flexed elbow.
o   Two classification systems have been proposed when categorizing Galeazzi fractures. The first classifications were based on the position of the distal radius:
    ▪ *Type I*: Dorsal displacement
    ▪ *Type II*: Volar displacement

IMAGING:

o   If a forearm fracture and dislocation are suspected, radiographs are warranted. An anteroposterior and lateral view will usually identify the injury.
o   An additional oblique view may help better classify the injury.

MANAGEMENT:

o   These injuries should be referred for reduction and internal fixation.

6. PAEDIATRIC INJURIES

A. SUPRACONDYLAR FRACTURES

MECHANISM OF INJURY:

o Supracondylar fractures of the humerus are the most frequent fractures of the paediatric elbow, with a peak incidence at the ages of five to eight years. Children are more prone to supracondylar fracture than adults due to the relatively thin trabeculae of the coronoid and olecranon fossae in this population.

o Extension-type fractures represent 97% to 99% of cases. Posteromedial displacement of the distal fragment is the most frequent; however, the radial and median nerves are equally affected. Flexion-type fractures are more commonly associated with ulnar nerve injuries.

IMAGING:

o Standard anteroposterior (AP) and true lateral radiographs of the elbow are usually sufficient to characterize the fracture.

o Presence of **fat pads** and **loss of normal anterior humeral alignment**.

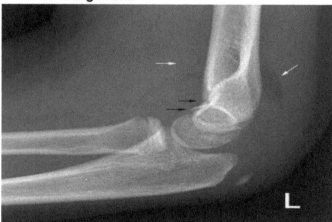

Supracondy fracture - From Wikiradiography.net

GARTLAND CLASSIFICATION OF SUPRACONDYLAR FRACTURES

Type I   Type II   Type III

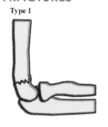 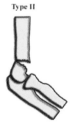 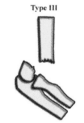

Type 1	*Undisplaced Fracture*
Type 2	*Anterior displacement with an intact Posterior Cortex.*
Type 3	*Complete cortical disruption with anterior and posterior displacements.*

MANAGEMENT:

• Analgesia and a search for associated neurovascular complications.

  o **Undisplaced fractures:**
    ▪ Collar and cuff and can be followed up in fracture clinic.
    ▪ If there is significant pain, a back slab may be a better option.

  o **Displaced fractures:**
    ▪ Should all be referred for manipulation,
    ▪ Urgently if circulation is compromised.

COMPLICATIONS INCLUDE:

• Anterior interosseous nerve (AIN) neurapraxia (branch of median n.)
• Radial nerve palsy
• Ulnar nerve palsy
• *Brachial artery injury (due to stretch and posterior displacement)*
• Ipsilateral distal radius fractures
• *Volkmann's ischaemic contracture (due to compartment swelling)*

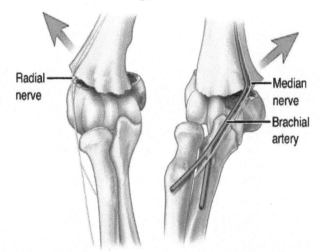

Neurovascular damage – Source musculoskeletalkey.com

B. LATERAL EPICONDYLE AVULSION INJURY

MECHANISM OF INJURY:

o Fractures of the lateral epicondyle are commonly seen in the pediatric population but are rare injuries in adults[94].

o This is the second most common elbow fracture seen in children, usually between the ages of **4 and 10**. It results from a varus force applied through the extended elbow, normally due to a fall on an outstretched hand. It is commonly displaced **by the action of the forearm extensors.**

---

[94] Sanchez-Sotelo J (2009) Lateral collateral ligament insufficiency. In: Morrey BF (ed) The elbow and it's disorders, 4th edn. WB Saunders Company, Philadelphia, pp 669–677. ISBN No 978-1-4160-2902-1

IMAGING:

o Appearance on x-ray may be subtle so an awareness of the possibility of this injury is necessary when interpreting films.

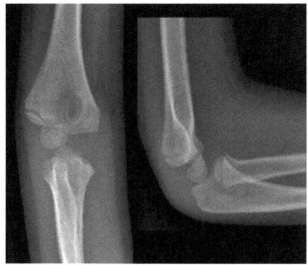

Lateral condyle fracture of the humerus - from rch.org.au

MANAGEMENT:

o **Undisplaced fractures:** Backslab with orthopaedic follow up.
o **Displaced fractures:** often need reduction

C. MEDIAL EPICONDYLE AVULSION INJURY

- Medial epicondyle fractures are common and account for 10% of all elbow fractures in children. They occur between the ages of 7-15 years.
- They are usually a result from an avulsion (pull off) injury caused by a valgus stress at the elbow and contraction of the flexor muscles.
- There may be associated **ulna nerve** damage and sometimes dislocation.
- Undisplaced avulsions can be managed conservatively while displaced fragments should be referred for reduction.

D. RADIAL NECK FRACTURE (CHILD)

- Radial neck fractures in children are a relatively common traumatic injury that usually affects the radial neck (metaphysis) in children 9-10 years of age.
- These injuries are more common in children due to weak metaphyseal bone and, as with radial head fractures, may be difficult to spot on an x-ray.
- Treatment is similar to that of radial head fractures and orthopaedic referral is recommended if there is greater than 30 degrees of angulation.

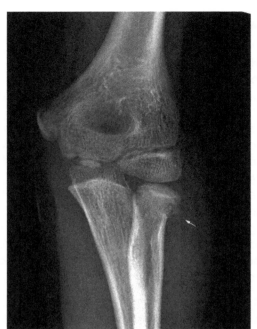

Radial Head and Neck Fractures - Pediatric - From Orthobullets

E. PULLED ELBOW

- This is also sometimes known as "**Nursemaids Elbow**".
- Nursemaid's elbow often occurs when a caregiver holds a child's hand or wrist and pulls suddenly on the arm to avoid a dangerous situation or to help the child onto a step or curb.
- The injury may also occur during play when an older friend or family member swings a child around holding just the arms or hands.
- The child will not be using the arm.
- It results from **subluxation of the radial head** from its normal position encircled by the annular ligament.
- Because moving the injured arm may be painful, the primary symptom of nursemaid's elbow is that the child will hold the arm still at his or her side, and refuse to bend or rotate the elbow, or use the arm.
- The x-ray is normal and therefore not necessary if clinical suspicion is high prior to attempted manipulation.
- Traditional treatment is usually by closed reduction with either a supination or a hyperpronation technique **flexing the elbow to 90 degrees and then fully supinating or pronating the forearm**, there may often be an associated click and the child will begin using the arm a short time later.

V. WRIST INJURIES

1. UNDISPLACED FRACTURE OF DISTAL RADIUS

A. GREEN STICK FRACTURE

- A greenstick fracture is a partial thickness fracture where only cortex and periosteum are interrupted on one side of the bone but remain uninterrupted on the other[95].
- They occur most often in long bones, including the fibula, tibia, ulna, radius, humerus, and clavicle.
- Most commonly, they occur in the forearm and arm involving either the ulna, radius or humerus.
- Greenstick fractures can take a long time to heal because they tend to occur in the middle, more slowly growing parts of bone.

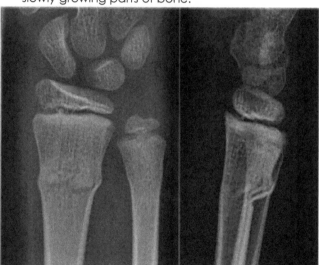

Buckle and Greenstick Fractures- from thesgem.com

B. TORUS/BUCKLE FRACTURE

- Torus fractures, or **buckle fractures**, are extremely common injuries in children.
- They are incomplete fractures of the shaft of a long bone that is characterized by bulging of the cortex.
- These injuries tend to heal much more quickly than the similar greenstick fractures.

MANAGEMENT

- Backslab and sling and Refer to the Fracture Clinic

2. FRACTURES OF THE ULNAR STYLOID

- No active treatment required; Backslab for comfort, sling and Fracture Clinic

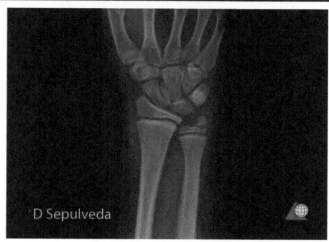

Ulnar styloid fracture- from aofoundation.org

3. SCAPHOID INJURIES

MECHANISM OF INJURY:

- o Scaphoid fractures usually result from a fall with wrist hyperextension past 95°[96].
- o A fall on an outstretched hand causes longitudinal loading of the scaphoid and a fracture occurs as the volar cortex fails in tension.
- o The force extends to the dorsal cortex, which fails in compression.

IMAGING:

- o Plain radiographs should be obtained in any patient with clinical suspicion for a scaphoid fracture. Preferred views include posteroanterior (PA), lateral, and oblique wrist films.

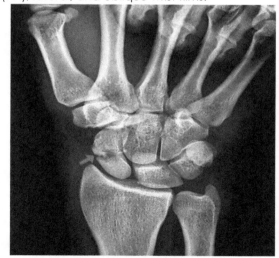

Scaphoid Fracture- from msdmanuals.com

---

[95] Chasm RM, Swencki SA. Pediatric orthopedic emergencies. Emerg. Med. Clin. North Am. 2010 Nov;28(4):907-26.

[96] Weber ER, Chao EY. An experimental approach to the mechanism of scaphoid waist fracture. J Hand Surg [Am] 1978;3:142–8. doi: 10.1016/S0363-5023(78)80062-8.

o Radiographic views specific for viewing the scaphoid include scaphoid (palm flush with cassette and ulnar wrist deviation) and clenched-fist PA view.

o Scaphoid fractures are not visible on initial plain radiographs in up to **25% of patients**[97].

o Typically patients are placed into a short arm thumb spica cast and follow-up in 10–14 days for repeat radiographs.

CLINICAL SIGN:

o Thumb compression pain

o Scaphoid tubercle

o Snuff box tenderness

o Ulnar deviation pain

o **Clamp sign**: ask patient "exactly where does it hurt?". The patient will form a clamp with the opposite thumb and index finger on both sides of the thumb.

o **Pain with resisted supination:** Hold the injured hand with forearm in neutral position. Patient attempts supination = pain when examiner resists

o Radiologically confirmed fractures should be treated by **Colles cast and referral to the Fracture Clinic.**

   o **Refer for ORIF if:**

      ▪ More than 1mm displacement of fragments,

      ▪ Angulation of 15%,

      ▪ Fracture comminution

o Check x-rays for signs of **ruptured scapholunate ligament** (Terry Thomas sign)

o If seen, confirm again no evidence of carpal dislocation and treat as a scaphoid fracture.

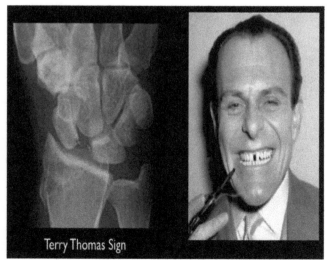

Terry Thomas sign - from slideshare.net

MANAGEMENT OF SCAPHOID FRACTURES

Adapted from GEMNet: Management of Suspected Scaphoid Fractures in the ED (September 2013)/RCEM Website[98]

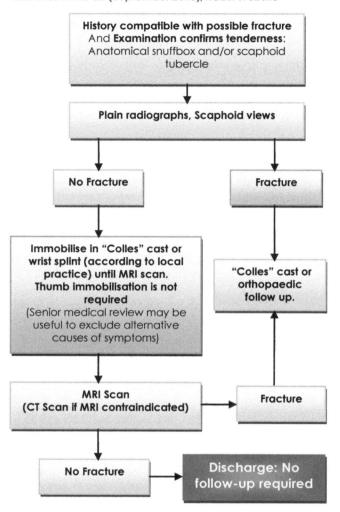

4. COLLES' FRACTURE

MECHANISM OF INJURY:

o A Colles Fracture is a complete fracture of the radius bone of the forearm close to the wrist resulting in an upward (posterior) displacement of the radius and obvious deformity[99].

o Most Colles fractures are secondary to a fall on an outstretched hand (FOOSH) with a pronated forearm in dorsiflexion (the position one adopts when trying to break a forward fall).

o Colles fractures are the most common type of distal radial fracture and are seen in all adult age groups and demographics. They are particularly common in patients with osteoporosis and as such, they are most frequently seen in **elderly women**.

[97] Geissler WB, Slade JF. Fractures of the carpal bones. In: Wolfe SW, Hotchkiss RN, Pederson WC, Kozin SH, editors. Green's Operative Hand Surgery, Sixth ed. Elsevier; 2011.

[98] RCEM Guideline for the Management of Suspected Scaphoid Fractures in the Emergency Department.pdf- p25

[99] http://www.handandwristinstitute.com/colles-fracture/

o The relationship between Colles fractures and osteoporosis is strong enough that when an older male patient presents with a Colles fracture, he should be investigated for osteoporosis because his risk of a hip fracture is also elevated.

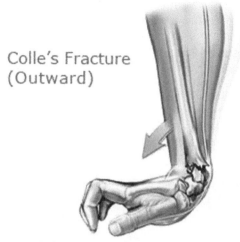

Colle's fracture - from pinterest.com

CLINICAL:

o The clinical presentation of Colles fracture is commonly described as a dinner fork deformity.
o A distal fracture of the radius causes posterior displacement of the distal fragment, causing the forearm to be angled posteriorly just proximal to the wrist. With the hand displaying its normal forward arch, the patient's forearm and hand resemble the curvature of a dinner fork.
   ▪ "Dinner Fork" Deformity
   ▪ History of fall on an outstretched hand
   ▪ Dorsal wrist pain
   ▪ Swelling of the wrist
   ▪ Increased angulation of the distal radius
   ▪ Inability to grasp object
o **Signs and Symptoms**- Pain, numbness, tenderness, bruising, deformity of wrist.

IMAGING:

o A careful history including the mechanism of injury establishes suspicion for a Colles fracture.
o Diagnosis is most often made upon interpretation of pasteroanterior and lateral views alone[100].
o The classic Colles fracture has the following characteristics:
   ▪ Transverse fracture of the radius
   ▪ 2.5 cm (0.98 inches) proximal to the radio-carpal joint
   ▪ Dorsal displacement and dorsal angulation, together with radial tilt

o Other characteristics on plain radiographs may include:
   ▪ Radial shortening
   ▪ Loss of ulnar inclination
   ▪ Radial angulation of the wrist
   ▪ Comminution at the fracture site
   ▪ Associated fracture of the ulnar styloid process in more than 60% of cases.

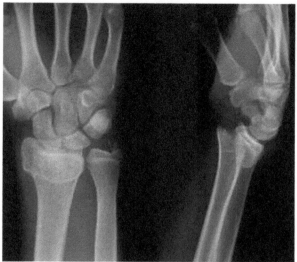

Colle's fracture - from researchgate.net

COMPLICATIONS OF COLLE'S FRACTURE:

o **Median Nerve Palsy**
o **EPL tendon tear**
o Malunion resulting in **Dinner fork deformity**
o Post traumatic **carpal tunnel syndrome**
o **Reflex Sympathetic Dystrophy**
o **Secondary Osteoarthritis**, more frequently seen in patients with intra-articular involvement

FRYKMAN CLASSIFICATION[101]

• **Type I:** transverse metaphyseal fracture
• **Type II:** type I + ulnar styloid fracture
• **Type III:** fracture involves the radiocarpal joint
• **Type IV:** type III + ulnar styloid fracture
• **Type V:** transverse fracture involves distal radioulnar joint
• **Type VI:** type V + ulnar styloid fracture
• **Type VII:** comminuted fracture with the involvement of both the radiocarpal and radioulnar joints
• **Type VIII:** type VII + ulnar styloid fracture

MANAGEMENT:

o **If stable:**
   ▪ Apply POP backslab and sling.
   ▪ Refer to the Fracture Clinic

---

[100] Adam, Greenspan,. _Orthopedic imaging : a practical approach._ Beltran, Javier (Professor of radiology), (Sixth edition ed.). Philadelphia.

[101] Frykman, G. (1967). "Fracture of the distal radius including sequelae–shoulder-hand-finger syndrome, disturbance in the distal radio-ulnar joint and impairment of nerve function. A clinical and experimental study." _Acta Orthop Scand_: Suppl **108**:103+.

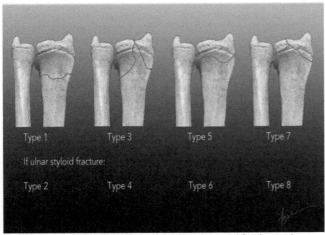

Frykman classification - from faculty.washington.edu

REFER TO ORTHO IF:

- More than 10° dorsal angulation (tilt)
- Radial shortening more than 3 mm
- Radial shift more than 2 mm
- Dorsal displacement more than 2 mm
- These "rules" may not apply in some (elderly e.g.) patients

5. SMITH'S FRACTURE

MECHANISM OF INJURY:

- Also known as a **Goyrand fracture** in the French literature, This describes the **volar angulation** of the distal fragment of an **extra-articular fracture** of the distal radius (the reverse of a Colles fracture), with or without volar displacement.
- This type of fracture is caused by landing on the dorsal surface of the wrist and are much less common.

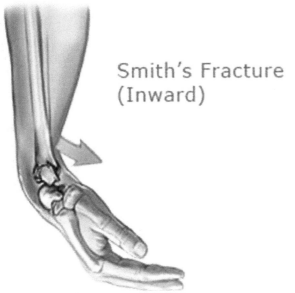

Smith's Fracture (Inward)

Smith's fracture - from pinterest.com

- Smith fractures usually occur in one of two ways:
  o A fall onto a flexed wrist
  o Direct blow to the back of the wrist
- Classically, these fractures are extra-articular transverse fractures and can be thought of as a **reverse Colles fracture**.
- The term is sometimes used to describe intra-articular fractures with volar displacement (a **reverse Barton fracture**) or juxta-articular fractures.

EPIDEMIOLOGY

- Smith fractures account for less than 3% of all fractures of the radius and ulna and have a bimodal distribution: **young males (most common) and elderly females**.

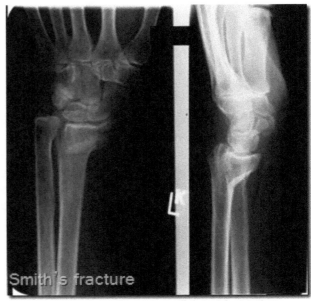

Smith's fracture - from abcradiology.blogspot.com

IMAGING:

o A wrist radiograph series is adequate for the characterization of a distal wrist fracture and can differentiate between a Colles and Smith fracture. Typically, orthogonal views (AP, lateral) are adequate.

o The fracture line is usually evident, although in undisplaced of mildly impacted fractures it can be difficult to see and subtle cortical breaches / buckling should be sought.

MANAGEMENT

o Usually internally fixed and so should be referred to on-call Orthopaedic Team.

o If not **manipulate under LA or GA by disimpaction, supination, extension and ulnar deviation and apply ventral POP slab.**

o Provide sling and refer to the Fracture Clinic.

6. BARTON'S FRACTURE

- **Barton fractures** are **intra-articular** fractures of the distal radius with **associated dislocation** of the radio-carpal joint.
- A Barton fracture can be described as volar (more common) or dorsal (less common), depending on whether the volar or dorsal rim of the radius is involved.
  - o **Volar-type Barton's** is a fracture-dislocation of the volar rim of the radius. This type is the most common.
  - o **Dorsal-type Barton's** is a fracture-dislocation of the dorsal rim of the radius.
- Patient's with Barton fractures will typically present to the urgent care or emergency department with acute wrist pain and deformity following a recent trauma.
- A younger patient commonly will describe a sporting injury or motor vehicle accident while older patients may report a lower energy trauma such as fall from standing.
- These fractures have a great tendency for redislocation and malunion.
- They usually require operative treatment.

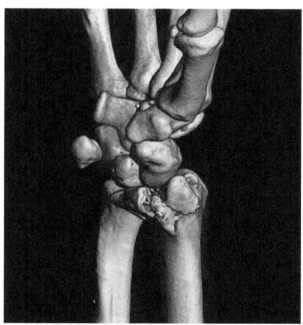

Barton's fracture - from wikipaedia.com

MANAGEMENT:
- o Often requires **MUA** under **Bier's block**.
- o Beware neurovascular compromise - **always check median nerve function** and advise immediate return if symptoms.
- o If reduction not ideal - refer to on-call Orthopaedic Team.

7. CHAUFFEUR'S FRACTURE

- An isolated fracture of the radial styloid process is also called a **Hutchinson's or chauffeur's fracture**.
- Displacement of the fragment is uncommon.
- There can be associated injury to the scapholunate ligament.
- In most cases a fracture of the radial styloid process is part of a comminutive intraarticular fracture.

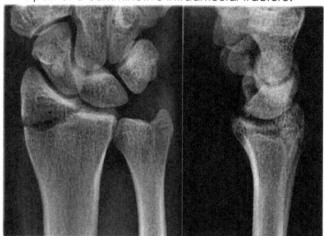

Chauffeur's fracture - from radiologyassistant.nl

8. LUNATE & PERILUNATE DISLOCATION

8.1. SPILLED TEACUP SIGN
- The **spilled teacup sign** : abnormal volar displacement and tilt of a dislocated lunate on lateral radiographs of the wrist.
- In lunate dislocations, the lunate's articulations with both the radius and capitate are disrupted displacing the lunate volarly creating a **"spilled teacup"**.

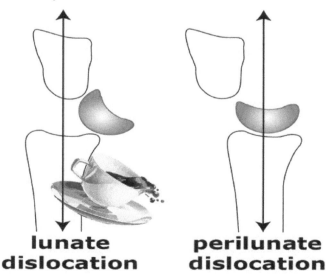

Lunate & Perilunate dislocations - from startradiology.com

- It is an important sign to help differentiate lunate dislocation from perilunate dislocation.
- In the latter, the lunate remains in articulation with the distal radius and therefore does not appear to 'spill' forward.

8.2. PIECE OF PIE SIGN
- **The piece of pie sign**: an abnormal triangular appearance of the lunate on a **PA image** of the wrist indicating lunate dislocation or perilunate dislocation.
- **A lateral image** will help differentiate whether there is lunate or perilunate dislocation with lunate dislocation demonstrating a spilled teacup sign.

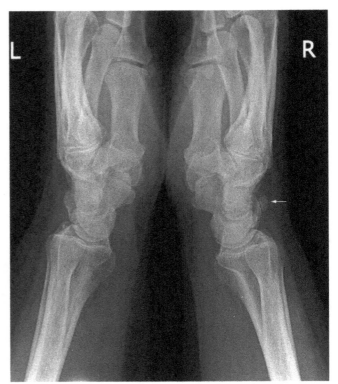

Triquetal fracture - from wikiradiography.net

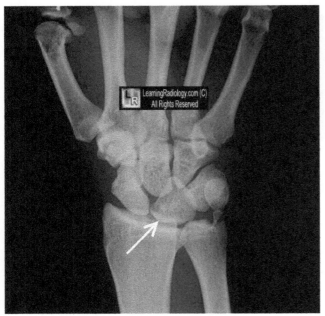

The piece of pie sign - from lerningradiology.com

9. FLAKE TRIQUETRAL FRACTURE
- The **triquetrum** is the most commonly **fractured** carpal **bone**.
  Isolated **fractures** are rare; most **triquetral fractures** are associated with other carpal injuries, such as perilunate transtriquetral dislocation. Two types of **triquetral fractures** occur, dorsal cortical **fractures** and **fractures** through the **triquetral** body.
- Commonest is **flake triquetral fracture** seen on dorsum carpus lateral view.
- Immobilise in backslab, sling and refer to the Fracture Clinic.
- Triquetral complication: **Deep branch ulnar nerve**: beware early ulnar motor signs.

VI. HAND & FINGER INJURIES

1. BENNETT & ROLANDO FRACTURES

- A **Bennett fracture-dislocation** is an Intra-articular *two-part* fracture of the base of the first metacarpal with carpometacarpal joint involvement. Thumb fracture usually sustained with forced abduction of the first metacarpal.

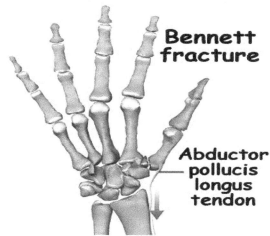

Bennet fracture - from sites.google.com

- A **Rolando fracture** is a three part or comminuted intra-articular fracture-dislocation of the base of thumb (proximal first metacarpal). It can be thought of as a **comminuted Bennett fracture.**

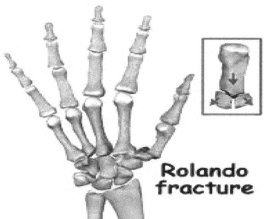

Rolando fracture - from sites.google.com

RADIOGRAPHIC FEATURES
o Routine views of the thumb adequately define the nature of the fragment(s).
o CT scans may be performed as part of the definitive management work-up.

MANAGEMENT:
o Treatment goals are to achieve articular congruity and stability of the thumb carpo-metacarpal joint.

Initial management
o RICE
o thumb spica splint

Definitive management options[102]
o Closed reduction alone is unlikely to be successful as CMC stability is compromised by the pull of APL
o Closed reduction with percutaneous pinning (most common)
o Open reduction and internal fixation (this is also the usual treatment of a Rolando fracture, although external fixation may be performed depending on the size of the fragments).

2. GAMEKEEPER'S THUMB

- Skier's thumb, also known as Gamekeeper's thumb, is an injury to the ulnar collateral ligament (UCL), which is located in the metacarpophalangeal (MCP) joint where the thumb meets the hand.
- The purpose of the UCL is to keep the thumb stable in order to pinch objects. An injury to the UCL can be painful and result in a loss of function and pinch strength. Most often, these injuries are caused by accidents or falls.

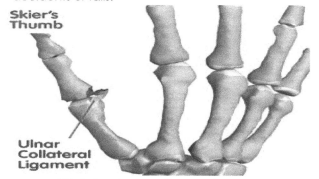

Skier's thumb - from sites.google.com

PLAIN RADIOGRAPH
- Before any manipulation of the thumb, obtain standard anteroposterior, lateral, and oblique radiographs to exclude metacarpal fractures and gamekeeper's fractures.
- Small, nondisplaced avulsion fractures that are associated with rupture of the insertion point of the UCL are not contraindications to manipulation.
- If displacement of these fractures did not take place at the time of injury and greatest stress, it is believed that they are stable enough for the manipulation of stress testing.

---

[102] *https://litfl.com/bennett-fracture-eponymictionary/*

- **Stress radiographs:** Radiographs obtained with the thumb in the flexed and extended positions and with valgus stress at the MCP joint can help the physician to determine the degree of instability of partial tears of the UCL.
- **Stener lesion:** a type of traumatic **injury** to the thumb. It occurs when the aponeurosis of the adductor pollicis muscle becomes interposed between the ruptured ulnar collateral ligament (UCL) of the thumb and its site of insertion at the base of the proximal phalanx.

ULTRASOUND

- Helpful in identifying not only the tear but also whether or not a **Stener lesion is present**.
- Clearly this requires a knowledge of local anatomy and use of a high frequency probe.

MRI

- To investigate the degree of UCL displacement in order to create a simple classification to aid in determining which UCL injuries require surgery.
- MRI is increasingly used to assess x-ray occult injuries to the ulnar collateral or to attempt to identify **a Stener lesion**.

TREATMENT AND PROGNOSIS

- Refer to ortho on duty.
- Treatment depends on classification, but essentially boils down to whether there is displacement or instability: if there is, surgical fixation is required.
- For small, nondisplaced avulsion fractures of the proximal phalanx that are found to be stable on stress testing, nonoperative treatment by a spica-type cast for 4 weeks can be completed with good result. The presence of a **Stener lesion** an indication for surgery.

3. BOXER FRACTURES

MECHANISM

- Boxer fracture ia a fracture of the forth or fifth metacarpal neck with volar displacement of the metacarpal head. One of the most common injuries seen in the ED, and occurs in 20% of patients that punch a hard object.
- The typical symptoms of a boxer's fracture are pain or tenderness centered in a specific location on the hand corresponding to one of the metacarpal bones, around the knuckle.
- The patient may be reluctant to disclose the mechanism of injury related embarrassment, or fear or repercussions if they disclose it occurred in a fight. A high clinical suspicion should be used when assessing these injuries. If injury occurred during a fight, look for other injuries as well.

PLAIN RADIOGRAPHS

- AP and Oblique view should be obtained; lateral views can help with assessing angulation and other injuries in the carpometacarpal area.
- It is usually angulated in a volar direction.
- Spiral fractures or angulation in other directions are also sometimes encountered.

TREATMENT AND PROGNOSIS

- A short arm **gutter-splint** is applied, with flexion of the metacarpophalangeal joint, typically for 2-3 weeks followed by buddy-strapping.
- Prolonged immobilisation can lead to stiffness.
- **Check rotational deformity**
- Fracture Clinic Follow up
- Severely displaced fractures may benefit from K-wire.
- Fractures of the fourth metacarpal neck can be treated in a similar fashion, whereas the second and third metacarpals usually require internal fixation.

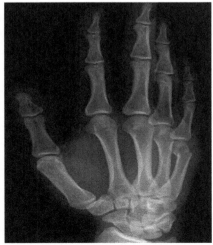

Boxer's fracture- from lifeinthefastlane

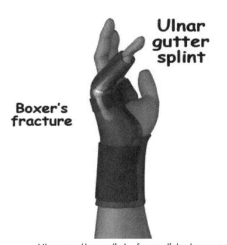

Ulnar gutter splint - from slideshare.net

4. PROXIMAL METACARPAL INJURIES

- Divided into fractures of metacarpal head, neck, shaft. Treatment based on which metacarpal is involved and location of fracture
- Acceptable angulation varies by location
- No degree of malrotation is acceptable
- Most are stable injuries if sustained with a clenched fist (no rotation at the time of injury).
- As with most other limb view **scrutinises the lateral view** for deformity or unusual appearance.

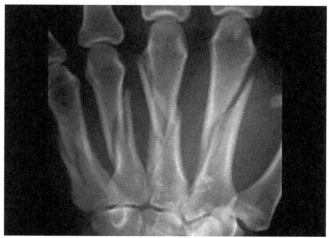

Metacarpal fractures – from orthobullets.com

5. DISLOCATION OF PIP & DIP JOINTS

- Confirm with X-ray (exclude fracture).
- Reduce under LA.
- Assess stability (AP side-to-side).
- **If stable**, apply a **Bedford splint**, **sling** and refer to the fracture clinic.
- **If unstable**, refer to the on-call orthopaedic Team.
- Always do a post reduction x-ray

6. VOLAR PLATE INJURIES

- A **volar plate injury** is commonly called a "jammed finger" or "sprain." This happens when the finger is bent backward too far (hyperextended).
- It often happens to athletes.
- The middle joint of the finger is affected.
- Forced, sudden hyperextension and occasionally crush injuries of the PIPJ can result in partial or complete volar plate and collateral rupture.
- Volar plate injury occurs more commonly in younger patients, particularly those involved in hand/contact sports. In most instances, volar plate rupture occurs distally, at the weaker fusion with the middle phalanx, whereas the proximal stronger checkrein ligaments rarely rupture.

- Volar plate injury can occur with an avulsion fracture, most commonly at the volar base of the middle phalanx.
- Subluxation/dislocation of the PIPJ may also occur[103].
- **Neighbour strap** and encourage early joint mobilisation. Refer to fracture clinic.

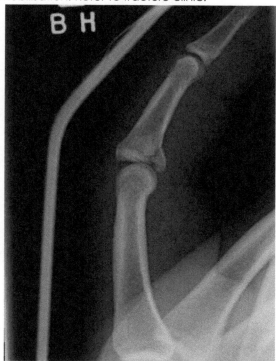

Volar Plate fracture – from Bone School

7. PHALANGEAL FRACTURES

- Phalangeal fractures of the hand are usually the result of a direct trauma, crush or twisting injury.
- The fracture will cause severe pain and swelling in the finger. Usually you will see a doctor or specialist nurse in A&E who will examine you and arrange an X-ray if they suspect you have broken a bone.
- **Transverse fractures** of the proximal phalanges are unstable (often need fixing)
- **Spiral fractures** are also unstable and particularly prone to rotation.
- **ANY rotation deformity** must be corrected and splinted in a position of anatomical function before discharge from the department.
- **All spiral** fractures are followed up in the next fracture clinic.
- Refer to on-call ortho if reduction not achieved
- **Displaced finger** fractures involving the joint should be referred to the orthopaedic team on call.

---

[103] Rettig AC. Athletic injuries of the hand, part II: overuse injuries of the wrist and traumatic injuries to the hand. Am J Sports Med. 2004;32(1):262–73

- **Open fractures** other than those of the tuft require immediate referral. Those of the tuft require wound toilet and anti-staphylococcal antibiotics.

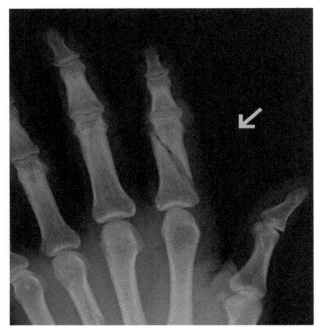

Phalangeal fracture – from orthobullets.com

8. MALLET FINGER

- **Mallet finger** is an injury to the thin tendon that straightens the end joint of a **finger** or thumb.
- Although it is also known as "baseball **finger**," this injury can happen to anyone when an unyielding object (like a ball) strikes the tip of a **finger** or thumb and forces it to bend further than it is intended to go.
- X-ray to look for avulsion fracture (better chance of healing). With a large fragment check that the DIP joint is not subluxed.
- Check that PIPJ is not going into hyperextension (occurs in small % of those with mallet) - will need to be treated if present.
- **General management includes:**
  o   Apply a **mallet (stack) splint** full-time for 6 weeks, then at night for 2 weeks.
  o   Ortho/GP/Plastic follow up (depending on your local guidelines).
- Follow 2-week rule - if extension lag at any time then return to splint full time for another fortnight.
- If splint is removed the finger must be kept straight even when washing.
- It is important that the mallet splint allows for full flexion at the PIP joint and patients are encouraged to mobilize at the PIPJ level.
- If the joint is subluxed please refer to the on-call orthopaedic team.

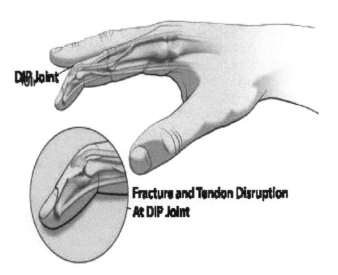

Mallet finger injury – from Medscape.com

9. BOUTONNIÈRE FINGER

- Boutonnière deformity is a deformity in which the middle finger joint is bent in a fixed position inward (toward the palm) and the outermost finger joint is bent excessively outward (away from the palm).
- Finger extensor tendon normally has **two lateral slips** (inserting into distal phalanx) and a **middle slip** inserting into the base of the intermediate phalanx.
- If this middle slip ruptures the patient may have point tenderness as the site of the rupture and a "**button hole**" or **Boutonniere deformity** ensues.
- **Patients will be unable to extend the PIPJ flexed over the edge of a table (and will have hyperextension of the DIPJ).**
- Apply splint to hold the PIPJ straight and refer to the next fracture clinic.

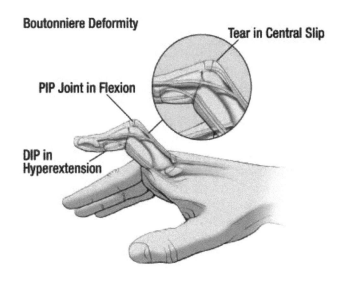

Boutonnière deformity – from Medscape.com

10. SWAN NECK DEFORMITY

- Swan-Neck Deformity (SND) is a deformity of the finger, in which the distal interphalangeal joint (DIP) and the metacarpal phalangeal (MCP) is in flexion.
- While the proximal interphalangeal (PIP) is in hyperextension; it is caused by abnormal stress on the volar plate, the ligament around the middle joint of the finger (PIP joint)[104], plus some damage to the attachment of the extensor tendon.

  o Hyperextension of the proximal interphalangeal (PIP) joints
  o Compensatory flexion of the distal interphalangeal (DIP) joints

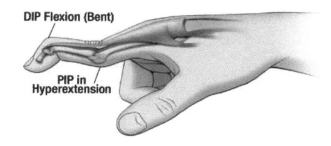

Swan-Neck Deformity – from Medscape.com

11. SUBUNGUAL HAEMATOMA

- Crush injury
- X-Ray for fracture if significant force / pain
- Trephine & drain haematoma if > 25% nail
- Nail removal not indicated
- Non-adherent dressing
- GP follow up
- No antibiotics for uncomplicated subungual haematoma
- Antibiotics if fracture and wound open / intervention

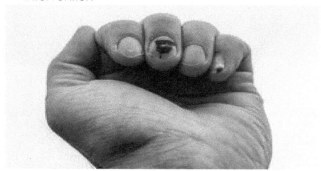

Subungual hematoma – from Medscape.com

12. PARONYCHIA / FELON

- Acute paronychia develops over a few hours when a nail fold becomes painful, red and swollen.
- Throbbing pain indicated presence of pus
- Usually staphylococcus
- F: M = 3:1
- Ask about background **Immunosuppression, Diabetes, Raynaud's or fungal** infections.
- Acute case: treat with incision / elevation nail fold (image right) rather than antibiotics.
- Recurrent paronychia or if nail bed involvement best treated by removing whole nail

- **PARONYCHIA DDX INCLUDES**
  - Felon
  - Herpetic whitlow
  - Malignant tumours
  - Fungal infection
  - Pemphigus vulgaris23
  - Splinters, foreign body

- **FELON**
  o A felon is an abscess of the distal pulp or phalanx pad of the fingertip[105]. The pulp of the fingertip is divided into small compartments by 15 to 20 fibrous septa that run from the periosteum to the skin.
  o Risk of osteomyelitis of distal phalanx
  o Treat with I&D - longitudinal incision parallel with nail.

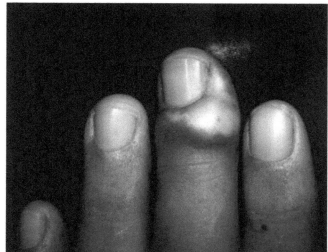

Paronychia– from emergencymedicinecases.com

---

[104] MedicalNewsToday. What's to know about swan neck deformity. Available from: https://www.medicalnewstoday.com/articles/318642.php

[105] Jebson PJ. Infections of the fingertip. Paronychias and felons. Hand Clin. 1998;14:547–55.

VII. PELVIC TRAUMA

- **Pelvic fractures** can be simple or complex and can involve any part of the **bony pelvis**.
- Pelvic fractures can be fatal, and an unstable pelvis requires immediate management.

EPIDEMIOLOGY

o Pelvic fractures can be seen in any group of patients.
o Like much trauma, there is a bimodal distribution with younger male patients involved in high-energy trauma and older female patients presenting after minor trauma.

CLINICAL PRESENTATION

o Patients tend to present following trauma with pelvic/hip pain.
o They will often be immobilised by ambulance crews on arrival and potentially have other life-threatening conditions associated with high-energy trauma.

PATHOLOGY

o Most pelvic fractures result from trauma:
  - Motor vehicle collision (~50%)
  - Pedestrian vs. Motor vehicle (~30%)
  - Fall from height (~10%)
  - Motorbike collisions (~4%)
  - Other e.g. Sports injury, low-energy fall
  - Pelvic insufficiency fractures are common in the elderly.
o The type of fracture that occurs is a result of the type of injury (impact or compression), the energy involved and the strength of the bones.
o The potential morbidity associated with these fractures is related to the involvement of the pelvic ring. Injuries that result in disruption of the pelvic rings result in a significantly worse prognosis.
o Direct impact low-to-moderate energy injuries usually result in a solitary and localised fracture.
o Compression injuries tend to cause fractures that involve the pelvic ring and are unstable.

CLASSIFICATION

o Four main forces have been described in high-energy blunt force trauma that results in unstable pelvic fractures:
  - **Anteroposterior compression:** result in an **open book** or **sprung pelvis fractures**
  - **Lateral compression:** result in a **windswept pelvis**
  - **Vertical shear:** results in **bucket handle fracture**

- **Combined mechanical:** occur when two different force vectors are involved and results in a complex fracture pattern
- Isolated stable pelvic fractures can also occur in the context of lower energy mechanisms or sporting injuries:
  o Acetabular fracture
  o Pubic ramus fracture
  o Iliac wing fracture (**Duverney fracture**)
  o Avulsion fractures (e.g. ASIS, iliac crest, ischial tuberosity)

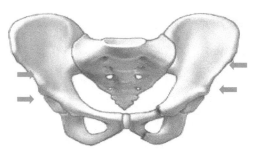

Lateral compression (closed) 60-70% frequency

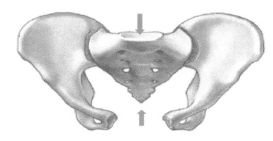

Anterior-posterior compression (open book) 15-20% frequency

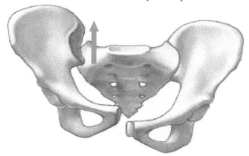

Vertical shear 5-15% frequency

ASSOCIATED INJURIES

o Pelvic fractures carry a significant risk of uncontrolled pelvic bleeding and exsanguination from pelvic fractures is a real possibility.
o This may result in pelvic, thigh and/or **retroperitoneal haemorrhage**.

o Pelvic angio-embolisation should be considered in patients with evidence of persistent blood loss with no evidence of intra-abdominal bleeding prior to surgical fixation.

OTHER COMPLICATIONS INCLUDE:
o Bladder rupture
o Urethral rupture

RADIOGRAPHIC FEATURES
o The radiographic features are varied and even for serious and severe injuries can be subtle on plain radiographs.
o **X-ray**
  ▪ X-ray is a quick and simple test that will detect the majority of pelvic fractures.
  ▪ They can be difficult to assess because of the complexity of the shape of the sacrum, pelvis and proximal femora.
o **CT**
  ▪ CT is the modality of choice for accurately depicting complex acetabular or pelvic ring fractures.
  ▪ After an initial plain radiograph, a CT is often required to make an accurate assessment of the fracture.

TREATMENT AND PROGNOSIS
o Treatment and prognosis depend on the type of injury:
  ▪ **Simple ramal fractures** are treated by immobilisation.
  ▪ **Multi-part acetabular fractures** require reconstruction by an experienced operator.
  ▪ **Complex pelvic ring fractures** may require external fixation. In these patients, their prognosis is partly dependent on their comorbidities and other related injuries.
o Pelvic fractures carry a significant mortality and morbidity.
o It has been reported that ~75% of pre-hospital deaths from motor vehicle collisions are secondary to pelvic fractures.

ED MANAGEMENT OF PELVIC INJURIES
o Generic trauma management principles apply.
o Assessment of the pelvis occurs during 'C' assessment in the primary survey.
o **A pelvic X-ray** is part of the trauma series of X-rays and should be performed as an adjunct to the primary survey.
o Patients should be X-rayed in the resuscitation room to identify fractures.
o Manipulation of the pelvis to determine instability is not recommended.

o The log roll should be delayed until the pelvis has been 'cleared'. Excessive movement may disrupt clots that have formed.
o If a pelvic fracture is identified, the patient should be **scooped** for transfer and not log rolled.
o **Pelvic splinting** may be used for unstable fractures to close the increased volume of the pelvis.
o If no splint is available, **a sheet** can be used as a temporary holding measure.
o The sheet should be wrapped around the pelvis at the level of the anterior superior iliac spines and the legs internally rotated and secured in this position.
o The aim is to reduce the volume of the pelvis and allow tamponade of bleeding points.
o Patients should be **referred early to the trauma surgeons.**
o If the patient is haemodynamically unstable, **a FAST** should be performed to determine the need for laparotomy as well as pelvic fixation.
o Pelvic injuries may be managed operatively (internal or external fixation/ packing) or by interventional radiology (angiography /embolization).

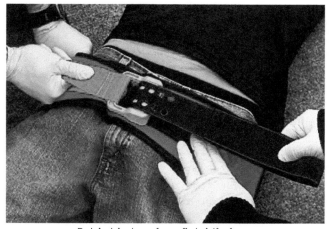

Pelvic binder – from firstaidfrofree.com

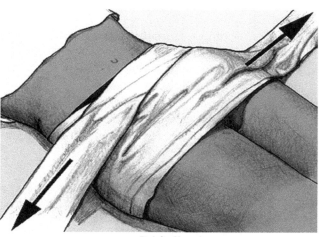

Pelvic Sheet

1. SACRAL FRACTURES

o Sacral fractures can be difficult to identify on X-ray, alignment of the sacral alar and the sacroiliac joints should be carefully assessed.

o **Sacral nerve roots** may be damaged, so check **bladder and bowel function, saddle sensation, and lower limb function.**

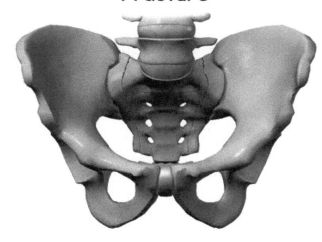

Sacral fracture – from concordortho.com

2. ACETABULAR FRACTURES

o Acetabular fractures are uncommon, with a reported frequency of three fractures per 100,000 trauma patients[106].

o Acetabular fractures result from either high-energy trauma or low-energy trauma in the elderly, with one meta-analysis reporting that 80.5% of acetabular fractures result from motor vehicle accidents and 10.7% result from falls[107].

o Usually associated with traumatic posterior hip dislocation (e.g. from knees hitting the dashboard in a RTC).

o In major trauma, resuscitate and prioritize other injuries, as required.

o Massive haemorrhage may be a problem.

o Risk of damage to the **sciatic nerve.**

o Later problems with **arthritis** are likely.

o Once the patient is stable, **dedicated Judet views (45° oblique)** or **CT of acetabulum** will help guide operative management.

---

106 Laird A, Keating JF. Acetabular fractures: a 16-year prospective epidemiological study. **J Bone Joint Surg Br** 2005; 87(7):969–973.

107 Dakin GJ, Eberhardt AW, Alonso JE, Stannard JP, Mann KA. Acetabular fracture patterns: associations with motor vehicle crash information. **J Trauma** 1999;47(6):1063–1071.

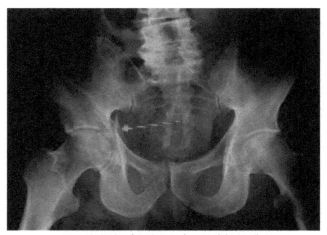

Acetabular fracture – from wikipaedia.org

3. COCCYGEAL FRACTURES

o May result from a heavy fall on to the bottom.

o Check for **rectal tears/damage** (refer if present).

o X-ray is rarely required, diagnosis is clinical.

o Majority are managed conservatively with advice (sit on ring cushion) and analgesia.

o If grossly displaced, may require manipulation (with anaesthetic) by orthopaedic team.

4. NECK OF FEMUR FRACTURE

BACKGROUND

o Stress fractures of the femoral neck are uncommon injuries.

o In general, these injuries occur in 2 distinct populations:

▪ **Young**, active individuals with unaccustomed strenuous activity or changes in activity, such as **runners or endurance athletes**

▪ **Elderly** individuals with **osteoporosis**.

o Elderly individuals may also sustain femoral neck stress fractures; however, hip fractures are much more common and are often devastating injuries.

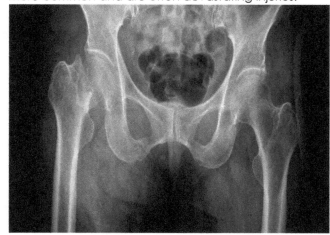

Right Neck of Femur fracture – from orthobullets.com

CAUSES OF NOF FRACTURE:

o **Neck of femur fractures** are typically caused either by:

- **Low energy injuries** – such as a fall in frail older patient; or
- **High energy injuries** – such as a road traffic collision, affecting the ipsilateral side.

o The neck of the femur is around 130 degrees to the shaft (also anteverted by roughly 10 degrees), with the femoral head sitting within the **acetabulum.**

o The femoral head's **blood supply is primarily uni-directional**, most arriving from the medial femoral circumflex artery* (arising from the deep femoral artery). The medial femoral circumflex artery lies directly on the femoral neck and is thus **vulnerable to damage** in a fracture.

o Other causes:

- Osteoporosis
- Metastases
- Paget's disease
- Osteomalacea
- Hyperparathyroidism

RISK FACTORS

RISK FACTORS FOR OSTEOPOROSIS	• Age • Inactivity • Current smoking • Excessive alcohol intake • BMI <18.5 • Heredity.
RISK FACTORS FOR FALLS	• Age ≥ 75 years • History of previous falls • Fear • Acute illness • Neuromuscular disorders • Multiple medications • Home hazards • Gait deficit • Balance deficit • Visual impairment • Mobility impairment • Cognitive impairment • Decreased hearing • Urinary incontinence • Living alone

CLINICAL ASSESSMENT

- A patient will typically present with a history of a recent fall or trauma, with significant pain (in the groin, over the hip, in the thigh, or the knee) and an inability to weight bear. There may be an associated history of chronic metabolic problems such as osteoporosis or renal failure

- On examination, the leg is characteristically shortened and externally rotated (due to the pull of the short external rotators), with pain on pin-rolling the leg and axial loading. The patient will be unable to straight leg raise.

- Fortunately, distal neurovascular deficits are rare in isolated neck of femur fractures. However, a full neurovascular examination of the limb is essential, with any deficits urgently acted on accordingly.

DIAGNOSIS OF THE TYPE OF FRACTURE

- Neck of femur fractures can be classified by the fracture line in relation to the joint capsule:

  o **Intracapsular** – either subcapital (through the junction of the head and neck) or basocervical fracture (through the base of femoral neck)

  o **Extracapsular** – either intertrochanteric (between the two trochanters) or subtrochanteric (<5cm distal to the lesser trochanter)

- The importance of this classification is that a large proportion of the blood supply to the head of the femur comes via the capsule, so in intracapsular fractures, there is a risk of **non-union and avascular necrosis.**

- For this reason, **arthroplasty** (either hemiarthroplasty or total hip replacement) may be indicated for these fractures.

- **Intracapsular fractures** can be further divided according to their site into:

  o **Subcapital fractures**
  o **Transcervical fractures**
  o **Basal fractures**

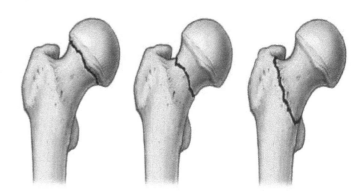

Subcapital fracture   Transcervical fracture   Basal fracture

- Basal fractures are, technically, intracapsular injuries but behave like extracapsular injuries and for prognosis purposes are usefully classified as such.

- **Extracapsular fractures** include:

  o **Trochanteric fractures**
  o **Transtrochanteric fractures**
  o **Subtrochanteric fractures**

DIFFERENTIAL DIAGNOSIS

- **Fractures** of the pelvis (especially pubic ramus fractures), acetabulum, femoral head and femoral diaphysis all need to be considered.
- **Pathological fractures** should be considered if there is not a significant history of trauma.

INVESTIGATION STRATEGIES

- **Initial radiographic imaging** should include antero-posterior (AP) and lateral views of the affected hip, as well as an AP pelvis (useful to assess the contralateral normal hip for pre-operative planning and templating).
- Obtain full length femoral views if there is suspicion of a pathological fracture.
- Basic **routine blood tests**, including FBC, U&Es, and coagulation screen, are required alongside a Group and Save; if a long lie time could have occurred, a creatinine kinase level would be recommended to assess for any rhabdomyolysis.
- A urine dip, chest radiograph (CXR), and ECG are all useful in **complete assessment** of the older patient group, especially for pre-operative assessment and peri-operative management.

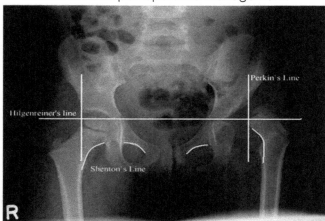

Hip Radiographic lines- from researchgate.net

Imaging

- **X-ray** of the hip should be performed rapidly.
- Protocols should be in place to enable all preoperative imaging (e.g. chest x-rays if indicated) to be completed at the time of initial x-ray to minimise patient transport/transfers and delays within the ED[108].
- A normal x-ray does not exclude a hip fracture. Where there is doubt regarding the radiological diagnosis or the patient is unable to mobilise or weight bear on the affected leg without pain, further imaging should be advised.

- **AP pelvis.** This shows both hips for comparison and will also show other fractures (e.g. pubic rami) that may also occur in a fall.
- **Lateral of the hip.** This is essential as not all fractures will show on an AP X-ray
- Fractures are commonly missed.
- To avoid missing fractures, look for:
  o **Shenton's Line:** is a curve that can be drawn on an AP view of the pelvis. This line continues from the inferior border of the femoral neck to the inferior border of the pubic ramus. This should be smooth.
  o If there is any interruption in the line then this is suggestive of an abnormal position of the femoral head.
  o Follow the trabeculae along the neck of the femur and ensure that they are intact.
  o A sclerotic line across the neck of the femur may indicate an impacted fracture
  o Look for steps in the cortex.
- **Magnetic resonance imaging (MRI)** is the modality of choice where there is doubt regarding diagnosis but as it is often not routinely available within 24 hours, CT is an acceptable alternative.

- If the X-ray is thought to be normal, there are two possibilities:
  o Most likely is that the X-ray is normal. However, fractures are not always easy to see and it is possible that there is a fracture that has been missed. If the clinical features suggest a fracture but the X-ray appears normal, it is important that the X-ray is re-examined and consider obtaining a second opinion.
  o In the majority of cases, a normal X-ray means that there is no bony injury but about 1% of hip fractures are not visible on initial X-rays.
  o There are no validated guidelines on the management of patients with hip pain following a fall but with no obvious fracture visible on an X-ray. A pragmatic approach to the problem would be:
    ▪ Give analgesia and try to mobilise the patient.
    ▪ If the patient walks well, there is no fracture and they can be discharged.
    ▪ If the patient cannot walk, they will need admission
    ▪ Try again to mobilise the patient the following day: if they are still immobile, they will need further imaging to exclude an occult fracture.

---

[108] *IAEM CG Management of Patients with Suspected Hip Fracture in the Emergency Department Version 1, September 2018*

ED MANAGEMENT OF NOF[109]

a. Analgesia:

- All patients who require analgesia should receive it in a timely manner.
- IV opiates are often necessary and, if deployed, should be administered by careful titration starting with small doses.
- The recommended analgesia for patients with hip fracture are:
  - o **Ultrasound-guided nerve block:** All patients with confirmed hip fracture should be consider for nerve block as part of their pain management, unless contraindicated.
  - o **Paracetamol 1 gram PO, PR or IV** every 6 hours, unless contraindicated. In adult < 50 kg, the dosage is 15mg/kg.
  - o **Opiates**, such as morphine 0.1-0.2 mg/kg IV, titrating the dose slowly to achieve desired response.
  - o **Non-steroidal anti-inflammatory drugs (NSAIDs)** – caution in older people, due to the gastrointestinal, renal and cardiovascular side effects, as well as drug-drug interaction and effects on other comorbidities. Avoids NSAIDS in patients with asthma, renal impairment and previous or known peptic ulcer disease.
- Adjunctive measures for pain management should be considered for each patient. These include:
  - o Minimal movement of the patient, e.g. if the patient has to be transferred onto an x-ray table from a "trolley", consider transferring them to a bed with a soft mattress from x-ray if an obvious fracture is identified.
  - o Traction is not routinely recommended.
  - o Patients should have adequate analgesia upon arrival and reevaluation within 30 minutes. Pain should be under control before transfer from the ED trolley or prior to ward admission.
- Optimisation of patient physiology including oxygenation, fluid balance, electrolyte status etc.
- Recheck response to analgesia within 30 minutes.
- If not already performed, an ultrasound-guided nerve block should be performed by trained personnel.
- Warfarin reversal if indicated.
- Take blood for the following tests: Full blood count, renal and bone profile, Group and Hold and INR (if indicated). Other blood tests as indicated by individual circumstances.
- Commenced IV fluid early-Start 1 litre of 0.9% saline solution over 12 hours.

- Exercise caution in patients on fluid restriction, or patients with symptoms of heart failure

b. Refer to ortho[110]:

- o Admission to acute orthopaedic care - All patients with a hip fracture should be admitted to a specialist orthopaedic ward without avoidable delays. Delayed admission has been shown to correlate with increased hospital stay.
- o A target time of 2 hours from ED arrival is Rapid transfer to an orthopaedic ward is recommended but all patients should be admitted within 4 hours of arrival at the ED to which they first presented.
- o ED assessment and patient transfer to the ward should be completed within this timeframe.
- o Ward admission should not be delayed for completion of non-urgent clinical investigations in the ED, other than initial x-rays. However, ED clinicians should ensure appropriate communication/handover across the ED/ward interface.

PROGNOSIS & FOLLOW-UP STRATEGIES

- While the prognosis following a hip, fracture is very dependent on the degree of frailty before the injury and the pre-existing medical problems, there are some statistics that may act as a guide:
  - o **The 30 days in hospital mortality** is **about 10%.**
  - o **The 12-month mortality is about 30%**
  - o **Risk of DVT** up to **91%.**
  - o **Risk of pulmonary embolus (PE):** is **10-14%** (but the incidence of clinically apparent PE is only about 1% and the incidence of death due to PE is about 0.5%).
  - o Other complications include:
    - Haematoma formation,
    - Superficial and deep infection,
    - Loosening of prostheses,
    - Peri-prosthetic fracture.
  - o **Pressure sores** are common but should be avoidable

SURGICAL TREATMENT	INDICATION
Internal fixation	Physiologically young and active patients < 60years
Total hip replacement	Active, independent patients > 60years
Hemiarthroplasty	Elderly patients with functional limitations and dependent living status

---

[109] *IAEM CG Management of Patients with Suspected Hip Fracture in the Emergency Department Version 1, September 2018*

[110] *IAEM CG Management of Patients with Suspected Hip Fracture in the Emergency Department Version 1, September 2018*

5. FEMUR FRACTURE

PREHOSPITAL CARE

- Treatment of a patient who complains of hip pain should include immobilization on a stretcher.
- If the patient is a victim of multiple traumas, **address the ABCs and immobilize the cervical spine as appropriate.**
- If fracture or deformity of the femur is obvious, **apply a traction splint** and **place an intravenous (IV) line for hydration.**
- If the patient is hypotensive or tachycardic, initiate **crystalloid fluid bolus and place patient on supplemental oxygen.**

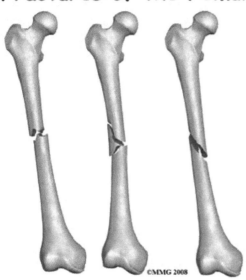

Femur fractures – from fyzical.com

EMERGENCY DEPARTMENT CARE

- Attend to the ABCs first and conduct a thorough search for other possible injuries.
- In cases of obvious femur fracture:
  - Immobilize the patient,
  - Place 2 large-bore IV lines for hydrations and possible transfusion,
  - Restrict the patient's oral intake to nothing by mouth (NPO),
  - Obtain specimens for preoperative labs if necessary.
  - Orthopaedic treatment decisions vary significantly among different practitioners, thus early consultation for all hip fractures is recommended.
- Initiate appropriate parenteral analgesia as soon as possible.

- Ultrasound-guided **femoral nerve blocks** or **Fascia Iliaca Compartment Block (FICB)** may also be used to achieve adequate analgesia.
- **A muscle relaxant** also may be necessary.
- Administer **antibiotics to cover skin flora** (i.e., cefazolin sodium)
- Tetanus immunization, as necessary, in open fractures.

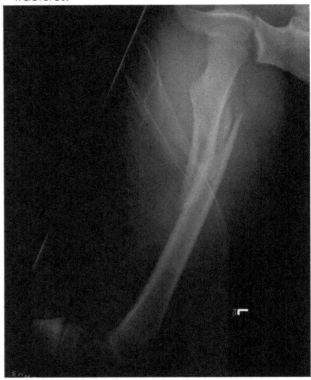

Pediatric Femur Fractures – From Core EM

A. FEMORAL HEAD FRACTURES

- **For type 1 femoral head fractures**, orthopaedic consultation in the ED should be obtained.
- Treatment is to reduce dislocated femoral head and fracture fragment as soon as possible to avoid avascular necrosis.
- Small fracture fragments may need to be removed.
- If a single attempt at closed reduction fails, then open reduction and internal fixation (ORIF) is the next treatment of choice.
- **For type 2**, early orthopaedic consultation for admission and arthroplasty is recommended.

VIII. KNEE / LEG INJURIES

OTTAWA KNEE RULE[111]

- A Knee X-ray series is only required for knee injury patients with any of these findings:
  - o Age ≥ 55
  - o Isolated tenderness of the patella (no bone tenderness of the knee other than the patella).
  - o Tenderness at the head of the fibula.
  - o Inability to flex to 90°.
  - o Inability to bear weight both immediately and in the ED (4 steps; unable to transfer weight twice onto each lower limb regardless of limping).

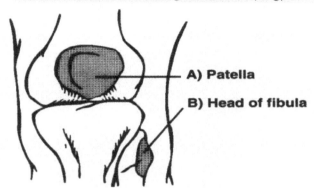

A) Patella

B) Head of fibula

1. PATELLAR FRACTURES

- The patella is the largest sesamoid bone and serves several important functions. It improves the mechanics of knee extension, protects the knee joint from direct trauma, and assists in providing nourishment for the articular cartilage of the distal femur[112]. Patella fractures account for approximately 1 percent of all skeletal injuries in both adults and children.

CLINICAL PRESENTATION

- o An individual who has sustained a patella fracture usually presents with pain in the affected knee. The history reveals a direct blow to the knee, a fall, or a combination of the two.
- o Overlying abrasions, ecchymosis over the anterior aspect of the knee, or both may be present.
- o An accompanying intra-articular effusion may be present, which, if aspirated, will reveal fat globules. If the fracture is displaced, a defect is palpable at the fracture site.

---

[111] Stiell IG, Greenberg GH, Wells GA, McDowell I, Cwinn AA, Smith NA, Cacciotti TF, Sivilotti MLA. Prospective validation of a decision rule for the use of radiography in acute knee injuries. JAMA 1996;275-8:611-615.

[112] Harris, RM. Fracture of the patella. In: Rockwood and Green's Fractures in Adults, Bucholz, RW, Heckman, JD (Eds), Lippincott Williams & Wilkins, Philadelphia 2002. p.1775.

- o The extensor mechanism must always be evaluated. As a result of the pain associated with the injury and hemarthrosis, the patient may be unable to perform a straight leg raise.

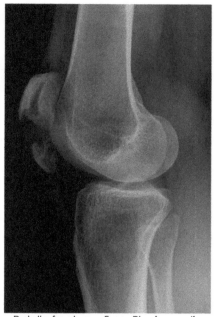

Patella fracture – From Physiopaedia

MECHANISM OF INJURY

- o Direct blow to patella, e.g. Dashboard injury
- o Severe forces by extensor mechanism
- o After anterior cruciate ligament reconstruction
- o After total knee reconstruction
- o Pathological fracture

MORPHOLOGY

- o Transverse fracture in mid-patella (most common)
- o Comminuted fracture
- o Vertical fracture (rare)
- o Osteochondral defect usually from medial facet
- o Patellar sleeve fracture in children

Undisplaced   **Transverse**   **Lower or upper pole**   **Comminuted undisplaced**

Comminuted displaced   **Vertical**   **Osteochondral**

Patella Fractures | From Emergency Care Institute

DIFFERENTIAL DIAGNOSIS

- Bipartite patella: well corticated

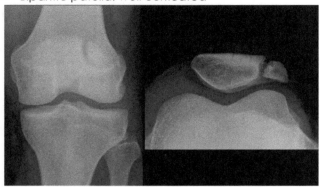

Bipartite Patella - Pediatrics - Orthobullets

MANAGEMENT IN ED

o **If undisplaced**: apply POP backslab and refer to the Fracture Clinic

o **If displaced**: refer to the on-call Orthopaedic Team.

o Most need internal fixation as quads tone distracts the fragments

o For the treatment of transverse fractures, the classic method is the tension band.

2. DISLOCATED PATELLA

- A patellar dislocation occurs by a **lateral shift** of the patella, leaving the trochlea groove of the femoral condyle. This mostly occurs as a disruption of the medial patellofemoral ligament[113].

EPIDEMIOLOGY

o The incidence for acute primary patellar dislocations are 2-3%[114]. Patellar disolocations are often associated with athletes, and is most common in females in the second decade of life.

o Redislocation rates after conservative management is estimated betweeen 15 and 44%.

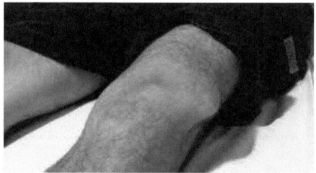

Patella Dislocation | From orangecountyfl.net

---

113 Frobell R, Cooper R, Morris H, Arendt, H. Acute knee injuries. In: Brukner P, Bahr R, Blair S, Cook J, Crossley K, McConnell J, McCrory P, Noakes T, Khan K. Clinical Sports Medicine: 4th edition. Sydney: McGraw-Hill. p.626-683.

114 Kirsch MD, Fitzgerald SW, Friedman H, Rogers LF. Transient lateral patellar dislocation: diagnosis with MR imaging. AJR Am J Roentgenol 1993;161:109–113.

MECHANISM

o **Non-contact**: Twisting of the leg, with internal rotation of the femur on a fixed foot and tibia. Often associated with valgus stress (strong lateral force then dislocates the patella).

o **Traumatic**: A direct blow to the knee (lateral or medial)

RADIOGRAPHIC FEATURES

- **X-rays**: To exclude associated fractures (osteochondral, avulsion); sublaxation will be seen on lateral view

- **CT**: To measure tuberosity tibia-trochlea groove distance

- **MRI**: To differentiate degree of tear; to rule out osteochondral fractures. Indicated in young patients with primary dislocations[115].

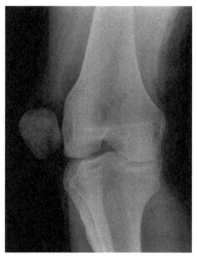

Patellar dislocation - Wikipedia

DIFFERENTIAL DIAGNOSIS

o **Acute ACL tear**: no medial patella contusion in this injury

o **Direct trauma to lateral knee**: normally no patellar contusion

MANAGEMENT:

o Usually reduced before presentation - if not, reduce by extending hip (Entonox)

o X-ray to exclude fracture

o If first episode, treat conservatively in preference to surgery

o If first episode, apply cricket bat splint in preference to POP cylinder

o Refer to the Fracture Clinic

o **Consider prophylactic anticoagulation** (LMWH) if high risk of VTE or prior DVT.

---

115 Frobell R, Cooper R, Morris H, Arendt, H. Acute knee injuries. In: Brukner P, Bahr R, Blair S, Cook J, Crossley K, McConnell J, McCrory P, Noakes T, Khan K. Clinical Sports Medicine: 4th edition. Sydney: McGraw-Hill. p.626-683.

3. KNEE DISLOCATION

RELEVANT ANATOMY

o The knee complex is stabilized by 6 main ligamentous or cartilaginous structures as well as several muscles and tendons. Anterior and posterior tibial translations are prevented by the anterior cruciate ligament (ACL) and posterior cruciate ligament (PCL), respectively. The popliteal artery attaches proximally to the adductor hiatus and distally to the fibrous arch of the soleus muscle[116].

o Inside the popliteal fossa, the popliteal artery gives off 5 genicular arteries: paired superior and paired inferior arteries and the middle genicular artery[117].

o Also supplying collateral circulation to the knee are the lateral femoral circumflex and anterior tibial arteries.

o Knee dislocations are typically classified in terms of tibial displacement with respect to the femur.

o Knee dislocations occur in 5 main types: anterior, posterior, medial, lateral, and rotary.

IMAGING

o **Plain X-rays:** Should be obtained if patient has good peripheral pulses. Used to confirm the clinical findings and document associated fractures (femur and tibial).

▪ Check for asymmetric / irregular joint space

▪ Check for avulsion fractures

▪ **Segond sign** – lateral tibial condyle avulsion fracture.

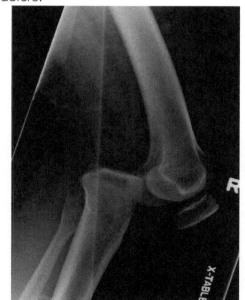

Posterior knee dislocation - Radiology at St. Vincent's University

---

[116] *Cole BJ, Harner CD. The multiple ligament injured knee. Clin Sports Med. 1999;18:241–262.*

[117] *Reckling FW, Peltier LF. Acute knee dislocations and their complications. J Trauma. 1969;9:181–191.*

o **Standard angiography:** Standard of care modality.

o **CT angiography:** Provides accurate non-invasive assessment of vascular injury and is most commonly used in place of standard angiography.

o **Color flow Doppler ultrasonography:** Gaining acceptance as an alternative to standard angiography in select groups of low-risk patients.

o **MRI:** Helps determine extent of injury, will identify ligamentous injury, joint capsule, meniscus, and articular cartilage integrity. Rarely used in acute management of knee dislocations.

CLASSIFICATION

o Classification is based on the position that the **tibia is displaced relative to the femur.**

o There are five general types of knee dislocations in order of frequency:

▪ **Anterior:** most common dislocation (50-60%) and occurs from hyperextension of the knee resulting in tearing of the posterior structures. This injury drives the distal femur posterior to the proximal tibia.

▪ **Posterior:** most commonly associated with **popliteal artery injury.** Usually results from direct blow to the proximal tibia displacing it posterior to the distal femur.

▪ **Lateral**

▪ **Medial**

▪ **Rotatory:** There are 2 types of rotator dislocations with posterolateral being the most important, although rare. Posterolateral dislocations cannot be reduced by closed reduction. These results from the body rotating in opposite direction of the remainder of the lower leg.

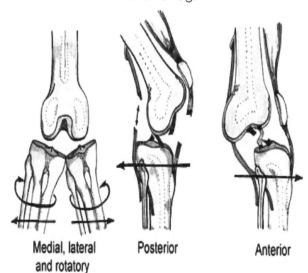

Medial, lateral and rotatory   **Posterior**   **Anterior**

Picture of knee dislocations plus ligament and artery damages. SOURCE: Medscape

MANAGEMENT

o Once the patient has reached the emergency room, the dislocation should be reduced immediately and the neurovascular status reassessed, especially if neurovascular compromise exists, without radiographs[118].

o **Neurovascular status** should be documented **before and after attempting reduction.**

o Prior to reduction evaluate the patient for signs of a posterolateral dislocation (i.e. "**Dimple sign**"), as these dislocations are not amenable to closed reduction.

o An anteromedial skin furrow, or "**dimple sign**" at the medial joint line, is suggestive of a posterolateral dislocation, which are **irreducible.**

o Attempts at closed reduction may compromise the thin veil of skin overlying the prominent femoral condyle in posterolateral dislocations leading to **skin necrosis.**

o Longitudinal traction to tibia[119]
  - **Anterior:** lift distal femur and posteriorly push tibia
  - **Posterior:** Lift tibia anteriorly and put pressure on distal tibia
  - **Rotational:** Rotate tibia towards natural position
  - **TKA dislocations:** while rare, more commonly posteriorly, associate neurovascular injury with difficult reduction due to vertical post, consult ortho

o Check pulses and ABIs after reduction

o After reduction, the knee should be immobilized in a long leg posterior splint with the knee in 15-20 degrees of flexion.

COMPLICATIONS

o **Short-term complications:**
  - Popliteal artery injury
  - Compartment syndrome of leg
  - Common peroneal nerve injury (**Foot Drop**)
  - Associated fracture or ligamentous injury
  - DVT

o **Long-term complications:**
  - Pseudoaneurysm
  - Early osteoarthritis
  - Stiffness
  - Chronic pain

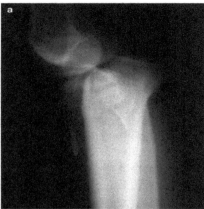

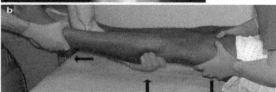

Dislocation(s)/Reduction(s) | From SpringerLink

CLINICAL PEARLS

- Occurs in both high energy traumas as well as low energy mechanism in the obese
- Lift extended leg to assess for hyperextension in a spontaneously reduced knee
- Distal pulses can be present even if vascular damage as occurred
- If hard signs of vascular damage present, immediately precede to the OR
- Admit for serial evaluations with high risk of compartment syndrome

4. FRACTURES OF THE TIBIAL SHAFT

- Beware compartment syndrome in all (even apparently simple fractures).
- Record neurovascular status.
- Analgesia, above knee POP and Refer to the on-call Orthopaedic Team

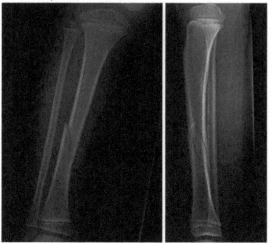

Pediatric Tibial Shaft Fractures | SpringerLink

---

[118] *Windsor RE. Dislocation. In: Insall JN, editor. Surgery of the Knee. 2nd ed. New York, NY: Churchill Livingstone; 1993. pp. 555–560.*

[119] *Voos JE, Heyworth BE, Piasecki DP, Henn RF, MacGillivray JD. Traumatic bilateral knee dislocations, unilateral hip dislocation, and contralateral humeral amputation: a case report. HSS J. 2009;5(1):40-44. doi:10.1007/s11420-008-9100-9*

5. SEGOND FRACTURE

- It is an **avulsion fracture of the knee** that involves the lateral aspect of the tibial plateau and is very frequently (~75% of cases) associated with disruption of the **anterior cruciate ligament (ACL) tear**.

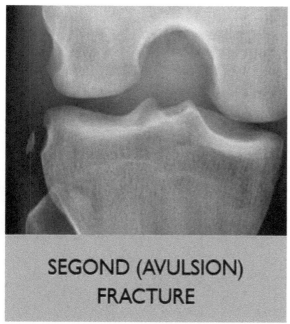

Segond fracture - Google Search | Pinterest

6. FRACTURES SHAFT OF FIBULA

- Ensure no ankle diastasis by requesting ankle X-rays.
- Check **common peroneal nerve.**
- If no other abnormality bandage or plaster for comfort and refer to the Fracture Clinic.

7. ANTERIOR CRUCIATE LIGAMENT INJURY

- **Pathology**
  - o The ACL is the most commonly disrupted ligament of the knee, especially in athletes who participate in sports that involve rapid starting, stopping, and pivoting (e.g. soccer, basketball, tennis, netball and snow skiing).
- **Associations**
  - o **O'Donoghue's unhappy triad**
- **Radiographic features**
  - o An avulsion of the tibial attachment may be seen in younger patients.
- **Radiograph**
  - o Deep lateral sulcus sign
  - o Anterior tibial translocation sign
  - o Segond fracture
  - o Arcuate fracture
  - o Joint effusion

- **CT arthrography**
  - o Considered to have high specificity and sensitivity in detecting ACL disruption.
  - o CT is helpful in characterising the avulsion bone fragment, when it is present.
- **MRI**
  - o Imaging of ACL tears should be divided into primary and secondary signs.
  - o **Primary signs** are those that pertain to the ligament itself.
  - o **Secondary signs** are those which are closely related to ACL injuries.

8. LARGE EFFUSION OR HAEMARTHROSIS

- Aspirate under full aseptic conditions, unless immediate referral or surgery intended because of severity of injury.
- **If frank blood in the joint:**
  - o Immobilise in POP knee backslab and refer to Fracture Clinic
  - o Refer to on-call Orthopaedic Team
  - o There is no evidence to support early MRI in acute traumatic knee haemarthrosis with normal x-rays.

9. LOCKED KNEE

- The knee will flex but will not fully extend.
- Refer to the on-call Orthopaedic Team.

10. COLLATERAL LIGAMENT TEAR

- Tenderness and pain on stressing the ligament.
- If there is definite laxity and marked bruising/swelling obtain an opinion from consultant.
- Complete ligament rupture can be masked by muscle spasm. If little laxity or pain is evident, apply tubigrip and refer to the physiotherapist.

11. POSSIBLE MENISCAL TEAR

- If **not** locked, apply a double tubigrip and provide crutches.
- Refer ED physio clinic.
- **Possible torn cruciate ligaments:** Rest, crutches, physiotherapy referral and GP follow up.
- ACL rupture patients are NOT routinely referred to the fracture clinic or orthopaedic follow up as conservative management gives similar functional results to (early or late) surgery.
- These patients should NOT be referred to the ED clinic.

IX. ANKLE & FOOT INJURIES

THE OTTAWA ANKLE & FOOT RULES[120]

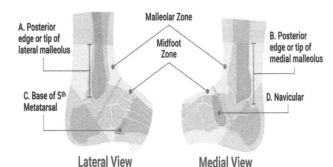

An ankle X-Ray series is required only if there is any pain in malleolar zone and any of these findings:
Bone tenderness at Posterior edge or tip of lateral malleolus **(A)**
Bone tenderness at Posterior edge or tip of medial malleolus **(B)**
Inability to bear weight both immediately and in ED.

A foot X-Ray series is required only if there is any pain in midfoot zone and any of these findings:
Bone tenderness at the base of the 5th metatarsal **(C)**
Bone tenderness at the navicular **(D)**
Inability to bear weight both immediately and in ED.

SPECIFIC MANAGEMENT IN THE ED

1. ANKLE FRACTURES

- Ankle fractures can be caused by excessive strain to the ankle joint as well as by blunt trauma[121].

DIAGNOSIS

- **History**
  - o History is an integral part of any medical evaluation. In addition to the standard history (setting, chronology, location, quality, quantity, aggravating/alleviating factors, associated symptoms), it is important to ask specific questions targeted toward an ankle injury.
  - o Medical comorbidities such as diabetes, peripheral vascular disease and smoking, which can complicate wound and fracture healing.
  - o A social history should be taken to identify the patient's pre-injury level of mobility, home situation and regular activities as well as their future functional aspirations.

[120] **Stiell IG**, McKnight RD, Greenberg GH, McDowell I, Nair RC, Wells GA, Johns C, Worthington JR. Implementation of the Ottawa Ankle Rules. JAMA 1994;271:827-832.

[121] Barile A, Bruno F, Arrigoni F, Splendiani A, Di Cesare E, Zappia M, Guglielmi G, Masciocchi C. Emergency and Trauma of the Ankle. Semin Musculoskelet Radiol. 2017 Jul;21(3):282-289.

- **Examination**
  - o Always examine the contralateral un-injured ankle first, as it helps to establish a baseline ankle examination (what it looked like before injury). It is also vital to examine the tibia, fibula, knee, and foot as well.
  - o Look, feel and Move
  - o The neurovascular status of the limb should be checked before and after reduction.

RADIOLOGICAL FEATURES

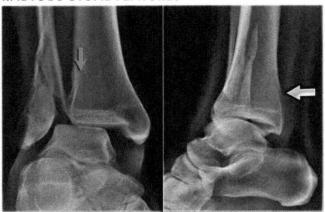

Ankle fracture | Radiologyassistant.nl

Ankle x-ray: 3-view

- o **AP view:** assess for soft tissue swelling that may lead to the discovery of other more subtle fractures
- o **Mortise view:** taken with the foot in 15 degrees of internal rotation, evaluates talus positioning and syndesmosis widening
- o **Lateral view:** assess for anterior and/or posterior avulsion fractures assess for an effusion of ankle joint
- o If proximal leg tenderness is present or medial clear space widening with no obvious fibular fracture, radiographs of the tibia and fibula should be obtained to rule out the presence of a Maisonneuve injury.
- o A Maisonneuve fracture is a proximal fibula spiral fracture with concomitant disruption of the distal fibular syndesmosis and interosseous membrane.
- o More complex axial imaging is rarely necessary; exceptions include triplane and pilon fractures.
- o Posterior malleolus fractures usually require a **CT** as the plain film underestimates the degree of impaction.
- o **Weight-bearing radiographs** not indicated in the acute ankle fracture in the emergency department, usually used for more stable injuries in outpatient settings

o **MRI** although rarely emergently indicated is used to assess soft tissue, cartilaginous, or ligamentous injuries. It can also help to detect occult fractures.

o **Ultrasound** can be used to assess for fractures as well a ligament and tendon injuries; however, results are user-dependent[122].

WEBER CLASSIFICATION ANKLE FRACTURES[123]

o **Type A** - Infrasyndesmotic

o **Type B** – Transsyndesmotic

o **Type C** - Suprasyndesmotic

WEBER A

- Occurs below the syndesmosis, which is intact. According to **Lauge-Hansen**, it is the result of an adduction force on the supinated foot.
- **Stage 1** - Tension on the lateral collateral ligaments results in rupture of the ligaments or avulsion of the lateral malleolus below the syndesmosis.
- **Stage 2** - Oblique fracture of the medial malleolus.

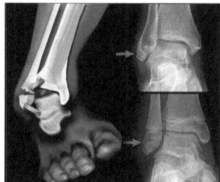

Weber A Ankle fracture | Radiologyassistant.nl

WEBER B

- This is a Transsyndesmotic fracture with usually partial - and less commonly, total - rupture of the syndesmosis.
- According to Lauge-Hansen, it is the result of an exorotation force on the supinated foot.

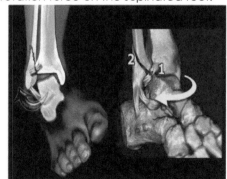

Weber B Ankle fracture | Radiologyassistant.nl

- **Stage 1** - Rupture of the anterior syndesmosis
- **Stage 2** - Oblique fracture of the fibula (this is the true Weber B fracture)
- **Stage 3** - Rupture of the posterior syndesmosis or – fracture of the malleolus tertius
- **Stage 4** - Avulsion of the medial malleolus or - rupture of the medial collateral bands

WEBER C

- This is a fracture above the level of the syndesmosis.
- Usually there is a total rupture of the syndesmosis with instability of the ankle.
- According to Lauge-Hansen, it is the result of an exorotation force on the pronated foot.

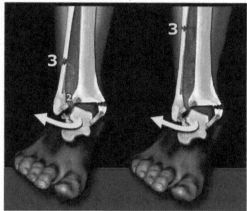

Weber C Ankle fracture | Radiologyassistant.nl

- **Stage 1** - Avulsion of the medial malleolus or - ligamentous rupture
- **Stage 2** - Rupture of the anterior syndesmosis
- **Stage 3** - Fibula fracture above the level of the syndesmosis (this is the true Weber C fracture)
- **Stage 4** - Avulsion of the malleolus tertius or - rupture of the posterior syndesmosis
- These fractures are identical to the fractures described by **Lauge-Hansen** as supination-adduction, supination-exorotation and pronation-exorotation

TREATMENT

- **Analgesia**
- **If displaced:**
  o Reduction and immobilisation in a splint or cast.
  o **Check neurovascular status pre-and post-reduction**
  o **Control X-ray post reduction**
  o Refer to ortho on call

- **If undisplaced:**
  o Below knee plaster of Paris.
  o Crutches
  o Advice on elevation
  o Referral to fracture clinic for follow up.

---

122 *Barile A, Bruno F, Arrigoni F, Splendiani A, Di Cesare E, Zappia M, Guglielmi G, Masciocchi C. Emergency and Trauma of the Ankle. Semin Musculoskelet Radiol. 2017 Jul;21(3):282-289.*

123 *Mcrae, Ronald; Esser, Max. Practical Fracture Treatment (Fifth ed.). p. 382.*

2. MAISONNEUVE FRACTURE

- **Maisonneuve fracture** is the combination of a spiral fracture of the **proximal fibula** and **unstable ankle injury** which could manifest radiographically by widening of the ankle joint due to distal **tibiofibular syndesmosis** and/or **deltoid ligament** disruption, or fracture of the medial malleolus.
- It is caused by pronation external-rotation mechanism.
- It requires **surgical fixation.**

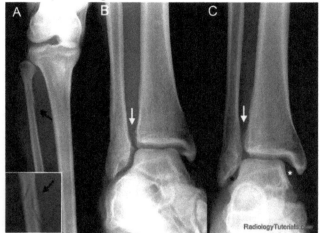

There is a spiral, comminuted fracture of the **proximal fibula** (A, black arrows). There is also widening of the **distal tibio-fibular syndesmosis** (white arrows) and disruption of the ankle mortise with widening of the **tibio-talar joint** (white asterisk) and **talo-fibular joint** (black asterisk) which is compatible with a **Maisonneuve fracture.** (Source: Radiologytutorials.com)

3. FRACTURED CALCANEUM

- Calcaneus fractures are rare but potentially debilitating injuries. The calcaneus is one of seven tarsal bones and is part of the hind-foot which includes the calcaneus and the talus.
- The hindfoot articulates with the tibia and fibula creating the ankle joint.
- The subtalar or calcaneotalar joint accounts for at least some foot and ankle dorsal/plantar flexion.
- Calcaneal fractures most commonly occur during high energy events leading to axial loading of the bone but can occur with any injury to the foot and ankle[124].
- Falls from height and automobile accidents are the predominant mechanisms of injury, although jumping onto hard surfaces, blunt or penetrating trauma and twisting/shearing events may also cause injury.

- Fractures may not be obvious on the **lateral X-ray** and it is important to obtain an **axial view.**
- On the lateral X-ray, look at **Bohler's angle** which should be approximately 140° (or between 20°-40°)
- Flattening of this angle suggests a fracture.
- Calcaneal fractures can be classified into two general categories[125].
  - o **Extraarticular fractures** account for 25 % of calcaneal fractures. These typically are avulsion injuries of either the calcaneal tuberosity from the Achilles tendon, the anterior process from the bifurcate ligament, or the sustenaculum tali.
  - o **Intraarticular Fractures** account for the remaining 75%. The talus acts as a hammer or wedge compressing the calcaneus at the angle of Gissane causing the fracture.
- **There are two main classification systems of extraarticular fractures:**

1. Essex-Lopresti:
- Joint depression type with a single verticle fracture line through the angle of Gissane separating the anterior and posterior portions of the calcaneus.
- Tongue type which has the same verticle fracture line as a depression type with another horizontal fracture line running posteriorly, creating a superior posterior fragment.

2. Sanders Classification:
- Based on reconstituted CT findings.
  - o **Type I fractures:** 1 nondisplaced or minimally displaced bony fragment
  - o **Type II fractures:** 2 bony fragments involving the posterior facet. Subdivided into types A, B, and C depending on the medial or lateral location of the fracture line.
  - o **Type III fractures:** 3 bony fragments including an additional depressed middle fragment. Subdivided into types AB, AC, and BC, depending on the position and location of the fracture lines.
  - o **Type IV fractures:** 4 comminuted bony fragments.

A. EXTRA-ARTICULAR CALCANEAL FRACTURES
- **Types:** They include fractures of:
  - o The medial tubercle
  - o The anterior process
  - o The tuberosity
  - o The sustenaculum tali
  - o The body of the calcaneum posterior to the subtalar joint.

124 Hordyk PJ, Fuerbringer BA, Roukis TS. Clinical Management of Acute, Closed Displaced Intra-Articular Calcaneal Fractures. Clin Podiatr Med Surg. 2019 Apr;36(2):163-171.

125 Jiménez-Almonte JH, King JD, Luo TD, Aneja A, Moghadamian E. Classifications in Brief: Sanders Classification of Intraarticular Fractures of the Calcaneus. Clin. Orthop. Relat. Res. 2019 Feb;477(2):467-471.

MANAGEMENT OF EXTRA-ARTICULAR CALCANEAL FRACTURES:

- o Treatment is usually conservative unless there is significant displacement, in which case open reduction and internal fixation (ORIF) will be undertaken.
- o **Treatment in the ED includes:**
  - Analgesia
  - If there is any doubt about whether the fracture involves the subtalar joint, a **CT may be requested.**
  - **If displaced**, refer for orthopaedic opinion.
  - Otherwise:
    - **Support bandage** (e.g. wool and crepe) or **below-Knee plaster of Paris.**
    - **Crutches**
    - **Advice on elevation**
    - Referral to **fracture clinic** for follow up.
- o Avulsion fractures of the Achilles tendon will need **ORIF.**
- o **Prognosis:** These fractures are relatively minor and have a good prognosis

B. INTRA-ARTICULAR CALCANEAL FRACTURES

- Intra-articular calcaneal fractures are usually caused by a fall from a height onto the heel.
- In older patients with osteoporosis, the height may be as little as half a metre.
- Extra-articular fractures of the body and the medial tubercle are also caused by the same mechanism, though with lesser degrees of force.

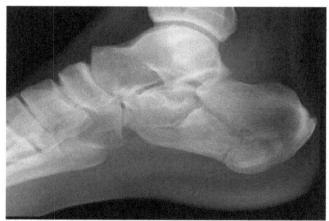

Intra-articular fracture of the calcaneum.
This image shows an intra-articular fracture of the calcaneum; the bone texture is abnormal and there are lucencies suggestive of a fracture but there are no obvious breaks in the cortex. Bohler's angle is grossly flattened. (Source: The Bone School)

- **Bilateral fractures are common** and, as discussed above, **calcaneal fractures may be associated with lumbar spine fractures.**

- There are several patterns of fracture but the exact patterns need not be known by emergency physicians as all these injuries will be referred to orthopaedic surgeons for further management.

MANAGEMENT OF INTRAARTICULAR CALCANEAL FRACTURE:

- o Analgesia
- o Elevation foot
- o Patients will usually be admitted and investigated **further by CT.**
- o There are a variety of treatment options including reconstructive surgery.
- o **Prognosis:**
  - There is usually severe disruption of the subtalar joint and stiffness and arthritis of this joint requiring further surgery is very common.

⎯ *If you suspect a fractured calcaneum, ask for* **specific calcaneal views**.
⎯ *When looking at a lateral ankle or foot X-ray,* **always evaluate Bohler's angle.**

4. FRACTURED TALUS

- Fractures of the talus are uncommon, accounting for approximately 0.1% of all fractures. The talus is the second most common tarsal bone to be injured after the calcaneus[126].
- **Avulsion fractures of the talus** and **fractures of the talar dome** are classified as ankle injuries and are discussed in a different session.
- The commonest cause for this is a road crash in which the car-driver's foot is forced backwards in a head-on collision.
- Injuries can also occur in a fall from a height.

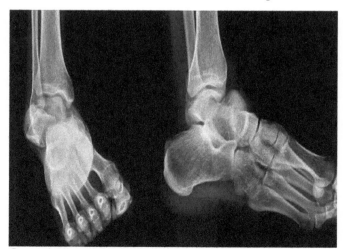

Coronal plane talar body fracture associated with subtalar and talonavicular dislocations – from semanticscholar.org

---

126 Fortin PT, Balazsy JE J Am Acad Orthop Surg. 2001 Mar-Apr; 9(2):114-27.

Fractures of the neck of the talus are classified as:

o **Type I:** undisplaced

o **Type II:** displaced (however little) and associated with subluxation or dislocation of the subtalar joint

o **Type III:** displaced with dislocation of the talus from the ankle joint

- Imaging is initially undertaken with plain radiography. The views required are anterior-posterior, lateral and mortise. Plain radiographs may detect talar neck fractures but there is a high false negative rate. A study of 132 talar fractures found that 93% had additional fracture information on Computerised Tomography (CT) scanning that was not found on initial plain radiography[127].
- As they are high velocity injuries, they may be associated with life-threatening injuries of the head and trunk and may be overlooked.
- Dislocation of the talus can occur with or without an associated fracture.

ED MANAGEMENT OF TALAR FRACTURES

- Fractures of the talus are high energy injuries and the patient may often present as a polytrauma with life or limb threatening injuries.
- In some situations, life and limb saving treatments take priority, but as soon as is safe to do so, this injury should be assessed and managed.
- Treatment of fractures of the talus depends on the location of the fracture[128].
- **Truly undisplaced fractures:** can be treated in a below knee POP.
- All others need to be **referred to an orthopaedic surgeon** as an anatomical reduction is needed and this usually requires ORIF.
- If the skin is tight over the fracture, this is urgent.
- The major complication of these injuries is **avascular necrosis of the proximal part of the bone.**

5. FRACTURED NAVICULAR

- Fractures of the tarsal navicular bone are most commonly the result of either traumatic injury or undue stress, with the latter having a higher incidence in younger individuals and athletes.
- Even though midfoot fractures are relatively uncommon injuries, tarsal navicular stress fractures represent up to one-third of all stress fractures[129].

- Minor avulsion fractures are common, often in association with a sprain of the ankle, and usually require no specific treatment.
- **Isolated fractures** of the navicular are uncommon. If they are undisplaced, they will normally be treated conservatively;
- **Displaced fractures** will need an orthopaedic opinion for consideration of ORIF.
- Fractures of the navicular may occur in association with dislocations of the mid-foot.
- Any significant injury in this area requires a lateral X-ray of the foot in addition to normal foot X-rays.
- If there is suspicion of a dislocation, **CT evaluation** is required.

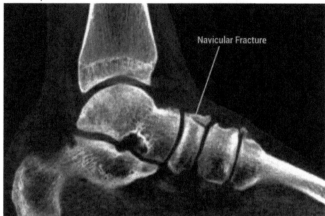

Navicular fracture

6. FRACTURED CUBOID

- Minor avulsion fractures are common and usually require no specific treatment.
- Most fractures are **undisplaced** and will be treated conservatively.
- **Displaced fractures** may be part of a more complex foot injury and will need an orthopaedic review.

7. SUBTALAR DISLOCATION

- Isolated subtalar dislocations are rare injuries. Subtalar dislocations occur typically in combination with fractures of the adjacent bones such as malleoli, talus, and calcaneus.
- The subtalar joint is the joint between the talus and the calcaneum. If this joint dislocates, the forefoot stays attached to the calcaneum and so the talo-navicular joint also dislocates.
- Subtalar dislocation occurs in excessive inversion or eversion and can occur medially or laterally.
- It may be associated with a fracture of the lateral malleolus.

[127] Dale JD, Ha AS, Chew FS AJR Am J Roentgenol. 2013 Nov; 201(5):1087-92.

[128] Fortin PT, Balazsy JE J Am Acad Orthop Surg. 2001 Mar-Apr; 9(2):114-27.

[129] Ramadorai MU, Beuchel MW, Sangeorzan BJ. Fractures and Dislocations of the Tarsal Navicular. J Am Acad Orthop Surg. 2016 Jun;24(6):379-89

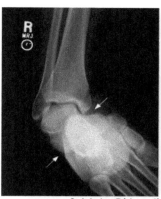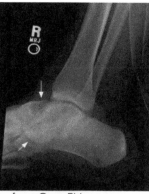

Subtalar Dislocation – from Core EM

MANAGEMENT

- Ideally the ankle and foot should be X-rayed to confirm the diagnosis. However, if there is neurovascular impairment or if the skin is stretched and there is concern that tightness of the skin may risk skin necrosis, it is common practice to try to reduce significantly displaced ankle and foot injuries before X-ray.
- If a displaced fracture is reduced before X-ray, the fracture is still visible and so a diagnosis is still possible but if a dislocation is reduced before X-ray, the subsequent X-ray may be normal and it may be difficult to establish the true diagnosis.
- These injuries should be **reduced under sedation or general anaesthesia** and **immobilised in a below knee POP**. They should be followed up by an orthopaedic surgeon.

8. MIDTARSAL DISLOCATION

- The midtarsal joint, also known as the **Chopart** or the transverse tarsal joint, is composed of the talonavicular and calcaneocuboid articulations[130].
- Midtarsal joint dislocations are rare injuries given the strong periarticular ligamentous support. In a midtarsal dislocation, the cuboid and navicular dislocate from the talus and calcaneum.
- The joint may dislocate medially (with an adduction force) or laterally (with an abduction force).
- These dislocations may be associated with fractures of the tarsal bones (particularly the navicular) or with smaller avulsion fractures.
- In major foot injuries always obtain a lateral X-ray of the foot in addition to the usual AP and oblique views.
- Following diagnosis with plain radiographs or CT scan, the joints should be promptly reduced and any open wounds irrigated and dressed.

9. LISFRANC INJURY or TARSO-METATARSAL DISLOCATION

- The tarso-metatarsal joint is also known as the **Lisfranc joint** and so dislocations at this site are also known as **Lisfranc injuries**.
- Lisfranc joint complex injury can occur as a result of direct or indirect trauma[131].
- Direct trauma occurs when an external force strikes the foot. With indirect trauma, force is transmitted to the stationary foot so that the weight of the body becomes a deforming force by torque, rotation or compression.
- Apart from a crush injury with marked swelling and radiographic changes, the Lisfranc joint injury can be difficult to diagnose. Gross subluxation or lateral deviation of the forefoot is rare[132].
- Swelling in the midfoot region and an inability to bear weight may be the only findings that suggest the diagnosis.
- Lisfranc joint injury should be suspected when the mechanism of injury is consistent with this traumatic injury and soft tissue edema or pain in the foot persists five or more days after the initial injury.
- There is often an area of **plantar medial ecchymosis**.

MANAGEMENT:

o These injuries need orthopaedic referral.
o Most will be investigated with a **CT** and require internal fixation.
o Not all injuries at this joint are obvious on initial X-rays.
o If it is suspected clinically but X-rays are normal, the patient should be kept under review and consideration given for a CT.

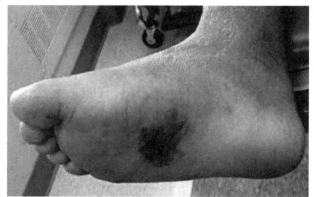

Lisfranc injuries - AO Surgery Reference

[130] Melão L., Canella C., Weber M., Negrão P., Trudell D., Resnick D. Ligaments of the transverse tarsal joint complex: MRI-anatomic correlation in cadavers. AJR Am J Roentgenol. 2009;193(3):662–671.

[131] Arntz CT, Hansen ST Jr. Dislocations and fracture dislocations of the tarsometatarsal joints. Orthop Clin North Am. 1987;18:105–14.

[132] Englanoff G, Anglin D, Hutson HR. Lisfranc fracture-dislocation: a frequently missed diagnosis in the emergency department. Ann Emerg Med. 1995;26:229–33.

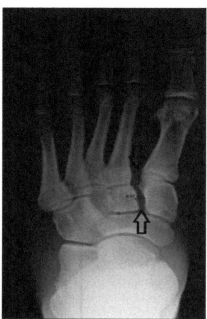

Ligamentous Lisfranc Injuries – From ScienceDirect

10. FRACTURES OF THE 5th METATARSAL

- Metatarsal fractures are frequently encountered injuries of the foot[133]. Approximately five to six percent of fractures encountered in the primary care setting are metatarsal fractures.
- Fractures of the 5th metatarsal base in association with an inversion injury of the ankle are avulsion fractures occurring at the insertion of the tendon of **peroneus brevis**.
- They are normally treated symptomatically with either a supportive bandage or plaster, with or without crutches (depending on the patient's mobility). Most fractures heal quickly but occasionally go to non-union.
- **This only needs treatment if it is symptomatic.**
- These fractures must also be differentiated from fractures at the base of the shaft.
- These are usually **stress fractures** and are commonly called **Jones fractures** though they can occur as a result of direct trauma. These are important as there is a significant incidence of non-union and so they are normally treated in plaster and should be referred for orthopaedic follow-up.
- The apophysis at the base of the 5th metatarsal in children may be mistaken for a fracture. However, the apophyseal line is longitudinal (**parallel to the metatarsal**) whereas fractures are transverse (**perpendicular to the metatarsal**).

---

133 *DeLee JC, Evans JP, Julian J. Stress fracture of the fifth metatarsal. Am J Sports Med. 1983;11:349–353.*

- The apophysis may be fragmented i.e. an apophysis and a fracture can co-exist.
- Fractures of the shaft of the metatarsal are treated symptomatically.

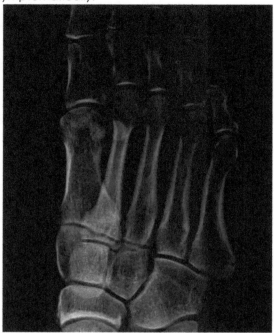

Base of 5th Metatarsal Fracture | The Bone School

11. JONES FRACTURE

- Transverse fracture of shaft of little metatarsal.
- Very different to pull off fracture as above.
- **Unstable** as peroneus (brevis) tendons distract fracture and mal/non-union likely.
- Treat in POP and refer fracture clinic.

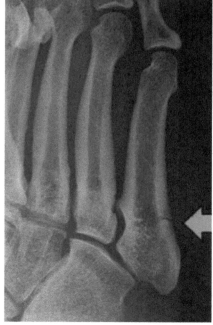

Jones Fractures | Resurgens Orthopaedics

12. STRESS FRACTURES

- **Stress fracture** is a fatigue-induced **fracture** of the bone caused by repeated **stress** over time.
- Instead of resulting from a single severe impact, **stress fractures** are the result of accumulated trauma from repeated submaximal loading, such as running or jumping.
- Sports related insideous onset midfoot pain;
- Point tender over dorsum navicular **("N spot")**
- Tender or medial plantar arch (less specific);
- Pain with passive eversion and active inversion.
- Difficult to see on plain views (? bone scan or CT)
- **Management:**
  - o Strict non-weight bearing POP and Fracture Clinic Referral
  - o Analgesia, physio rehab back to sports

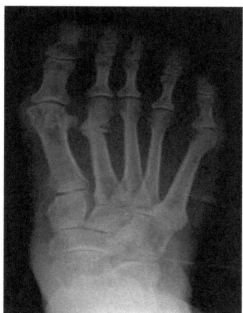
Stress fracture – from Wikipedia.org

13. FRACTURES OF OTHER METATARSALS

- Fractures of a single metatarsal (2nd, 3rd or 4th) are usually well splinted by the other, intact, metatarsals and require symptomatic treatment only.
- However, fractures of the 1st metatarsal may displace and **need internal fixation.**
- If there are multiple metatarsal fractures, this allows each fracture to displace.
- These patients need orthopaedic admission both for elevation and treatment of the associated soft tissue swelling and for consideration of internal fixation of the fractures.
- Fractures at the bases of the metatarsals (except for 5th) may be associated with injuries of the tarso-metatarsal joint.

14. TOES INJURIES

- Most toe fractures will be caused either by dropping a weight on the foot or by stubbing the toe.
- **An undisplaced fracture** requires no specific treatment but will usually be treated with neighbour strapping for a few weeks and advice on analgesia and footwear. Most patients seem more comfortable in sandals but some prefer wearing walking boots or similar as they are less likely to knock their toe.
- **Displaced fractures** may require manipulation followed by neighbour strapping. Displaced fractures of the big toe are more serious than injuries of the other toes. These **may need internal fixation.**
- It has been argued that X-rays of clinically undisplaced injuries of the toe are unnecessary as they do not alter treatment.
- This is only true as long as the toe is examined carefully as it is important not to miss a dislocation of the toe as these need reduction.

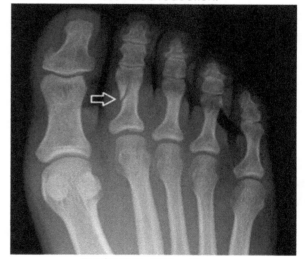
Toe fracture- From aafp.org

15. SUBUNGUAL HAEMATOMA

- A subungual haematoma is usually caused by a weight falling onto the toe which may also cause a fracture. The pressure from it often causes significant pain and this can be significantly relieved by trephining the nail to allow the release of blood. However, there is no evidence that this treatment is better than no treatment.
- It is sometimes argued that patients with an underlying fracture should be given antibiotics as the act of trephining converts a closed fracture to an open one. There is no evidence to support this approach.

16. DISLOCATION OF THE TOES

- Dislocations usually occur at the metatarso-phalangeal joint or the inter-phalangeal joint of the big toe.
- They should be reduced under local anaesthesia and a post reduction X-ray obtained.

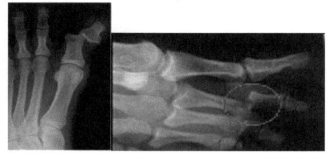

17. ACHILLES TENDON RUPTURE

- **RISK FACTORS**
  - o Steroid or Quinolone use
  - o Rheumatoid arthritis/ SLE/ Gout
  - o Renal failure
  - o Hyperparathyroidism
  - o Hyperlipoproteinaemia

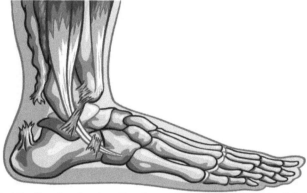

Achilles Tendon Rupture Treatment | Johns Hopkins Medicine

CLINICAL

- o Observe fracture foot may not rest in natural plantar-flexion
- o **Palpable step** in Achilles Tendon
- o **Thompson test** - lie prone and calf squeeze produces plantar flexion in normal individuals.

DIFFERENTIAL

- o Server's (calcaneal apophysitis) in teenagers
- o Peroneal tendinopathy or dislocation
- o Retrocalcaneal bursa,
- o Os trigonum syndrome
- o Ankle OA,
- o Systemic arthritis (check other side)
- o Sural neuroma (or referred pain from sacral roots)

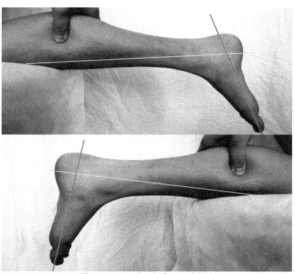

Thompson test- From BMJ

- o **Matles test** - lie prone, knees flexed 90°, gravity makes fracture side ankle more dorsiflexed.

MANAGEMENT

- o Refer to on call orthopaedic team
- o Operative repair is preferable to conservative management
- o If conservative Mx consider prophylactic anticoagulation (LMWH) particularly if high risk of VTE or prior DVT.

18. SALTER HARRIS FRACTURES

- The Salter Harris Classification of Paediatric fractures is as follow:

TYPE	CHARACTERISTICS
I	Separation through the physis, usually through areas of hypertrophic and degenerating cartilage cell columns.
II	Fracture through a portion of the physis that extends through the metaphysis
III	Fracture through a portion of the physis that extends through the epiphysis and into the joint.
IV	Fracture across the metaphysic, physis and epiphysis.
V	Crush injury to the physis

The Salter-Harris Classification of Growth Plate Injuries

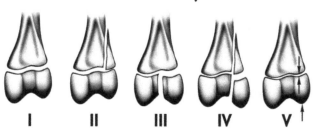

Salter-Harris classification – From saem.org

12. Wound Management
I. APPROACH TO A WOUND IN ED

1. INITIAL MANAGEMENT

- While the temptation may be to focus solely on the injury itself, it is very important to assess the whole person.
- Begin with a **primary survey**: airway, breathing, circulatory volume and level of consciousness.
- If this survey is overlooked, a potentially life-threatening injury may be missed.
- A patient with a bleeding laceration should have gentle pressure applied with a sterile dressing to control the haemorrhage, and the affected area should be elevated.
- If the patient feels or looks faint, they should be asked to lie down.
- Analgesia should be given as appropriate.
- Avoid anti –inflammatory medication as it may interfere with the body's natural responses to injury.
- The removal of a large foreign body, such as a knife, should only be undertaken in theatre.
- This reduces the risk of uncontrolled bleeding and allows any serious underlying damage to be treated immediately.

HISTORY-TAKING

- Once the patient has been stabilised, a more detailed history should be taken.
- **Details should include:**
  - **How did the injury occur?** The mechanism of the injury is vital to the assessment and care of the patient, as it provides clues to the type and amount of tissue damage.
  - **Where was the wound sustained?** This is important as wounds sustained in an unclean environment are at a very high risk of contamination with bacteria, fungi and spores - for example, Clostridium tetani.
  - **When did the wound occur?** Research indicates that the greater the time between wounding and good wound care, the greater the chance of infection
  - **Why did the wound occur?** The reason why the wound occurred should be established, as it may be an outward manifestation of abuse or underlying medical disorder.

WHEN INTERVENTION IS REQUIRED

Wound assessment should note the environment where the injury occurred, and include a holistic assessment of the individual. You should consult with senior colleagues if any of the following present:

- **Vascular damage**: arterial bleeding from wound, loss of pulse, or poor perfusion distal to the injury.
- **Nerve damage**: loss of light touch or motor function distal to the injury.
- **Tendon injury**, including injury to the sheath.
- **Facial lacerations** for which a good cosmetic repair is important, particularly lacerations crossing the margins of lips, nose, or ears.
- **Lacerations of palm of hand** with any signs of infection.
- Lacerations associated with marked cellulitis over a joint.
- **Possible foreign body** remaining in the wound after cleaning, including all injuries caused by glass.
- **Complex**, widely gaping, or extensively devitalized lacerations.
- **Burns**

EXAMINATION

- Examine to detect individual structures that could be damaged (e.g. tendons, nerves), for the presence of dirt, foreign bodies and the displacement and loss of tissue. (e.g. use "DP" or "FDS" not "tendons" intact)
- Check the skin edge of viability.
- If a skin flap has been raised record the dimension in terms of width, length and orientation of the base of the flap.
- Make an accurate record of your clinical findings.
- **All Wounds caused by glass must always be x-rayed.**

TREATMENT

- Thorough mechanical cleaning is essential for all wounds, e.g. for dirty hands get the patient to use tap water, Hibiscrub himself or Swarfega if grease is present. Remember to use scrubbing/toothbrushes if necessary.
- Local anaesthesia will probably be required to assess and clean the wound thoroughly.

o Wounds may be closed by:
- **Primary suture**: for clean wounds less than 6 hours old and for clean incised wounds that can be closed tension free.
- **Delayed primary suture**: 3-4 days for wounds that are potentially infected - daily dressings required.

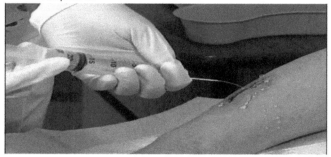

o Wounds should not be closed if they are dirty, old, if there is a possibility of a foreign body, crush injury, cannot be closed without tension or are due to a bite (except on the face)
o Use DELAYED primary closure.
o Clean and dress the wound and review it at 48 hours. If it is not infected, then close it between days 2 and 5.

SUTURING

Wound	Suture	Removal days
Scalp	3/0 4/0	7
Face	5/0 6/0	4 - 5
Anterior trunk	4/0	7 - 10
Posterior trunk	3/0	7 - 10
Upper limbs	4/0	7 - 10
Hands	5/0	7
Lower limbs	3/0	10 - 14
Extensor surface joints	3/0	14

- The wound should be sutured so that at the end it is completely closed throughout its depth and length.
- **Avoid any dead space.** (Achieved with vertical mattress stitches without tension) with 5/0 Vicryl.
- **Interrupted suture** should always be used.
- The knots should be placed to one or other side of the wound and must not be tied tightly to allow for swelling.
- Knots should be placed at least **2 mm from the skin edge and 3 mm apart** (hand).
- All suturing is the responsibility of the SHO / ENP treating the patient.
- When medical students or dental students suture, the assessment of the wound and suggestion for suturing must be made by the SHO / ENP who will also need to check the wound after suturing.

- Remember sutures on extensor surfaces of joints need to stay in longer and the joint may need immobilisation to produce a good scar.
- Record the number of sutures inserted as this helps nurses/patients when they remove them.
- If the patient is referred back to the GP's Practice Nurse for removal of sutures, the number, type and date of removal must be indicated in the GP letter given to the patient.

2. TYPES OF ACUTE WOUND

1. Avulsion:
- Made by strong shearing forces and friction that can result in significant tearing and destruction of tissues.

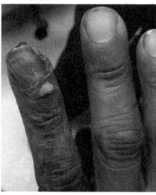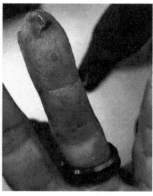

2. Laceration:
- Made by an object that tears tissues, producing jagged, irregular edges, such as glass, jagged wire, or a blunt knife.

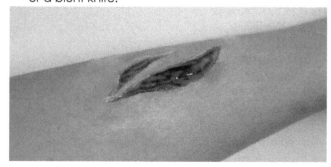

3. Contusion:
- Made by blunt force causing tissue damage with bruising and swelling, typically not breaking the skin.

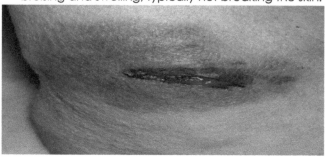

4. Puncture Wound:
- Made by a pointed instrument, such as an ice pick, bullet, or nail.

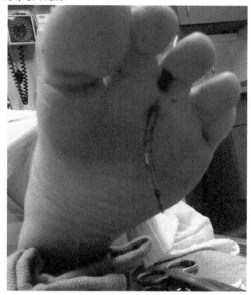

5. Burn:
- Caused by thermal, chemical, or electrical injury to the skin.

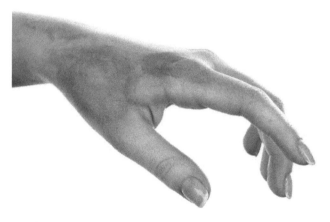

6. Abrasion:
- Injury where a superficial layer of tissue is removed.

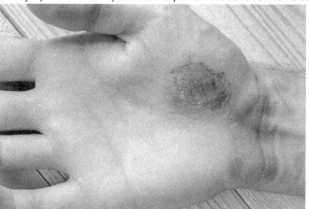

3. RISK OF INFECTION

It is important the wound is managed according to the level of risk of infection. There are 3 broad categories:
- **Low Risk:** A wound that is assessed not to be infected or at high risk of infection.
- **High Risk:** A wound that has been assessed as not being infected, but is at high risk of infection.
- **Infected:** A dirty-infected wound is one that retains devitalised tissue or involves preoperatively-existing infection or perforated viscera.

1. LOW RISK LACERATIONS
A Low Risk laceration may be defined as:
- A wound that is assessed not to be infected or at high risk of infection.
- The wound will not be contaminated with soil, faeces, bodily fluids, or pus.
- It may present as a sharp neat, usually shallow cut, typically made in a straight, single slash.
- Classically these are caused by knives but can be due to falling through glass, accidents with sheet metal, in fact anything with a sharp, cutting edge.
- If these edges can be approximated easily, blood loss can be minimised and the **risk of infection is minimal.**
- Indiscriminate use of prophylactic antimicrobials in low risk wounds is not warranted.

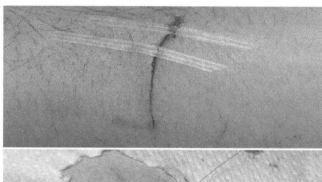

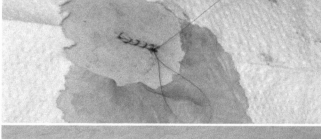

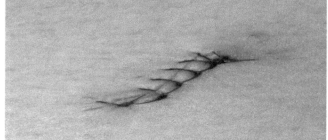

1. CLEANING THE WOUND

- Disinfect the skin around the wound with an antiseptic if necessary, but avoid getting antiseptic into the wound.
- Keep hair out of the wound. Cut hair along the wound edge and flatten it away from the wound with ointment.
- Debride devitalized tissue and pick out as much foreign material as possible — if there may be glass in the wound, **refer for radiography**.
- Irrigate the wound with normal saline, drinking-quality water, or cooled boiled water. Low-pressure irrigation using a syringe is sufficient for lacerations that are not visibly contaminated.

2. CLOSING THE WOUND

- **Sutures** are the preferred method of closing lacerations that are longer than 5 cm long, or those 5 cm or shorter when:
  - Deep dermal sutures are required, to allow low-tension apposition of the wound edges.
  - The wound is subject to excessive flexing, tension, or wetting.
  - **Local anaesthetic** is required before suturing.

- **Tissue adhesives and adhesive strips** are equally preferred to sutures to close wounds 5 cm or shorter when:
  - There are no risk factors for infection *and*
  - The wound edges are easily apposed without leaving any dead space *and*
  - The wound is not subject to excessive flexing, tension, or wetting.

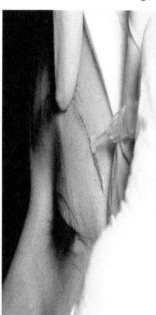
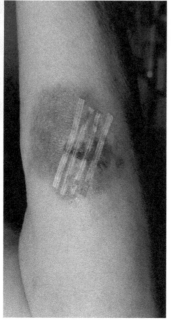

- **Adhesive strips** are preferred to **tissue adhesives** to close wounds 5 cm or shorter when:
  - The laceration is a pretibial flap *or*
  - There are any risk factors for infection *and*
  - The wound edges are easily apposed without leaving any dead space *and*
  - The wound is not subject to excessive flexing, tension, or wetting.

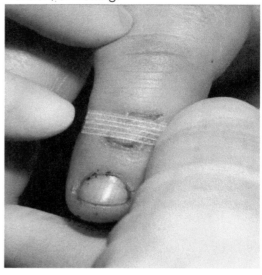

3. DRESSING THE WOUND

- Apply a dressing after closing the laceration:
  - For lacerations with minimal exudate, dress with a clear vapour-permeable dressing(a).
  - For lacerations with modest exudate, dress with a low-adherence, absorbent, perforated dressing with an adhesive border(b).

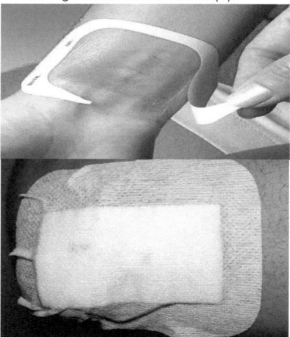

4. FOLLOW UP

- **If symptoms and signs of infection develop** after closure of the laceration:
  - o Remove sutures or adhesive strips and incise if it is not draining.
  - o Incise through tissue adhesive to allow drainage.
  - o Take swabs from any discharge for microbiological investigation, and start empirical antibiotics while awaiting results.

- **Remove sutures after:**
  - o 3–5 days on the head.
  - o 10–14 days over joints.
  - o 7–10 days at other sites.

- **Remove adhesive strips after:**
  - o 3–5 days on the head.
  - o 7–10 days at other sites.

- **Tissue adhesive** does not need to be removed; it will slough off naturally after 7–10 days.

- **Removal of dressings:**
  - o Keep the laceration dressed until sutures or adhesive strips are due to be removed.
  - o Low–adherence absorbent dressings should be replaced if exudate has caused significant wetting of the dressing.

5. ADVICE TO PATIENTS

- o Seek medical attention if infection develops.
- o Look out for increasing pain, redness, or swelling spreading from the laceration.
- o Report fever or general malaise.
- o Take simple analgesia, such as paracetamol or ibuprofen, if the wound is painful.
- o Keep the wound dry.
- o Waterproof dressings, such as vapour-permeable dressings, allow light wetting (as from showering) without the dressing separating or the wound becoming wet.

2. HIGH RISK LACERATION

A High-Risk laceration may be defined as:

- A wound that has been assessed as not being infected, but is at high risk of infection.
- The wound may be contaminated with soil, faeces, bodily fluids, or pus.
- People may have additional risk factors. These include:
  - o Diabetes.
  - o Oral steroid therapy and other causes of immunosuppression.
  - o Age older than 65 years.
  - o Foreign body present before cleaning of wound.
  - o Stellate shape or jagged wound margins.

- o Visible contamination with substances other than soil, faeces, saliva, or pus.
- o Presentation longer than 6 hours after injury.
- o Wounds longer than 5 cm.

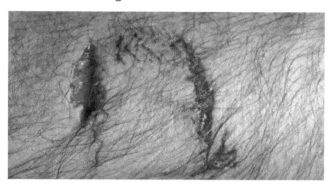

1. CLEANING THE WOUND

- Disinfect the skin around the wound with an antiseptic, but avoid getting antiseptic into the wound.
- Keep hair out of the wound.
- Cut hair along the wound edge and flatten it away from the wound with ointment.
- Debride devitalized tissue and pick out as much foreign material as possible — if there may be glass in the wound, refer for radiography.
- Irrigate the wound with normal saline, drinking-quality water, or cooled boiled water.
- High-pressure irrigation should be used to remove visible debris from the wound, using a syringe and a **green needle**.

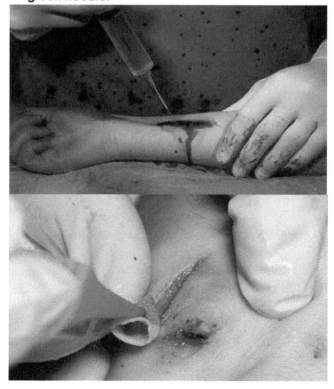

2. DRESSING THE WOUND

Important: Wounds that are of High Risk of Infection are dressed but not closed.

- Prevent apposition of the wound edges by packing with a non-adherent dressing.
- Cover all lacerations at high risk of infection with a non-adherent, absorbent dressing.
- For lacerations with small quantities of exudate, dress with a non-adherent or topical iodine dressing.

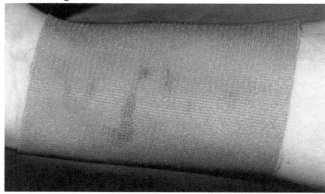

- For lacerations with more exudate, cover with a non-adherent or hydrofibre dressing (good for cavities), or a foam dressing.

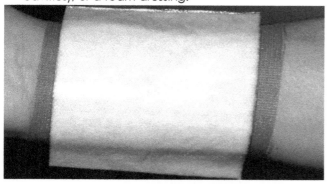

- Arrange review 3–5 days after initial presentation.

3. ANTIBIOTIC THERAPY AND TETANUS

- Treat lacerations that may be contaminated with soil, faeces, saliva, or purulent exudates with co-amoxiclav.
- If the person is **allergic** to penicillin, treat with **erythromycin** combined with **metronidazole**.
- Treat lacerations that are **not** obviously contaminated with **flucloxacillin**. Use **erythromycin** if the person is **allergic** to penicillin.
- Refer people with a tetanus-prone wound which is at high risk of **contamination** with **human tetanus immunoglobulin**, regardless of tetanus immunization status.
- Check the person's tetanus immunization status and

administer an opportunistic booster dose of tetanus vaccine if they are not up to date. A fully immunized person will have had a primary course of three vaccines followed by two boosters spaced 10 years apart.

4. CLOSING THE WOUND FOLLOWING THE 3 DAY REVIEW.

- **Review and close the laceration 3–5 days after presentation** if there are **no signs** of infection.
- If infection is present, see Managing an infected laceration.
  - **Tissue adhesives are not recommended** for delayed closure of lacerations at high risk of infection because they are not easily removed to allow drainage.
  - **Skin closure strips are recommended** because they are easily removed if infection develops and have been shown to be an effective method of closing simple lacerations in children compared with tissue adhesives.
- Review and close the laceration 3–5 days after presentation; if there are no signs of infection. (see Low Risk Lacerations -Closing the wound)
- Apply a dressing after closing the laceration. (see Low Risk Lacerations -Dressing the wound)

5. FOLLOW-UP POINTS

See Low Risk Lacerations – Follow up

6. ADVICE TO PATIENTS

See Low Risk Lacerations – Advice

3. INFECTED LACERATIONS

- An Infected laceration may be defined as one that retains devitalised tissue or involves preoperatively-existing infection or perforated viscera.
- An infected laceration may present with:
  - Erythema spreading from the laceration
  - Heat at site
  - Cellulitis
  - General malaise
  - Fever
  - Discharge (serous exudate with pus, seropurulent or haemopurulent
  - Abnormal smell
  - Friable granulation tissue
  - Pain and tenderness at the site
  - Delayed healing (compared with expected rate for site and condition)

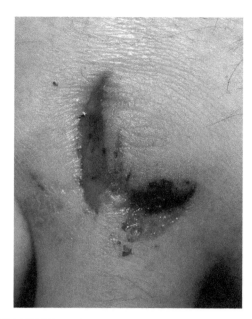

1. CLEANING THE WOUND

- Before cleaning the laceration, **take swabs for microbiological investigation** from deep within the infected wound.
  - o Disinfect around the wound area with antiseptic, but avoid getting antiseptic into the wound.
  - o Keep hair out of the wound.
  - o Anaesthetize the laceration before cleaning if debridement or exploration of the wound for foreign bodies is necessary and is likely to be painful.
  - o Debride devitalized tissue and pick out as much foreign material as possible —if there may be glass in the wound, refer for radiography.
  - o Irrigate the wound with normal saline, drinking-quality water, or cooled boiled water.

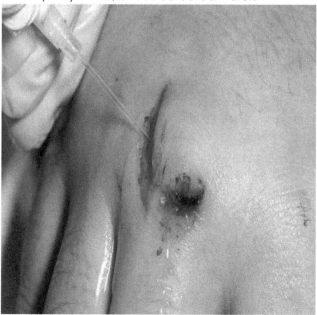

2. DRESSING THE WOUND

- Prevent apposition of the wound edges by packing with a non-adherent dressing.
- Cover all lacerations at high risk of infection with a non-adherent, absorbent dressing:
  - o For lacerations with small quantities of exudate, dress with a non-adherent or topical iodine dressing.
  - o For lacerations with more exudate, cover with a hydrofibre (good for a cavity) dressing or a foam dressing.
  - o Consider topical anti-microbials.
- Arrange review 3–5 days after initial presentation.

3. ANTIBIOTIC THERAPY AND TETANUS

- Take a detailed history and ascertain whether the wound was originally contaminated with high-risk material (soil, faeces, bodily fluids, or purulent exudates):
  - o Treat contaminated lacerations with **co-amoxiclav.** If the person is allergic to penicillin, treat with **erythromycin combined with metronidazole.**
  - o **Metronidazole** provides additional coverage for anaerobes that are not susceptible to erythromycin. It is licensed for various deep soft-tissue infections in which anaerobes are likely to proliferate.
- If the wound has not improved and bacteria culture indicates resistance to the first-choice antibiotic, change to a suitable antibiotic guided by the results of sensitivity testing. Check your local policy regarding anti-biotic therapy.
- Refer urgently if the person has signs or symptoms of **tetanus** (generalized rigidity and spasm of skeletal muscles, including lockjaw) and has had a laceration in the previous days or weeks.
- Refer people with a tetanus-prone wound which is at high risk of contamination to hospital for treatment with **human tetanus immunoglobulin**, regardless of tetanus immunization status.
- Check the person's tetanus immunization status and administer a booster dose of tetanus vaccine if needed.

4. CLOSING THE WOUND

- **Review 3–5 days after presentation:**
  - o **Close the laceration** if there are **no signs of infection**.
  - o If signs of infection persist, review the swab results, change the antibiotics if indicated, and arrange further review.

- Review and close the laceration 3–5 days after presentation if there are no signs of infection. (see Low Risk Lacerations -Closing the wound)
- Apply a dressing after closing the laceration. (see Low Risk Lacerations -Dressing the wound)

5. FOLLOW-UP POINTS
See Low Risk Lacerations – Follow up

6. ADVICE TO PATIENTS
See Low Risk Lacerations – Advice

4. BITES WOUNDS
1. BACKGROUND
- **Dog bites** are the most common bite injury (account for 80-90% of presentations).
- **Cats bites** become more frequently infected then dogs.

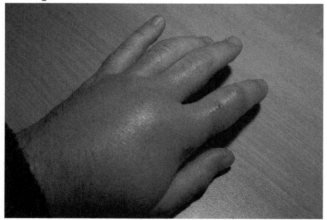

- **Human bite** wounds account for 2-3% of bite presentations.
- **Clenched fist injuries**
  o Are the most severe of human bite injuries.
  o Commonly present as a small wound over the MCPJ of the dominant hand (patient striking another person's teeth)
  o Human bite wounds to the hand more commonly develop bacterial infection than human bites at other sites, with clenched fist injuries conferring the highest risk, particularly because of the potential for breaching the MCP joint space to produce **septic arthritis** or **osteomyelitis**.
  o Clinical examination should focus on the possibility of **extensor tendon injury** and **joint penetration**.
  o Extensor tendon retracts when the hand is opened, so evaluation needs to be done with the hand in both the open and the clenched positions.

Elements to ask when taking history:
- Source of bite
- Time of injury
- Site, number, and depth of bite
- Tetanus and hepatitis status (hepatitis status only in human bites)
- Immunodeficiency

Elements to include during this patient's initial assessment:
- Location of wound
- Size and depth of the wound
- Degree of injury (devitalized tissue, nerve or tendon damage, involvement of bones, joints or blood vessels) Presence or absence of infection
- Foreign body

Criteria to classify a bite wound as high risk:
- Bite wound > 24 hours old at presentation
- Wound in immunocompromised patients
- Signs of infection
- Wound involving bone, tendon or joint
- Hand wound
- Puncture wound

Criteria to classify a bite wound as low risk:
- Bite wound < 24 hours
- No sign of infection
- No bone, tendon or joint involvement
- No puncture wound
- Does not involve the hand
- Immunocompetent

To close or not to close?
- Some elements of wound care remain standard – vigorous irrigation, debridement of nonviable tissue, and antibiotic coverage when appropriate.
- The classic teaching is that bite wounds should not be closed due to concern for infection; however, several studies have challenged this dogma, particularly in low-risk wounds and patients.
- Here is the crux of the issue: should this wound be closed? It is widely accepted that wound closure will improve the cosmetic outcome, but what is the **increased risk of infection associated with closing a dog bite injury?**

Wounds NOT to close
- Crush injuries involving damage to deep structures such as muscles and tendons
- Puncture wounds: these have an increased risk of infection due to penetration of deep structures
- Bites involving the hands and feet (due to high infection rates and easily damaged complex structures)
- Wounds more than 12 hours old (or potentially 24 hours old on the face)

- Cat or human bites (consider risk/benefit in facial wounds)
- Wounds in immunocompromised patients

2. ED MANAGEMENT OF BITES WOUNDS

- Intact skin surrounding dirty wounds can be scrubbed with a sponge and 1% iodine solution.
- **Copious irrigation** (warmed solution 33-37°C) of the wound with normal saline using a **19-G syringe** is necessary.
- Wounds that are dirty and contain **devitalized tissue** should be cleaned with gauze and **debrided.**
- Fresh head and neck wounds can generally be primarily closed. **Bite wounds to the hand or feet should be left open** for delayed primary closure or secondary intention.
- Non-puncture wounds elsewhere may be safely treated by primary closure after thorough cleaning.
- Complete management of bite injuries should include consideration of **tetanus immunisation.**
- For potential hepatitis exposure cases, please see needlestick section below.

3. PROPHYLACTIC ANTIBIOTICS

- Use of oral antibiotics for all types of dog bite wounds reduces the risk of infection by nearly half.
- Prophylaxis is generally given for 5-7 days.

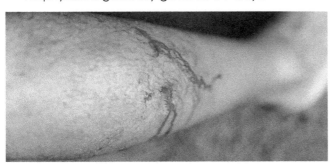

DOG AND CAT BITES
o Use **Co-Amoxiclav.**
o In penicillin allergy use **Erythromycin or clindamycin plus Ciprofloxacin,** or **clindamycin plus trimethoprim-sulfamethoxazole.**

HUMAN BITES
o Use **Co-Amoxiclav.**
o In penicillin allergy use - **clindamycin plus either Ciprofloxacin** or **trimethoprim/sulfamethoxazole** or **doxycycline** (to treat Eikenella corrodens).

- Wounds of low risk (face, scalp, ears or mouth, large, clean lacerations) should be re-evaluated in **2 days' time.** High risk (all other parts of the body, puncture wounds, immunocompromised patients) should be re-evaluated **in 1-day time.**

PREVENTION OF COMPLICATION IN FUTURE
- Perform x-ray if Suspected radio-opaque foreign body or Joint involvement (Look out for air)
- Check tetanus status**
- Prescribe prophylactic antibiotic

5. TETANUS-PRONE WOUND
- The following wounds are considered tetanus-prone[134]:
  o Wounds contaminated with soil, faeces, saliva or foreign bodies
  o Puncture wounds, avulsions, burns or crush injuries
  o Wounds or burns requiring surgical treatment which has been delayed for more than 6 hours
  o Compound fractures.
- Occasionally, apparently trivial injuries can result in tetanus.

DOSE AND ROUTE OF ADMINISTRATION
- Tetanus immunoglobulin for prophylaxis is 250 IU (1 ml) IMI into the anterolateral thigh.
- This dose is doubled to 500 IU (2ml) when any of the following situations exist:
  o The injury occurred more than 24 hours previously.
  o The patient weighs more than 90 kg.
  o The wound is heavily contaminated.
  o The wound is infected or involves a fracture

Indications for Prophylaxis with tetanus immunoglobulin
- Tetanus-prone wounds who[135]:
  o Have not received at least 3 doses of tetanus vaccine and their last dose within 10 years or
  o Are immunocompromised, even if fully immunised.

TETANUS IMMUNIZATION SCHEDULE
Primary immunizations
- The primary tetanus immunizations are given with Diphtheria, pertussis, polio, and Hib vaccines at the following intervals:
  o 2 months old.
  o 3 months old.
  o 4 months old.

Reinforcing immunizations
- Tetanus boosters are combined with diphtheria, pertussis, and polio vaccines.
  o 1st booster—between ages 3½ to 5 years (ideally 3 years after completion of primary course).
  o 2nd booster—between ages 13 and 18 years (ideally 10 years after the 1st booster).

---

[134] www.hse.ie/eng/health/immunisation/hcpinfo/guidelines/chapter21.pdf p.3-4

[135] www.hse.ie/eng/health/immunisation/hcpinfo/guidelines/chapter21.pdf p.3-4

Risk assessment of wounds for use of vaccination and tetanus immunoglobulin (TIG)

Vaccination status	Clean wound	Tetanus prone wound	
Fully immunised (5 doses of tetanus vaccine at appropriate intervals)	Nil	No vaccine required unless more than 10 years since previous tetanus vaccine	Consider TIG*
Primary immunisation and age appropriate boosters complete	Nil	Nil	Consider TIG*
Primary immunisation or age appropriate boosters incomplete	Age appropriate tetanus vaccine and complete vaccine schedule	Age appropriate tetanus vaccine and complete vaccine schedule	TIG
Unimmunised or unknown vaccine status	Age appropriate tetanus vaccine and complete vaccine schedule	Age appropriate tetanus vaccine and complete vaccine schedule	TIG

*Consider TIG for fully vaccinated patients who are immunocompromised Refer to GP for follow-up vaccines. If both TIG and vaccine are required these should be administered at separate sites.

PRETIBIAL LACERATION

- Pre-tibial lacerations are becoming common as the number of older women increases and they can be troublesome.
- Minor cuts in the skin, or where only a small amount of skin has been lifted up to form a 'flap' of skin can often be treated in the casualty department with a supportive dressing and a period of resting the leg up at home, but more extensive lacerations or if the flap of skin is large, can mean that some of the skin will not survive and requires to be trimmed away (debrided) and the area of missing skin repaired with a skin graft.

CAUSES OF DELAY HEALING OF THIS WOUND

- **Age** of the patient,
- **Co-existent disease processes:** diabetes, peripheral vascular disease, venous hypertension, cardiac failure or renal impairment

- The fact that the pre-tibial region is naturally **poorly vascularised.**
- **Hematoma formation:** The use of anticoagulants increases the risk of bleeding and haematoma formation.
- Infection

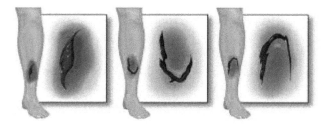

Pretibial laceration (Source magonlinelibrary.com)

ASSESSMENT THE VIABILITY OF THE SKIN FLAP

- The time and circumstances of the injury are important, as the resultant flap may remain viable for up to **six hours post-injury**.
- Viability is usually determined by colour - a dark flap or one with a dusky blue edge is likely to be unviable.

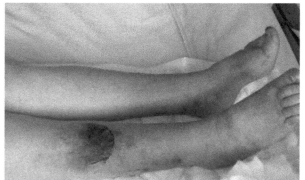

Pretibial laceration (Source semanticscholar.org)

ED MANAGEMENT

- **Wound cleaning with normal saline:** The aim of cleansing is to remove debris, devitalised skin and haematoma, as their presence will delay healing by prolonging the inflammatory response and increasing the risk of infection.
- **Debridement:** While irrigation will remove debris and contaminants, devitalised tissue is best removed using sharp debridement.
- **Steristrips:** the use of adhesive tapes to secure the flap is preferable to sutures because of the fragility of the skin
- **Silicone-based dressing** such as **Mepitel** can be used to secure it. This dressing is thought to be non-adherent to the wound bed but gently adherent to skin and is atraumatic on remova
- Recall for the first dressing change should be around **day five.**

15. Needlestick Injury

1. OVERVIEW

- **Approach**
  - First aid
  - Quantify risk
  - Post procedure prophylaxis
  - Quality assurance
  - Education

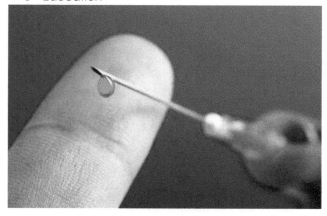

2. HAZARDS OF NEEDLESTICK & SHARPS INJURIES

- These injuries transmit infectious diseases, especially blood-borne viruses. Concern includes the Human Immunodeficiency Virus (HIV) which leads to AIDS (Acquired Immune Deficiency Syndrome), hepatitis B, and hepatitis C.
- Incidental punctures by contaminated needles can inject hazardous fluids into the body through the skin. There is potential for injection of hazardous drugs, but contact with infectious fluids, especially blood, is by far the greatest concern. Even small amounts of infectious fluid can spread certain diseases effectively.
- Sharps can create a cut in the skin which allows contact between blood, or fluids.
- The risk of infection after exposure to infected blood varies by bloodborne pathogen.

3. MANAGEMENT

- **Stop the procedure**
  - Ensure patient and proceduralist are safe
  - Take over care if required
- **First aid**
  - Express blood from wound
  - Wash wound immediately with soap and water (2% chlorhexidine wash)
  - Dress

4. RISK STRATIFICATION

- Identify source patient and test for HIV, Hep B and C
- Test exposed staff member
- Type injury – Depth, Type, Location, Barriers to transmission (double, single gloved),
- Blood on needle

- **Low risk:**
  - Contact with saliva, urines or feces
  - Bite with no donor blood
  - Blood onto intact skin

- **Moderate risk:**
  - Needlestick: solid needle, Hollow needle with no visible blood in hub/syringe
  - Small amount of blood onto mucosa or non-intact skin
  - Superficial bite with donor blood

- **High Risk:**
  - Hollow needle with visible blood
  - Deep bite with donor blood on wound
  - Large amount of blood on mucosa or non-intact skin

- **Notify patient and family**
  - Open disclosure
  - Consent for testing

- **Occupational health involvement**
  - Initiate the injury reporting system used in workplace (in hours vs out of hours)
  - Counselling required with specific risk depending on depth of injury, whether there is visible blood on needle, needle placement in vein or artery, lower risk if solid needle vs hollow
  - Document the exposure in detail

- **Advice on:** safe sex and no blood donation until testing complete

5. POST-EXPOSURE PROPHYLAXIS

  - Discuss with Infectious Disease
  - **HIV +ve** -> post-exposure prophylaxis within 2 hours
  - **Hep B +ve** -> Hep B immunoglobulin
  - **Hep C +ve** -> no treatment recommended currently

- **Systems analysis to look at prevention of further events:**
  - Document thoroughly

o   Identify factors that may have led to exposure and could prevent further exposures

o   A unit policy may be appropriate

6. FOLLOW UP

o   Follow up post exposure testing @ six weeks, 3 months and 6 months +/- 1 year

o   If post exposure prophylaxis prescribed -> monitor for toxicity

o   Take precautions (safe sex) to prevent exposing others until follow up testing complete

o   Review of technique with proceduralist.

7. PREVENTION

Preventing injuries is the most effective way to protect workers. A comprehensive sharps injury prevention program would include:

• Recommended guidelines.

• Improved equipment design.

• Effective disposal systems.

• Employee training.

• Safe recapping procedures, where necessary.

• Surveillance programs.

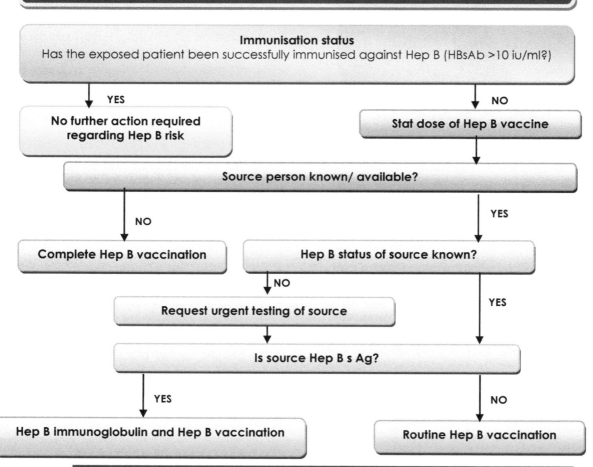

POTENTIAL HBV EXPOSURE

Immunisation status
Has the exposed patient been successfully immunised against Hep B (HBsAb >10 iu/ml?)

YES → **No further action required regarding Hep B risk**

NO → **Stat dose of Hep B vaccine**

Source person known/ available?

NO → **Complete Hep B vaccination**

YES → **Hep B status of source known?**

NO → **Request urgent testing of source** → **Is source Hep B s Ag?**

YES → **Is source Hep B s Ag?**

Is source Hep B s Ag?
YES → **Hep B immunoglobulin and Hep B vaccination**
NO → **Routine Hep B vaccination**

Hepatitis B virus prescribing details

o   **HBV Vaccine:** Engerix B 1ml IMI (Deltoid) or B Vax II 1ml IMI (Deltoid); will need 2 further injections to complete the course.

o   **HBV Immunoglobulin:** Hepatect CP 0.16-0.2ml/Kg IV infusion at rate of 0.1ml/kg for 10 minutes

Further reading:

o   *Needle stick injuries - Nottingham University Hospitals, April 2015).pdf*

o   *The College of Emergency Medicine-Emergency Department care of patients who have been potentially exposed to blood borne viruses by needlesticks.pdf*

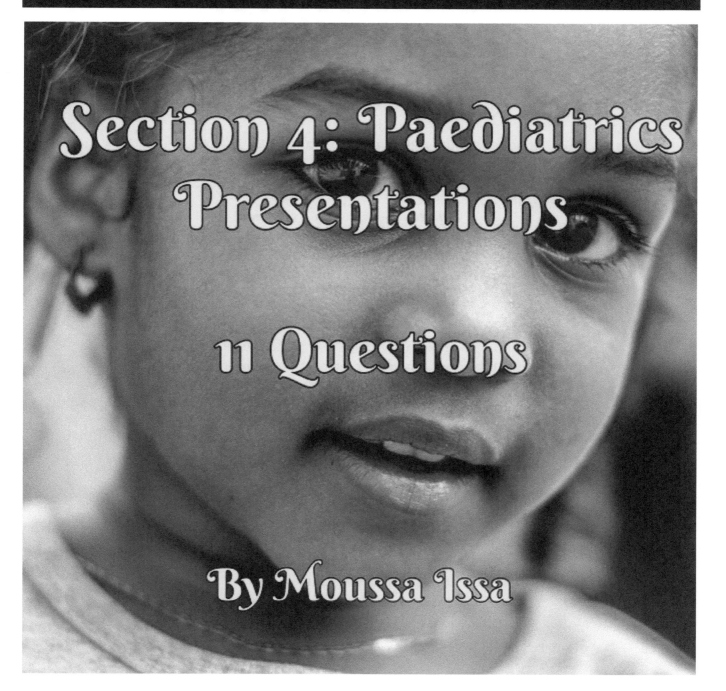

Section IV. Paediatric Competences

Section 4: Paediatrics Presentations

11 Questions

By Moussa Issa

Ebook for only £3/month!

Get our Reading App for your Android smartphone or tablet to start enjoying the Moussa Issa eBookstore discovery and digital reading experience.

Download our APP on your Smart device Now.

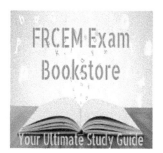

FRCEM Exam eBookstore

FRCEM Exam Bookstore   Books & Reference

PEGI 3

Offers in-app purchases

This app is compatible with all of your devices.

Installed

A static eBook with little interactivity cannot draw your attention any more. Thus it is essential to engage readers with interactive reading experience.
Moussa Issa eBookstore proves to be on top of the interactive eBook game, enabling readers to watch integrated videos related to the subject directly on the page.
The additional flipping effect makes the eBook fully interactive and dynamic.

Customize your experience with multiple font and page styles and social sharing tools.

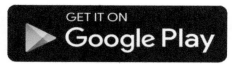
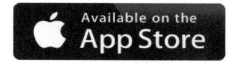

Distributed by Moussa Issa Bookstore Ltd
Website: www.moussaissabooks.com
Email: info@moussaissabooks.com
eBook subscription: www.moussaissabooks.com/read-ebook-online

1. Apnoea, Stridor & Airway Obstruction

I. APPROACH TO THE CHILD WITH WHEEZE

1. THE CHILD WITH ASTHMA

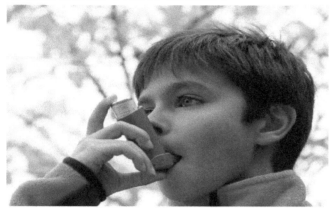

Asthma in children- From Prescriber.com

- Pediatric asthma is the most commonly encountered childhood chronic disease, occurring in approximately 13.5% of children[136].
- The two common causes of lower respiratory obstruction are:
  - **Acute severe asthma or episodic viral wheeze.**
  - **Bronchiolitis.**
- Bronchiolitis is mostly confined to the under 1-year-olds and asthma is much more commonly diagnosed in the over 1-year-olds.

APPROACH SUMMARY
- It can be difficult to assess the severity of an acute exacerbation of asthma.
- Clinical signs correlate poorly with the severity of airway obstruction.
- Some children with acute severe asthma do not appear distressed, and young children with severe asthma are especially difficult to assess.
- Historical features associated with more severe or life-threatening airway obstruction include:

- o A long duration of symptoms and symptoms of regular nocturnal awakening
- o Poor response to treatment already given in this episode
- o A severe course of previous attacks, including the use of intravenous therapy, and those who have required admission to an intensive care unit.

- The BTS guidelines on acute asthma in children recommend that **oral steroids** should be given early in the treatment of acute asthma attacks.
- The following is advised:
  - o Use a dose of:
    - **Children < 2 years: 10mg Prednisolone**
    - **Children aged 2–5 years: 20 mg Prednisolone**
    - **Children >5 years: 30–40 mg Prednisolone**
  - o Those already receiving maintenance steroid tablets should receive **2 mg/kg prednisolone up to a maximum dose of 60 mg.**
  - o **Repeat the dose** of prednisolone in children who vomit and consider intravenous steroids in those who are unable to retain orally ingested medication.
  - o Treatment for **up to three days** is usually sufficient, but the length of course should be tailored to the number of days necessary to bring about recovery.
  - o Tapering is unnecessary unless the course of steroids exceeds 14 days.

INDICATIONS FOR INTUBATION
- o Increasing exhaustion
- o Progressive deterioration in:
  - Clinical condition
  - SpO2 – decreasing and/or oxygen requirement increasing
  - PCO2 – increasing.

---

[136] *US Department of Health and Human Services. Centers for Disease Control and Prevention. Asthma and Schools.*

Available at: www.cdc.gov/healthyschools/asthma/index.htm.

MANAGEMENT ASTHMA BETWEEN 2 – 5-YEAR-OLD

The below flow diagram was copied from the joint BTS/SIGN guidelines 2019[137]

Assess Asthma Severity

MODERATE ASTHMA
- SpO2 ≥92%
- No features of acute severe asthma

NB: If a patient has signs and symptoms across categories, always treat according to their most severe features

SEVERE ASTHMA
- SpO2 <92%
- Too Breathless to talk
- Resp rate >40/min
- Heart rate >140/min
- Use of accessory neck muscles

LIFE-THREATENING ASTHMA
SpO$_2$ <92% plus any of:
- Silent chest,
- Poor resp effort
- Agitation
- Cyanosis
- Altered consciousness

Oxygen via face mask/ nasal prongs to achieve SpO2 94-98%

(Moderate)
- **β2 agonist** 2-10 puffs via spacer ± facemask (given one at a time single puffs, tidal breathing and inhaled separately)
- Increase **β2 agonist** dose by 2 puffs every 2 minutes up to 10 puffs according to response
- consider soluble **oral Prednisolone 20mg**

Reassess within 1 hour

(Severe)
- **β2 agonist** 10 puffs via spacer ± facemask or nebulised **Salbutamol** 2.5mg or **Terbutaline** 5mg.
- Soluble **Prednisolone 20mg** or **IV Hydrocortisone 4mg/kg**
- Repeat β2 agonist up to every 20-30min according to response
- if poor response, add **0.25mg nebulised Ipratropium bromide**

(Life-threatening)
- Nebulised **β2 agonist:**
- **Salbutamol** 2.5 mg or **Terbutaline** 5mg + **Ipratropium bromide** 0.25mg nebulised.
- Oral **Prednisolone 20mg** or **IV Hydrocortisone 4mg/kg** if vomiting.
- Discuss with senior clinician, PICU team or paediatrician.
- Repeat bronchodilators every 20-30minutes

ASSESS RESPONSE TO TREATMENT
Record RR, HR and Oxygen saturation every 1-4hours

RESPONDING
- Continue bronchodilators 1-4hours prn
- Discharge when stable on 4 hourly treatment
- Continue oral Prednisolone for up to 3 days

At Discharge
- Unsure stable on 4 hly inhaled treatment
- Review the need for regular treatment and the use of inhaled steroids
- Review inhaler technique
- Provide a written asthma action plan for treating future attacks
- Arrange follow up according to local policy

NOT RESPONDING
- Arrange **HDU/PICU** transfer

Consider
- CXR and Blood gases
- IV Salbutamol 15mcg/Kg bolus over 10min followed by **continuous infusion 1-5mcg/kg/min (dilute to 200mcg/ml)**
- IV Aminophylline 5mg/Kg loading dose over 20min (omit in those receiving oral theophylline) followed by continuous infusion 1mg/kg/hour.

---

[137] *Summary of the diagnosis and pharmacological management of asthma in children (from the British guideline on the management of asthma)*

By SIGN and BTS (16 September 2019)

MANAGEMENT ASTHMA >5-YEAR-OLD

The below flow diagram was copied from the joint BTS/SIGN guidelines 2019[138]

ASSESS ASTHMA SEVERITY

MODERATE ASTHMA
- SpO2 ≥92%
- PEF >50% Best or predicted
- No features of acute severe asthma

NB: If a patient has signs and symptoms across categories, always treat according to their most severe features

SEVERE ASTHMA
- SpO2 <92%
- PEF 33-50% best or predicted
- Resp rate >30/min
- Heart rate >125/min
- Use of accessory neck muscles

LIFE-THREATENING ASTHMA
SpO2 <92% plus any of:
- PEF < 33% best or predicted
- Silent chest,
- Poor resp effort
- Cyanosis
- Altered consciousness

Oxygen via face mask/ nasal prongs to achieve SpO2 94-98%

MODERATE
- **β2 agonist** 2-10 puffs via spacer
- Increase **β2 agonist** dose by 2 puffs every 2 minutes up to 10 puffs according to response
- Oral **Prednisolone** 30-40 mg

Reassess within 1 hour

SEVERE
- **β2 agonist** 10 puffs via spacer or nebulised **Salbutamol** 2.5 - 5mg or **Terbutaline** 5 -10mg.
- Oral **Prednisolone** 30-40mg or IV **Hydrocortisone** 4mg/kg
- Repeat β2 agonist up to every 20-30min according to response
- if poor response, add 0.25mg nebulised **Ipratropium bromide**

LIFE-THREATENING
- Nebulised **β2 agonist:**
- **Salbutamol** 5 mg or **Terbutaline** 10mg + **Ipratropium bromide** 0.25 mg nebulised.
- Oral **Prednisolone** 30-40mg or IV **Hydrocortisone** 4mg/kg if vomiting.
- Discuss with senior clinician, PICU team or paediatrician.
- Repeat bronchodilators every 20-30minutes

ASSESS RESPONSE TO TREATMENT
Record RR, HR, Oxygen saturation and PEF/FEV every 1-4hours

RESPONDING
- Continue bronchodilators 1-4hours prn
- Discharge when stable on 4 hourly treatment
- Continue oral Prednisolone for up to 3 days

At Discharge
- Unsure stable on 4 hly inhaled treatment
- Review the need for regular treatment and the use of inhaled steroids
- Review inhaler technique
- Provide a written asthma action plan for treating future attacks
- Arrange follow up according to local policy

NOT RESPONDING
- Arrange **HDU/PICU** transfer

Consider
- **CXR and Blood gases**
- **IV Salbutamol** 15mcg/Kg bolus over 10min followed by continuous infusion 1-5mcg/kg/min (dilute to 200mcg/ml)
- **IV Aminophylline** 5mg/Kg loading dose over 20min (omit in those receiving oral theophylline) followed by continuous infusion 1mg/kg/hour.

---

[138] *Summary of the diagnosis and pharmacological management of asthma in children (from the British guideline on the management of asthma)*

By *SIGN and BTS* (16 September 2019)

2. THE CHILD WITH BRONCHIOLITIS

INTRODUCTION

o Bronchiolitis is the most common disease of the lower respiratory tract during the first year of life.

o Bronchiolitis is typically caused by a virus.

o **Respiratory syncytial virus (RSV)** is the most common cause.

o It usually presents with **cough** with **increased work of breathing**, and it often **affects a child's ability to feed**.

o In primary care, the condition may often be confused with a common cold, though the presence of lower respiratory tract signs (wheeze and/or crackles on auscultation) in an infant in mid-winter would be consistent with this clinical diagnosis.

o The symptoms are usually mild and may **only last for a few days**, but in some cases the disease can cause severe illness. There are several individual and environmental risk factors that can put children with bronchiolitis at increased risk of severe illness.

Healthcare professionals should be aware of the increased need for hospital admission in infants with the following:

• Pre-existing lung disease, congenital heart disease, neuromuscular weakness, immune-incompetence

• Age < 6 weeks (corrected)

• Prematurity

• Family anxiety

• Re-attendance

• Duration of illness is less than 3 days and Amber-may need to admit

SIGNS AND SYMPTOMS CAN INCLUDE:

• Rhinorrhoea (Runny nose)

• Cough

• Poor feeding

• Vomiting

• Pyrexia

• Respiratory distress

• Apnoea

• Inspiratory crackles ± wheeze

• Cyanosis

DIAGNOSTIC CRITERIA

o Diagnose bronchiolitis if the child has:

▪ **A coryzal prodrome** lasting 1 to 3 days, followed by:

• Persistent **cough** and either

• **Tachypnoea** or **chest recession** (or both) and either

• **Wheeze** or **crackles** on chest auscultation (or both).

o When diagnosing bronchiolitis, take into account that the following symptoms are common in children with this disease[139]:

▪ **Fever** (in around 30% of cases, usually of less than 39°C)

▪ **Poor feeding** (typically after 3 to 5 days of illness).

o When diagnosing bronchiolitis, take into account that young infants with this disease (in particular those under 6 weeks of age) may present **with apnoea without** other clinical signs.

o Consider a diagnosis of **Pneumonia** if the child has:

▪ Bronchiolitis in children: high fever (over 39°C) and/or

▪ Persistently focal crackles.

o Think about a diagnosis of **viral-induced wheeze** or **early-onset asthma** rather than bronchiolitis in older infants and young children if they have:

▪ Persistent wheeze without crackles or

▪ Recurrent episodic wheeze or

▪ A personal or family history of atopy.

o Take into account that the above conditions are unusual in children under 1 year of age

ADMISSION CRITERIA

o Admit to hospital if **life threatening symptoms** (RED FLAGS):

▪ Unable to rouse

▪ Apnoea (observed or reported)

▪ Persistent SPO2 <92% when breathing air

▪ Inadequate oral fluid intake: < 50% fluid intake over 2-3 feeds

▪ Significant reduced urine output

▪ Persisting severe respiratory distress: grunting, marked chest recession, or a respiratory rate of over 70 breaths/minute, cyanosis

▪ Pale, mottled skin with CRT > 3sec

▪ Presence of risk factors

ED MANAGEMENT

o The management of bronchiolitis depends on the severity of the illness.

o In most children bronchiolitis can be managed at home by parents or carers.

o Do not use any of the following to treat bronchiolitis in children: antibiotics, hypertonic saline, adrenaline (nebulised), salbutamol, montelukast, ipratropium bromide, systemic or inhaled corticosteroids.

---

[139] *Bronchiolitis in children: diagnosis and management*
NICE guideline [NG9. Published date: June 2015

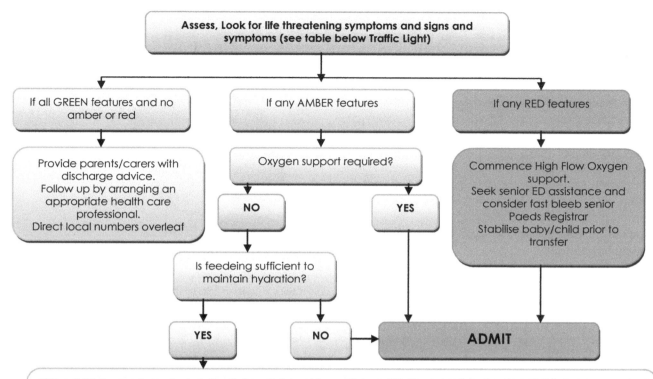

If the child does not need admission to hospital provide a safety net for the parents/carers by using one or more of the following:
- Provide parent/carer with a written or verbal information on warning symptoms and accessing further healthcare
- Arrange appropriate follow-up
- Liaise with other professionals to ensure parent/carer has direct access to further assessment

TRAFFIC LIGHT SYSTEM FOR IDENTIFYING SEVERUTY OF ILLNESS

	GREEN-LOW RISK	AMBER-INTERMEDIATE RISK	RED-HIGH RISK
Behaviour	• Alert • Normal	• Irritable • Not responding normally to social cues • Decreased activity • No smile	• Unable to rouse • Wakes only with prolonged stimulation • No response to social cues • Weak, high pitched or continuous cry • Appears ill to a healthcare professional.
Skin	• CRT ≤2secs • Normal colour skin, lips & tongue	• CRT 2-3secs • Pale/Mottled • Pallor colour reported by parent/ carer • Cool Peripheries	• CRT over 3 secs • Pale/mottled/ ashen blue • Cyanotic lips and tongue
Resp rate	< 12mths: <50bpm > 12 mths: < 40bpm No respiratory distress	< 12mths: 50-60bpm > 12 mths: 40-60bpm	All ages > 60bpm
SATS in air	95% or above	92-94%	<92%
Chest recession	None	Moderate	Severe
Nasal flaring	Absent	May be present	Present
Grunting	Absent	Absent	Present
Feeding/ Hydration	• Normal • No vomiting	• 50-75% fluid intake over 3-4 feeds ± vomiting. • Reduced urine output	• < 50 % fluid intake over 2-3 feeds ± vomiting. • Significantly reduced urine output
Apnoea	Absent	Absent	Present

II. APPROACH TO THE CHILD WITH STRIDOR

INTRODUCTION

- **Stridor** is derived from the Latin word "stridulus," which means creaking, whistling or grating. Stridor is a harsh, vibratory sound of variable pitch caused by partial obstruction of the respiratory passages that results in turbulent airflow through the airway. Stridor is a sign of upper airway obstruction. In children, laryngomalacia is the most common cause of chronic stridor, while croup is the most common cause of acute stridor.
- **Wheeze** is predominantly expiratory from lower airway obstruction.
- **An expiratory grunt** may suggest small airway closure or alveolar filling, such as found in pneumonia or pulmonary oedema.

DIFFERENTIAL DIAGNOSIS OF ACUTE STRIDOR

CAUSES OF STRIDOR (UK Incidence)	
Very common	
- Croup or viral Laryngo-tracheo bronchitis	Coryzal, Barking cough, Mild fever, Hoarse voice
Uncommon	
- Foreign body aspiration	Sudden onset, History of choking
- Epiglottitis	Drooling, muffled voice, Septic appearance, Absent cough
Rare	
- Bacterial tracheitis	Harsh cough, Chest pain, Septic appearance
- Trauma	Crepitus, Bruising, Neck swelling,
- Retropharyngeal abscess or Peritonsillar abscess	Drooling, Septic appearance
- Inhalation of hot gases	Facial burns, Peri-oral soot
- Infectious mononucleosis	Sore throat, Tonsillar enlargement
- Angioneurotic oedema	Itching, facial swelling, Urticarial rash
- Diphtheria	Travel to endemic area, Unimmunised

1. THE CHILD WITH CROUP

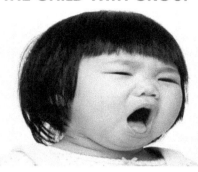

- The most common cause of acute stridor in childhood is laryngotracheobronchitis, or viral croup. it is a syndrome consisting of a **"barking" cough, stridor, hoarseness** and varying degrees of difficulty breathing.
- The condition is caused most commonly by parainfluenza virus, but it can also be caused by influenza virus types A or B, respiratory syncytial virus and rhinoviruses[140].
- Other viruses that cause croup are: Adenovirus, Measles, Coxsackie, Echovirus, Reovirus and Influenza A and B. Croup usually occurs in children six months to six years of age, with a peak incidence in the second year of life.
- The male-to-female ratio is approximately 3:2. Croup is usually preceded by an upper respiratory tract infection of several days' duration.
- A low-grade fever, barking cough, inspiratory stridor and hoarseness then develop. Symptoms are characteristically worse at night and are aggravated by agitation and crying..

CLINICAL PRESENTATION OF CROUP
THE WESTLEY CROUP SCORE [141]

Croup scoring system of Westley et al[1]					
Symptoms	Croup score				
	0	1	2	3	5
Stridor at rest	None	Audible with stethoscope	Audible without stethoscope	–	–
Retractions	None	Mild	Moderate	Severe	–
Air entry	Normal	Decreased	Severely decreased	–	–
Cyanosis	None	With agitation	At rest	–	–
Level of consciousness	Normal	–	–	–	Altered

---

140 Skolnik N. Croup. J Fam Pract. 1993;37(2):165–70.

141 Westley CR, Cotton EK, Brooks JG. Nebulized racemic epinephrine by IPPB for the treatment of croup: a double-blind study. Am J Dis Child. 1978 May;132(5):484-7.

- Children with croup can be divided into four levels of severity:
  o **Mild**: croup score 0-2
  o **Moderate**: croup score 3-5
  o **Severe**: croup score 6-11
  o **Impending respiratory failure**: croup score 12-17
- 85% of children have mild croup.
- 5% of children are admitted into hospital and of these 1-3% require intubation.
- Uncommon complications include **pneumonia** and **bacterial tracheitis**.

INVESTIGATION STRATEGIES

- Croup is essentially a **clinical diagnosis** and no investigations are required to make a diagnosis;
- ABG analysis and chest x-ray may be helpful in assessing severity and potential complications.

MANAGEMENT OF CROUP IN THE ED[142]

- Make the child **comfortable** (avoid agitating the child).
- **Maximal medical therapy**:
  o This consists of high-flow oxygen together with nebulised adrenaline (epinephrine) 5mg (5 ml 1:1000) and oral steroids.
  o If dexamethasone (0.15 mg/kg) cannot be taken then nebulised budesonide (2mg) should be given. Paediatric and anaesthetic support should be summoned immediately.
  o If there is no improvement then the adrenaline nebuliser can be repeated while preparations are made for induction and intubation.
- **Medical therapy:**
  o This consists of high-flow oxygen together with oral steroids (dexamethasone 0.15 mg/kg).
  o 2 hours of observation (monitoring P, RR and SaO_2) should be undertaken prior to reassessment of severity
- **Oral steroids:** Dexamethasone 0.15 mg/kg orally.
- Both can be repeated after 12 hours if clinically indicated.
- **Nebulised Adrenaline** is only used in children with severe and life-threatening croup: **Adrenaline 1: 1,000 0.4ml/kg Nebs** maximum 5 mL.
- **Antibiotics not indicated** (mostly viral aetiology).
- A very small proportion of children admitted to hospital with croup require tracheal intubation.
- The decision to intubate is a clinical one based on increasing tachycardia, tachypnoea and chest retraction, or the appearance of cyanosis, exhaustion or confusion.

- The respiratory rate, work of breathing, oxygen saturation and pulse rate should be carefully monitored.
- The work of breathing, respiratory rate, volume of stridor and pulse rate should decrease if the treatment is working.

DISPOSAL

- **Mild croup**: Discharge home **following a single dose of dexamethasone**
- **Moderate croup**: observe for a **minimum of four hours** following a dose of dexamethasone and then re-assessed.
- **Severe croup**: must be admitted into hospital.
- In children discharged home advice must be given to a parent and documented in the notes.

2. THE CHILD WITH FOREIGN BODY ASPIRATION

PRESENTATION

- Foreign body aspiration is a common cause of acute stridor. The peak incidence is between one and two years of age.
- The foreign body is usually food. A history of aspiration or choking can be obtained in 90 percent of cases. The most common symptoms of laryngotracheal foreign bodies are cough, stridor and dyspnea, whereas those of bronchial foreign bodies are cough, decreased breath sounds, wheezing and dysphagia. Stridor may occur because of direct compression of the trachea by large objects lodged in the postcricoid region, paraesophageal inflammation, abscess formation or direct extension of the inflammatory process into the trachea by ulceration and fistula formation.

INVESTIGATIONS

- An inspiratory **chest x-ray** may be normal, whilst an expiratory film may demonstrate air trapping.

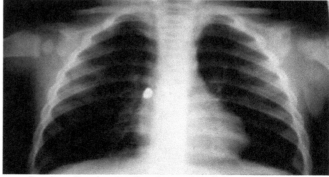

Trachea Foreign Bodies: From eMedicine Medscape

TREATMENT: It is by removal of the foreign body by bronchoscopy under general anaesthetic.

[142] RCEM Website- available at: https://www.rcem.ac.uk/docs/Local%20Guidelines_Paediatric/12cXii.%20Croup %20(Central%20Manchester%20University%20Hospitals,%202009).doc

3. THE CHILD WITH ANGIOEDEMA

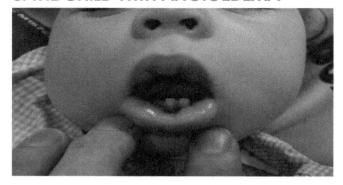

o Angioedema, with or without urticaria, is classified as allergic, hereditary, or idiopathic.
o Airway compromise is caused by vasodilatation and associated oedema.
o Treatment of allergic and idiopathic angioedema is with IM adrenaline, oxygen, steroids, H1 and H2 blockers, IV fluids and consideration of intubation.
o If adrenaline is required, then all children must be admitted for observation due to the risk of re-occurrence after six hours.
o On discharge children, should be referred to an allergy specialist, receive training on the use of an adrenaline auto-injector (e.g. Epipen or Anapen) and be discharged with two adrenaline auto-injectors, one of which should be kept at school.
• **In Hereditary angioedema (HAE)** (autosomal dominant disorder of C1 esterase inhibitor):
  o Oedema formation is related to the reduction or dysfunction of C1 inhibitor which results in the release of bradykinin and C2-kinin mediators.
  o This enhances vascular permeability and leads to extra-vascular fluid shifts.
  o Approximately 40% of people with HAE present with the first episode before the age of 5 years and 75% present before age 15 years.
  o **Treatment of HAE:**
    ▪ **C1 inhibitor concentrate** is the treatment of choice.
    ▪ Clinical improvement is seen within 15-60 min.
    ▪ A repeat dose may be required if symptoms are not relieved within an hour or progress.

Dose of C1 inhibitor concentrate	
Weight	Dose
<50Kg	10 U/Kg
50-100Kg	1000 U
>100Kg	1500 U

    ▪ If C1 inhibitor concentrate is not available, then **fresh frozen plasma** or solvent detergent treated plasma (**Octaplex**) can be used.
    ▪ **HAE does not respond to adrenaline.**

4. THE CHILD WITH RETROPHARYNGEAL ABSCESS

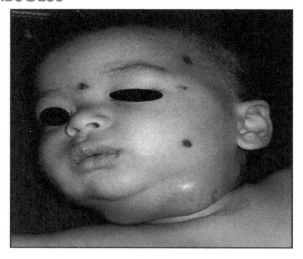

o A retropharyngeal or peritonsillar abscess may cause stridor as edema of the hypopharynx develops. Although both may present with fever, drooling and dysphagia, the child with a peritonsillar abscess may have difficulty opening the mouth (trismus) because of spasm of the pterygoid muscles, while the child with a retropharyngeal abscess often keeps the neck hyperextended.
o In retropharyngeal abscess, the bacteria most commonly identified are **streptococcus pyogenes, staphylococcus aureus, haemophilus influenzae and Neisseria species and anaerobes.**
o In stable patients **lateral soft tissue x-rays** can show an enlarged prevertebral soft tissue shadowing.
o Children with airway compromise must be admitted for close monitoring with **urgent I&D** of the abscess.

5. THE CHILD WITH EPIGLOTTITIS

o Following the introduction of the Haemophilus influenza type b (Hib) vaccination in 1992, childhood epiglottitis has become rare.
o In children, epiglottitis is almost always caused by *Haemophilus influenzae* type b[143]. In recent years, the occurrence of epiglottitis has been reduced dramatically by the widespread use of the *H. influenzae* type b vaccine. Epiglottitis usually occurs in children two to seven years of age, with a peak incidence in three-year-olds[144].
o The male-to-female ratio is approximately 3:2.

[143] Leung AK, Jadavji T. Polysaccharide vaccine for prevention of Haemophilus influenzae type b disease. J Roy Soc Health. 1988;108:180–1.

[144] Orenstein DM. Acute inflammatory upper airway obstruction. In: Nelson WE, Behrman RE, Kliegman RM, Arvin AM, eds. Nelson Textbook of pediatrics. Philadelphia: W.B. Saunders, 1996:1201–5.

o The disease is characterized by an abrupt onset of high fever, toxicity, agitation, stridor, dyspnea, muffled voice, dysphagia and drooling. The older child may prefer to sit leaning forward with the mouth open and the tongue somewhat protruding. There is no spontaneous cough.

o An edematous, cherry red epiglottis, visualized in a controlled environment, is the hallmark of epiglottitis.

o Management of this condition remains controversial:

- The cornerstone is **not to distress** the child as this can precipitate complete airway obstruction.
- **Oxygen** should be administered if the child is hypoxic.
- In the first instance, intravenous antibiotics should be administered, if IV access can be achieved without distressing a younger child.
- **A third-generation cephalosporin** is a reasonable choice.
- Children under six years of age require **urgent intubation**, ideally in theatre by an experienced anaesthetist with an ENT surgeon present.
- If there is no time to transfer the child to theatre, then a difficult intubation trolley and cricothyroidotomy kit must be accessible.
- In those over the age of six years observation may be an option following consultation with an ENT and PICU consultant.

o The average time for children to remain intubated is **48 to 96 hours.**

o Extubation occurs when direct visualisation of the epiglottis confirms that the inflammation of the epiglottis and surrounding tissues has resolved.

6. THE CHILD WITH BACTERIAL TRACHEITIS

- **Bacterial tracheitis** or **Pseudomembranous croup** is an uncommon but life-threatening form of upper airway infection. It is usually caused by *Staphylococcus aureus*, although it can also be caused by *H. influenzae* **type b** and *Moraxella catarrhalis.* Most patients are younger than three years of age.
- Bacterial tracheitis usually follows an upper respiratory tract infection.
- The patient then becomes seriously ill with high fever, toxicity and respiratory distress.
- The child appears toxic, with a high fever and the signs of progressive upper airway obstruction.
- The croupy cough, absence of drooling and a longer history help distinguish this condition from epiglottitis.

- **Radiography: Steeple sign**: a radiologic **sign** found on a frontal neck radiograph where subglottic tracheal narrowing produces the shape of a church **steeple** within the trachea itself. The presence of the **steeple sign** supports a diagnosis of croup, usually caused by paramyxoviruses.

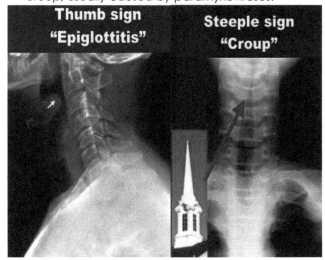

Thumb sign & Steeple sign: From pinterest.com

- Over 80% of children with this illness need intubation and ventilatory support to maintain an adequate airway, as well as intravenous antibiotics (cefotaxime or ceftriaxone plus flucloxacillin).

7. THE CHILD WITH LARYNGOMALACIA

- Laryngomalacia is the commonest congenital laryngeal abnormality and a relatively common cause of stridor in infancy. It is the most common cause of chronic stridor in children younger than two years. It has a male-to-female ratio of approximately 2:1 [145]. The condition is due to an intrinsic defect or delayed maturation of supporting structures of the larynx. The airway is partially obstructed during inspiration by the prolapse of the flaccid epiglottis, arytenoids and aryepiglottic folds.
- The inspiratory stridor is usually worse when the child is in a supine position, when crying or agitated, or when an upper respiratory tract infection occurs [146].
- The stridor is often described as being '**high-pitched**' or '**crowing**'.
- The stridor can be worsened by a co-existing coryza and tends to initially worsen before spontaneously resolving within the **first 18-14 months of life**.
- The diagnosis can be confirmed by **flexible laryngoscopy** and treatment is rarely required.

---

[145] *Simon NP. Evaluation and management of stridor in the newborn. Clin Pediatr. 1991;30:211–6.*

[146] *Clough J. Managing stridor in children. Practitioner. 1995;239(1557):724–8.*

III. APPROACH TO WHOOPING COUGH

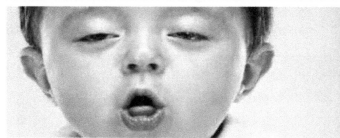

Whooping Cough – From Tom Liberman

INTRODUCTION

- Pertussis, also known as whooping cough, is an acute respiratory tract infection that presents as a chronic cough in most patients. Up to 17% of patients who develop a cough lasting more than two weeks have pertussis[147].

- Most cases of pertussis are caused by **Bordetella pertussis**, but other species (*Bordetella parapertussis* and *Bordetella bronchiseptica*) have also been implicated[148] and is a notifiable disease.

- This disease is preventable by childhood immunisation. It is a highly infectious bacterial disease of the respiratory tract and spread by droplet transmission.

- The incubation period of pertussis is **7 to 10 days**, longer than the typical one- to three-day period for most viral upper respiratory tract infections.

- Patients then develop a presentation that can vary from asymptomatic to a mild respiratory tract infection to a persistent, severe cough.

- Much of this variation is due to patient age and the degree of immunity to *B. pertussis*.

- The highest incidence is in infants who are not immunized or too young to be fully protected.

- School children are often the source of infection for younger siblings at home. Infection can also occur in adolescents and adults, even if previously immunized, because immunity wanes over time.

VACCINATION

- In the UK accellular pertussis vaccine is given in the primary course with diphtheria, tetanus, polio and Hib (as DtaP/IPV/Hib), given at aged 2, 3, & 4 months of age.

- A further booster dose is given with the preschool boosters between the ages of 3 & 5.

---

[147] *Dempsey AF, Cowan AE, Broder KR, Kretsinger K, Stokley S, Clark SJ. Diagnosis and testing practices for adolescent pertussis among a national sample of primary care physicians. Prev Med. 2009;48(5):500–504.*

[148] *Altunaiji S, Kukuruzovic R, Curtis N, Massie J. Antibiotics for whooping cough (pertussis). Cochrane Database Syst Rev. 2007;(3):CD004404.*

CLINICAL PRESENTATION

- Initial symptoms include coryza and cough.

- Gradually the cough progresses to severe coughing bouts which can be prolonged.

- Not all children have the characteristic 'whoop' (inspiratory noise) at the end of a coughing bout, and some cough spasms may be followed by periods of vomiting.

- These coughing episodes can be severe and may result in **subconjunctival and periorbital haemorrhages.**

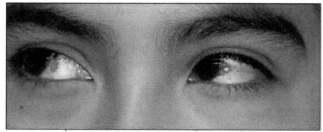

subconjunctival and periorbital haemorrhages.

COMPLICATIONS

- Pneumonia,
- Seizure,
- Encephalopathy,
- Weight loss and
- Death.

- Complications are most likely to occur in young infants among who the most common cause of pertussis related deaths is **secondary bacterial pneumonia.**

- Pertussis can occur in previously immunized and infected individuals, but immunization and prior infection attenuate the clinical picture.

INVESTIGATION

- Confirmation of the diagnosis is via **PCR** and **serological testing** because the viral culture lacks sensitivity. Other investigations should be directed as for a suspected pneumonia.

MANAGEMENT OF PERTUSSIS IN THE ED

- Antibiotic prophylaxis may be of value for unvaccinated household contacts of cases, particularly in infants <6 months of age, **if given within 21 days of onset of the first case.**

- **Macrolide antibiotics** (azithromycin, clarithromycin, and erythromycin) are recommended for the treatment of pertussis in people aged ≥1 month.

- For infants aged <1-month, **Azithromycin** is the preferred antibiotic.

2. Cardio-Respiratory Arrest
I. APPROACH TO CARDIAC LIFE SUPPORT

1. PAEDIATRIC BLS AND ACLS (adapted from APLS manual, 6th Edition)

Basic life support algorithm

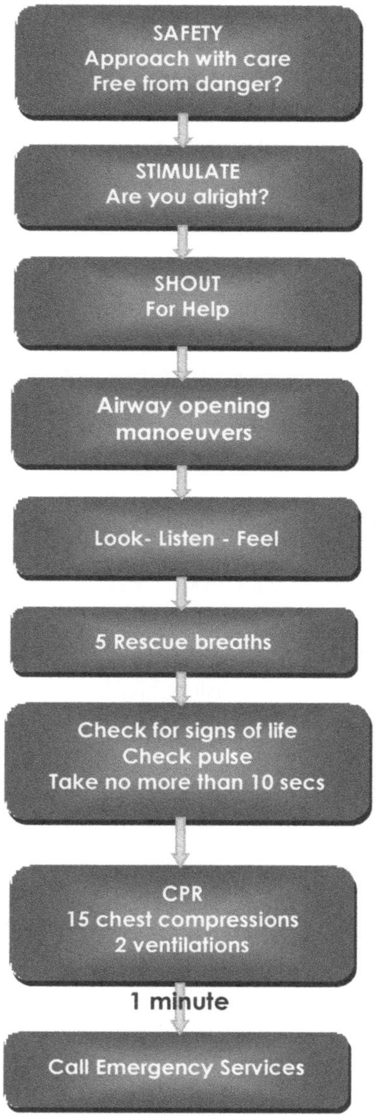

SAFETY
Approach with care
Free from danger?

STIMULATE
Are you alright?

SHOUT
For Help

Airway opening manoeuvers

Look- Listen - Feel

5 Rescue breaths

Check for signs of life
Check pulse
Take no more than 10 secs

CPR
15 chest compressions
2 ventilations

1 minute

Call Emergency Services

o **A newborn** is a child just after birth.
o **A neonate** is a child in the first 28 days of life.
o **An infant** is a child under 1 year.
o **A child** is between 1 year and puberty.

Cardiac arrest algorithm

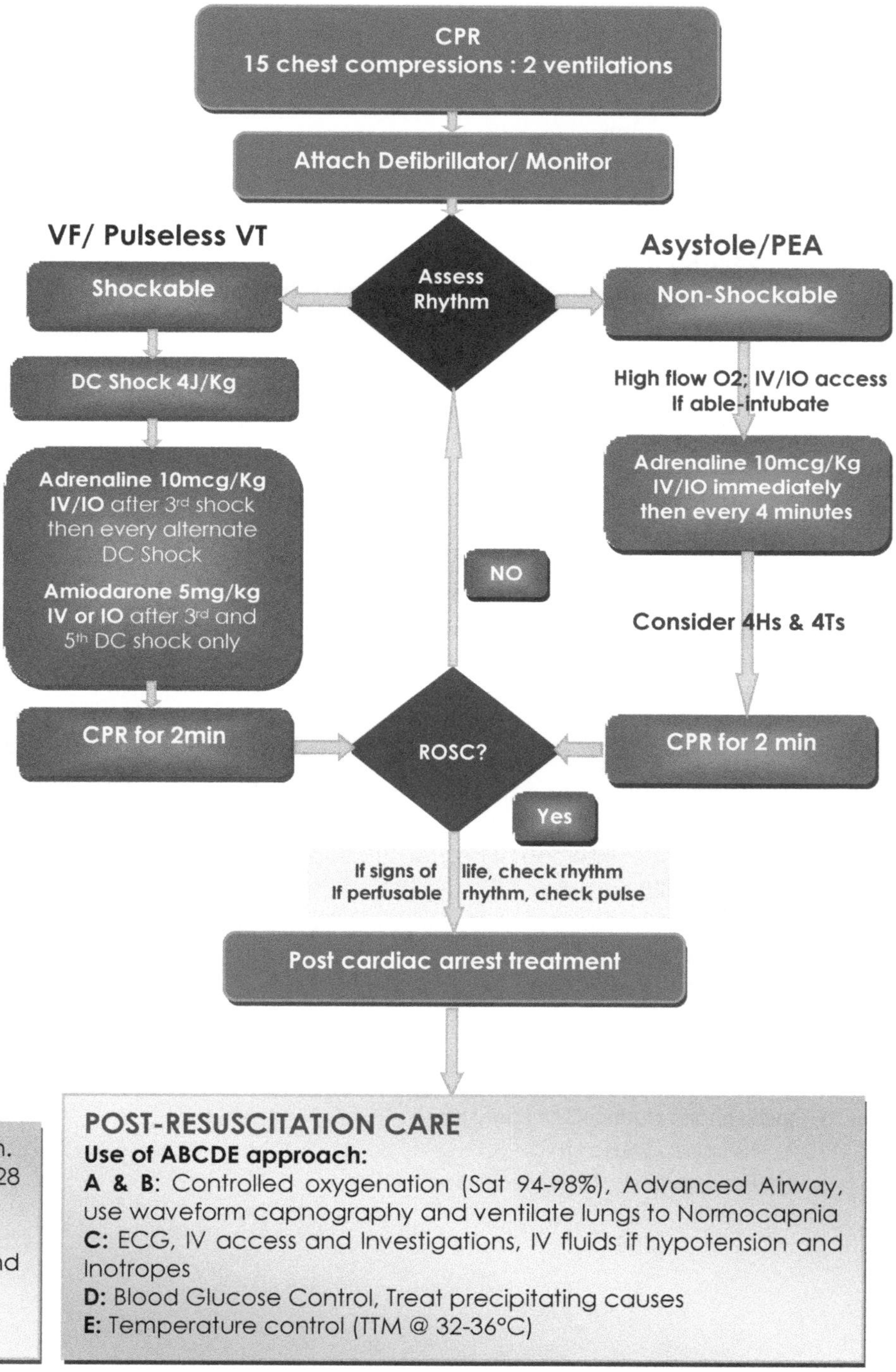

CPR
15 chest compressions : 2 ventilations

Attach Defibrillator/ Monitor

Assess Rhythm

VF/ Pulseless VT

Shockable

DC Shock 4J/Kg

Adrenaline 10mcg/Kg IV/IO after 3rd shock then every alternate DC Shock

Amiodarone 5mg/kg IV or IO after 3rd and 5th DC shock only

CPR for 2min

NO

Asystole/PEA

Non-Shockable

High flow O2; IV/IO access
If able-intubate

Adrenaline 10mcg/Kg IV/IO immediately then every 4 minutes

Consider 4Hs & 4Ts

CPR for 2 min

ROSC?

Yes

If signs of life, check rhythm
If perfusable rhythm, check pulse

Post cardiac arrest treatment

POST-RESUSCITATION CARE
Use of ABCDE approach:
A & B: Controlled oxygenation (Sat 94-98%), Advanced Airway, use waveform capnography and ventilate lungs to Normocapnia
C: ECG, IV access and Investigations, IV fluids if hypotension and Inotropes
D: Blood Glucose Control, Treat precipitating causes
E: Temperature control (TTM @ 32-36°C)

DRUGS USED IN CPR

1. ADRENALINE
o Adrenaline 1:1,000=1mg/ml;
o Adrenaline 1:10,000= 0.1mg/ml or 100mcg/ml or 1mg/10ml
o **Children CPR dosage: IV/IO Adrenaline 10mcg/kg =** (0.1 ml/kg of 1: 10,000).
o Subsequent doses of adrenaline are given **every 3–5 min**.
o Do not use higher doses of IV adrenaline in children, it may worsen outcome.

2. AMIODARONE
o Amiodarone 150mg/3ml= **50mg/ml** (450mg/9ml and 900mg/18ml)
o **Children CPR dosage:** In the treatment of shockable rhythms:
   ▪ Initial **IV** bolus dose of **Amiodarone 5mg/kg after the third defibrillation**.
   ▪ Repeat the dose after the **fifth shock if still in VF/pVT**.
   ▪ If defibrillation was successful but VF/pVT recurs, amiodarone can be repeated (unless two doses have already been given) and a continuous infusion started.
o Amiodarone can cause **thrombophlebitis** when injected into a peripheral vein and, ideally, should be delivered via a central vein.
o If central venous access is unavailable (likely at the time of cardiac arrest) and so it has to be given peripherally, flush it liberally with **0.9% sodium chloride or 5% glucose.**

3. ATROPINE
o Atropine is effective in increasing heart rate when bradycardia is caused by excessive vagal tone (e.g. after insertion of nasogastric tube).
o The dose is **20 mcg/kg.**
o There is no evidence that atropine has any benefit in asphyxial bradycardia or asystole and its routine use has been removed from the ALS algorithms.

4. MAGNESIUM
o **Indications during CPR (only if):**
   ▪ Hypomagnesaemia
   ▪ Polymorphic VT (torsade de pointes).

5. CALCIUM
o **Indications during CPR (only if):**
   ▪ Hyperkalaemia,
   ▪ Hypocalcaemia
   ▪ Overdose of calcium-channel-blocking drugs

o High plasma concentrations achieved after intravenous injection may be harmful to the ischaemic myocardium and may also impair cerebral recovery.

6. SODIUM BICARBONATE
o **8.4% NaHCO3⁻ 1 mEq/mL => 50 mL Single Dose vial (50mEq/50ml); 1 mEq = 84mg NaHCO3⁻**
o Cardiorespiratory arrest results in combined respiratory and metabolic acidosis, caused by cessation of pulmonary gas exchange and the development of anaerobic cellular metabolism respectively.
o The best treatment for acidaemia in cardiac arrest is a combination of effective chest compression and ventilation (high quality CPR).
o The routine use of sodium bicarbonate in CPR is not recommended.

o **Indications during CPR (only if):**
   ▪ Hyperkalaemia
   ▪ Arrhythmias associated with TCA overdose

RISK OF ADMINISTRATION OF SODIUM BICARBONATE:
▪ It generates carbon dioxide, which diffuses rapidly into the cells, exacerbating intracellular acidosis if it is not rapidly cleared via the lungs.
▪ It produces a negative inotropic effect on an ischaemic myocardium.
▪ It presents a large, osmotically active, sodium load to an already compromised circulation and brain.
▪ It produces a shift to the left in the oxygen dissociation curve, further inhibiting release of oxygen to the tissues.

PAEDIATRIC FORMULAS AND DRUG DOSES FOR ARREST AND PERI-ARREST SCENARIOS "WET FLAGS"

WET FLAG FORMULA

Weight	• **1–12 months =** (0.5 × age months) + 4 = ½age in months +4 • **1–5 years =** (2 × age years) + 8 • **6–12 years =** (3 × age years) + 7
Electricity	• **Defibrillation** 4 J/kg (single shocks) • **Cardioversion** 1 J/kg then 2 J/kg then amiodarone and repeat

Tube: Endotracheal tube (ETT)	• **Length:**
	  ○ Oral ETT = **Age/2 + 12**
	  ○ Nasal ETT = **Age/2 + 15**
	• **Children aged over 1 year:**
	  ○ Diameter in mm: **Age/4 + 4**
	• **Children under 1 year the following sizes should be used:**
	  ○ Neonates under 3 kg – size **3.0 or 3.5 mm**
	  ○ Age 6 months – size **4.0 mm**
	  ○ Age 1 year – size **4.5 mm**

Fluids	• Boluses are **20ml/Kg** of Normal saline • Trauma: **10ml/Kg (Blood: 10ml/kg)** • DKA: **10 ml/kg.** • Burns: % burn × weight × 3 (½ given in first 8 h, ½ given over next 16 h)
Lorazepam	**0.1mg/kg IV/IO**

Adrenaline	• Cardiac arrest: **0.1 mg/kg IV/ IO** (0.1 ml/kg of 1: 10,000)
	• Anaphylaxis:
	  ○ Age >12 years 0.5 mg IM.
	  ○ Age 6–12 years 0.3 mg IM.
	  ○ Age <6 years 0.15 mg IM.
	• Croup: 0.4ml/kg (max. 5 ml) of 1:1000 nebulized

Glucose	• Dextrose **10% 2 ml/kg**

DRUG DOSES AND INDICATIONS

Amiodarone	• Shockable cardiac arrest rhythms (VF/pVT) • 5 mg/kg IV (after 3rd shock)
Atropine	• 0.02 mg/kg (minimum dose 0.1 mg, maximum 0.6 mg) • Use pre-intubation or for bradycardia secondary to vagal stimulation. • Not recommended in cardiac arrest.
Budesonide	• Croup: 2 mg nebulizer
Ceftriaxone or cefotaxime	• Meningitis: 80 mg/kg IV (avoid ceftriaxone in neonates)
Dexamethasone	• Croup: 0.15–0.6 mg/kg
CPR	• Ratio 15:2 (5 rescue breaths first) • Rate: 100–120 per min • Hand positioning: Lower ½ of sternum (locate as 1 finger-breadth above xiphisternum) • Depth of compression: At least 1/3 depth of chest • Technique: Infant 2 fingers (or encircling technique with 2 thumbs). • Child 1 or 2 hands.

II. APPROACH TO NEONATAL RESUSCITATION

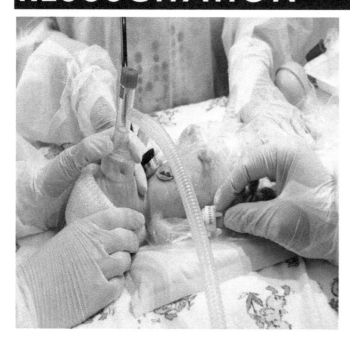

- The structured approach is outlined below.
- In reality the first four steps (up to and including assessment) are completed simultaneously.
- After this, appropriate intervention can begin following an ABC approach.
  - Call/shout for help
  - Start the clock or note the time
  - Dry and wrap the baby in warmed dry towels.
  - Maintain the baby's temperature
  - Assess the situation
  - Airway
  - Breathing
  - Chest compressions
  - Drugs/vascular access

- **CALL FOR HELP**
  - Ask for help if you expect or encounter any difficulty or if the delivery is outside the labour suite.

- **START THE CLOCK**
  - Start the clock, if available, or note the time of birth.

- **AT BIRTH**
  - **There is no need to rush to clamp the cord at delivery.**

- It can be left unclamped while the following steps are completed.
- **Dry the baby quickly and effectively.**
- Remove the wet towel and wrap the baby in a fresh, dry, warm towel.
- **Assess the baby during and after drying**: decide whether any intervention is going to be needed.
  - *If your assessment suggests that the baby is in need of resuscitation, clamp and cut the cord.*
  - *If the baby appears well, **wait for at least 1 minute from the complete delivery of the baby before clamping the cord.** (FRCEM Intermediate exam question)*

- **KEEP THE BABY WARM**
  - The normal temperature range for a newborn baby is **36.5–37.5°C.**
  - For each 1°C decrease in admission temperature below this range in otherwise healthy term newborn babies there is an associated increase in mortality of 28%.
  - Eliminate any draughts from the room (close window and doors where possible) and heat the room to above 23°C (term babies) or 25°C (preterm babies).
  - Once delivered, dry the baby immediately and then wrap in a warm, dry towel.
  - In addition to increased mortality risk, a cold baby has an increased rate of oxygen consumption and is more likely to become hypoglycaemic and acidotic.
  - If this is not addressed at the beginning of resuscitation it is often forgotten.
  - Babies of all gestations born outside the normal delivery environment may benefit from placement in a food-grade polyethylene bag or wrap after drying and then swaddling.
  - Alternatively, well, newborn babies of more than 30 weeks' gestation who are breathing may be dried and nursed with skin-to-skin contact (or kangaroo mother care) to maintain their temperature whilst they are transferred.
  - Exposed skin should be covered to protect against cooling draughts.

NEWBORN LIFE SUPPORT ALGORITHM *(Adapted from APLS 6th Edition book)*

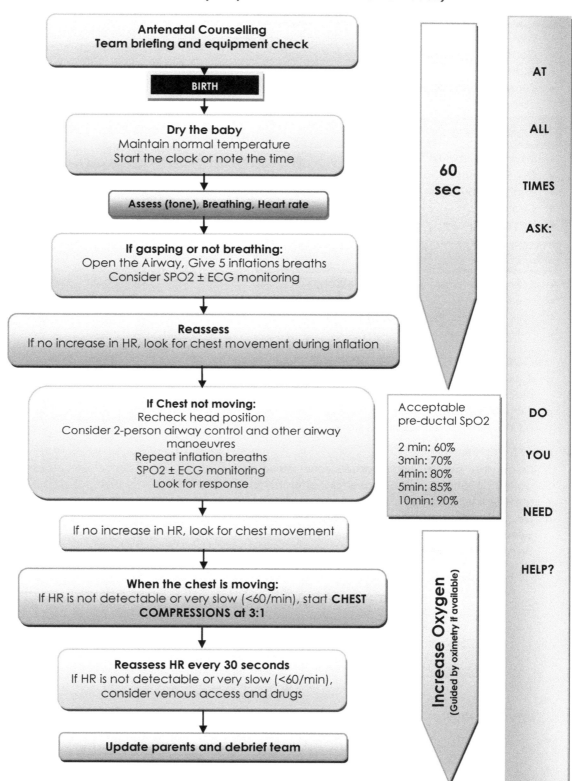

Antenatal Counselling
Team briefing and equipment check

BIRTH

Dry the baby
Maintain normal temperature
Start the clock or note the time

Assess (tone), Breathing, Heart rate

If gasping or not breathing:
Open the Airway, Give 5 inflations breaths
Consider SPO2 ± ECG monitoring

Reassess
If no increase in HR, look for chest movement during inflation

If Chest not moving:
Recheck head position
Consider 2-person airway control and other airway manoeuvres
Repeat inflation breaths
SPO2 ± ECG monitoring
Look for response

If no increase in HR, look for chest movement

When the chest is moving:
If HR is not detectable or very slow (<60/min), start **CHEST COMPRESSIONS at 3:1**

Reassess HR every 30 seconds
If HR is not detectable or very slow (<60/min), consider venous access and drugs

Update parents and debrief team

Maintain temperature

60 sec

Acceptable pre-ductal SpO2

2 min: 60%
3min: 70%
4min: 80%
5min: 85%
10min: 90%

Increase Oxygen (Guided by oximetry if available)

AT

ALL

TIMES

ASK:

DO

YOU

NEED

HELP?

III. APPROACH TO THE CHOKING CHILD

GENERAL SIGNS OF CHOKING

- Witnessed episode
- Coughing or choking
- Sudden onset
- Recent history of playing with or eating small objects

SEVERE AIRWAY OBSTRUCTION:
Ineffective coughing

- Unable to vocalise
- Quiet or silent cough
- Unable to breathe
- Cyanosis
- Decreasing level of consciousness

MILD AIRWAY OBSTRUCTION:
Effective cough

- Crying or verbal response to questions
- Loud cough
- Able to take a breath before coughing
- Fully responsive

- **UNCONSCIOUS CHILD WITH CHOKING**
  - If the choking child is, or becomes, unconscious place him on a firm, flat surface.
  - Call out, or send, for help if it is still not available.
  - Do not leave the child at this stage.

- **AIRWAY OPENING**
  - Open the mouth and look for any obvious object. If one is seen, make an attempt to remove it with a single finger sweep.
  - **Do not attempt blind or repeated finger sweeps** – these can push the object more deeply into the pharynx and cause injury.

- **RESCUE BREATHS**
  - Open the airway and attempt 5 rescue breaths.
  - Assess the effectiveness of each breath: if a breath does not make the chest rise, reposition the head before making the next attempt.
  - **Attempt 5 rescue breaths** and if there is no response, proceed immediately to chest compression regardless of whether the breaths are successful.

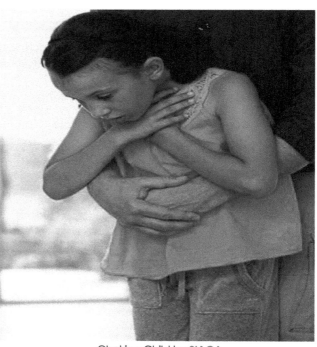

Choking Child by SIAGA

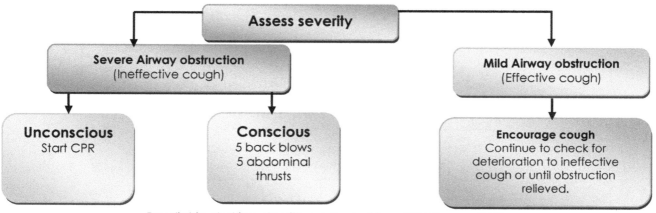

Paediatric choking algorithm-adapted from RESUS council UK

Infants < 1 year: Chest thrusts and infants >1-year abdominal thrusts.

3. Paediatric Trauma
I. APPROACH TO THE CHILD WITH TRAUM

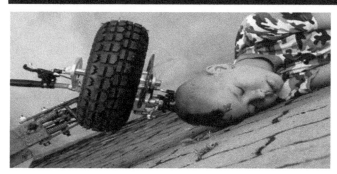

INITIAL ACTIONS

- Always start with the primary survey
- Address any problems found before moving on with your evaluation
- Log roll the patient and get them off the backboard when able
- Secondary survey with FAST exam and x-rays
- If the patient begins to deteriorate, reassess the patient and restart your evaluation with the ABC's.
- Remember this is likely a very terrified child and this can alter your exam.
- When able, always include family members to help calm and comfort the child.

TEAM LEADER ACTIONS: ASSIMILATE INFORMATION – ATMISTER

- o **A**: Age/sex
- o **T** : Time of incident
- o **M**: Mechanism of injury
- o **I** : Injury suspected
- o **S** : Signs including vital signs, Glasgow Coma Scale
- o **T** : Treatment so far
- o **E** : Estimated time of arrival to emergency department
- o **R** : Requirements, i.e. bloods, specialist services, tiered response, ambulance call sign

STRUCTURED APPROACH

- **Immediate**
  - o Primary survey (immediate life threats)
  - o Resuscitation
- **Focused**
  - o Secondary survey (key features)
  - o Emergency treatment
- **Detailed review**
  - o Reassessment (system control)
  - o Continuing stabilisation and definitive care

1. PRIMARY SURVEY

- During the primary survey life-threatening problems should be treated as they are identified.
- **<C> ABCDE**
  - o **<C**atastrophic external haemorrhage>
  - o **A**irway (with cervical spine control)
  - o **B**reathing with ventilatory support
  - o **C**irculation with haemorrhage control
  - o **D**isability with prevention of secondary insult
  - o **E**xposure with temperature control

C. CATASTROPHIC EXTERNAL HAEMORRHAGE

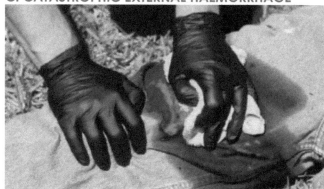

- In major trauma <C>ABC has become the established approach.
- Obvious external exsanguinating haemorrhage becomes the immediate priority.
- Simple direct pressure, specialised haemostatic dressings or a tourniquet must be applied instantly in these circumstances.
- ***Tranexamic acid should be given 15 mg/kg as soon as possible.***

A. AIRWAY AND CERVICAL SPINE IMMOBILISATION

- Look for anything compromising the airway.
  - o Material in the lumen (blood, vomit, teeth or a foreign body)
  - o Damage to or loss of control of the structures in the wall (the mouth, tongue, pharynx, larynx or trachea)
  - o External compression or distortion from outside the wall (e.g. compression from a pre-vertebral haematoma in the neck or distortion from a displaced maxillary fracture)

- Problems can develop after the primary survey e.g. bleeding or progressive swelling in facial trauma or burns. A child with a GCS score of 8 or less is unlikely to be adequately protecting their airway.
- The commonest cause is from occlusion by the tongue in an unconscious, head-injured child.

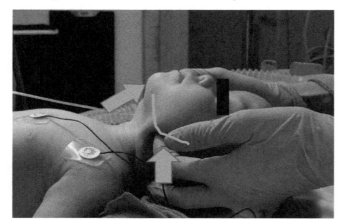

AIRWAY MANAGEMENT SEQUENCE

o Jaw thrust
o Suction/removal of foreign body under direct vision
o Oro-/nasopharyngeal airways
o Tracheal intubation
o Surgical airway

- Head tilt/chin lift is not recommended following trauma, because this manoeuvre can move the cervical spine and may exacerbate an injury.
- For any mechanism of injury capable of causing spinal injury (or in cases with an uncertain history), the cervical spine is presumed to be at risk, until it can be cleared.
- If protection is considered necessary, start with **manual in-line stabilisation (MILS)** by a competent assistant or, if this is not possible, consider using a **head block and appropriate strapping**.
- Rigid immobilisation of the head risks increasing leverage on the neck as the child struggles.
- Minimise anxiety by avoiding unnecessary interventions and encouraging the parents to remain at the bedside.
- Vomiting poses an obvious threat to the unprotected airway, especially if there is also a risk of spinal injury.
- Before providing airway suction, **tilt the patient trolley head down**, ensuring they are secure.
- The child should be taken off the scoop stretcher as soon as possible, using the 20° tilt method, and placed directly onto a trauma board or an emergency department trolley.
- If the spine has not been cleared, manual-in-line immobilisation will be needed for intubation if indicated.

- If the child is paralysed, sedated and ventilated the cervical spine cannot be cleared, and spinal immobilisation needs to be maintained until definitive imaging and neurological examinations can take place.

B. BREATHING

- Adequacy of breathing is checked in three domains: **Effort**, **Efficacy** and **Effects** on other organ systems.
- When examining the chest, look, listen and feel:
  o **Look and listen** – remembering asymmetry and asymmetrical movement (flail chest)
  o **Feel** – remember to check for crepitus (surgical emphysema), tracheal deviation, and percuss to distinguish a tension pneumothorax from a massive haemothorax

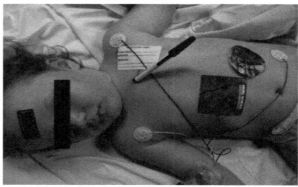

CONDITIONS IDENTIFIED

- By the end of the primary survey, the following conditions may have been recognised and treatment should be initiated as soon as they are found: "**ATOM FC**"
  o **A**irway obstruction
  o **T**ension pneumothorax
  o **O**pen pneumothorax
  o **M**assive haemothorax
  o **F**lail chest
  o **C**ardiac tamponade
- If breathing is inadequate, commence ventilation with a bag–mask and prepare for intubation, which is likely to be required.

INDICATIONS FOR INTUBATION & VENTILATION

o Persistent airway obstruction
o Predicted airway obstruction, e.g. inhalational burn
o Loss of airway reflexes
o Inadequate ventilatory effort or increasing fatigue
o Disrupted ventilatory mechanism, e.g. severe flail chest
o Persistent hypoxia despite supplemental oxygen
o Controlled ventilation required to prevent secondary brain injury

C. CIRCULATION

- Circulatory assessment in the primary survey involves the rapid assessment of heart rate and rhythm, pulse volume and peripheral perfusion including colour, temperature and capillary return and blood pressure.
- Circulatory assessment must take into account the fact that resting heart rate, blood pressure and respiratory rate vary with age.

Recognition of clinical signs indicating blood loss requiring urgent treatment:

SIGN	INDICATOR
Heart rate	Marked or increasing tachycardia or relative bradycardia
Systolic blood pressure	Falling
CRT (normal <2 sec)	Increasing
Respiratory rate	Tachypnoea unrelated to thoracic problem
Mental state	Altered conscious level unrelated to isolated head injury

- Additionally, in trauma:
  - Check peripheral pulses in limb injury
  - Look for internal haemorrhage (chest, abdomen, pelvis and femurs), including consideration of bleeding from multiple sites and progressive deterioration
  - Apply pressure to significant external haemorrhage (if appropriate)
  - Remember that exposure to cold prolongs the capillary refill time in healthy people
  - Check lactate and haemoglobin as early indicators of circulatory compromise
  - All seriously injured children require vascular access to be established urgently using two relatively large intravenous cannulae.
  - *If the child is stable with no signs of shock, an immediate fluid bolus is not required.*
  - *The principles behind this are **'the first clot is the best clot'**.*

- Major haemorrhage following injury is not common in children.
- Its management requires an understanding of concepts that have become standard in adult trauma care:
  - Use of tranexamic acid (dose 15 mg/kg)
  - Effective use of adjuncts (e.g. tourniquets, pelvic splints)
  - Implementation of massive haemorrhage protocols (MHP)

- Avoidance of hypothermia using airflow heating devices
- Maintenance of an adequate haematocrit used to aid clotting
- Damage control interventions, involving surgery and interventional radiology

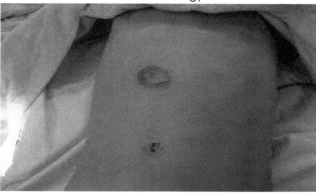

Handlebar injury

- *If abdominal haemorrhage is suspected, CT with contrast should be performed.*
- *In children, FAST (focused abdominal with sonography for trauma) has very limited application and there is limited evidence of its worth in detecting abdominal haemorrhage.*
- The child's condition should be constantly reassessed and surgical intervention considered.

D. DISABILITY

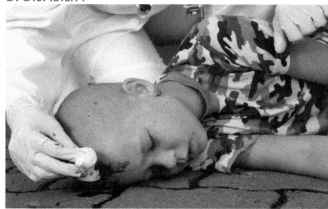

- The assessment of disability during the primary survey consists of a brief neurological examination to determine the conscious level and to assess pupil size and reactivity.
- The conscious level is described by the child's response to voice and (where necessary) to pain.
- The **AVPU** method describes the child as **A**lert, responding to **V**oice, responding to **P**ain or **U**nresponsive and is a rapid, and simple, assessment.
- A children's GCS score should be performed as soon as possible.

- Agitation in a child may suggest cerebral hypoxia.
- If the GCS score is less than 8 and/or AVPU equivalent of 'P' or 'U', immediate intervention is necessary. Remember that the GCS is modified in the smaller child.

E. EXPOSURE

- In order to assess a seriously injured child fully, it is necessary to take their clothes off.
- Children become cold very quickly, and may be acutely embarrassed when undressed in front of strangers.
- Although exposure is necessary the duration should be minimised, and a blanket provided at all other times.
- Ensure that the child's temperature is maintained and hypothermia.
- This is achieved by having a warm resuscitation area and tasking one or more of the nursing team members to keep the child covered with a blanket or hot air warming device at all times and to warm all fluids given.

INVESTIGATIONS

- When venous access is achieved and blood is taken for cross-matching, samples for other investigations should be taken at the same time, including:
  - Full Blood Count,
  - Clotting screen,
  - Amylase/Trypsinogen,
  - Urea and Electrolytes and
  - Clotting
  - Glucose: especially in adolescents (who are prone to both injury and hypoglycaemia after drinking alcohol) and in very small children.
  - Blood gas: lactate and β-human chorionic gonadotrophin should also be taken in adolescent females.

NASOGASTRIC TUBE PLACEMENT

- Acute gastric dilatation is common in children and the stomach should be decompressed.
- If there is evidence or suspicion of base of skull fracture, the tube should not be passed by the nasal route.
- In the intubated patient, the oral route is a simple alternative.
- Gastric stasis is a frequent consequence of major trauma.

ANALGESIA

- Analgesia can usually be administered just after completing the primary survey and resuscitation.

2. SECONDARY SURVEY

The secondary survey is a thorough head to toe, front to back examination searching for key anatomical features of injury. It is helpful to think in terms of **"SOCE"**:
- **Surface** (head to toe, front and back)
- **Orifice** (mouth, nose, ears, orbits; rectum, genitals)
- **Cavity** (chest, abdomen, pelvic cavity, retro-peritoneum)
- **Extremity** (upper limbs including shoulders; lower limbs including pelvic girdle)
- Occasionally, a full secondary survey may be delayed if immediate life-saving interventions are required. Ensure that this decision is clearly documented and a secondary survey carried out at a later stage.
- Throughout this stage of management, the vital signs and neurological status should be continually reassessed, and any deterioration should lead to an immediate return to the primary survey.

HISTORY

- History should be sought from the child, ambulance personnel, relatives and witnesses of the accident.
- An AMPLE history can be used to obtain relevant information pertaining to:
- In addition, consider the mechanism of injury.
- The following should cause concern and increase the likelihood of significant injury:
  - Death or serious injury of an occupant of the vehicle
  - Ejection from vehicle
  - Prolonged extrication
  - >40 mph head-on collision

SPECIAL CONSIDERATIONS IN INJURY

- Perform otoscopy (for haemotympanum) and ophthalmoscopy (for retinal haemorrhage)
- Inspect the mouth inside and out – intraoral bruising may represent fractures
- Palpate the teeth for looseness
- Assess for nasal septal haematoma
- Assess for midface stability
- Look for signs of base of skull injury (panda eyes, mastoid bruising)
- Perform a full neurological examination
- Inspect neck veins and pulses if there is a neck injury; Observe for movement
- Inspect for any external evidence of injury – tyre marks, bruising, lacerations and swelling
- Note unusual injury and bruising patterns suggesting non-accidental injury
- Inspect the perineum and external urethral meatus for blood

3. THE CHILD WITH SPECIFIC INJURIES

1. THE CHILD WITH TRAUMATIC BRAIN INJURY

- A key aim of head injury management is to prevent or minimise secondary brain injury.

PRIMARY DAMAGE

o **Injury to neural tissue:**
  - Focal cerebral contusions and lacerations (direct impact and contrecoup)
  - Diffuse axonal injury (shearing injury)

o **Injury to intracranial blood vessels:**
  - Extradural haematoma (especially middle meningeal artery)
  - Subdural haematoma (especially dural bridging veins)
  - Intracerebral haematoma
  - Subarachnoid haemorrhage

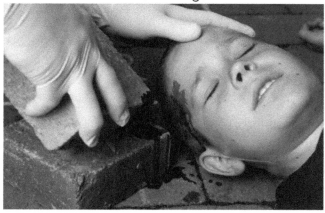

SECONDARY DAMAGE

- This may result from either the direct secondary effects of cerebral injury or from the cerebral consequences of associated injuries and stress.

  o **Ischaemia from poor cerebral perfusion secondary to raised intracranial pressure:**
    - Expanding intracranial haematoma (exacerbated by coagulopathy)
    - Cerebral swelling/oedema

  o **Ischaemia secondary to hypotension and anaemia:**
    - Haemorrhage with hypovolaemia or dilutional anaemia
    - Other causes of hypotension (spinal cord injury, drug-induced vasodilatation or later sepsis)

  o **Hypoxia:**
    - Airway obstruction
    - Inadequate respiration (loss of respiratory drive or mechanical disruption of chest wall or diaphragm)
    - Shunt from pulmonary contusion or later respiratory failure

o **Hypoglycaemia and hyperglycaemia**
o **Fever**
o **Convulsions**
o **Later infection**

RAISED INTRACRANIAL PRESSURE

- Once sutures have closed at 12–18 months of age, the child's cranial cavity behaves like an adult with a fixed volume.
- If cerebral oedema worsens or if intracranial haematomas increase in size, the pressure within the cranium increases.
- Initial compensatory mechanisms include diminution in the volume of cerebrospinal fluid and venous blood within the cranial cavity.
- When these mechanisms fail, ICP rises, compromising cerebral perfusion:

$$CPP = MAP - ICP$$
$$CPP\downarrow \rightarrow CBF\downarrow$$

- Normal cerebral blood flow is **50 ml of blood per 100 g** brain tissue per minute.
  o A fall in cerebral perfusion pressure decreases cerebral blood flow.
  o A flow below **20 ml/100 g brain tissue/min** will produce ischaemia.
  o This in turn increases cerebral oedema, causing a further rise in ICP.
  o A cerebral blood flow of below **10 ml/100 g brain tissue/min** leads to electrical dysfunction of the neurones and loss of intracellular homeostasis.

- A generalised increase of ICP in the supratentorial compartment initially causes transtentorial (uncal) herniation, leading to transforaminal (central) herniation and death.
  o **In uncal herniation,** the third nerve is nipped against the free border of the tentorium, causing **ipsilateral pupillary dilatation** secondary to loss of parasympathetic constrictor tone to the ciliary muscles.
  o **In central herniation,** also known as **coning,** the cerebellar tonsils are forced through the foramen magnum.

- In childhood, the most common cause of raised ICP following head injury is **cerebral oedema.**
- Children are especially prone to this problem.
- They may, of course, also have expanding extradural, subdural or intracerebral haematomas that require prompt surgical treatment.
- Depending on the aetiology of the raised ICP, treatment is either aimed at preventing it rising further or removing its cause (by surgical evacuation of haematomas).

- There are special considerations in infants with head injuries. Unfused sutures allow the cranial volume to increase initially.
- Large extradural or subdural bleeds may occur before neurological signs or symptoms develop.
- Such infants may show a significant fall in haemoglobin concentration.
- In addition, the infant's vascular scalp may bleed profusely, causing shock.
- In children aged over 1 year with shock associated with head injury, serious extracranial injury should be sought as the cause of the shock.

FACTORS INDICATING A POTENTIALLY SERIOUS INJURY

- History of substantial trauma such as involvement in a road traffic accident or a fall from a height
- A history of loss of consciousness
- Children who are not fully conscious and responsive
- Any child with obvious neurological signs/symptoms such as headache, convulsions or limb weakness.

PRIMARY SURVEY AND RESUSCITATION

- The first priority is to assess and stabilise the **Airway, Breathing** and **Circulation** as discussed earlier.
- Head injury may be associated with cervical spine injury, and stabilisation must be achieved as previously described.
- Pupil size and reactivity should be examined and a rapid assessment of conscious level should be made.
- In the first place, the AVPU classification may be used. In a time-limited situation, it is not essential to work out the numerical Glasgow Coma Scale (GCS) score immediately, although the EMV (eye, motor, verbal) responses will have been noted.
- But it is important to note the response to voice or pain (if not responding to voice) in more detail using the GCS before proceeding with neurological resuscitation.
- The assessment serves as a baseline for continuing care and as a key indicator of the need to intervene immediately.
- Resuscitation of a child with a traumatic brain injury requires good coordination and you should have a low threshold for calling the trauma team.
- Throughout the resuscitation process, **the team leader** must be aware of the need for urgent neurosurgical intervention or the timely transfer to a neurosurgical centre (within the first hour of a child's attendance).
- During the primary survey assessment of **Disability**, evidence of decompensating head injury will have been recognised.

- In the severely injured child, extra information from blood gas sampling will be obtained during the resuscitation phase or ongoing monitoring.

INDICATIONS FOR IMMEDIATE INTUBATION AND VENTILATION

- Coma – not obeying commands, not speaking, not eye opening (equivalent to a **GCS score of <8**)
- Loss of protective laryngeal gag reflexes
- Ventilatory insufficiency as judged by blood gases: Hypoxaemia (**PaO2 <9 kPa** (68 mmHg) on air or **<13 kPa** (98 mmHg) with added oxygen) or hypercarbia (**PaCO2 >6 kPa** (45 mmHg))
- Spontaneous hyperventilation (causing PaCO2 <3.5 kPa (26 mmHg))
- Respiratory irregularity
- Significantly deteriorating conscious level
- Unstable facial fractures
- Copious bleeding into the mouth
- Seizure

SECONDARY SURVEY AND LOOKING FOR KEY FEATURES
Examination

- The head should be carefully observed and palpated for bruises and lacerations to the scalp and for evidence of a depressed skull fracture.
- Look for evidence of a basal skull fracture, such as blood or CSF from the nose or ear, haemotympanum, panda eyes or Battle's sign (bruising behind the ear over the mastoid process).
- The conscious level should be reassessed using the modified GCS if the child is less than 4 years old, or using the standard scale in older children.
- It should be noted that the coma scales reflect the degree of brain dysfunction at the time of the examination. Assessment should be repeated frequently – every few minutes if the level is changing.
- Communication with the child's care-givers is required to establish the child's best usual verbal response. A 'grimace' alternative to verbal responses should be used in pre-verbal or intubated patients.
- The pupils should be re-examined for size and reactivity. A dilated, non-reactive pupil indicates third nerve dysfunction due to an ipsilateral intracranial haematoma until proven otherwise.
- The fundi should be examined using an ophthalmoscope.
- Papilloedema will not be seen in acute raised ICP, but **the presence of retinal haemorrhage may indicate non-accidental injury** in a young infant.

- Motor function should be assessed.
- This includes examination of extraocular muscle function and facial and limb movements.
- Limb tone, movement and reflexes should be assessed and any focal or lateralising signs noted.

INVESTIGATIONS

- **Blood tests**
  o Blood for full blood count, clotting, glucose, urea and electrolytes should already have been taken during the immediate care phase.
  o Blood for cross-matching should have been sent off at the same time.
  o Blood gases should be taken in head-injured patients to allow careful control of $PaCO_2$ and PaO_2, as well as to check pH and base deficit or lactate. End-tidal CO_2 should also be monitored.

- **Imaging**
  Indications for performing an emergency head CT scan within 1 hour:
  o For children who have sustained a head injury and have any of the following risk factors, perform a CT head scan within 1 hour of the risk factor being identified:
    - Suspicion of non-accidental injury
    - Post-traumatic seizure but no history of epilepsy
    - On initial emergency department assessment GCS score <14, or for children under 1-year GCS (paediatric) score<15
    - At 2 hours after the injury, GCS score <15
    - Suspected open or depressed skull fracture or tense fontanelle
    - Any sign of basal skull fracture (haemotympanum, panda eyes, cerebrospinal fluid leakage from the ear or nose, Battle's sign)
    - Focal neurological deficit
    - For children under 1 year, presence of bruise, swelling or laceration of more than 5 cm on the head.
  o For children who have sustained a head injury and have more than one of the following risk factors, perform a CT head scan within 1 hour of the risk factors being identified;
    - Loss of consciousness lasting more than 5 minutes
    - Abnormal drowsiness
    - Three or more discrete vomiting episodes
    - Dangerous mechanism of injury
    - Amnesia retrograde or antegrade lasting more than 5 minutes.

MANAGEMENT OF PAEDIATRIC HEAD INJURY

- The initial aim of management for a child with a traumatic brain injury is **prevention of secondary brain damage.**
- The key aims are to maintain oxygenation, ventilation and circulation, and institute neuro-protective measures, to avoid rises in intracranial pressure.
- These can best be achieved by paying attention to the <C>ABCs.
  o If the airway is at risk, it should be secured.
  o Children with a GCS score of 8 or less or who appear agitated/combative should be **intubated and ventilated** without delay.
  o There is good evidence to suggest that **ketamine and rocuronium should be the induction agents of choice** as they offer a degree of neuro-protection and avoid the risk of sudden hypotension.

  o **Capnography** must be used immediately after intubation to confirm endotracheal tube placement, to serve as a disconnection monitor, and to help maintain normocapnia or mild hypocapnia if there is evidence of a raised ICP.
  o Remember that the end-tidal CO_2 level may differ significantly from the arterial level, especially in the shocked child – it is essential to check the PCO_2 level with a blood gas sample.

  o The PaO_2 should be maintained at a level greater than 13 kPa (98 mmHg) with an oxygen saturation >98%.

  o **Hypotension** should be treated vigorously to avoid hypoperfusion of the brain, initially with normal saline; consider early inotropic support and the use of blood products.
  o A systolic blood pressure above the 95th centile for age should be maintained to ensure adequate cerebral pressure.
  o Tranexamic acid **(15 mg/kg)** may be useful in preventing progressive intracranial haemorrhage in traumatic brain injuries; however further trials are ongoing to evaluate its use.

SYSTOLIC BLOOD PRESSURE	TARGETS (AGE SPECIFIC)
<1 year	>80 mmHg
1–5 years	>90 mmHg
5–14 years	>100 mmHg
>14 years	>110 mmHg

MEASURES TO INCREASE CEREBRAL PERFUSION TEMPORARILY

o Nurse in the 30° head-up position and head in midline to help venous drainage

o Ventilation to achieve a PaCO2 of 4.0–4.5 kPa (30–34 mmHg) *

o Infusion of intravenous mannitol 0.25–0.5 g/kg or 3% hypertonic saline (3 ml/kg)

o Combat hypotension if present with crystalloid/blood infusion and inotropes if necessary

o **A loading dose of phenytoin** may be useful to avoid any risk of convulsion or seizure activity.

o It is important to keep the child **normothermic** throughout avoiding any dramatic changes in core temperature.

o Following initial assessment, **sufficient analgesia** should be administered by careful titration.

o There have been concerns that opioid analgesic agents will lower the conscious level, cause respiratory depression and conceal pain in the abdomen and elsewhere. However, withholding analgesia may contribute to deterioration of the child's condition by leading to a rise in ICP.

• Failing to control pain will leave the child agitated and uncooperative, making any assessment of the pain more difficult, rather than easier.

• **INDICATIONS FOR REFERRAL TO A NEUROSURGEON**

o Persisting coma (GCS score <8) after initial resuscitation

o Unexplained confusion lasting for more than 4 hours

o Deteriorating conscious level (especially motor response changes)

o Focal neurological signs

o Seizure without full recovery

o Definite or suspected penetrating injury

o A cerebrospinal fluid leak

• **Examples of neurological deterioration prompting urgent reappraisal**

o Development of agitated or abnormal behaviour

o A sustained (>30 minutes) drop of 1 point in the GCS (especially in the motor score)

o Any drop of 2 points in the GCS

o Severe/increasing headache/vomiting

o New neurological signs

TRANSFER TO DEFINITIVE CARE

• Children with a traumatic brain injury often require time-critical transfers for timely surgical intervention.

2. THE CHILD WITH SPINAL TRAUMA

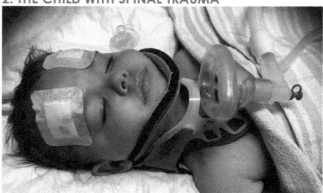

IMMOBILISATION

• If the child is unconscious, uncooperative or has had a significant mechanism of injury that makes it possible to have a spinal injury, the head and neck should be stabilised initially by manual immobilisation.

• **Head block and tape** should be considered to assist with stabilisation of the neck and to provide staff and carers with a visual indicator that the neck has not been cleared.

• An injured child may be uncooperative for many reasons including fear, pain or hypoxia.

• Manual immobilisation should be maintained and the contributing factors addressed.

• Too rigid immobilisation of the head in such cases may increase leverage on the neck as the child struggles.

• Children being transported between institutions may require additional immobilisation. This may involve **head blocks**, **sand bags** or a **vacuum mattress**, where possible axial loading must be avoided. Spinal boards should only be used in the short term for extrication: scoop stretchers should be used to assist with transportation and transfer.

• If guidelines for clinically clearing the cervical spine are met, indicating a low risk of cervical spine injury, the patient should be asked **to rotate their neck 45° to the left and right.**

• If any of these manoeuvres cause midline posterior pain the neck should be immobilised again and the spine imaged. If there is no pain on movement, immobilisation is no longer required.

NEXUS GUIDELINES FOR CLINICALLY CLEARING A CERVICAL SPINE (NSAID)

o No focal **N**eurological deficit

o No midline **S**pinal (cervical) tenderness on direct palpation

o Normal **A**lertness

o No **I**ntoxication

o No painful **D**istracting injuries

A. INJURIES OF THE CERVICAL SPINE

- Injuries to the cervical spine are rare in children; however, they are associated with substantial levels of impact.
- **The upper three vertebrae are usually involved –** injury is more common in the lower segments of an adult.

CERVICAL SPINE IMAGING

- Imaging must be taken in all children who cannot have their spine cleared clinically.
- Children with a GCS score of 15 who need imaging and have no features suggestive of cord or nerve root injury can generally be imaged with **plain spinal radiographs** initially.
- These children should have a full cervical spine series including lateral, anteroposterior and odontoid peg views (the latter only if they can open their mouth).
- Injury must be presumed until excluded radiologically and clinically.
- Spinal injury may be present even with a normal radiograph.
- **Pseudosubluxation of C2 on C3 and of C3 on C4** occurs in approximately 9% of children; particularly those aged **1–7 years.**
- Interpretation of cervical radiographs can therefore be difficult even for the most experienced (50% sensitivity) and there is growing support for just ordering MRI scans in preference to plain films or CT.
- Indirect evidence of trauma can be detected by assessing **retropharyngeal swelling**:
  - At the inferior part of the body of C3, the pre-vertebral distance should be **one-third the width of the body of C2.**
  - This distance varies during breathing and is increased in a crying child.
- Proceed to an MRI scan if the plain views are abnormal or inadequate.
- Children with a **GCS score of <13 require a CT scan of the entire cervical spine,** as well as a head CT scan.
- After a high-energy mechanism of injury, if there is evidence of a serious trunk injury or cardiorespiratory instability, a **CT scan from the occiput to the pelvis** should be considered, irrespective of the conscious level. This will encompass the entire spine.
- Plain spinal films are not then required.
- If there are features suggestive of cord or nerve root injury an **MRI scan is indicated**. The timing is a matter of clinical judgement by a spinal injury specialist.

INJURY TYPES

- **Atlantoaxial rotary subluxation**: It is the most common injury to the cervical spine. The child presents with torticollis following trauma. Radiological demonstration of the injury is difficult, and CT or MRI may be necessary.
- Other injuries of C1 and C2 include:
  - **Odontoid epiphyseal separations** and
  - **Traumatic ligament disruption.**
- Significant cervical cord injuries have been reported with no radiological evidence of trauma.

B. INJURIES OF THE THORACIC AND LUMBAR SPINE

- They are rare in children; they are most common in the multiply injured child.
- In the second decade, 44% of reported injuries result from sporting and other recreational activity.
- Some spinal injuries may result from non-accidental injury. When an injury does occur, it is not uncommon to find multiple levels of involvement because the force is dissipated over many segments in the child's mobile spine. This increased mobility may also lead to neurological involvement without significant skeletal injury.
- The most common mechanism of injury is **hyperflexion**, and the most common radiographic finding is a **wedge- or beakshaped vertebra** resulting from compression. The most important clinical sign is a **sensory level.**
- Neurological assessment is difficult in children, and such a level may only become apparent after repeated examinations. Because of the difficulties of assessment, a child with multiple injuries should be assumed to have spinal injury, and therefore their spines should remain protected.
- If injury is confirmed, further treatment is similar to that in adults. Unstable injuries may require open reduction and stabilisation with fusion.

C. SPINAL CORD INJURY WITHOUT RADIOGRAPHIC ABNORMALITY (SCIWORA)

- SCIWORA is said to have occurred when the spinal cord has been injured without an obvious accompanying injury to the vertebral column.
- The cervical spine is affected more frequently than the thoracic spine. Because the upper segments of the cervical spine have the greatest mobility, the upper cervical cord is most susceptible to this injury.
- Children who are seriously injured should have immobilisation of the spine maintained until such time as a full neurological assessment can be carried out since normal X-rays do not exclude a cord injury.
- If there is any doubt, **MRI scans should be obtained.**

3. THE CHILD WITH CHEST TRAUMA

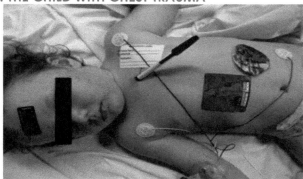

o Children have thoracic anatomic and physiologic differences from adults:
  ▪ Compliant chest wall
  ▪ Fewer rib fractures
  ▪ Mediastinum is more mobile
o Compliance can mask underlying injuries and minimize external signs of trauma. Though increased compliance leads to fewer rib fractures, it also leads to increased **pulmonary contusion.**
o The physical exam evaluating the chest is similar in children compared to adults.
  ▪ **Inspection:** nasal flaring, chest wall injuries, bruising, seat belt sign (shoulder belt), paradoxical chest wall movement
  ▪ **Palpation:** crepitus and/or tenderness
  ▪ **Auscultation:** muffled heart sounds, abnormal lung sounds (absent, muffled); least reliable finding of the three
o Isolated thoracic injury is uncommon in children.
o It is more likely to result with a significant injury causing concomitant injuries.
o Children will have injuries similar to adults.
  ▪ **Pneumothorax / Haemothorax**
  ▪ **Pulmonary contusion**
    • Responsible for ~ 10% of all paediatric trauma admissions
    • Mild to severe hypoxia depending on the extent of contused lung
    • Always be vigilant because it can worsen over time as contusion evolves
    • CXR findings may lag behind injury but if abnormal, represents a significant injury
  ▪ **Flail chest**: Results from two or more fractures in contiguous ribs.
  ▪ **Rib fractures**
  ▪ **Traumatic asphyxiation**
    • Due to increased compliance of the paediatric chest wall.
    • Occurs after direct compression of the chest and deep inspiration against a closed glottis with a crush injury.

• This increases pressure in the superior and inferior vena cava and leads to facial/neck hemorrhage, cyanosis, and facial swelling.
• Treat by addressing associated injuries and elevating the head of the bed.

  ▪ **Commotio cordis**:
    • Almost solely a paediatric traumatic injury.
    • This is a combination of direct anterior chest injury leading to ventricular fibrillation and sudden cardiac death.
    • Treatment consists of rapid recognition and use of an automated external defibrillator by by-standers or first responders.

4. THE CHILD WITH ABDOMINAL INJURY

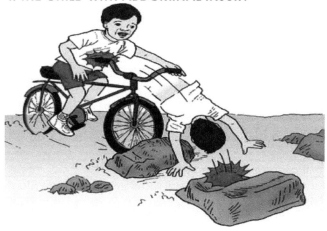

INTRODUCTION

• Blunt trauma causes the majority of abdominal injuries in children.
• Most occur because of accidents on the roads, although a significant number happen during recreational activities.
• It is important to consider non-accidental injury.
• A high index of suspicion is necessary if some injuries are not to be missed.
• The abdominal contents are susceptible to injury in children for a number of reasons:
  o The abdominal wall is thin and offers relatively little protection
  o The diaphragm is more horizontal than in adults, causing the liver and spleen to lie lower and more anteriorly
  o The ribs, being very elastic, offer less protection to these organs
  o The bladder is intra-abdominal, rather than pelvic, and is therefore more exposed when full.

• The management of children with abdominal injury may be complicated by respiratory compromise because of diaphragmatic irritation or splinting.

HISTORY

- A precise history of the mechanism of injury may help in diagnosis.
- Rapid deceleration, such as experienced during road accidents, causes abdominal compression or sheering of fixed organs. The solid organs and duodenum especially are at risk from such forces.
- Direct blows, such as those caused by punching (consider non-accidental injury if history is not compatible) or impact with bicycle handlebars, readily injure the underlying solid organs.
- Injury to the pancreas or duodenum is a particular feature of handlebar injury due to their fixed position anterior to the spine.
- Finally, straddling injuries associated with a significant perineal haematoma or urethral bleeding suggests urethral injury.

ASSESSMENT OF THE INJURED ABDOMEN

- Initial assessment and management must be structured and directed to the care of the airway, breathing and circulation as discussed earlier.

EXAMINATION

- If shock is not amenable to fluid replacement during the primary survey and resuscitation, and no obvious site of haemorrhage exists, then intra-abdominal injury may be the cause of blood loss.
- The abdomen should be assessed urgently to establish whether early surgical or interventional radiological management is necessary.
- In other circumstances, the abdominal examination is carried out during the secondary survey.
- The abdomen should be inspected for bruising, lacerations and penetrating wounds.
- Although major intra-abdominal injury can occur without obvious external signs, visible bruising increases the likelihood of significant injury.
- A high index of suspicion and frequent, repeated clinical assessment is appropriate in such cases.
- The external urethral meatus should be examined for blood. Gentle palpation should be carried out.
- This will reveal areas of tenderness and rigidity.
- Care should be taken not to hurt the child because his or her continued cooperation is important during the repeated examinations that form an important part of management. Rectal and vaginal examinations are rarely required in the injured child.

GASTRIC DRAINAGE

- Air swallowing during crying with consequent acute gastric dilatation is common in children.
- Early passage of a nasogastric/orogastric tube of an appropriate size is essential.

- If there is a possibility of a basal skull fracture this should be by the oral rather than nasal route.
- The tube should be aspirated regularly and left on free drainage at other times.
- A massively distended stomach can mimic intra-abdominal pathology needing laparotomy, and cause serious diaphragm splintage with consequent respiratory compromise.

URINARY CATHETERISATION

- Catheterisation of a child should only be performed if the child cannot pass urine spontaneously or if continuous accurate output measurement is required.
- The route (urethral or suprapubic) will depend on factors related to signs of urethral, bladder, intra-abdominal or pelvic injury (such as blood at the external meatus, or bruising in the scrotum or perineum).
- If a boy requires urethral catheterisation, urethral damage must be excluded first.
- The catheter should be silastic and as small as possible in order to reduce the risk of subsequent urethral stricture formation.

INVESTIGATIONS

- **Blood Tests**
  - Intravenous access will have already been secured during the primary survey and resuscitation, and at that time blood will have been drawn for baseline blood counts, urea and electrolytes and cross-matching.
  - **Amylase/tryptase** estimation should be requested and can usually be performed on the sample sent for urea and electrolytes.
  - Repeated monitoring of blood parameters may be appropriate in some patients.

- **Imaging**
  - There is no place for FAST scanning in the emergency department resuscitation room in children.
  - A formal radiologist USS of the abdomen can be helpful however.
  - Most imaging of the abdomen will be by **CT with contrast** but only if specific criteria are met:
    - Lap belt injury/bruising
    - Abdominal wall bruising
    - Abdominal tenderness in a conscious patient
    - Abdominal distension
    - Clinical evidence of persistent hypovolaemia
    - Blood from the rectum or nasogastric tube
    - Significant handle bar injuries

5. THE CHILD WITH PELVIC TRAUMA

o Pelvic injuries are uncommon in children.
o Children should still be inspected and palpated for signs of pain or pelvic instability. If there is concern, pelvic films should still be ordered.
o If there is concern for instability and a pelvic fracture, compression with a wrapped sheet or a pelvic binder should still be placed.

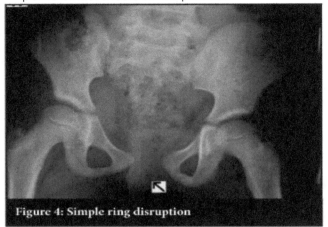

Figure 4: Simple ring disruption

6. THE CHILD WITH GENITAL, PERINEAL, AND RECTAL TRAUMA

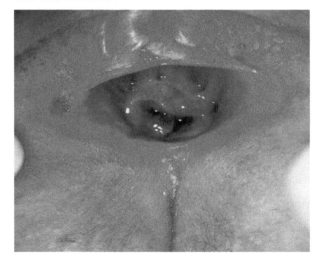

o Any signs of genital hematomas, blood at the urethral meatus, or lacerations should be evaluated further.
o If there is concern for blood, a rectal exam should still be performed.
o Often times, visualized rectal tone (anal wink) is sufficient unless neurologic injury (spinal shock) is a concern and then a digital rectal exam should be performed.

7. THE CHILD WITH MUSCULOSKELETAL TRAUMA

o A thorough extremity exam is always needed.
o Evaluate the neurovascular status.
o Patients with a gross deformity or point tenderness will need x-rays to evaluate for fracture.
o Splint deformed extremities to help prevent further injury and alleviate pain.

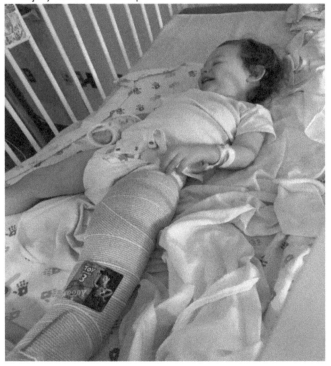

II. APPROACH TO THE CHILD WITH BURNS

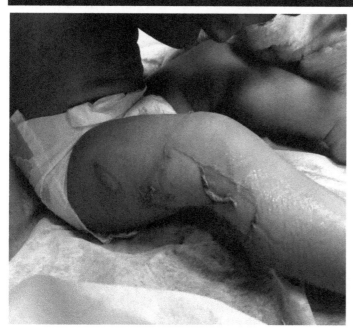

- The same principles apply for the management of burns in children as in adults.
- **The possibility of non-accidental injury** must always be considered in a child with burns and appropriate safeguarding action taken.
- Suspicious patterns of burn include **cigarette burns**, **immersion-type injuries** (glove and stocking pattern or buttocks), or **burns to the dorsum of the hands**.
- Scalds from pulling hot drinks off surfaces are common accidental injuries.
- Advice should be given about how to prevent future similar injuries occurring.

MANAGEMENT OF BURNS IN CHILDREN
1. PRIMARY SURVEY AND RESUSCITATION
A. AIRWAY AND CERVICAL SPINE
- The airway may be compromised either because of inhalational injury and oral scalds or because of severe burns to the face.
- The latter is usually obvious, whereas the former two may not be and a high index of suspicion is required. The presence of inhalation injury is directly related to mortality.

INDICATIONS OF INHALATIONAL INJURY
- *History of exposure to smoke in a confined space*
- *Deposits around the mouth and nose*
- *Carbonaceous sputum*
- Because oedema occurs following thermal injury, the airway can deteriorate rapidly.

- Thus, even suspicion of airway compromise, or the discovery of injuries that might be expected to cause problems with the airway at a later stage, should lead to immediate consideration of **tracheal intubation**.
- This procedure increases in difficulty as oedema progresses; it is therefore important to perform it as soon as possible.
- All but the most experienced should seek expert help urgently, unless apnoea requires immediate intervention.
- *If there is any suspicion of cervical spine injury, or if the history is unobtainable, appropriate precautions to immobilise the neck should be taken until such injury is excluded.*

B. BREATHING
- Once the airway has been secured, the adequacy of breathing should be assessed.
- Signs that should arouse suspicion of inadequacy include abnormal rate, abnormal chest movements and cyanosis (a late sign).
- Circumferential burns to the chest or abdomen (the latter in infants) may cause breathing difficulty by mechanically restricting chest movement.
- All children who have suffered significant burns should be given **high-flow oxygen**.
- If there is evidence of increased work of breathing then senior anaesthetic help should be sought and intubation and ventilation should be considered.

C. CIRCULATION
- In the first few hours following injury signs of hypovolaemic shock are rarely attributable to burns. Therefore, any such signs should raise the suspicion of bleeding from elsewhere, and the source should be actively sought.
- Intravenous access should be established with two cannulae during resuscitation, and fluids started.
- If possible, drips should be put up in unburnt areas, but burned skin (eschar) can be perforated if necessary.
- Remember that the intraosseous route can be used to administer fluid and drugs.
- Blood should be taken for
  - Blood glucose,
  - Carboxyhaemoglobin level,
  - Haemoglobin,
  - Electrolytes and urea
  - Cross-matching.

D. DISABILITY

o Reduced conscious level following burns may be due to **hypoxia** (remember smoke-filled rooms may contain little oxygen), **head injury** or **hypovolaemia**.

E. EXPOSURE

o Exposure should be complete remembering that burned children lose heat particularly rapidly, and should be kept in a warm environment and covered with blankets when not being examined.

o Remove all jewellery including piercings as soon as possible prior to digit and/or limb swelling.

2. SECONDARY SURVEY AND LOOKING FOR KEY FEATURES

- As well as being burned, children may suffer the effects of blast, be injured by falling objects or may fall while trying to escape from the fire.

- Thus, other injuries are not uncommon and a thorough head-to-toe secondary survey must be carried out. Any injuries discovered, including the burn, should be treated in order of priority.

ASSESSING THE BURN

- The severity of a burn depends on its relative surface area and depth.

1. SURFACE AREA

o The surface area is usually estimated using burns charts. It is particularly important to use a paediatric chart when assessing burn size in children, because the relative surface areas of the head and limbs change with age.

o Another useful method of estimating relative **surface area** relies on the fact that the patient's palm and adducted fingers cover an area of approximately 1% of the body surface.

o This method can be used when charts are not immediately available, and is obviously already related to the child's size.

o Note that **the 'rule of 9s'** cannot be applied to a child who is less than 14 years old.

o There are a number of apps available to help assess BSA and these include the Mersey Burns app.

2. DEPTH

o Burns are classified as being superficial epidermal, superficial dermal, mid-dermal, deep dermal, partial thickness and full thickness.

o **SUPERFICIAL DERMAL BURNS** present with pale pink skin with blisters;

o **MID-DERMAL BURNS** have sluggish capillary refill, are dark pink in colour and sensation to touch may be decreased;

o **DEEP DERMAL BURNS** have blotchy, red skin and may or may not have blisters and the hallmark of these burns is the loss of capillary blush phenomenon.

o **PARTIAL-THICKNESS BURNS** cause some damage to the dermis, blistering is usually seen and the skin is pink or mottled.

o **DEEPER, FULL-THICKNESS BURNS** damage both the epidermis and dermis, and may cause injury to deeper structures as well. The skin looks white or charred, and is painless and leathery to the touch.

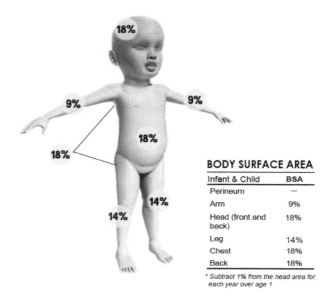

BODY SURFACE AREA	
Infant & Child	BSA
Perineum	—
Arm	9%
Head (front and back)	18%
Leg	14%
Chest	18%
Back	18%

Subtract 1% from the head area for each year over age 1

3. SPECIAL AREAS

o **Burns to the face and mouth** have already been dealt with above.

o **Burns involving the hands or feet** can cause severe functional loss if scarring occurs.

o **Perineal burns** are prone to infection and present particularly difficult management problems.

o **Circumferential, full- or partial-thickness burns of the limbs or neck** may require urgent incision to relieve distal ischaemia.

o Similarly, **circumferential burns to the torso may restrict** ventilation and also require urgent incision. This procedure is called **escharotomy** and usually needs to be done before transfer to a burns centre.

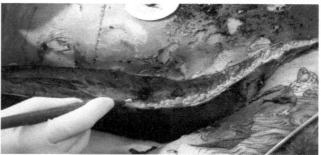

EMERGENCY TREATMENT

1. ANALGESIA

o Most children with a burn will be in severe pain, and this should be dealt with urgently. Older children may manage to use Entonox®, but most will not.

o Any child with more than a minor burn should be given **intranasal diamorphine** initially and then further pain can be controlled with **intravenous morphine at a dose of 100 micrograms/kg (<1 year: 80 micrograms/kg)**, if needed, as soon as possible.

o Further doses are often required.

2. FLUID THERAPY

o Two cannulae should already have been sited during the primary survey and resuscitation and therapy for shock (10 + 10 ml/kg) commenced if indicated. **Children with burns of 10% body surface area or more** will require intravenous fluids as part of their burns care. This fluid is in addition to their normal maintenance fluid requirement.

o The additional fluid (in ml) required per day to treat the burn can be estimated using the following **MODIFIED PARKLAND FORMULA**

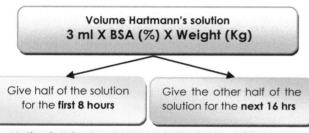

Volume Hartmann's solution
3 ml X BSA (%) X Weight (Kg)

Give half of the solution for the **first 8 hours**

Give the other half of the solution for the **next 16 hrs**

o Half of this should be given in the first 8 hours following the time of their burn.

o Remember that this is only an initial guide; subsequent therapy will be guided by urine output, which should be kept at **1 ml/kg/h or more**; in children who have sustained greater than 15% burns it should be **2 ml/kg/h or more**.

o **Urethral catheterisation** should be considered early to help with fluid management.

3. WOUND CARE

o Infection is a significant cause of mortality and morbidity in burns victims, and wound care should start as early as possible to reduce this risk.

o Furthermore, appropriate wound care will reduce the pain associated with air passing over burned areas. The burned area should be cooled immediately for 20 minutes.

o Although **cold compresses** and **irrigation with cold water** may reduce pain and can be useful for several hours after the injury, it should be remembered that burned children lose heat rapidly.

o Children should never be transferred with cold soaks in place. Burns should then be covered with non-adhesive sterile towels or cling film.

o **Cling film** is often used as a sterile dressing, and can be applied loosely onto the burned area.

o No additional ointments or creams should be applied. Unnecessary re-examination should be avoided and blisters should be left intact.

o Photographs taken prior to applying the dressing can aid this process and allow others to assess the burn without disturbing the child.

o Provide **tetanus prophylaxis** if required.

4. MANAGEMENT OF CO POISONING

• During a fire, burning of organic compounds in a low-oxygen environment produces carbon monoxide. Inhalation by the victim induces the production of COHb, which has a 200-fold greater affinity for oxygen molecules than haemoglobin.

• A high level will therefore cause cellular hypoxia as oxygen will not be given up to cells. Children who have been in house fires should have their blood carboxyhaemoglobin measured.

• **Note:** most pulse oximeters show the oxygen saturation, regardless of haemoglobin concentration, i.e. normal SpO2 does not exclude carbon monoxide poisoning.

• **Levels of 5–20%** are treated with oxygen (which speeds up the removal of CO). Levels over 20% should prompt consideration of hyperbaric oxygen chamber treatment – discuss with the paediatric burns service. In some environments the burning of plastics, wool and silk can produce **cyanide**.

• Assessment and treatments are complex. Be aware of the possibility of cyanide poisoning and consider it in a child from a house fire who is in a coma or presents with a severe metabolic acidosis without apparent cause. In general, antidotes are used when blood levels of **cyanide are > 3 mg/l**.

• Discuss treatment immediately with a poisons centre if cyanide poisoning is suspected as other factors such as the concomitant presence of COHb are contraindications for some antidotes.

TRANSFERRAL CRITERIA TO A BURN CENTRE

o Burns > 5 % TBSA in a Child
o Full thickness burns > 5% TBSA
o Burns of face, hands, feet, perineum, genitalia, and major joints
o Circumferential burns
o Chemical or electrical burns
o Burns in the presence of major trauma or significant co-morbidity
o Burns in the very young patient
o Suspicion of Non-Accidental Injury

III. APPROACH TO THE CHILD WITH DROWNING

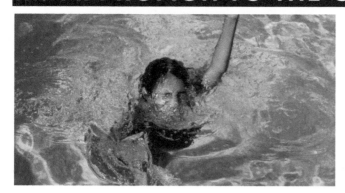

INTRODUCTION

- The International Liaison Committee on Resuscitation (ILCOR) defines drowning as 'a process resulting in primary respiratory impairment from submersion/immersion in a liquid medium'.
- The term **'near drowning'** and **'wet' or 'dry' drowning** are no longer official terms, mainly because they have been used differently worldwide, which has caused confusion.

1. PRIMARY SURVEY OF DROWNING

- The first priority is to move the victim from the water as quickly as possible without risk to the rescuer in order to allow cardiopulmonary resuscitation and ABC stabilisation without delay.
- Immobilisation of the neck should be instigated as soon as practicable until injury is excluded, although cervical spine injury is uncommon except after diving or traffic accidents.
- Rescue of the victim in a vertical position may lead to cardiovascular collapse due to venous pooling.
- However, horizontal rescue or cervical spine immobilisation in the water must not be allowed to delay the rescue.
- The initiation of early and effective basic life support (BLS) reduces the mortality drastically and is the most important factor for survival.
- **Rescue breaths** must be commenced as early as possible even in shallow water if this can be done without risk to the rescuer. Mouth-to-nose ventilation may be easier in this situation.
- BLS then proceeds according to the standard paediatric algorithm even in hypothermia.
- The presence of cardiac arrest can be difficult to diagnose as pulses are difficult to feel. If in doubt chest compressions should be given and continued.
- If an automatic external defibrillator (AED) is used it is vital to first dry the chest before applying the electrodes.

- Following a submersion episode, the stomach is usually full of swallowed water. The risk of aspiration is therefore increased and the airway must be secured as soon as possible, usually by **endotracheal intubation using a rapid sequence induction**. Following this an **oro- or nasogastric tube** should be inserted.
- Ventilate the child to achieve an SpO2 of 94–98% using additional oxygen and positive end-expiratory pressure (PEEP) as required.
- Respiratory deterioration can be delayed for 4–6 hours after submersion and even children who have initially apparently recovered should be observed for at least 8 hours.
- Chest X-ray changes may occur even later.

1. HYPOTHERMIA

- A core temperature reading **(rectal or oesophageal)** should be obtained as soon as possible and further cooling prevented.
- Hypothermia is common following drowning and adversely affects resuscitation attempts unless treated.
  - o Not only are arrhythmias more common but some, such as ventricular fibrillation, may be refractory at temperatures below 30°C, **when defibrillation should be limited to three shocks** and **inotropic or antiarrhythmic drugs should not be given**.
  - o If unsuccessful the patient should be warmed to **above 30°C** as quickly as possible, when further defibrillation may be attempted.
  - o **The dose interval for resuscitation drugs is doubled between 30°C and 35°C.**
  - o Resuscitation should be continued **until the core temperature is at least 32°C** or cannot be raised despite active measures.
  - o If a child requires endotracheal intubation, the advantages outweigh the small risk of precipitating malignant arrhythmias.
- Rewarming strategies depend on the core temperature and signs of circulation.
  - o **External rewarming** including a warm air system is usually sufficient if the core temperature is above 30°C.
  - o **Active core rewarming** should be added in patients with a core temperature of less than 30°C.
  - o **Extracorporeal warming** is the preferred method in circulatory arrest.

2. REWARMING

- **External rewarming**
  - o Remove cold, wet clothing
  - o Supply warm blankets
  - o Warm air system
  - o Heating blanket
  - o Infrared radiant lamp
- **Core rewarming**
  - o Warm intravenous fluids to 39°C to prevent further heat loss
  - o Warm ventilator gases to 42°C to prevent further heat loss
  - o Gastric or bladder lavage with normal (physiological) saline at 42°C
  - o Peritoneal lavage with potassium-free dialysate at 42°C, 20 ml/kg with a 15-minute cycle
  - o Pleural or pericardial lavage
  - o Endovascular warming
- **Extracorporeal blood rewarming** (i.e. extracorporeal membrane oxygenation or bypass)

2. SECONDARY SURVEY AND LOOKING FOR KEY FEATURES IN DROWNING

- During the secondary survey, the child should be carefully examined from head to toe.
- Any injury may have occurred during the incident that preceded immersion, including spinal injuries.
- Older children may have ingested alcohol and/or drugs.

INVESTIGATIONS

- o Blood glucose, ABG and lactate
- o U&Es, Coagulation status
- o Blood and aspirate cultures
- o CXR, ECG, C- Spine imaging, if indicated

ED TREATMENT & STABILISATION

- Monitor the vital functions closely.
- Early suggestions of respiratory insufficiency, haemodynamic instability or hypothermia are indications for admission to the intensive care unit.
- Prophylactic antibiotics have not been shown to be helpful but are often given after immersion in severely contaminated water.
- Fever is common during the first 24 hours but is not necessarily a sign of infection, which usually becomes manifest later. **Gram-negative organisms**, especially **Pseudomonas aeruginosa**, are common and **Aspergillus** species have been reported.
- When an infection is suspected broad-spectrum intravenous antibiotic therapy (such as **cefotaxime**) should be started after repeating blood and sputum cultures.

- Signs of raised intracranial pressure may develop as a result of a post-hypoxic injury, and this should be treated, although aggressive treatment to lower a raised ICP has not been shown to improve the prognosis. Unless obvious, a careful search should be made for a precipitating cause of the drowning such as a channelopathy, particularly **long QT-syndrome**. The duration of resuscitation efforts may not be a helpful prognostic factor.
- The decision to discontinue resuscitation attempts is particularly difficult in cases of drowning, and should be taken only after all the prognostic factors discussed above have been considered carefully.
- Resuscitation should only be discontinued out of hospital if there is clear evidence of futility such as **massive trauma or rigor mortis.**

OUTCOME OF DROWNING

- 70% of children survive drowning when BLS is provided at the scene, whereas only 40% survive without early BLS, even with maximum therapy.
- Of those who do survive, having required full CPR in hospital, ≈ 70% will make a complete recovery and 25% will have a mild neurological deficit.
- The remainder will be severely disabled or remain in a persisting vegetative state.

PROGNOSTIC INDICATORS IN DROWNING	
Immersion time	• Most children who have been submerged for more than 10 minutes have a very small chance of intact neurological recovery or survival. • Details of the incident are therefore vital
Time to Basic Life Support	• Starting BLS at the scene greatly reduces mortality, whereas a delay of more than 10 minutes is associated with a poor prognosis
Time to first respiratory effort	• If this occurs within 3 min after the start of basic cardiopulmonary support, the prognosis is good. • If there has been no respiratory effort after 40 minutes of full CPR, there is little or no chance of survival unless the child's respiration has been depressed (e.g. by hypothermia, medication or alcohol)
Core temperature	• Pre-existing hypothermia and rapid cooling after submersion also seem to protect vital organs and can improve the prognosis. • A core T°< 33°C on arrival and a water T°< 10°C have been associated with increased survival. This effect is more pronounced in small children because of their large surface area to weight ratio
Persisting coma	• A persistent GCS score of less than 5 indicates a bad prognosis
Arterial blood pH	• If this remains below 7.1 despite treatment, the prognosis is poor
Arterial blood PO2	• If this remains below 8.0 kPa (60 mmHg) despite treatment, the prognosis is poor
Type of water	• Whether the water was salt or fresh has no bearing on the prognosis

4. Paediatric Shock
I. APPROACH TO THE SHOCKED CHILD

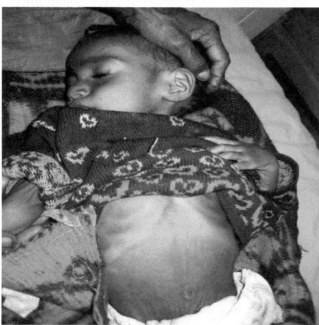

Shocked child

INTRODUCTION

- Shock is a term used to describe inadequate oxygen delivery to the tissues that cannot keep up with metabolic demand. This creates a state of hypoperfusion.
- It may be uncompensated, meaning there is hypotension and inability to maintain normal perfusion, or it may be compensated, meaning that blood pressure and perfusion are maintained for the time being.
- There are several different types of shock (below) and shock is often thought of as being "warm" or "cold." This can be useful in helping to differentiate the type of shock, but there are several other factors that need to be considered when defining the type of shock and there are often mixed pictures so take the "warm" and "cold" shock differentiation with a grain of salt.
- Inadequate tissue perfusion resulting in impaired cellular respiration (i.e. shock) may result from defects of the heart pump (cardiogenic), loss of fluid (hypovolaemic), abnormalities of vessels (distributive), flow restriction (obstructive) or inadequate oxygen-releasing capacity of blood (dissociative).

CAUSES OF SHOCK	
Hypovolaemic	• Haemorrhage • Gastroenteritis, stomal losses • Intussusception, volvulus • Burns • Peritonitis
Distributive	• Septicaemia • Anaphylaxis • Spinal cord injury (Neurogenic) • Vasodilating drugs
Cardiogenic	• Arrhythmias • Heart failure (cardiomyopathy, myocarditis) • Valvular disease • Myocardial contusion
Obstructive	• Congenital cardiac (coarctation, hypoplastic left heart, aortic stenosis) • Tension/haemopneumothorax • Flail chest • Cardiac tamponade • Pulmonary embolism
Dissociative	• Profound anaemia • Carbon monoxide poisoning • Methaemoglobinaemia

- Shock is a progressive state which can be divided into three phases: **compensated, uncompensated and irreversible.**
  - **Uncompensated,** meaning there is hypotension and inability to maintain normal perfusion
  - **Compensated,** meaning that blood pressure and perfusion are maintained for the time being.
  - **Irreversible:** If the shock goes untreated, it progresses to an irreversible stage where the cellular damage cannot be reversed even if cardiovascular function is restored to adequate levels. Despite haemodynamic correction, multiple organ failure occurs.

KEY FEATURES OF THE CHILD IN SHOCK

- While the primary assessment and resuscitation are being carried out, a focused history of the child's health and activity over the previous 24 hours and any significant previous illness should be gained.

- Certain key features that will be identified from this – and the initial blood test results – can point the clinician to the likeliest working diagnosis for emergency treatment.
  - A history of vomiting and/or diarrhoea points to fluid loss either externally (e.g. gastroenteritis) or into the abdomen (e.g. volvulus, intussusception, ruptured appendix). The presence of fever and/or rash points to **septicaemia**.
  - The presence of urticaria, angioneurotic oedema or history of allergen exposure points to **anaphylaxis**.
  - The presence of cyanosis unresponsive to oxygen or a grey colour with signs of heart failure in a baby under 4–6 weeks points to **duct-dependent congenital heart disease.**
  - The presence of heart failure in an older infant or child points to **cardiomyopathy or myocarditis.**
  - A history of sickle cell disease or a recent diarrhoeal illness and a very low haemoglobin points to **acute haemolysis.**
  - A history of sickle cell disease, abdominal pain and enlarged spleen points to **Acute Splenic Sequestration.**
  - An immediate history of major trauma points to **blood loss** and, more rarely, **tension pneumothorax, haemothorax, cardiac tamponade or spinal cord transection.**
  - The presence of severe tachycardia and an abnormal rhythm on the ECG points to a **cardiac cause for shock.**
  - A history of polyuria and the presence of acidotic breathing and a very high blood glucose points to **Diabetes Ketoacidosis.**
  - A history of drug ingestion points to **Poisoning.**

INITIAL ACTIONS

- **Primary Survey:**
  - **ABC's** are the critical first step in a patient with shock! Place the child on the **monitor, pulse oximeter, and obtain blood pressure.**
  - **A&B:** Start supplemental oxygen and consider **early intubation** if the child will require ventilatory assistance, significant help with oxygenation, or airway protection.
  - **C:** Obtain IV/IO access; give a **20 ml/kg bolus** of IV crystalloid.
    - This may be repeated twice up to a total fluid administration of **60 ml/kg.**
    - If the child remains in shock, this is considered refractory shock and it would then be prudent to consider adding **vasopressor support**, often in the form of **Norepinephrine (α1 effect) or Dopamine (β1 effect).**

- If a child has risk factors for adrenal insufficiency, consider administering stress-dose steroids as adrenal insufficiency can also lead to a refractory shock state.
- If the child is suffering from haemorrhagic shock, **blood should be administered** after the initial crystalloid bolus and the site of hemorrhage should be managed appropriately.

  - THEN identify the type of shock, which may not always be easy in mixed shock states (see Differential Diagnosis).

CARDIOGENIC SHOCK

- It is a special type of shock in which there is failure of the pump due to malformation, overload, obstruction, or non-perfusing rhythm.
- Fluid may still be given in this instance but at a lower bolus **(5-10 ml/kg) and over a longer period of time (up to 20 minutes)** to prevent exacerbation of the failure state and worsening pulmonary edema.
- Closely monitor fluid and respiratory status during fluid administration in this instance.
- If suspicious for a **ductal-dependent cardiac lesion or anomaly**, which can cause an obstructive shock picture with cardiogenic shock, you should also consider administering **prostaglandin** in this instance to open the ductus arteriosus which can ease the amount of vascular congestion and fluid backing up into the lungs.
- Discuss with paediatric cardiologist and/or paediatric cardiothoracic surgeon.

GOALS FOR RESUSCITATION SHOULD INCLUDE:

- **Blood pressure** (systolic pressure at least fifth percentile for age: 60 mmHg <1 month of age, 70 mmHg + [2 x age in years] in children 1 month to 10 years of age, 90 mmHg in children 10 years of age or older)
- **Quality of central and peripheral pulses** (strong, distal pulses equal to central pulses)
- **Skin perfusion** (warm, with capillary refill <2 seconds)
- **Mental status** (normal mental status)
- **Urine output** (≥1 mL/kg per hour, once effective circulating volume is restored)
- **Clearance of lactate** (hope to see down trending and preferably cut in half after initial resuscitation)

1. THE CHILD WITH HYPOVOLEMIC SHOCK

CLINICAL FEATURES OF DEHYDRATION AND SHOCK

Dehydration (5%)

- Appears 'unwell'
- Normal HR or tachycardia
- Normal RR or tachypnoea
- Normal peripheral pulses
- Normal or mildly ↑ CRT
- Normal blood pressure
- Warm extremities
- Decreased urine output
- Reduced skin turgor
- Sunken eyes
- Depressed fontanelle
- Dry mucous membranes

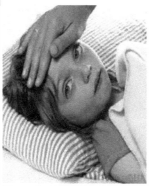

Clinical Shock (10%)

- Pale, lethargic, mottled
- Tachycardia
- Tachypnoea
- Weak peripheral pulses
- Prolonged CRT
- Hypotension
- Cold extremities
- Decreased urine output
- Decreased LOC

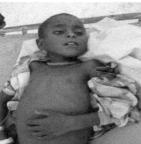

- This is the most common cause of shock worldwide in infants; most often secondary to diarrhoea (Other examples include **blood loss, vomiting, heat stroke, or burns).** It is important to realize the stages of shock, especially in children who can compensate for a larger percentage of losses than adults and then rapidly decompensate. The intravascular volume of an infant is approximately **80 ml/kg.** In older children, the intravascular volume is approximately **70 ml/kg.** Dehydration in itself does not cause death, but shock does. S0hock can occur with losses of **20 ml/kg** from the intravascular space, while clinical dehydration is only evident after total losses of greater than **25 ml/kg.**

- The maintenance fluid requirements for well, normal children are summarized in the table below:

Body weight	Daily fluid requirement	Hourly fluid requirement
First 10 kg	100 ml/kg	4 ml/kg
Second 10 kg	50 ml/kg	2 ml/kg
Subsequent kg	20 ml/kg	1 ml/kg

- Generally speaking, a child with clinical signs of dehydration but no evidence of shock can be assumed to be **5% dehydrated.**
- 5% dehydration implies that the body has lost 5 g per 100 g body weight i.e. **50 ml/kg of fluid.**
- If shock is also present that 10% dehydration of greater can be assumed to have occurred.

2. THE CHILD WITH DISTRIBUTIVE SHOCK

o Distributive shock often results from vasodilation and a decrease in systemic vascular resistance.

o It is associated with normal to increased cardiac output.

o Given the vasodilation, the extremities are warm, making this an example of "warm shock."

o **CAUSES OF DISTRIBUTIVE SHOCK INCLUDE:**

- **SEPSIS**
  - Most common aetiology in children
  - Infection causes significant vasodilation
  - Think about in a child with fever and other signs of infection

- **ANAPHYLAXIS**
  - Think about in a child with wheezing, urticaria, angioedema, or stridor.

- **NEUROGENIC**
  - Spinal cord injury resulting in loss of sympathetic tone. This results in vasodilation as well as bradycardia.
  - Think about in trauma patients with neurological deficits and paradoxical bradycardia in the setting of hypotension

3. THE CHILD WITH CARDIOGENIC SHOCK

o Cardiogenic shock results from pump failure and depressed cardiac output.

o This decreased cardiac output results in cool extremities, another example of "cold shock.".

o The most common causes of cardiogenic shock in children are as follows:

- **STRUCTURAL DISORDERS** – often present a picture of obstructive shock
  - Hypoplastic left heart syndrome, tetralogy of Fallot, coarctation of the aorta and other structural disorders can result in systolic heart failure
  - Think about in children with hepatomegaly, signs of pulmonary edema, JVD, or murmur

- **CARDIOMYOPATHIES**
  - **Infections** such as myocarditis, familial causes such as hypertrophic obstructive cardiomyopathy.
  - **Infiltrative causes** such as hemochromatosis can cause myocardial dysfunction and failure.
  - Think about in children with recent infection, murmur, chest pain, or signs of heart failure.

- **ARRHYTHMIAS**
  - Prolonged SVT or ventricular dysrhythmias can cause substantial decrease in stroke volume and thus cardiac output, also leading to failure.

II. FLUID & ELECTROLYTE MANAGEMENT

FLUID BALANCE

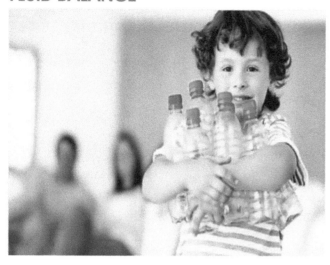

- Normally fluid balance is tightly controlled by thirst, hormonal responses and renal function.
- In critical illness or injury some or all of these mechanisms may be profoundly disrupted, and fluid therapy has to be tailored to the needs of the specific child.
- In the presence of anuria due to acute renal failure, fluid requirements may fall below **30 ml/kg/day**, while in high-output diarrhoea requirements may be as high as **400 ml/kg/day**.
- Fluid intake is required to replace fluid losses and to enable the excretion of various waste products through the urine.
- **Insensible losses** (via respiration and sweat) generally amount to between **10 and 30 ml/kg/day**.
- The actual volume of insensible fluid loss is related to the caloric content of the feeds, ambient temperature, humidity of inspired air, presence of pyrexia and quality of the skin.
- Insensible losses from a child on a ventilator in a cool environment with minimal caloric intake may be minimal.
- Usually between 0 and 10 ml/kg/day are lost in the stool (this will increase markedly in diarrhoea, where losses in excess of 300 ml/kg/day are not uncommon).
- **Urinary losses** are between 1 and 2 ml/kg/h (i.e. approximately 30 ml/kg/day).

- Fluid requirements in well, normal children.

Body weight	Daily fluid requirement	Hourly fluid requirement
First 10 kg	100 ml/kg	4 ml/kg
Second 10 kg	50 ml/kg	2 ml/kg
Subsequent kg	20 ml/kg	1 ml/kg

- These formulae are based on an assumption of 100 kcal/kg/day of caloric intake, 3 ml/kg/hour of urine output and normal stool output.
- The intravascular volume of an infant is **80 ml/kg**, and of an older child 70 ml/kg.
- A rapid loss of 25% of this volume (i.e. 20 ml/kg) will cause shock unless that volume is replaced from the interstitial fluid at a similar rate.
- Clinical signs of dehydration are only detectable when the patient is 2.5–5% dehydrated.
- 5% dehydration implies that the body has lost **5 g per 100 g body weight**, i.e. **50 ml/kg**.
- *Clearly, shock may occur in the absence of dehydration, dehydration may occur in the absence of shock, or both may occur together – all dependent on the rate of fluid loss and the rate of fluid shifts.*

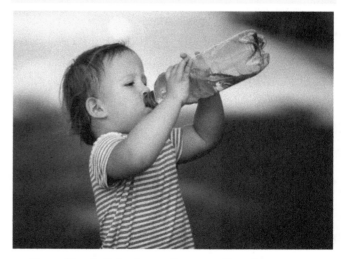

- **The critical clinical questions are therefore:**
  o Is the patient shocked?
  o Is the patient dehydrated?
  o Does the patient have a significant acid–base abnormality?
  o Are there significant electrolyte problems?

III. APPROACH TO GASTROENTERITIS

INTRODUCTION

- Pediatric acute gastroenteritis remains an important clinical illness commonly encountered by family physicians. Its attendant problems of vomiting, diarrhea and dehydration continue to present significant risks to children and are responsible for considerable health care expenditures.
- Vomiting: A forceful ejection of stomach contents up to and out of the mouth
- Diarrhoea: Passage of liquid or watery stools.
- In most cases there is an associated increase in frequency and volume.
- A uniform definition of acute gastroenteritis does not exist. The AAP defines acute gastroenteritis as "diarrheal disease of rapid onset, with or without accompanying symptoms or signs such as nausea, vomiting, fever or abdominal pain." [149] The hallmark of the disease is increased stool frequency with alteration of stool consistency.

CAUSATIVE ORGANISMS

- **Viruses (30-57%)**
  - o Rotavirus (most common)
  - o Enteric adenovirus
  - o Norwalk virus
  - o Calicivirus
  - o Astrovirus
  - o Parvovirus

- **Bacteria (6-14%)**
  - o Salmonella (most common)
  - o Toxigenic Escherichia coli
  - o Shigella (second most common)
  - o Campylobacter jejuni
  - o Yersinia enterocolitica (more common in Europe and Canada)
  - o Hemorrhagic E. coli O157:H7
  - o Clostridium difficile (iatrogenic)
- **Protozoa (~1%):**
  - o Giardia lamblia (most common)
  - o Cryptosporidium

RISK STRATIFICATION

- **The following children are at increased risk of dehydration:**
  - o *Young age (<1 year of age)*
  - o *Infants with low birth weight*
  - o *Those with signs of malnutrition*
  - o *Frequent symptoms (>5 diarrhoeal stools or >2 vomits within the previous 24 hours)*
  - o *Those who are not offered supplementary fluids or stopped breastfeeding prior to presentation.*

ASSESSMENT OF DEHYDRATION/NICE CG84 April 2009

Suspect hypernatraemic dehydration if there are any of the following[150] :

- Jittery movements
- Increased muscle tone
- Hyperreflexia
- Convulsions
- Drowsiness or coma.

INVESTIGATIONS

- **Stool Culture**

Consider performing stool microbiological investigations if:

- the child has recently been abroad **or**
- the diarrhoea has not improved by day 7 **or**
- there is uncertainty about the diagnosis of gastroenteritis.

Perform stool microbiological investigations if:

- you suspect septicaemia **or**
- there is blood and/or mucus in the stool **or**
- the child is immunocompromised.

LABORATORY MEASURES

- NICE guideline suggests the following[151] :
  - o Do not routinely perform blood biochemical testing.
  - o Measure plasma sodium, potassium, urea, creatinine and glucose concentrations if:
    - intravenous fluid therapy is required **or**
    - there are symptoms and/or signs that suggest hypernatraemia.
  - o Measure venous blood acid–base status and chloride concentration if shock is suspected or confirmed.
  - o Take **blood cultures** if starting antibiotics
  - o In children with Shiga toxin-producing *Escherichia coli* (STEC) infection, seek specialist advice on monitoring for haemolytic uraemic syndrome.

---

[149] American Academy of Pediatrics. Practice parameter: the management of acute gastroenteritis in young children. Pediatrics. 1996;97:424–35..

[150] NICE CG 84

[151] NICE CG 84

1. THE CHILD WITH NO CLINICAL DEHYDRATION

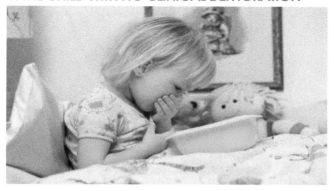

In children with gastroenteritis but without clinical dehydration[152]:

- Continue breastfeeding and other milk feeds
- Encourage fluid intake
- Discourage the drinking of fruit juices and carbonated drinks, especially in those at increased risk of dehydration.
- Offer ORS solution as supplemental fluid to those at increased risk of dehydration.
- Discharge home from the ED
- Reassure parents and carers that most cases can be safely managed at home
- If increased risk of dehydration, offer low osmolality **ORS** (i.e. Dioralyte®, Electrolade®) as a supplemental fluid.
- Seek advice from a healthcare professional if symptoms of dehydration develop.
- Advise on the typical duration of symptoms and to seek advice if they do not resolve within these timeframes.
- Provide verbal advice
- **Normal duration of symptoms**
  - o **Vomiting:** 1-2 days, most stop within 3 days
  - o **Diarrhoea:** 5-7 days, most stop within 2 weeks
- In children who are not clinically dehydrated do not perform an in hospital 'fluid challenge'.

2. THE CHILD WITH CLINICAL DEHYDRATION

In children with clinical dehydration, including hypernatraemic dehydration[153] :

- Use low-osmolarity ORS solution (240–250 mOsm/l) [154] for oral rehydration therapy
- Give 50 ml/kg for fluid deficit replacement over 4 hours as well as maintenance fluid
- Give the ORS solution frequently and in small amounts

---

[152] _NICE CG 84_

[153] _NICE CG 84_

[154] _The 'BNF for children' (BNFC) 2008 edition lists the following products with this composition: Dioralyte, Dioralyte Relief, Electrolade and Rapolyte._

- Consider supplementation with their usual fluids (including milk feeds or water, but not fruit juices or carbonated drinks) if they refuse to take sufficient quantities of ORS solution and do not have red flag symptoms or signs.
- Consider giving the ORS solution via a nasogastric tube if they are unable to drink it or if they vomit persistently
- Monitor the response to oral rehydration therapy by regular clinical assessment.

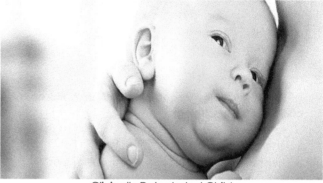

Clinically Dehydrated Child

- The measured weight loss or percentage dehydration:
  - o **5 % dehydration**= loss of 5ml of fluid per 100g body weight, or **50ml / kg**
  - o **10% dehydrated**= loss of 10ml of fluid per 100g body weight, or **100ml / kg**

A. ORAL REHYDRATION

- Continue to breastfeed (if applicable)
- Otherwise use low osmolality **ORS 50 ml/kg** (deficit replacement) plus maintenance fluid **over 4 hours**
- **Daily maintenance fluid** can be calculated using the child's body weight using the following formula:
- **Total Daily Maintenance (TDM):**
  - o **100 ml/kg** for the 1st 10 kg
  - o **50 ml/kg** for 2nd 10kg
  - o **20 ml/kg** for every subsequent 1 kg

- ORS should be given often and in small amounts
- Actual volumes needed clearly depends upon requirement
- If ORS is refused by the child and **there are no 'red flags'**:
  - o Consider other fluids (i.e. milk, water)
  - o Avoid fruit juices and carbonated drinks
  - o Consider NGT placement if the child is unable to drink and/or vomits persistently
  - o Monitor response to oral fluids
- **If oral fluid is tolerated:**
  - o Discharged home from ED
  - o Reassure parents or carers that oral rehydration is usually possible

- **Provide verbal advice:**
  - o Complete the remainder of the 4-hour fluid challenge at home
  - o Administer the fluid in small, frequent amounts
  - o Do not give other fluids unless advised
  - o Do not give solid foods
  - o Seek advice if the child refuses to drink or vomits persistently

- **Discuss with the paediatric team if:**
  - o Electrolyte imbalance (including hypernatraemic dehydration)
  - o An NGT is required
  - o There is an indication for IV fluids

B. IV FLUID [155]

- **IV fluids are only recommended in children with clinical dehydration if:**
  - o Evidence of deterioration during ORS therapy **and**
  - o Evidence of Red flags symptoms/signs **or**
  - o The child persistently vomits ORS

- **If IV fluids are required:**
  - ▪ Obtain urgent expert advice on fluid management
  - ▪ Commence isotonic fluids for deficit correction and maintenance (0.9% saline or 0.9% saline and 5% glucose)
  - ▪ Rehydrate slowly (normally over 48 hours)
  - ▪ Monitor serum sodium level frequently
  - ▪ Aim for a reduction of less than 0.5 mmol/l per hour

- **During IV fluid therapy**
  - ▪ Gradually attempt to introduce oral fluids early
  - ▪ If tolerated, complete rehydration with oral fluid therapy

- **In cases of suspected hypernatraemic dehydration:**
  - o Obtain baseline U&Es and blood glucose, Rapid correction can be dangerous
  - o Ideally **oral rehydration** should be used.

APPLICATION OF FLUID THERAPY

- Reassess clinical status and weight at 4–6 hours, and if satisfactory continue. If the child is losing weight increase the fluid rate, and if the weight gain is excessive decrease the fluid rate.
- Start giving more of the maintenance fluid as oral feeds if the child is tolerating the fluids.

3. THE CHILD WITH CLINICAL SHOCK

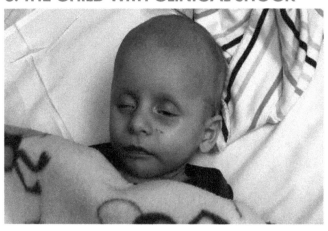

- **ABC DEFG** approach
- Ensure patient airway, give high flow oxygen
- Obtain urgent IV access
- Measure baseline U&Es, blood glucose and VBG
- Give a fluid bolus of **20 ml/kg 0.9% saline**
- **If remains shocked after bolus:**
  - o Give a further bolus
  - o Consider other causes for shock
  - o In the context of severe sepsis there is some concern about the use of fluid boluses for resuscitation.
  - o It seems reasonable to continue with fluid bolus administration with careful monitoring of the patient's response.
  - o Unless there is evidence of cardiac dysrhythmia or neurological abnormality, electrolyte abnormalities should be corrected gradually.
- **If remains shocked after 2nd bolus;** Consider discussion with paediatric ICU team
- **Once symptoms and signs of shock have resolved:**
  - o Calculate daily maintenance requirement
  - o Add **100 ml/kg** deficit to fluid calculations
  - o Commence isotonic fluids for deficit and maintenance
  - o 0.9% saline or 0.9% saline and 5% glucose
  - o Consider adding potassium to fluids once serum level is known
  - o Monitor clinical and laboratory response to fluid therapy, adjust subsequent fluids as appropriate.
  - o Discuss with paediatric team.
- **Children who have hypernatraemic dehydration**
  - o May be shocked at presentation
  - o Fluid resuscitation guidelines should be followed
  - o Rehydration should be managed as per the guidance for those children who are clinically dehydrated.

---

155 NICE CG 84

WORKED EXAMPLE

- *A 30-kg girl responded to a 20 ml/kg fluid bolus and is no longer shocked.*
- *What is his initial hourly IV fluid requirement?*
- *What type of fluid would you prescribe?*
- *Answer:*
  - o *Deficit = 100 ml/kg x 30 kg = 3000 ml*
  - o *Daily maintenance = (100ml/kg x 10kg) + (50ml/kg x 10kg) + (20 ml/kg x 10kg) = 1700 ml*
  - o *Hourly requirement = 3000 + 1700 ÷ 24 = 195 ml/hour*

- *A 8-kg boy is clinically shocked and 10% dehydrated as a result of gastroenteritis.*
  - o *Initial therapy*
    - ▪ *20 ml/kg for shock = 8 × 20 = 160 ml of 0.9% saline given as a rapid intravenous bolus*
  - o *Estimated fluid therapy over the next 24 hours*
    - ▪ *100 ml/kg for 10% dehydration = 100 × 8 = 800 ml*
    - ▪ *100 ml/kg for daily maintenance fluid = 100 × 8 = 800 ml*
    - ▪ *Rehydration + maintenance = 1600 ml*
    - ▪ *Therefore, start with an infusion of 1600/24 = 66 ml/h.*
- Start with **0.9% saline** or **0.9% saline and 5% glucose**
- Consider adding potassium once serum levels are known

4. THE CHILD WITH FLUID OVERLOAD AND OVERHYDRATION

- In the same way that fluid losses may cause shock, dehydration or both, excessive fluid administration can cause intravascular fluid overload, overhydration or both.
- **In the patient with nephrotic syndrome,** fluid has leaked out of the intravascular space and into the tissues because of a low serum albumin. Such children may be grossly overhydrated, with diffuse severe oedema. However, many patients with nephrotic syndrome have a contracted intravascular space, and attempts to diurese these patients without first expanding the intravascular space with albumin may result in shock.
- **By contrast the patient with myocardial dysfunction** may have an intravascular compartment that is grossly overfilled. The clinical signs of intravascular overload may be present, and yet the patient (particularly if they have been on diuretics) may actually be total body fluid depleted and may appear dehydrated.
- **Children with renal impairment** may present with a combination of intravascular and total body fluid overload. Administration of further fluid can worsen fluid overload leading to pulmonary oedema.

- The treatment of fluid overload can be complex and the non-specialist should seek expert advice.

5. ADDITIONAL THERAPIES[156]

- **Antibiotics**
  - o Do not routinely give antibiotics to children with gastroenteritis.
  - o Give antibiotic treatment to all children:
    - ▪ With suspected or confirmed septicaemia
    - ▪ With extra-intestinal spread of bacterial infection
    - ▪ Younger than 6 months with salmonella gastroenteritis
    - ▪ Who are malnourished or immunocompromised with salmonella gastroenteritis
    - ▪ With *clostridium* difficile-associated pseudomembranous enterocolitis, giardiasis, dysenteric shigellosis, dysenteric amoebiasis or cholera.
  - o For children who have recently been abroad, seek specialist advice about antibiotic therapy.

- **Anti-diarrheal agents**
  - o Do not use antidiarrhoeal medications·
- **Probiotics and Antiemetics**: No recommendations in NICE guidelines.

6. GASTROENTERITIS & PUBLIC HEALTH CONSIDERATIONS

- Advise parents, carers and children that[157]:
  - o Washing hands with soap (liquid if possible) in warm running water and careful drying are the most important factors in preventing the spread of gastroenteritis
  - o Hands should be washed after going to the toilet (children) or changing nappies (parents/carers) and before preparing, serving or eating food
  - o Towels used by infected children should not be shared
  - o Children should not attend any school or other childcare facility while they have diarrhoea or vomiting caused by gastroenteritis
  - o Children should not go back to their school or other childcare facility until at least 48 hours after the last episode of diarrhoea or vomiting
  - o Children should not swim in swimming pools for 2 weeks after the last episode of diarrhoea.

---

[156] *NICE CG 84*

[157] **Public Health England (2017)** *Health protection in schools and other childcare facilities*

IV. APPROACH TO ELECTROLYTES IMBALANCES

1. THE CHILD WITH SODIUM IMBALANCE

- **Severe hypernatraemia** may be associated with brain damage, because brain tissue shrinks as a result of intracellular dehydration and blood vessels may tear or clot up.

- Too rapid correction of hypernatraemia may lead to **cerebral oedema and convulsions**.

- Similarly, rapid correction of hyponatraemia may also be associated with **demyelination** and **permanent brain injury**.

- The electrolyte losses during dehydration depend on the reason for dehydration.

- In gastroenteritis, sodium losses in diarrhoea stool range from approximately **50 mmol/l (rotavirus)** to approximately **80 mmol/l (cholera and enteropathogenic Escherichia coli)**.

- In renal dysfunction sodium losses may be minimal (**diabetes insipidus**) or high (**renal tubular dysfunction**).

A. HYPERNATRAEMIA

- Hypernatraemia in the dehydrated patient may be the end result of:
  - **Excessive loss of water:** Diabetes insipidus, diarrhoea
  - **Excessive intake of sodium:** Iatrogenic poisoning, non-accidental injury
  - **Combination of both:** Children with gastroenteritis given excessive NaCl$^+$ in rehydration fluid.

- The electrolyte content of the replacement solution depends on the cause of the dehydration.

- Previously, 0.45% NaCl, containing 75 mmol/L NaCl, was considered a safe starting solution for intravenous rehydration. This was based largely on the electrolyte content of stool in diarrhoea.

- By contrast, patients with rare renal tubular dysfunction who lose excessive sodium and water through their kidneys may require 0.9% NaCl to replace the renal losses of sodium.

- Measurement of the sodium content of urine and stool may help direct replacement therapy.

- More recently, consensus guidelines have recommended starting with an isotonic solution such as 0.9% NaCl, or 0.9% NaCl with 5% glucose, for fluid-deficit replacement and maintenance for hypernatraemic dehydration due to a number of children developing a rapid fall in sodium with hypotonic solutions.

- **The principles in the treatment of hypernatraemia are:**
  - Treat shock first.
  - Calculate the maintenance fluid and estimate the fluid deficit carefully.
  - Aim to lower the serum sodium at a rate of **no more than 0.5 mmol/h**.
  - Check other electrolyte levels such as calcium and glucose.
  - Monitor the electrolytes frequently – obtain expert advice if correction is not improving.
  - Clinically assess hydration and weigh frequently.

B. HYPONATRAEMIA

- Hyponatraemia may be due to:
  - **Excessive water intake or retention**
  - **Excessive sodium losses**
  - **Combination of both**

- If the child is fitting from hyponatraemia, partial rapid correction of the serum sodium level will be necessary to stop the fitting.

- Administration of **4 ml/kg of 3% NaCl solution over 15 minutes** will raise the serum sodium by approximately 3 mmol and will usually stop the seizures.

- If hyponatraemia is due to excessive water intake or retention, and the patient is not symptomatic, **the restriction of fluid intake to 50% of normal estimated requirements** may be adequate therapy.

- If dehydrated and intravenous fluids are required then 0.9% NaCl is an appropriate fluid.

- **The principles in the treatment of hyponatraemia are:**
  - Treat the child's seizures with **hypertonic 3% NaCl** (seizure control should happen simultaneously).
  - Calculate the maintenance fluid and estimate the fluid deficit carefully.
  - Aim to raise the serum sodium at a rate of **no more than 0.5 mmol/h**
  - Check other electrolyte levels such as calcium and glucose.
  - Monitor the electrolytes frequently – obtain expert advice if correction is not improving.
  - Clinically assess hydration and weigh frequently.

2. THE CHILD WITH POTASSIUM IMBALANCE

- Causes of hypo- and hyperkalaemia

Hypokalaemia	Hyperkalaemia
• Diarrhoea	• Renal failure
• Alkalosis	• Acidosis
• Volume depletion	• Excessive K+ intake
• Primary hyperaldosteronism	• Adrenal insufficiency
• Diuretic abuse	• Cell lysis

- In the critically ill neonate, inadequate cardiac output must always be excluded as a cause.

A. HYPOKALAEMIA

- Hypokalaemia is rarely an emergency and is usually the result of **excessive potassium losses from acute diarrhoeal illnesses.**
- As total body depletion will have occurred, large amounts are required to return the serum potassium to normal.
- **Oral supplementation is the preferred route.**
- In cases where this is not suitable, intravenous supplements are required.
- However, strong potassium solutions are highly irritant and can precipitate cardiac arrhythmias, thus the concentration of potassium in intravenous solutions ought **not to exceed 40 mmol/l** except when given centrally with close cardiac monitoring.
- *Patients who are alkalotic or are receiving insulin or salbutamol will have high intracellular potassium stores.*
- *The hypokalaemia in these cases is the result of a redistribution of potassium into cells rather than potassium deficiency, and management of the underlying causes is indicated.*

B. HYPERKALAEMIA

- Hyperkalaemia is a dangerous condition.
- Although the normal range extends up to 5.5 mmol/l, **it is rare to get arrhythmias below 7.5 mmol/l.**
- Precise blood taking is critical as a squeezed sample lyses blood cells, raising potassium level spuriously.
- The most common cause of hyperkalaemia is **renal failure** – either acute or chronic.
- Hyperkalaemia can also result from **potassium overload, loss of potassium from cells** due to acidosis or cell lysis, or endocrine causes such as **hypoaldosteronism and hypoadrenalism.**

- If there is no immediate threat to the patient's life because of an arrhythmia then a logical sequence of investigation and treatment can be followed.
- **Beta-2 stimulants, such as salbutamol, are the immediate treatment of choice.**
  - They rapidly act within 30 minutes by stimulating the cell wall pumping mechanism and promoting cellular potassium uptake.
  - They are easily administered by a nebuliser.
  - The serum potassium will fall by about 1 mmol/l with these dosages.

APPROACH TO MANAGEMENT OF HYPERKALAEMIA IN CHILDREN

- **Monitoring:** continuous ECG (first signs are tented T-waves then loss of P-waves), SaO2, blood pressure, urine output, weight
- **Recheck urea and electrolytes urgently** – hours may have elapsed since last sample. Sample may have haemolysed
- **Consider the cause:** high K+ intake, high production or low output
- **Stop K+ intake:** Stop any potassium in diet and in any fluids being infused
- **Stop drugs that can cause hyperkalaemia:** ACE inhibitor, Angiotensin II blockers and β-blockers
- **Stabilise myocardium** with **10% calcium gluconate**
  - 0.5–1 ml/kg IV over 5 min, max. 20 ml; give undiluted
  - Give if ECG changes or K+ significantly above upper end of normal for age or rising
  - Effect occurs within minutes.
  - Duration of action approx. 1 h
  - Repeat within 5–10 min as necessary

- **Shift K+ into cells** with **Nebulised salbutamol**
  - <2 year: 2.5 mg or ≥2 years: 5 mg; repeat 2-hourly as necessary
  - Onset of action: within 30 min, max. effect at 60–90 min
  - Seek specialist advice

The following strategies can be used depending on clinical situation:
- **Shift K+ into cells**
  - **Sodium bicarbonate** 1–2 mmol/kg IV over 30 min (1 mmol = 1 ml of 8.4% NaHCO3, dilute 1:5 in 5% dextrose)
  - **Glucose + insulin:**
    - **Peripheral access:** 10% glucose 5–10 ml/kg/h
    - **Central access:** 20% glucose 2.5–5 ml/kg/h
    - Maintain blood glucose at 10–15 mmol/l.
    - Physiological homeostasis should increase endogenous insulin production.

- Add insulin after an hour if blood sugar >15 mmol/l: Make up a syringe of 50 units insulin in 50 ml 0.9% NaCl (=1 unit/ml); commence infusion at 0.05 ml/kg/h
- Maintain blood glucose at 10–15 mmol/l by adjusting infusion rate in 0.05 ml/kg/h steps
- Can cause severe hypoglycaemia.
- Measure blood sugar frequently (15 min after commencing or increase in dose, then every 30 min until stable)

- **Remove K+ from body**
  - **Calcium resonium:**
    - By rectum: 250 mg/kg (max. 15 g) 6-hourly, repeat if expelled within 30 min
    - By mouth: 250 mg/kg (max. 15 g) 6-hourly
  - Limited role for oral route as it is unpalatable.
  - Takes 4 h for full effect

3. THE CHILD WITH CALCIUM IMBALANCE

A. HYPOCALCAEMIA

- Hypocalcaemia can be a part of any severe illness, particularly septicaemia.
- Other specific conditions that may give rise to hypocalcaemia are:
  - Severe rickets,
  - Hypoparathyroidism,
  - Pancreatitis
  - Rhabdomyolysis
  - Citrate infusion (in massive blood transfusions).
  - Acute and chronic renal failure can also present with severe hypocalcaemia.

- In all cases, hypocalcaemia can produce weakness, tetany, convulsions, hypotension and arrhythmias.
- Treatment is that of the underlying condition.
- In the emergency situation, however, **intravenous calcium can be administered**.
- As most of the above conditions are associated with a total body depletion of calcium and because the total body pool is so large, acute doses will often only have a transient effect on the serum calcium.
- Continuous infusions will also often be required, and most appropriately given through a central venous line as calcium is irritant to peripheral veins.
- In renal failure, high serum phosphate levels may prevent the serum calcium from rising.
- The use of oral phosphate binders or dialysis may be necessary in these circumstances.

B. HYPERCALCAEMIA

- Hypercalcaemia usually presents as long-standing anorexia, malaise, weight loss, failure to thrive or vomiting.
- **Causes include:**
  - Malignancy,
  - Hyperparathyroidism,
  - Hypervitaminosis D or A,
  - Idiopathic hypercalcaemia of infancy,
  - Thiazide diuretic abuse
  - Skeletal disorders.

- Initial treatment is with volume expansion with **normal saline and furosemide diuretic**.
- Following this, investigation and specific treatment are indicated.

V. APPROACH TO THE CHILD WITH DKA

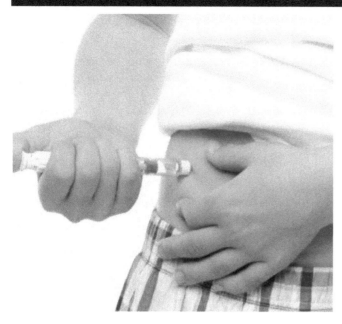

1. INTRODUCTION

- Diabetic ketoacidosis (DKA) is a condition in which a relative or absolute lack of insulin leads to an inability to metabolise glucose.
- This leads to hyperglycaemia and an osmotic diuresis. Once urine output exceeds the ability of the patient to drink, dehydration occurs.
- In addition, without insulin, fat is used as a source of energy, leading to the production of large quantities of **ketones and metabolic acidosis**.
- There is initial compensation for the acidosis by hyperventilation and a respiratory alkalosis but, as the condition progresses, the combination of acidosis, hyperosmolality and dehydration leads to coma.
- **DKA is often the first presentation of diabetes**; it can also be a problem in known diabetics who have decompensated through illness, infection or non-adherence to their treatment regimes.

2. HISTORY

- The history is usually of weight loss, abdominal pain, vomiting, polyuria and polydipsia, although symptoms may be much less specific in under 5-year-olds who also have an increased tendency to ketoacidosis.

3. EXAMINATION

- Children may be dehydrated with deep and rapid (Kussmaul) respiration.
- They may also be drowsy with the smell of ketones on their breath.

- **Salicylate poisoning** and **uraemia** are differential diagnoses that should be excluded.
- Whilst rare, infection often precipitates decompensation in both new and known diabetics.
- Fever is not part of DKA. Suspect sepsis in the presence of fever, hypothermia, hypotension and a refractory acidosis or lactic acidosis.

4. MANAGEMENT

- Assess A, B & C
- Give 100% oxygen
- Place on a cardiac monitor: observe for peaked T-waves from hyperkalaemia.
- Consider placement of a nasogastric tube
- Take blood for **Blood gases, Urea and electrolytes, creatinine, Glucose, Ketones**
- Take urine for **Sugar**
- Take other investigations only if indicated:
  o Full blood count (leucocytosis commonly occurs in DKA and is not necessarily a sign of infection)
  o Chest X-ray
  o Blood culture, CSF, Throat swab
  o Urinalysis, culture and sensitivity

- **The principles of management of diabetic ketoacidosis are:**
  o Fluid boluses are only to be given in DKA to reverse signs of shock and should be given slowly in **10 ml/kg aliquots.**
  o If there are no signs of shock, do not routinely give a fluid bolus.
  o If a second saline bolus is needed, specialist advice should be sought.
  o To rehydrate after signs of shock have been reversed **with 48 hours of replacement fluid.**
  o *The first 20 ml/kg of fluid resuscitation are given in addition to replacement fluid calculations and should not be subtracted from the calculations for the fluids for the next 48 hours.*
  o *Resuscitation volumes over 20 ml/kg should be subtracted from the fluid volume calculated for the 48-hour replacement.*
  o Discuss the use of inotropes with a paediatric intensive care specialist
  o To replace insulin; start an intravenous insulin infusion 1–2 hours after beginning intravenous fluid therapy.
  o Use a soluble insulin infusion at a dosage between **0.05 and 0.1 units/kg/h.**
  o To return the glucose level to that approaching normal.

- o To avoid hypokalaemia, hypoglycaemia and rapid changes in serum osmolarity.
- o To treat the underlying precipitating cause of the DKA.

- When calculating the fluid requirement for children and young people with DKA, assume:
  - o **Mild to Moderate DKA:** pH ≥7.1 = 5% fluid deficit (50ml/Kg)
  - o **Severe DKA:** pH <7.1= 10% fluid deficit (100ml/kg)

- Replace this **deficit over 48 hours**
- Calculate the maintenance fluid requirement for children and young people with DKA using the following 'reduced volume' rules:
  - o If they weigh less than 10 kg, give **2 ml/kg/h**
  - o If they weigh between 10 and 40 kg, give **1 ml/kg/h**
  - o If they weigh more than 40 kg, give a fixed volume of **40 ml/h**

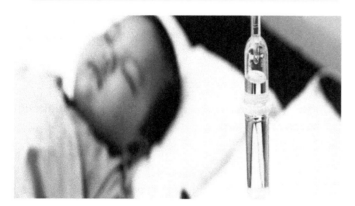

Body weight	Hourly fluid requirement
Less than 10 kg	2 ml/kg/hr
10 -40 kg	1 ml/kg/hr
More than 40kg	40 ml/**hr**

- These are lower than standard fluid maintenance volumes because large fluid volumes are associated with an **increased risk of cerebral oedema.**
- The total replacement fluid to be given **over 48 hours** is calculated as follows:

> **Hourly rate =**
> **(Deficit/48 hours) + Maintenance per hour**

- **If more than 20 ml/kg of fluid** has been given by intravenous bolus to a child or young person with DKA, **subtract any additional bolus volumes from the total fluid calculation for the 48-hour period.**

- **Work example:**
  - o **A 20 kg** 6-year-old boy who has a pH of **7.15**, who did not have a sodium chloride bolus, will require:
    - **Deficit 5 %** x 20 kg = 1000 mls **divide over 48 hours** = 21 ml/hr plus
    - **Maintenance** 1ml/kg/hr = 20 ml/hr
    - **Total** = 41 ml/hour
  - o **A 60 kg** 16-year-old girl with a pH of **6.9**, and who was given **30 ml/kg** 0.9% sodium chloride for circulatory collapse will require:
    - **Deficit** 10 % x 60 kg = 6000 mls
    - **Minus** 10ml/kg **Resuscitation Fluid** = - 600 ml
    - **Divide over 48 hours** = 113 ml/hr plus
    - **Maintenance** fixed rate = 40 ml/hr
    - **Total** = 153 ml/hour

5. MAJOR COMPLICATIONS OF DKA
- **Cerebral oedema**
  - o Most important cause of death and poor neurological outcome.
  - o Attempt to avoid by slow normalisation of osmolarity with attention to glucose and sodium levels, and hydration over 48h
  - o Monitor for headache, recurrence of vomiting, irritability, Glasgow Coma Scale score, inappropriate slowing of heart rate and rising blood pressure.
  - o Treat with **hypertonic (3%) saline 3 ml/kg** or **mannitol infusion (250–500 mg/kg over 20 min)**
  - o Hyperventilation has been associated with worse outcomes

- **Cardiac dysrhythmias**
  - o Usually secondary to electrolyte disturbances, particularly potassium

- **Pulmonary oedema**
  - o Careful fluid replacement may limit the occurrence of pulmonary oedema

- **Acute renal failure**
  - o Uncommon because of high osmotic urine flow

5. Unconscious Child

INTRODUCTION

- Coma is a state of unarousable unresponsiveness in which the subject lies with their eyes closed[158].
- At first glance, this definition imposes age-specific difficulties related to clinical diagnosis of coma in children, and especially in infants, [159] because the child's brain is less responsive than the adult brain.
- Conscious level ranges from full arousal to complete unresponsiveness. When communicating with other health professionals use the patient's GCS to describe conscious level; terms like coma, stupor and obtunded are less exact.

DIFFERENTIAL DIAGNOSIS

- Decreased consciousness is a non-specific sign with a wide differential diagnosis: **TIPS AEIOU**
  - o **T**rauma
  - o **I**ntracranial infection
  - o **P**oisoning
  - o **S**hock: hypovolaemic, distributive and cardiogenic
  - o **S**epsis
  - o **E**pilepsy
  - o **R**aised intracranial pressure
  - o **M**etabolic disease
  - o **H**ypertension

AVPU SCORE

- o **A: Alert**
- o **V:** Responsive to **verbal** stimuli
- o **P:** Responsive to **painful** stimuli
- o **U: Unresponsive**

HISTORY

- Exploring developmental milestones, past medical, travel, immunisation and family history including infant deaths further guides management. Non-accidental injury may be behind the cause of reduced consciousness, consider child protection issues. The key questions on presentation should explore prodromal events leading to decreased consciousness with reference to the wide differential diagnosis: any recent illness and length of symptoms:

Category	Symptoms
Shock	• Abdominal pain, excessive diarrhoea and vomiting may suggest fluid loss or surgical cause.
Sepsis	• Vomiting, headache, fever, rash and infectious exposure may suggest infection. • However recent antibiotic use may mask classical presentations of meningitis in the early phase. • A detailed history is recommended.
Trauma	• Trauma may or may not be evident particularly in the case of a **shaken baby.** • Inappropriate responses or inconsistencies and delays in seeking help arouse suspicion of non-accidental injury.
Intracranial	• History of ear pain is suggestive of otitis media; ask about frontal headaches, facial pains and purulent nasal discharge which are suggestive of sinusitis. • Intracranial extension can occur.
Epilepsy	• There may be a family history or prior seizures or a history of neuro developmental delay.
Poisoning	• No history may be given. • Examination may give clues to potential source.
Raised intracranial pressure	• If there is a past history of neuro-developmental problems, check whether a shunt has been inserted or if there is a history of hydrocephalus. • Make enquiries regarding recent head injuries.
Metabolic	• Recent weight loss, polydipsia or polyuria may suggest a metabolic cause. • A family history should be sought including if any consanguinity which may suggest inborn errors of metabolism.
Hypertension	• A review of medication history may give a clue to the cause.

---

[158] *Plum F, Posner JR: Diagnosis of Stupor and Coma (4th Edition). FA Davis, PA, USA (1995). Seminal and complete work on the states of impairment of consciousness.*

[159] *Shewmon DA: Coma prognosis in children: part I: definitional and methodological challenges. J. Clin. Neurophysiol. 17, 457–466 (2000).*

INVESTIGATIONS – MONITORING

- The following should be monitored: **MOVER (Monitor-Oxygen-Vitals-ECG-Resus)**
- **Core Blood and Urine Tests**
  - o **Bedside test: Capillary glucose** within 15 minutes of presentation.
  - o **Blood gas:** in all cases
  - o **Sepsis:** Urinalysis, FBC, CRP, Blood Culture
  - o **Metabolic**-specific cases: VBG/ABG, Glucose, Urines Ketones, LFT, U&E, Serum Ammonia
  - o **Overdose:** Plasma, serum and urine to be saved for later analysis of specific agents e.g. opiates, tricyclics.
- **Lumbar puncture**
  - o **Indications:**
    - ▪ Usually done in children's hospital Indicated if suspected intracranial infection
  - o **Contraindications:**
    - ▪ GCS 8 or less or deteriorating
    - ▪ Focal neurological signs or abnormal posture
    - ▪ Prolonged seizure lasting 10 minutes or more and a GCS of 12 or less
    - ▪ Shock, Systemic meningococcal disease
    - ▪ **Signs of raised ICP:**
      - • Unilateral or bilateral dilated pupils or sluggish pupillary reaction
      - • Bradycardia
      - • Hypertension,
      - • Abnormal breathing pattern.
- **Cerebral Imaging**
  - o **A CT scan** is indicated if:
    - ▪ Trauma
    - ▪ Signs of raised intracranial pressure
    - ▪ Focal neurological signs
    - ▪ Unknown cause

MANAGEMENT IN THE ED

- **General management is as per APLS guidelines.**
  - o **Airway and Breathing:**
    - ▪ **Oxygen** should be administered.
    - ▪ Open airway with manoeuvres/adjuncts
    - ▪ Intubate if not protecting airway
    - ▪ Consider intubation if GCS
    - ▪ Give oxygen if SpO2 <95%
  - o **Circulation**
    - ▪ If circulatory compromise give 20ml/kg fluid bolus In DKA or raised ICP give 10ml/kg instead

- o **Disability**
  - ▪ GCS and pupillary examination,
  - ▪ Assess fontanelle, tone and posture.
  - ▪ Perform BM – give 2ml/kg 10% dextrose if BM<3
  - ▪ Consider intubation to maintain PaCO2 4.5-5kPa if there is a clinical diagnosis of raised ICP
- o **Exposure**
  - ▪ Front/back examination is required to look for:
    - • A rash
    - • Evidence of trauma
    - • Drug use – check for powder residu

FEBRILE SEIZURES

- o Occur from the age of 12 months to around 5 years of age.
- o They should last less than 10 minutes and post-fit recovery should be relatively quick within 20 minutes, unless rescue medication has been given.
- o Delayed fit recovery may indicate a more sinister pathology.

NON-CONVULSIVE STATUS

- o Can occur and should be considered if the child's GCS is not improving. Careful examination may reveal intermittent gaze deviation, nystagmus or other subtle signs to suggest a continued seizure.
- o Use anticonvulsants as per protocol.

RAISED INTRACRANIAL PRESSURE

- o Bradycardia and hypertension
- o Papilloedema
- o Pupillary dilatation, inequality and loss of reaction to light (all late signs!)
- o 20 degree head up tilt
- o Consider mannitol Intubate and ventilate to PaCO2 4.5-5kPa
- o Discuss with PICU

INTRACRANIAL INFECTION

- Fever, photophobia, neck stiffness
- Signs raised ICP
- Unexplained fever and reduced consciousness
- Treat co-existing shock if present
- Cefotaxime (Amoxicillin+gentamycin if <6/52, Dexamethasone if >3/12)
- Aciclovir
- LP – usually at children's hospital
- CT – if focal neurology, reduced GCS, signs ICP

I. THE CHILD WITH MENINGITIS/ENCEPHALITIS

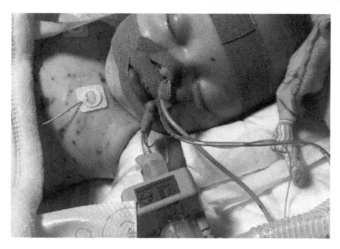

INTRODUCTION

- After the neonatal period, the commonest cause of bacterial meningitis is **Neisseria meningitidis (meningococcus).** There is still a mortality rate of around 5% and a similar rate of permanent serious sequelae.
- Infection with **Streptococcus pneumoniae** is less common and may follow an upper respiratory infection with or without otitis media. Long-term morbidity and mortality occur in up to 30% of cases.
- Widespread Hib vaccination has reduced the incidence of **Haemophilus influenzae** infection. A wide range of infections may also cause encephalitis.

DEFINITION

- **Meningococcal meningitis:** Inflammation of the pia and arachnoid mater, resulting from **meningococcal**
- **Meningococcal septicaemia:** Bacterial infection of the bloodstream by **Neisseria meningitides** with subsequent bacterial endotoxin release, and rapid progression to shock and circulatory collapse.
- The rate of confirmed meningococcal disease is highest in **the under-fives**, particularly among infants.
- Case fatality ratios in children are highest in teenagers older than 14, followed by infants less than 1 year of age.
- There is a marked seasonal variation in incidence, with case numbers peaking in the winter months and during outbreaks of viral respiratory infection.

- Approximately 10% of the population are asymptomatic carriers in the nasopharynx.
- Carriage rates vary from 2% in children < 5 years and peak to 25% in children between the ages of 15-19 years.
- The most common serogroups that cause disease are **A, B, C, W125, Y**
- Since the introduction of vaccines to control Hib, serogroup C meningococcus and pneumococcal disease, serogroup B meningococcus is now the most common cause of bacterial meningitis and septicaemia in children.

APLS GUIDELINE

1. MENINGITIS IN THE 3-YEAR-OLD CHILD AND UNDER

- o Bacterial meningitis is difficult to diagnose in its early stages in this age group.
- o The classic signs of neck rigidity, photophobia, headache and vomiting are often absent.
- o A **bulging fontanelle** is a sign of advanced meningitis in an infant, but even this serious and late sign will be masked if the baby is dehydrated from fever and vomiting.
- o Almost all children with meningitis have some degree of raised ICP, so that, in fact, the signs and symptoms of meningitis are **primarily those of raised ICP.**
- **The following are signs of possible meningitis in infants and young children:**
  - o *Coma*
  - o *Drowsiness (often shown by lack of eye contact with parents or doctor)*
  - o *High-pitched cry or irritability that cannot be easily soothed by parent*
  - o *Poor feeding*
  - o *Unexplained pyrexia*
  - o *Convulsions with or without fever*
  - o *Apnoeic or cyanotic attacks*
  - o *Purpuric rash*

2. MENINGITIS IN OLDER CHILDREN OF 4 YEARS AND OVER

- These children are more likely to have the classic signs of headache, vomiting, pyrexia, neck stiffness and photophobia.
- Some present with coma or convulsions.

- In all unwell children, and children with unexplained pyrexia, a careful search should be made for neck stiffness and for a purpuric rash.
- The finding of such a rash in an ill child is almost pathognomic of meningococcal infection, for which immediate treatment is required.

RASH IN MENINGOCOCCAL DISEASE

- Most patients with meningococcal septicaemia **develop a rash.** However, this will not always be a feature at initial presentation.
- The rash can range from scanty blanching macular or maculopapular lesions to a rapidly evolving haemorrhagic rash.
- The text-book **non-blanching rash** may be a very late sign, and the underlying meningitis or septicaemia is often very advanced by the time this rash appears.
- A generalised **petechial rash or purpuric rash** in any location, **in an ill child**, are strongly suggestive of meningococcal septicaemia and should prompt urgent treatment.

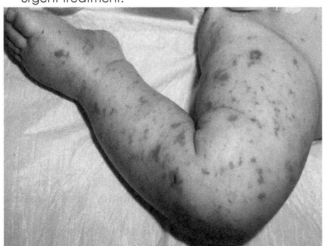

ED MANAGEMENT OF MENINGITIS

General Management

- All children with suspected Meningitis in the ED should be managed in the presence of full resuscitation facilities, with continuous cardiac and oxygen saturation monitoring.
- A senior member of the ED medical team and the duty paediatrician should be involved at an early stage.

A & B:

o **Oxygen** should be administered to all patients, and an anaesthetist immediately involved if there is any concern about the child's ability to maintain their own airway and adequately self-ventilate.

o Consider **Intubation** if GMSPS ≥ 8 or child requires **>40ml/Kg of fluid.**

C:

- **Two wide bore IV access (or IO)**
- Collect appropriate Blood tests
- **Fluids**
  - 0.9% Normal Saline **20 mls/kg** is recommended for the first fluid bolus
  - 0.9% Normal saline or 4.5% human albumen for subsequent boluses

o Repeated fluid boluses can be administered as needed, with the goal of attaining normal perfusion.

o If the child requires greater than **40 ml/kg** initial fluid resuscitation, or if they score **equal to or greater than 8** on the GMSPS (where used), it is important to consult with the local paediatric intensive care unit to consider elective intubation and ventilation, and rapid escalation of treatment with inotropic support and fluid management.

o In children suspected to have raised ICP secondary to meningitis, control the $PaCO_2$ within the normal range (4-4.5 kPa).

o All children requiring intensive care support should have **central venous access** and an **arterial line, NGT** and **urinary catheter** inserted.

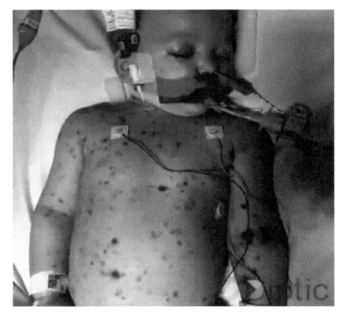

DRUGS:

o **Antibiotics:**
  - The NICE guideline recommends **CEFTRIAXONE 80 mg/kg OD in > 3-month-old.**
  - IV cefotaxime **(50 mg/kg)** should be used as initial treatment of previously well children over 3 months with a diagnosis of IMD.
  - **If < 3-month olds: Cefotaxime + Ampicillin or Amoxicillin** (active against listeria).

- Treat with **Acyclovir** and a **Macrolide** in a febrile, comatose child for the rare respective possibilities of **herpes simplex virus** and **Mycoplasma encephalitis.**
- Give **Dexamethasone** (150 micrograms/kg, max. 10 mg, four times/day) in suspected or confirmed bacterial meningitis, aiming **to start within 4 hours of antibiotics** (not later than 12 hours).
- Do not use in infants younger than 3 months, but in older infants and children
- Corticosteroids can reduce the rate of severe hearing loss and possibly other long-term neurological sequelae.

MENINGITIS WITH RAISED ICP

o This will require paediatric neuro-intensive care.
o Ensure normocapnia (PaCO$_2$ 4-4.5 kPa) and ensure adequate oxygenation.
o For acute raised ICP, diuretics (**Mannitol 0.25 g/kg over 5mins**, followed by **frusemide 1 mg/kg**) are recommended, and should be repeated if clinically indicated.
o Overaggressive fluid resuscitation in raised ICP will exacerbate cerebral oedema.
o Only children who are hypotensive secondary to septic shock require aggressive fluid replacement and inotropes to maintain cerebral perfusion pressure.
o The patient should be nursed with **their head elevated** as much as possible in the midline position, with regular monitoring of pupil size and reactivity.
o Keep normothermic, and treat seizures aggressively.

CLINICAL FEATURES OF MENINGITIS WITHOUT SHOCK OR SIGNS OF RAISED ICP

o Children with clinical features of suggestive of meningitis, but in the absence of shock or features of raised ICP should be treated empirically with:
- **IV Cefotaxime**, and closely monitored for any signs of disease progression.
- **Dexamethasone 0.4 mg/kg** administration as an adjunct to antibiotic therapy has been suggested to reduce neurological sequalae and hearing loss in children with meningitis, particularly if the pathogen proves to be H. Influenzae or S. Pneumonia.

MENINGITIS WITH RAISED ICP & SEIZURES

o Stepwise management of seizures:
- IV lorazepam 0.1 mg/kg or Midazolam IV or buccal (0.5 mg/kg)

- **Paraldehyde 0.4 ml/kg PR**
- **Phenytoin infusion 18 mg/kg over 30 mins** with ECG monitoring
- For persistent seizures **Thiopentone 4 mg/kg** (intubated patients only), or midazolam/thiopentone infusions should be considered with paediatric neuro-intensive care advice.

SEPTICAEMIA WITH SHOCK

- **INOTROPES**
  o The peripheral inotrope of choice is **Dopamine started at 10 mcg/Kg/min.**
  o **Adrenaline infusion** should be commenced if there is ongoing haemodynamic instability requiring large volume fluid resuscitation and escalation in inotrope dose.
  o This should be given centrally or intraosseously.

- **COAGULOPATHY**
  o Give **10 ml/Kg FFP or 5 ml/Kg cryoprecipitate** if fibrinogen less than 1 g/dL.
  o Consider **transfusing packed red cells to maintain Hb >10 g/dL.**

- **STEROIDS**
  o Corticosteroids are only indicated in meningococcal septicaemia **with shock refractory to inotropes at 60 minutes**, when **carefully titrated hydrocortisone** may be considered to cover for absolute adrenal insufficiency.

PROPHYLAXIS

- **Prophylaxis** should be given **within 24 hours** of diagnosis to:
  o **Household members** who have had prolonged close contact within 7 days before the onset illness (also consider child minders who may be looking after the child for a number of hours, pupils in a same dormitory)
  o **Kissing contacts** i.e. boyfriends/girlfriends
  o **Healthcare workers** who have had direct exposure to droplets/respiratory secretions prior to completion of 24 hours of antibiotics (not required in nurseries/schools with isolated cases unless close contact)

- **Dosage:**
  o **Rifampicin 600 mg every 12 hours for 2 days;**
  o **Children Rifampicin 10 mg/kg bd for 2 days;**
  o **Infants Rifampicin 5 mg/kg bd for 2 days**
  o Other alternatives for adults are **ciprofloxacin** and **ceftriaxone.**

II. THE CHILD POISONED WITH OPIATES

- These children are usually toddlers who have drunk the green liquid form of methadone.
- The sedative effect of the drug may reduce the conscious level sufficiently to put the airway at risk and cause hypoventilation.

EMERGENCY TREATMENT OF OPIATE POISONING

- **Reassess ABC**
- Following stabilisation of airway, breathing and circulation, the specific antidote is **Naloxone.**
- An initial bolus dose of **10 micrograms/kg** is used but some children need doses as high as 100 micrograms/kg, up to a maximum of 2 mg.
- Naloxone has a short half-life, relapse often occurring after 20 minutes.
- Further boluses, or an **infusion of 10–20 micrograms/kg/min**, may be required.
- It is important to normalise carbon dioxide before the naloxone is given because adverse events such as ventricular arrhythmias, acute pulmonary oedema, asystole or seizures may otherwise occur.
- This is because the opioid system and the adrenergic system are inter-related.
- **Opioid antagonists and hypercapnia stimulate sympathetic nervous system activity.**
- Therefore, if ventilation is not provided to normalise carbon dioxide prior to naloxone administration, the sudden rise in adrenaline concentration can cause arrhythmias.

III. THE CHILD WITH METABOLIC COMA

- The most common metabolic disorders that can result in encephalopathy are **hypoglycaemia** and **diabetic ketoacidosis** (see Chapter 4).
- Nevertheless, metabolic coma can arise from a variety of conditions, including a number of rare, inborn errors of metabolism.
- These illnesses often present with a rapidly progressive encephalopathy, vomiting, drowsiness and convulsions or coma.
- There may be associated hepatomegaly (from fatty change), hypoglycaemia, abnormal liver enzymes or hyperammonaemia.
- In a case of otherwise unexplained coma with a GCS of <12, a key urgent investigation is a **plasma ammonia**. Interpretation of the concentration can be difficult, as can specific treatment of the hyperammonaemia. In this event seek advice from a specialist in inherited metabolic disease and the paediatric intensive care unit.

IV. APPROACH TO THE CHILD WITH MALARIA

- **Plasmodium falciparum** causes 95% of deaths and most severe complications.
- It is transmitted by the bite of an infected Anopheles mosquito, and less commonly by infected blood transfusion, needle stick injuries or by the transplacental route.
- The clinical features of severe disease include reduced conscious level, convulsions, metabolic acidosis, hypoglycaemia and severe normocytic anaemia.
- Cerebral malaria may produce encephalopathy, rapid-onset coma and raised intracranial pressure.
- Diagnosis requires microscopy of a **thick film** (quick diagnosis) and **thin film** (species identification).
- Obtain a complete history for the laboratory, including the likely country or region of origination.

ED TREATMENT OF CEREBRAL MALARIA

- Reassess ABCDE
- **IV/IO artesunate** (2.4 mg/kg on admission, then at 12 and 24 hours, then OD) is the recommended treatment for severe P. falciparum malaria.
- **Quinine** is an acceptable alternative if artesunate is not available (loading dose **20 mg/kg over 4 hours in glucose 5% then 10 mg/kg every 8 hours**). Give with ECG monitoring.
- Consider antibiotics, e.g. **IV cefotaxime** since the risk of concomitant bacterial (Gram-negative) infections is high in children.
- **Monitor and treat hypoglycaemia** as needed.
- If there is evidence of life-threatening anaemia (haemoglobin <5 g/dl) consider transfusion, especially if there are signs of heart failure.
- Be cautious with fluid administration!

V. THE CHILD WITH SYNCOPE

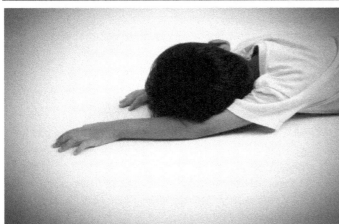

Paediatric Syncope- Image Source: blog.doctoroz.com

INTRODUCTION

- Syncope is defined as the temporary loss of consciousness resulting from a reversible disturbance of cerebral function. It is characterized by a loss of consciousness because of a lack of cerebral blood flow; rapid or sudden onset; falls by the patient if he or she is not supported; and transient attacks. In children, it is most often benign, but may sometimes herald a more serious and potentially life-threatening cause.

- Syncope is not an uncommon problem because it is estimated that 20% of all children will experience at least one episode of fainting before the end of adolescence[160]. Before the age of six years, syncope is unusual except in patients with seizure disorders, breath-holding episodes and primary cardiac dysrhythmias.

CAUSES

1. **Neurally mediated syncope (NMS) or Vasovagal syndrome**
2. **Cardiovascular syncope**
   o **Primary**
      - Left ventricular outflow obstruction
      - Right ventricular outflow obstruction
      - Pulmonary hypertension
      - Eisenmenger
      - Cardiomyopathy
   o **Arrhythmias**
      - **Tachyarrhythmias**
         - Long QT syndrome
         - Brugada syndrome (familial ventricular fibrillation)
         - Wolff-Parkinson-White syndrome
         - Supraventricular tachycardia
         - Ventricular tachycardia
            o Postoperative
            o Idiopathic
            o Right ventricular dysplasia
      - **Bradyarrhythmias**
         - Sick sinus syndrome
         - Heart block

3. Noncardiovascular syncope
   o Basilar migraine
   o Seizures
   o Vertigo
   o Hyperventilation
   o Situational (cough, micturition, stretch, hair grooming, defecation)
   o Breath-holding spells

- NMS, or vasovagal syncope, is the most common cause of syncope in young patients. It seems to be related to the beta-adrenergic hypersensitivity of baroreceptors in the vessels and the mechanoreceptors of the left ventricle after subtle changes in postural tone, circulating volume or the direct release of catecholamine from higher cerebral centres. This hypersensitivity results in an efferent response consisting of peripheral alpha-adrenergic withdrawal and enhanced parasympathetic tone.

- NMS is recognized by a constellation of signs and symptoms, beginning with a prodrome that lasts several seconds to minutes, progressing to a brief period of unconsciousness. The episode may be initiated by one of many provocative events that usually consist of emotional stress such as fear, anxiety or sudden change in posture.

- Other precipitating states include anemia, dehydration, hunger, physical exhaustion and a crowded or poorly ventilated environment.

- Premonitory symptoms include lightheadedness, dizziness, nausea, shortness of breath, pallor, diaphoresis and visual changes.

- Vasodepressor syncope that is associated with exercise has been well described in paediatric patients and most commonly occurs immediately after the termination of an activity.

- Cardiac syncope is less common than NMS, but a thorough evaluation is required to ensure the detection of potentially life-threatening diagnoses and to provide accurate prognostic information.

---

[160] Manolis AS. Evaluation of patients with syncope: Focus on age-related differences. J Am Coll Cardiol. 1994;3:13–8.

- Other situations or illnesses that can cause syncope or mimic syncope include:
  o Head injury
  o Seizure
  o Stroke
  o Inner ear problems
  o Dehydration
  o Low blood sugar
  o Breath holding episodes (Typically in children 6 month to 2 years of age)
  o Pregnancy
  o Anemia
  o Brain mass
  o Aneurysm or abnormality of the blood vessels of the brain
  o Urination
  o Having a bowel movement
  o Coughing

RISK FACTORS THAT SUGGEST CARDIAC SYNCOPE

Little or no prodrome

Prolonged loss of consciousness (longer than 5 min)

Exercise-induced syncope

Chest pain or palpitations

History of cardiac disease

Familial history of long QT syndrome, cardiomyopathy or sudden death

CLINICAL SYMPTOMS

- Some children will have symptoms before they faint.
- A child may have:
  o Dizziness
  o Lightheadedness
  o Nausea
  o Changes in his or her vision
  o Cold, damp skin
- There may be enough warning signs that your child will have time to sit or lie down before fainting occurs. This can prevent injuries that may happen because of falling during syncope, such as head injury.

INVESTIGATIONS

- **Should be aimed at suspected cause, but every patient presenting with syncope should at least have:**
  o ECG
  o Blood glucose
  o Lying and standing BP
  o Vital signs
  o Detailed systemic examination

- **Consider doing:**
  o Tilt test to confirm autonomic dysfunction.
  o Urine dipstix
  o FBC and electrolytes
  o Imaging: CXR, CT head
  o EEG

ED MANAGEMENT OF PAEDIATRIC SYNCOPE

- In NMS, the first line of treatment is behaviour modification.
- Conservative therapy is mandatory because there is a tendency for children to grow out of the propensity for syncope.
- It has been suggested that resolution is related to the recognition of prodromal symptoms and early interventions.
- The patient is advised to avoid dehydration, long periods of standing and irregular mealtimes. Other simple measures include water and table salt intake to increase plasma volume.
- When syncope persists despite behavioural changes, medical therapy can be used and usually includes a beta-blocker or fludrocortisone.
- Further therapy is rarely required. Avoidance of potentially toxic drugs is the rule; however, disopyramide has been used with success in some cases[161].
- Pacemaker therapy is rarely used.
- For cardiac syncope, the therapy is usually more clearly defined and directed to the underlying cause.
- It includes beta-blocker therapy in cases of long QT syndrome, medical therapy for some forms of cardiomyopathy, surgical resection for cardiac obstructive lesions and pacemaker therapy for a sick sinus or heart block.
- An implantable defibrillator is rarely required in cases of ressuscitated cardiac arrest or high risk familial disease (such as long QT syndrome, Brugada syndrome and hypertrophic cardiomyopathy).

---

[161] *A placebo-controlled trial of intravenous and oral disopyramide for prevention of neurally mediated syncope induced by head-up tilt.*

Morillo CA, Leitch JW, Yee R, Klein GJ, J Am Coll Cardiol. 1993 Dec; 22(7):1843-8.

6. Abdominal Pain

1. DIFFERENTIAL DIAGNOSIS OF AN ACUTE ABDOMEN BASED ON AGE GROUP

Age	Emergent	Non-Emergent
0-3 months	• Necrotizing enterocolitis • Volvulus • Testicular torsion • Incarcerated hernia • Trauma • Toxic megacolon • Tumor	• Colic • Acute gastroenteritis • Constipation
3 months - 3-year-old	• Intussusceptions • Testicular torsion • Trauma • Volvulus • Appendicitis • Toxic megacolon • Vaso-occlusive crisis	• Acute gastroenteritis • Constipation • Urinary tract infections • HSP

I. HYPERTROPHIC PYLORIC STENOSIS

- Hypertrophic pyloric stenosis (HPS) causes a functional gastric outlet obstruction as a result of hypertrophy and hyperplasia of the muscular layers of the pylorus.
- In infants, HPS is the most common cause of gastric outlet obstruction and the most common surgical cause of vomiting.

THE CLINICAL FEATURES INCLUDE:

o Typical presentation is onset of initially **nonbloody**, always **nonbilious** vomiting at **4-8 weeks of age.**

o Although vomiting may initially be infrequent, over several days it becomes more predictable, occurring at nearly every feeding.

o Vomiting intensity also increases until pathognomonic **projectile vomiting** ensues.

o **Slight hematemesis** of either bright-red flecks or a coffee-ground appearance is sometimes observed.

o Patients are usually not ill-looking or febrile; the baby in the early stage of the disease **remains hungry and sucks vigorously** after episodes of vomiting.

o Prolonged delay in diagnosis can lead to dehydration, poor weight gain, malnutrition, metabolic alterations, and lethargy.

o Parents often report trying several different baby formulas because they (or their physicians) assume vomiting is due to intolerance.

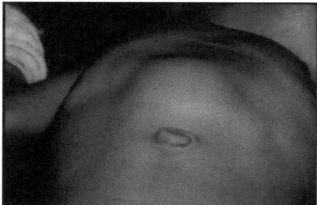

o An **olive-sized lump** may be palpable in the epigastrium (most prominent during a feed).

DIAGNOSIS:

o **Mainly clinical:** The child may develop **hypochloraemic alkalosis** and **hypokalaemia** due to recurrent vomiting of gastric contents.

o **Ultrasound**: Diagnostic of choice

o **Barium** upper GI study

o **Endoscopy**

ED MANAGEMENT

o Directed at correcting the fluid deficiency and electrolyte imbalance

o Base fluid resuscitation on the infant's degree of dehydration.

o Most infants can have their fluid status corrected within 24 hours; however, severely dehydrated children sometimes require several days for correction.

o If necessary, administer an initial fluid bolus **of 10 mL/kg with Hartmann's solution** or **0.45 isotonic sodium chloride solution**

o Keeping the infant nil by mouth.

o Correction of electrolyte abnormalities, including hypoglycaemia.

o Referral to the paediatric surgical team for **pylorotomy.**

II. THE CHILD WITH INTUSSUSCEPTION

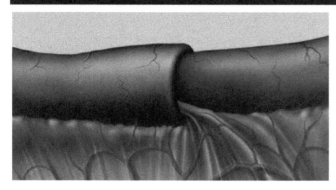

- Intussusception is the invagination of one segment of bowel into an adjacent lower segment, causing bowel obstruction.

- With early diagnosis, appropriate fluid resuscitation, and therapy, the mortality rate from intussusception in children is less than 1%. If left untreated, however, this condition is uniformly fatal in 2-5 days.

- It typically affects children aged between **6 months and 4 years.**

- It may affect the small or large bowel, but most cases are **ileocolic.**

- Intussusception can rapidly compromise the blood supply to the bowel making relief of this form of obstruction urgent.

- Usually no underlying cause is found although there is some evidence that viral infection leads to enlargement of Peyer's patches, which may form the lead point of the intussusception.

- Occasionally a Meckel's diverticulum, polyp, or lymphoma is the lead point.

CLINICAL FEATURES INCLUDE:

o **Vomiting:** Initially, vomiting is nonbilious and reflexive, but when the intestinal obstruction occurs, vomiting becomes bilious

o **Abdominal pain:** Pain in intussusception is colicky, severe, and intermittent

o **Passage of blood and mucus:** Parents report the passage of stools, by affected children, that look like "Redcurrant jelly' stool"; this is a mixture of mucus, sloughed mucosa, and shed blood;

o **Diarrheoa** can also be an early sign of intussusception

o **Lethargy:** This can be the sole presenting symptom of intussusception, which makes the condition's diagnosis challenging.

o **Palpable abdominal mass** and occasionally a "sausage-shaped" mass may be visible.

o **Dehydration and Pyrexia.**

o Occasionally the child presents **shocked** without an obvious cause.

DIAGNOSIS

o **Radiography:** Plain abdominal radiography reveals signs that suggest intussusception in only 60% of cases

o **Ultrasonography:** Hallmarks of ultrasonography include the **target sign** and "pseudokidney signs".

o **Barium enema:** This is the traditional and most reliable way to make the diagnosis of intussusception in children.

o A barium enema characteristically reveals a '**coiled spring' sign** or **sudden termination of the barium.** A barium enema is contraindicated if there is evidence of perforation, which requires surgical intervention.

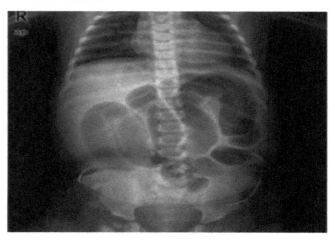

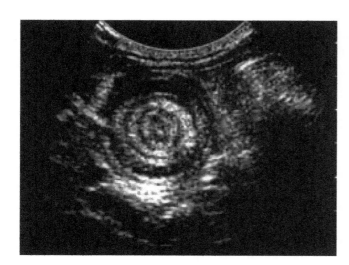

MANAGEMENT:

o IV Fluid resuscitation to Correct dehydration
o Initial blood tests and blood gas
o Analgesia
o Nil per month
o Nasogastric tube
o Refer to paediatric surgery

III. THE CHILD WITH VOLVULUS

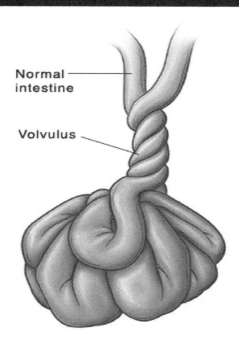

Normal intestine

Volvulus

ABDOMINAL RADIOGRAPHS

o Will show a large, dilated loop of colon, often with a few air-fluid levels.
o **Specific signs include:**
   ▪ **Coffee bean sign**
   ▪ **Frimann Dahl's sign** - three dense lines converge towards site of obstruction
   ▪ **Absent rectal gas**

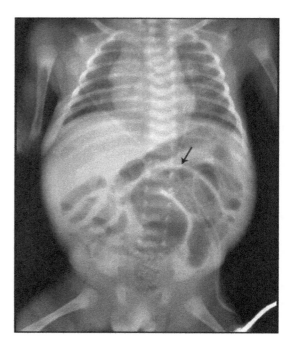

- Volvulus may be due to congenital malrotations, Meckel's diverticulum, or adhesions from previous surgery.
- Congenital malrotations are the most frequent and result from the abnormal movement of the intestine around the superior mesenteric artery during embryological development.

CLINICAL FEATURES INCLUDE:

o Abdominal pain.
o Vomiting.
o Abdominal distension.

7. BRUE, the New ALTE

Brief Resolved Unexplained Event – BRUE [162]

DEFINITION OF BRUE:

- Event lasting <1 minute in an infant <1 year of age that is associated with at least one of the following:
  - Cyanosis or pallor;
  - Absent, decreased, or irregular breathing;
  - Marked change in muscle tone (hypertonia or hypotonia);
  - Altered level of responsiveness
- Patient must otherwise be well-appearing and back to baseline health at the time of presentation, and, on evaluation, have no condition that could explain the event. The event occurs suddenly, lasts less than 30 to 60 seconds, and is frightening to the person caring for the infant.
- BRUE is present only when there is no explanation for the event after a thorough history and exam.
- An older name used for these types of events is an **apparent life-threatening event (ALTE).**

CAUSES OF BRUE

- It is unclear how often these events occur.
- BRUE is NOT the same as sudden infant death syndrome (SIDS). It is also NOT the same as older terms such as "near-miss SIDS" or "aborted crib deaths," which are no longer used.
- Events that involve a change in an infant's breathing, color, muscle tone, or behavior may be caused by an underlying medical problem.
- But these events would then NOT be considered a BRUE. Some of the causes for events that are NOT a BRUE include:
  - Reflux after eating
  - Severe infections (such as bronchiolitis, whooping cough)
  - Birth defects that involve the face, throat, or neck
  - Birth defects of the heart or lungs
  - Allergic reactions
  - A brain, nerve, or muscle disorder
  - Child abuse
  - Certain uncommon genetic disorders

A specific cause of the event is found about half the time. In healthy children who only have one event, the cause is rarely identified.

RISK FACTORS OF BRUE

The main risk factors for BRUE are:

- A prior episode when the child stopped breathing, turned pale, or had blue coloring
- Feeding problems
- Recent head cold or bronchitis
- Age younger than 10 weeks

Low birth weight, being born early, or second-hand smoke exposure also may be risk factors.

CRITERIA FOR DESIGNATING LOWER RISK:

- Age >60 days
- Gestational age ≥32 weeks and postconceptional age ≥45 weeks
- First BRUE
- No cardiopulmonary resuscitation (CPR) required by trained medical provider
- No features in the history of concern (e.g., possible child abuse, family history of sudden unexplained death, toxic exposures)
- No worrisome physical exam findings (e.g., bruising, cardiac murmurs, organomegaly).

ED MANAGEMENT OF BRUE

- In the ED, the clinician can monitor the low-risk patient briefly (1 to 4 hours) with continuous pulse oximetry and serial observations to ensure that vital signs and symptomatology remain stable.
- Physicians might also consider obtaining pertussis testing, as well as a 12-lead electrocardiogram to eliminate channelopathies, based on clinical suspicion. The most considerable change from previous practice is the emphasis on not admitting patients to the hospital merely for the purpose of cardiopulmonary monitoring and also on limiting overtesting.
- Performing no tests might be challenging to some physicians, especially under pressure from concerned caregivers. Nevertheless, the guidelines stress the lack of benefit of generic laboratory work in low-risk patients.
- Specific recommendations are not offered for patients who fall into a higher-risk category; it is likely that a more thorough evaluation and period of observation is appropriate for these infants.

---

[162] Tieder JS et al. Brief resolved unexplained events (formerly apparent life-threatening events) and evaluation of lower-risk infants. Pediatrics 2016 May; 137:e20160590. (http://dx.doi.org/10.1542/peds.2016-0590)

8. Blood Disorders

I. APPROACH TO HENOCH-SCHÖNLEIN PURPURA

CAUSES OF PURPURA INCLUDE

- *Meningococcal disease*
- *Henoch–Schönlein purpura*
- *Thrombocytopenia, e.g. ITP*
- *Leukaemia, Septic shock, or Aplastic anaemia*
- *Enteroviral infection*
- *Trauma*
- *Forceful coughing or vomiting.*

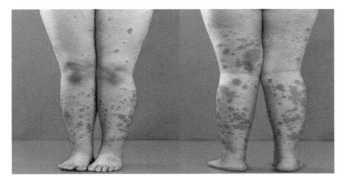

- **Henoch–Schönlein purpura** (also called **IgA vasculitis (IgAV))** is a vasculitic condition that affects the small arteries of the kidneys, skin, and gastrointestinal tract. It usually affects children between the **ages of 3 and 10 years old.**
- It is twice as common in boys, peaks during the winter months, and is often preceded by an upper respiratory tract infection.

1. CLINICAL FEATURES INCLUDE:

- **Rash:** erythematous macules develop into purpuric lesions, which are characteristically concentrated over the buttocks and extensor surfaces of the lower limbs.
- **Arthralgia:** particularly the knees and ankles.
- **Peri-articular oedema**
- **GIT:** Abdominal pain, N&V, Bloody diarrhoea
- **Haematuria:** due to glomerulonephritis

2. ED INVESTIGATIONS

- **Urinalysis:** which may reveal micro- or macroscopic haematuria, and/or proteinuria.
- **U&E:** occasionally nephrotic syndrome and renal failure develop.
- **Blood pressure:** hypertension is a risk factor for progressive renal disease.
- **FBC:** to ensure a normal platelet count and exclude thrombocytopenia as a cause.

3. COMPLICATIONS

- Renal failure: involvement occurs in 50% of older children but is only serious in approximately 10% of patients. Less than 1% of patients with HSP progress to end-stage kidney disease.
- Intussusception (in 2-3% of patients),
- Gastrointestinal bleeding,
- Bowel infarction,
- Myocardial infarction,
- Pulmonary haemorrhage,
- Pleural effusion,
- Seizures
- Mononeuropathies.

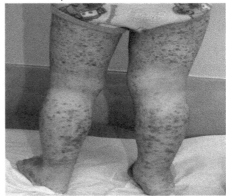

4. ED MANAGEMENT OF HSP

- **Mainly symptomatic:**
  - Adequate oral hydration/bed rest
  - Symptomatic relief of joint and abdominal pain:
    - **Naproxen 10 to 20 mg/kg** BD (maximum 1500 mg per day)
    - **Oral Prednisone 1 to 2 mg/kg per day** (maximum dose of 60 to 80 mg per day)
    - **IV Methylprednisolone 0.8 to 1.6 mg/kg per day (maximum dose of 64 mg/day)**
  - Paediatric referral.
- **Hospitalization is indicated in:**
  - Fail to maintain oral hydration and require the administration of intravenous fluids.
  - Patients who have significant gastrointestinal bleeding, severe abdominal pain, changes in mental status, severe joint involvement limiting ambulation and/or self-care, or evidence of significant renal disease (elevated creatinine, hypertension, or proteinuria).

II. APPROACH TO CHILD WITH SICKLE CELL

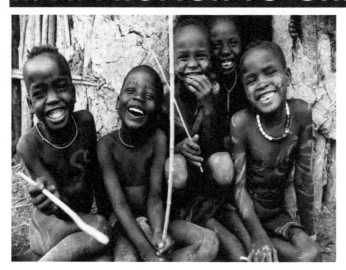

1. OVERVIEW
- Sickle cell disease is caused by **HbS hemoglobinopathy** which produces rigid, distorted and dysfunctional erythrocytes called sickle cells.

2. CAUSE
- **Types of sickle cell disease**
  - Sickle cell anaemia (homozygous SS genotype)
  - Sickle beta thalassemia
  - Sickle HbC disease

3. PRECIPITANTS
- **Commonly:**
  - Infection
  - Dehydration
  - Hypoxia
  - Drugs (e.g. Sedatives, local anaesthetics)
  - Functional asplenia typically develops in childhood.
- Prophylactic treatment with hydroxyurea can cause neutropenia and cardiomyopathy.
- Patients with sickle cell disease are at risk of infection due to underlying immunosuppression.

4. PRESENTATIONS
- Types of sickle cell crisis presentations:
  - Infections
  - Vaso-occlusive crisis
  - Acute chest syndrome
  - Acute splenic sequestration
  - Aplastic crisis
  - Stroke
  - Priapism
  - Bone pain: The long bones of the extremities are often involved, often due to bone marrow infarction

- Anaemia: Universally present, chronic, and haemolytic in nature
- Hand-foot syndrome: This is a **dactylitis** presenting as bilateral painful and swollen hands and/or feet in children
- Ophthalmologic involvement: Ptosis, retinal vascular changes, proliferative retinitis
- Cardiac involvement: Dilation of both ventricles and the left atrium
- GI involvement: Cholelithiasis is common in children; liver may become involved
- GU involvement: Kidneys lose concentrating capacity; priapism is a well-recognized complication of SCD
- Dermatologic involvement: Leg ulcers are a chronic painful problem

5. ASSESSMENT
- Always consider the presence of all types of sickle cell crisis, regardless of the dominant presentation:
  - Symptoms and signs of local and systemic infection
  - Respiratory signs and symptoms
  - Increasing spleen size
  - Shock and evidence of organ failure
  - Baseline and current Hb
  - CXR if fever, chest pain or hypoxia
  - CT Head if stroke suspected
  - Consider MSU, FBC, reticulocytes, bilirubin, haemolytic screen and cross-match
  - Abdominal ultrasound if crisis is in abdomen.
  - Blood film: sickle cells and evidence of hemolysis (e.g. target cells, schistocytes)

6. ED MANAGEMENT OF SICKLE CELL DISEASE
- **Immediate treatment in the ED**
  - **Assess pain and give analgesia:**
    - **Morphine**: Assess 20 min after administration.
    - If more than one dose is required, use a **Diamorphine 10 mcg/kg/hour** infusion pump.
    - Start with a high dose and reduce once pain control is achieved.
  - **Keep patient warm and well hydrated,** Reassure patient: **IV fluid: Dextrose-saline with KCL.**
  - **Assess O₂ saturation:** Use O₂ via face mask if necessary.
  - **Antibiotherapy:**
    - Is patient taking Penicillin regularly? If not, consider **IV Penicillin.**
    - Advise to **double dose of Penicillin** at sign of infection or start of crisis.

- If already taking Penicillin change antibiotic to **Cephalosporin**.
- If Penicillin and Cephalosporin not acceptable, then give **IV Erythromycin** - give <u>slowly</u> as it can be irritant to veins.
  - **Anti-emetic:** Metoclopramide.
  - **Reassess pain:** If pain settles after 1 hour, discharge home. Follow up with haematology.
  - **Admit if:**
    - The pain is not controlled after 1 hour, or is severe
    - Patient is pyrexial or signs of infection. (Most sickle cell crises are precipitated by infection.)

1. THE CHILD WITH ACUTE CHEST SYNDROME

- Acute chest syndrome is sequestration within the lungs. It is characterised by:
  - Pyrexia (The temperature > 38°C)
  - Chest pain or acute respiratory distress
  - Often bilateral lung consolidation
  - Tachycardia and tachypnoea.
  - Cough is a late symptom
- Hypoxia sets up a vicious cycle of sickling within the lungs.
- Very difficult to reverse, early prompt and effective treatment is vital.
- This is a haematological emergency and must be discussed with haematology.

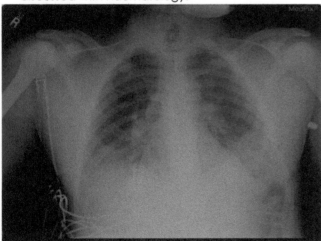

MANAGEMENT OF ACUTE CHEST SYNDROME
- Oxygen - monitor with pulse oximeter
- Blood gases
- Urgent CXR
- IV antibiotics - Penicillin and Cephalosporin
- IV fluids & Analgesia
- Inform Haematologist on duty as exchange transfusion may be indicated
- Inform Consultant Anaesthetist as ventilation may be necessary.

2. THE CHILD WITH APLASTIC CRISIS

- The production of red cells by the bone marrow may be reduced after an infection.
- An individual with sickle cell relies on the constant activity of the bone marrow to produce enough red cells to survive.
- The life span of their blood cells is 15 - 20 days, if there is a rapid fall in the Hb without reticulocyte response, this should be taken very seriously.
- Therefore, an aplastic crisis can be lethal.
- **Parvovirus** which presents like influenza is the usual cause of an aplastic crisis that follows an infection.
- Check: Hb, Reticulocyte count, Folate level, Parvovirus antigen & Antibody titre.
- **Transfuse** if no reticulocyte response, but inform Haematologist first.

3. THE CHILD WITH ACUTE SPLENIC SEQUESTRATION

- Acute splenic sequestration is caused by the spleen enlarging during the crisis and results from massive sickling in the spleen and hepatic sinuses.
- There is a precipitate fall in the patient's normal haemoglobin level of **more than 2 g/dl** from steady state and a marked increase of reticulocytes in the peripheral blood.
- Acute splenic sequestration is characterised by:
  - Sudden onset of tachypnoea,
  - Pallor,
  - Abdominal pain and Splenic enlargement.

- This may be precipitated **by fever, dehydration and hypoxia.** Rapid sequestration of the red cells leads to **sudden anaemia** and **death** from hypoxic cardiac failure with pulmonary oedema.
- This is most common in children and infants under the age of 5 years.
- It is useful to teach the parent(s) to palpate the spleen in these children so that if they become ill and the spleen enlarges, they know that they must get the child to hospital quickly.

INVESTIGATIONS:
- WBC, U&Es, Hb, Reticulocytes,
- Group and X-Match, Blood Cultures,

MANAGEMENT OF ACUTE SPLENIC SEQUESTRATION
- **IV access**
- **Packed red cells transfusion** without delay
- If shocked, **start colloid infusion** while waiting for blood
- **Broad spectrum antibiotics** - <u>IV Penicillin and Cephalosporin.</u> This should offer some protection against pneumococcus and haemophilus influenza
- If breathless - **urgent CXR**
- Inform Haematologist on-call.

4. THE CHILD WITH PRIAPISM IN SICKLE CELL DISEASE

- This is a painful persistent erection of the penis caused by intravascular sickling in the erectile tissue.
- If priapism persists for more than 12 hours this can lead to damage of the erectile tissue which results in the patient being unable to get an erection.
- This can lead **to permanent impotence.**

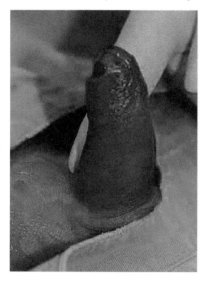

MANAGEMENT OF PRIAPISM IN SICKLE CELL SYNDROME

- Give **adequate analgesia**
- **Reassure** and keep the patient **warm**
- Re-hydrate - **IV fluids**
- Contact Urologist and Haematologist immediately
- Sedate? **IV Diazepam**
- **Group and save** - consult Haematologist before transfusing
- Surgical intervention may be necessary if there is no improvement
- **Do not use ice packs**

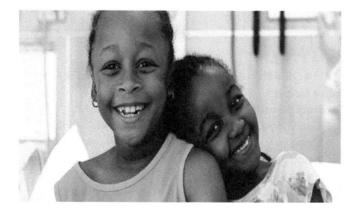

5. THE CHILD WITH OSTEOMYELITIS

- Consider particularly if any localised pain fails to resolve within 48 hours.
- Osteomyelitis most often results from infection with **Haemophilus, staphylococcus or salmonella.**
- If no resolution of fever or swelling **within 48 hours:**
  - Repeat Blood cultures
  - X-Ray affected area
  - Review antibiotics
  - Obtain an orthopaedic opinion.
- **Admission to ward from the ED**
  - Patients usually go to the haematology team
  - Inform Haematologist as soon as possible

6. THE CHILD WITH HAND FOOT SYNDROME: "DACTYLITIS"

- Early complication of SCD
- Highest incidence 6 months to 2 years
- Painful swelling of hands and feet
- Treatment involves fluids and pain medication
- Fevers treated as medical emergency

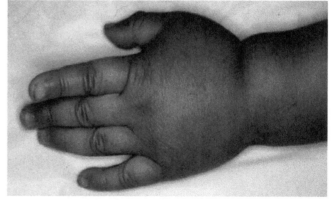

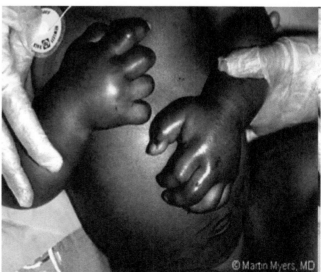

9. Concerning Presentations
I. APPROACH TO NON-ACCIDENTAL INJURIES

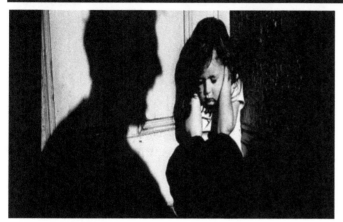

1. THE CHILD WITH PHYSICAL ABUSE

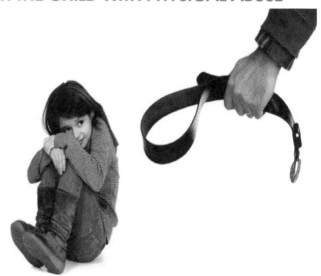

SUSCEPTIBILITY TO ABUSE

- The possibility of child ill treatment or abuse must be considered in the differential diagnosis of all children who have suffered injury.
- Child abuse/ill treatment occurs in all social classes.
- However, the possible features of parenting known to be associated with child ill treatment or abuse include:
  - Where the relationship between the parent and child does not appear loving and caring
  - Where one or both parents have been abused themselves as children
  - Parents who are young, single, unsupportive or substitutive
  - Parents with learning difficulties
  - Parents who have a poor or unstable relationship
  - Situations where there is domestic violence or drug or alcohol dependence
  - Parents who have mental illness or personality disorders
- **Factors in the child that make them vulnerable to abuse and ill treatment include:**
  - Prematurity
  - Separation and impaired bonding in the neonatal period
  - Physical or mental handicap
  - Behavioural problems
  - Difficult temperament or personality
  - Soiling and wetting past developmental age
  - Hyperactivity and attention deficit
  - Screaming or crying interminably and inconsolably

- A form of abuse that may involve hitting, shaking, throwing, poisoning, burning or scalding, drowning, suffocating or otherwise causing physical harm to a child.
- Physical harm may also be caused when a parent or carer fabricates the symptoms of, or deliberately induces, illness in a child.

RECOGNITION OF A CHILD WITH PHYSICAL ABUSE

- As highlighted above, abuse should always be considered as a potential differential diagnosis.
- It can often be rapidly excluded but if it is not thought about it will be missed.
- In emergency paediatrics consider the following key areas:
  - Asphyxial event: suffocation, hanging
  - Subdural haemorrhage
  - Poisoning and other induced illness (e.g. septicaemia)
  - Ruptured abdominal viscus
  - Cervical spine injury
  - Rib cage and long bone fractures
  - Drowning
  - Burns

PRESENTATIONS OF PHYSICAL ABUSE

1. HEAD INJURIES

o Fractures, intracranial injury: These may present as an acute life-threatening event with breathing difficulty or apnoea, or with raised intracranial pressure including symptoms or signs of poor feeding, vomiting, drowsiness and seizures

2. THE SHAKEN BABY SYNDROME

- Abusive head trauma, also known as **shaken baby syndrome**, is the most common cause of child abuse death, usually occurring during the first year of life.
- Shaking or blunt head trauma can result in cranial injuries such as **unilateral or bilateral subdural hemorrhage, diffuse retinal hemorrhage, and diffuse brain injury.**

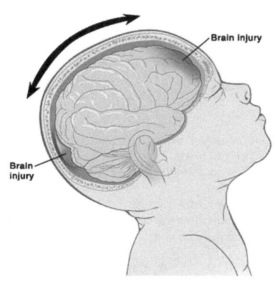

- **Retinal haemorrhages**, often multilayered, occur in 60-85 % of non-accidental head injuries and are uncommon in accidental head trauma.
- The diagnosis of abusive head trauma is often missed since often no history of head trauma is provided and the signs and symptoms may be non-specific, such as vomiting, poor feeding, irritability or lethargy.
- Some caregivers may only present for medical care if more severe symptoms arise such as seizure, apnea or coma.
- The majority of children have an abnormal neurological exam but many will have no external signs of injury

3. INTERNAL DAMAGE

o e.g. rupture of bowel

4. BURNS AND SCALDS

o 'Glove and Stocking' appearance for scalds, implement imprints for contact burns

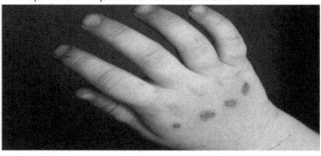

5. CUTS AND BRUISES

o Imprints of hands, sticks, whips, belts, bites, etc. may be present
o Bruising in a non-mobile infant

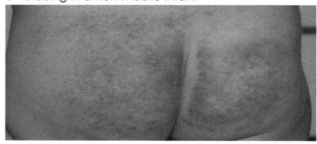

6. COLD INJURY

o Hypothermia,
o Frostbite

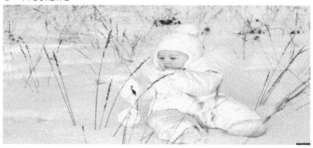

7. POISONING

o Drugs or household substances

8. SUFFOCATION

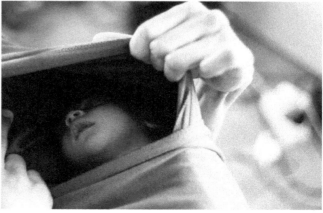

9. FRACTURES

- Any fracture in a young child should be concerning, especially if the child is not ambulating.
- If an infant is **pulled or wrenched**, the corner of the metaphysis can be torn, commonly referred to as a **"bucket handle" fracture**.

A. BUCKET HANDLE FRACTURES

o **Metaphyseal corner fractures**, also known as **classical metaphyseal lesions** (CML) or **bucket handle fractures**, are observed in young children, less than 2 years old.

o It is considered pathognomic for non-accidental injury (NAI).

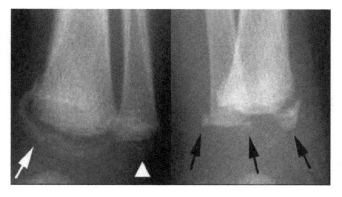

B. SPIRAL FRACTURES

o **Finding spiral fractures** in the bone shaft is indicative of a twisting injury rather than a transverse fracture from direct impact.

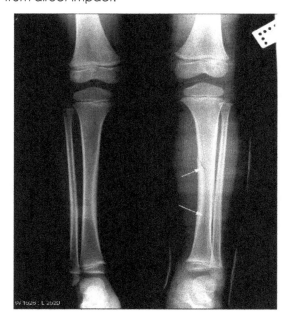

C. FEMUR FRACTURES

o **Femur fractures prior to the age of walking** are especially concerning, as are bilateral long-bone fractures.

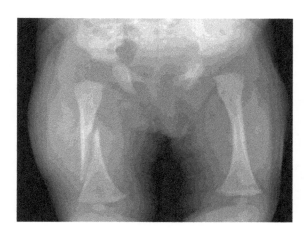

D. RIBS, STERNUM AND SCAPULA FRACTURES

o Violent squeezing of an infant's chest results in **anterior and/or posterior rib fractures** which are difficult to acquire with other injuries as children's ribs are flexible.

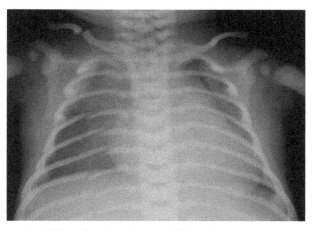

o Additionally, **fractures of the sternum, scapula, or spinous processes** are unusual in the paediatric population.

E. SKULL FRACTURES

o Result from a direct force on the calvarium and are very uncommon in children less than 18 months.

o In non-accidental trauma, they most commonly occur as linear fractures in the parietal bone and can often be complex in nature.

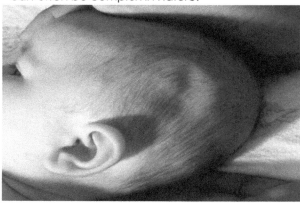

2. THE CHILD WITH SEXUAL ABUSE

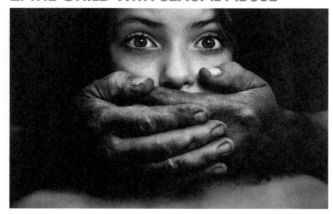

- Involves forcing or enticing a child or young person to take part in sexual activities, not necessarily involving a high level of violence, whether or not the child is aware of what is happening.
- The activities may involve physical contact, including assault by penetration (e.g. rape or oral sex) or non-penetrative acts such as masturbation, kissing, rubbing and touching outside of clothing.
- They may also include non-contact activities, such as involving children in looking at, or in the production of, sexual images, watching sexual activities, encouraging children to behave in sexually inappropriate ways, or grooming a child in preparation for abuse (including via the internet).
- Sexual abuse is not solely perpetrated by adult males. Women can also commit acts of sexual abuse, as can other children.

PRESENTATIONS OF SEXUAL ABUSE

o Disclosure by child
o Disclosure by witness
o Suspicion by third party because of the behaviour of the child, especially changes in behaviour. These include:
  - Insecurity;
  - Fear of men;
  - Sleep disorders;
  - Mood changes,
  - Tantrums and aggression at home;
  - Anxiety,
  - Despair,
  - Withdrawal and secretiveness;
  - Poor peer relationships;
  - Lying,
  - Stealing or arson;
  - School failure;
  - Eating disorders like anorexia and compulsive overeating;
  - Running away and truancy;

- Suicide attempts,
- Self-poisoning,
- Self-mutilation and abuse of drugs,
- Solvents and alcohol;
- Unexplained acquisition of money;
- Sexualised behaviour such as drawings with a sexual content;
- knowledge of adult sexual behaviour shown in speech, play or drawing;
- Apparent sexual approaches;
- Promiscuity.

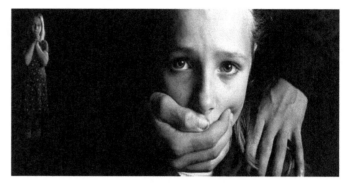

o Symptoms such as a sore bottom, vaginal discharge, bleeding per vagina in a pre-pubertal child, bleeding per rectum or inflamed penis that the care-giver believes is due to sexual abuse.
o Symptoms as above and/or signs (e.g. unexplained perineal tear and/or bruising, torn hymen or perineal warts), but the doctor is the first person to suspect abuse.
o Faecal soiling or relapse of enuresis
o Sexually transmitted disease
o Pregnancy where the girl refuses to name the putative father or even indicate the category, e.g. boyfriend, casual acquaintance
o Sexual intercourse with a child younger than 13 years is unlawful and therefore pregnancy in such a child means the child has been maltreated
o Female genital mutilation (FGM)

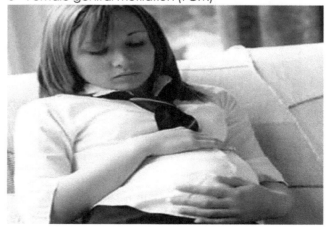

3. THE NEGLECTED CHILD

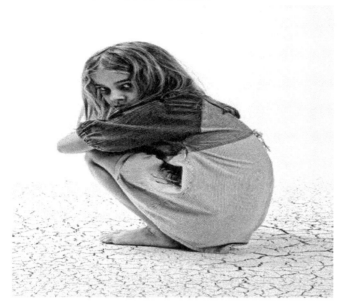

- The persistent failure to meet a child's basic physical and/or psychological needs, likely to result in the serious impairment of the child's health or development.
- Neglect may occur during pregnancy as a result of maternal substance abuse.
- Once a child is born, neglect may involve a parent or carer failing to:
  - Provide adequate food, clothing and shelter (including exclusion from home or abandonment)
  - Protect a child from physical and emotional harm or danger
  - Ensure adequate supervision (including the use of inadequate care-givers)
  - Ensure access to appropriate medical care or treatment
- It may also include neglect of, or unresponsiveness to, a child's basic emotional needs

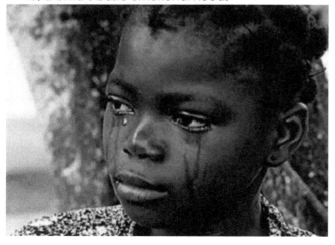

PRESENTATIONS OF NEGLECTED CHILD

  - Severe and persistent infestations, such as scabies or head lice.
  - A child's clothing or footwear is consistently inappropriate (e.g. for the weather or the child's size)
  - A child is persistently smelly and dirty, especially if seen at times of the day when it is unlikely that they would have had an opportunity to become dirty or smelly (e.g. early morning)

- Repeated observation or reports of the home environment being of a poor standard of hygiene that affects a child's health.
- The home environment is unsuitable for the child's stage of development and impacts on the child's safety or well-being.

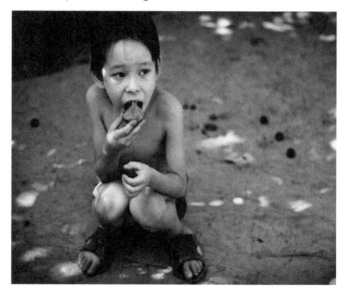

- It may be difficult to distinguish between neglect and material poverty. However, care should be taken to balance recognition of the constraints on the parents' or carers' ability to meet their children's needs for food, clothing and shelter with an appreciation of how people in similar circumstances have been able to meet those needs
- Child abandonment
- Non-organic failure to thrive
- Repeated non-attendances at appointments that are necessary for the child's health and well-being
- Parents or carers fail to administer essential prescribed treatment for their child
- Parents or carers fail to seek medical advice for their child to the extent that the child's health and well-being is compromised
- Poor/inadequate supervision which may lead/has led to injury

4. THE CHILD WITH EMOTIONAL ABUSE

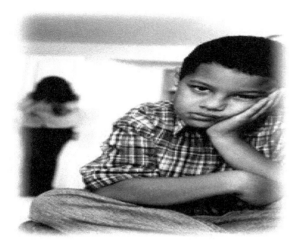

- The persistent emotional maltreatment of a child such as to cause severe and persistent adverse effects on the child's emotional development.
- It may involve conveying to a child that they are worthless or unloved, inadequate or valued only in so far as they meet the needs of another person.
- It may include not giving the child opportunities to express their views, deliberately silencing them or 'making fun' of what they say or how they communicate.
- It may feature age or developmentally inappropriate expectations being imposed on children. These may include interactions that are beyond a child's developmental capability, as well as overprotection and limitation of exploration and learning, or preventing the child participating in normal social interaction.
- It may involve seeing or hearing the ill treatment of another.
- It may involve serious bullying (including cyber bullying), causing children frequently to feel frightened or in danger, or the exploitation or corruption of children.
- Some level of emotional abuse is involved in all types of maltreatment of a child, although it may occur alone

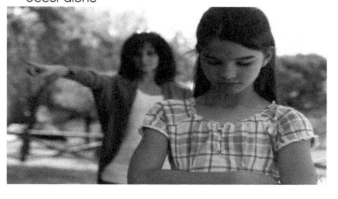

- **Below the list of other pointers to be aware of during history taking and examination:**
  - There is delay in seeking medical help or medical help is not sought at all.
  - The story of the 'accident' is vague, is lacking in detail and may vary with each telling and from person to person. Innocent accidents tend to have vivid accounts that ring true
  - The account of the accident is not compatible with the injury observed
  - The injury is not compatible with the child's level of development or of the level of development of another child alleged to have caused the injury
  - The parents' affect is abnormal. Note anything that appears abnormal to you in this regard
  - The parents' behaviour gives cause for concern. They may become hostile, rebut accusations that have not been made or leave before the consultant arrives
  - The child's appearance and his interaction with his parents are abnormal.
  - He may look sad, withdrawn or frightened.
  - There may be visible evidence of failure to thrive.
  - Full-blown frozen watchfulness is a late stage and results from repetitive physical and emotional abuse over a period of time

ASSESSMENT

- The assessment of all children should follow the standard ABCDE procedure and full medical assessment approach.
- Consent for examination is mandatory in all cases unless a serious life-threatening injury is suspected. This needs to be given by an adult with parental responsibility or the child if competent.
- Social care may need to get a court order if appropriate consent is not available or refused.
- This is also an aspect that will be subject to national laws, policies and procedures and you should familiarise yourself with those relevant to your practice using national guidance.

HISTORY

- A full history should be taken as in any medical assessment. There are some specific issues to consider if child abuse and neglect is on your list of differential diagnoses.
- Full details of the history of the incident(s) should be obtained from the child and the caregivers.
- If social workers and police officers have previously talked to the child, then taking this history from them may be appropriate, especially for alleged sexual offences.

- Frequent repetition of the details can be very disturbing to the child and can jeopardise evidence
  - In history related to the gastrointestinal tract remember to ask about soiling, constipation, rectal pain and rectal bleeding
  - In history related to the urogenital system remember to ask about wetting, vaginal bleeding, vaginal discharge and, when appropriate, menarche, cycle, sanitary protection and previous sexual intercourse
  - Personal history must start with pregnancy, birth, the neonatal period and subsequent developmental milestones. Then details of immunisations, drug history (including alcohol and street drugs) and allergies are obtained.
  - Information on the child's performance at nursery or school should include social factors
  - Enquiries are made about previous illnesses and injuries, with dates of attendance at hospital or the surgery of the family doctor.
  - Past records should be obtained and relevant information should be extracted
  - The traditional family history should include details of the natural parents, all co-habitees and any other people who regularly care for the child, e.g. relatives and childminders.
  - Parental illness should be discussed, particularly psychiatric illness.

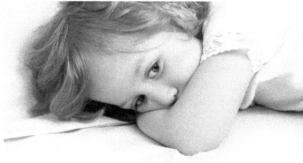

  - The presence of domestic abuse should be explored
  - Then the names, ages and medical histories of all siblings and half-siblings are obtained.
  - Any miscarriages, stillbirths or deaths of siblings are discussed sensitively
  - Familial illnesses that are particularly important are inherited skin or blood disorders
  - Remember to remain objective and show professional sensitivity.
  - Document who is present and their relationship to the child. Use open questions and avoid leading questions.
  - Full contemporaneous notes are essential.

  - If the child has been video-interviewed you may be able to obtain the transcript of this prior to examination to avoid unnecessary repetition.

EXAMINATION

- Ensure an appropriate **chaperone** is present.
- The general examination starts while the history is being taken. During that time the doctor observes the affect of the child, the relationships between the child, mother, father and others present, and any behavioural problems.
- If the child is reluctant to be examined, then playing with toys or the doctor's stethoscope often breaks the ice. No child should be examined against his or her will as this constitutes an assault.
- Examination under anaesthesia is rarely required.

- **General examination**
  - Full head-to-toe examination
  - Plot growth on growth chart including head circumference in younger children
  - Comment on general level of hygiene, clothing, etc.
  - Document any injuries on a body map
  - Comment on developmental level and interaction with carers

- **Sexual abuse examination**
  - This should be undertaken by a doctor with the necessary competences
  - Best practice is to use a colposcope for magnification and to take digital images
  - If there has been acute assault, then forensic examination taking forensic swabs will be needed – often this is as a joint examination with the paediatrician/forensic medical examiner
  - Need to consider post-coital contraception or screening for sexually transmitted infections

INVESTIGATIONS

- The investigations are dependent on the initial presentation and injuries.
- Young babies presenting with concerns about physical abuse all need:
  - Full blood count and clotting
  - Neuro-imaging
  - Fundoscopy
  - Skeletal survey – which should include a repeat chest X-ray 10–14 days later to exclude rib fractures
- Blood investigations to exclude differential diagnosis will also depend on clinical presentation and may include:
  - Blood cultures and Metabolic investigations
  - Renal, bone profile & Extended clotting studies

ED MANAGEMENT OF A CHILD WITH A CONCERNING PRESENTATION

- The immediate management should involve **ensuring the child is pain-free** and **treating any injuries or illness appropriately.**
- **Meticulous documentation is essential.** Notes should be factual (e.g. 4 × 1cm round bruises found on the medial aspect of the left upper arm) and not attribute blame or causation (e.g. finger imprints found on medial aspect of left upper arm).
- Documenting injuries in a diagram is a useful way to capture information.
- If sexual assault is suspected, a **genital examination should not be pursued in the ED**. This should be performed only once, by a senior clinician in child protection, in collaboration with a police surgeon (clinical forensic physician).
- Further information should be gathered about the child. For example: checking whether the child or any siblings are known to social services or whether they are subject of a Child Protection Plan; looking up previous ED attendances; contacting the GP to gain a past medical history for the child and background information on the family (e.g. parental mental health or substance misuse issues).
- Any suspicion of abuse should prompt early involvement of an expert senior doctor, e.g. ED consultant and/or paediatrician.
- Once information has been gathered and the case has been discussed/reviewed with a senior clinician the level of concern can be established e.g. **no concern; minor concern or unsure; more than a minor concern.**
- The level of concern determines the ongoing management:

No concern:
- A routine notification **letter of the child's ED attendance should be sent to the GP.**
- Plus, a letter of notification should be sent **to the midwife if the child is <10 days old (faxed urgently)**; the **Health Visiting Team**, if the child is aged 10 days—5 years (pre-school children); or the **School Nurse** for school children (within 5 days).
- This is the standard recommended by **Lord Laming's report in 2009** (The Protection of Children in England: a progress report), the Government's report Working Together to safeguard children 2006, and the College of Emergency Medicine Best Practice Statement for Safeguarding Children.

Minor concern or unsure:
- Should have **a senior Emergency Medicine opinion** and then be referred to the **ED Liaison Health Visitor the next working day.**

More than a minor concern:
- Should be referred **directly for a senior paediatric opinion** and **referred to social services** (the local Trust Child Protection Policy should be followed for this).

SIGNIFICANT HARM AND THRESHOLDS FOR INTERVENTION

- In addition to the areas listed above, also consider the following.
- **Grave concern**
  - This is described in children whose situations do not currently fit the above categories, but where social and medical assessments indicate that they are at significant risk of abuse.
  - These could include situations where another child in the household has been harmed or the household contains a known abuser, including situations where an adult is the subject of domestic abuse.
- **Organised abuse**
  - This characteristically involves multiple perpetrators, involves multiple victims and is a form of organised crime.
  - There are three subsections:
    - The first is **paedophile and/or pornographic rings**.
    - The second is **cult-based ritualistic abuse** in which the abuse has spiritual or social objectives.
    - The third is **pseudo-ritualistic abuse** in which the degradation of children is the end rather than the means.
  - The details of management of these many facets require a referral and a multiagency response.

- Doctors may be concerned about sharing information with other professionals because of the ethical consideration of confidentiality.
- In the UK, the General Medical Council (2012) gives the following advice.
  - *Ask for consent to share information unless there is a compelling reason for not doing so.*
  - *Information can be shared without consent if it is justified in the public interest or required by law.*
  - *Do not delay disclosing information to obtain consent if that might put children or young people at risk of significant harm.*
  - *Advice on consent will vary from country to country and you should be aware of your own national guidance and advice.*

II. LEGAL FRAMEWORK FOR CHILD PROTECTION

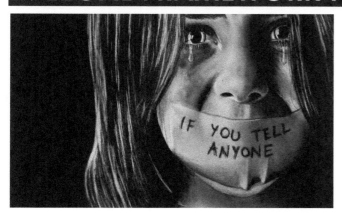

- Healthcare professionals must be familiar with the medicolegal aspects of their work.
- These may vary according to the jurisdiction where the clinician practices.
- They will in most cases cover the following:
  - Court orders to enable:
    - Emergency protection
    - Child assessment
    - Residence
    - Police protection
    - Consent to examination
- In some cases where there is involvement of either a criminal or family court, healthcare professionals may be required to write statements and/or present evidence.
- Everyone who deals with children is responsible for safeguarding and has a legal obligation to raise any concerns they may have about a child's welfare.
- The Children Act 1989 contains most of the relevant law relating to child protection.
- **Section 47 of the Children Act 1989** covers children at risk or suffering harm, from physical, sexual, or emotional abuse, or neglect.
- If there is significant concern that a child is at risk of harm, then social services will instigate **Section 47** and contact the police.
- Social services, the police, and the paediatricians will then formulate a joint strategy plan to decide if the child needs to be taken into care or can be discharged home.
- If it is felt that a child needs to be in a place of safety, the parents can voluntarily allow the child to be taken into care, which may be the hospital or a close relative (**Section 20 of the Children Act**).
- If the parents insist on taking the child out of hospital when there is concern for the child's welfare, the police should be informed.

- **Under Section 46 of the Children Act**, the police have the power to enforce a police protection order that can keep the child in a designated place of safety for **up to 72 hours**.
- The social worker can apply for an extension to this in the form of an emergency protection order (**Section 44 of the Children Act**).
- The Children's Act 2004 requires each local authority in England and Wales to promote cooperation between different agencies involved in the welfare of children.
- It also requires them to establish Local Safeguarding Children Boards of which NHS Trusts are statutory members.
- Every NHS Trust will have a named doctor for Child Protection who is responsible for promoting and advising on safeguarding issues.

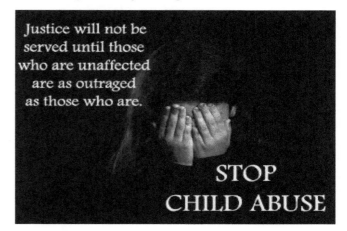

COURT REPORTS

- When preparing a written report on a child for the court, all healthcare professionals should keep in mind that the written report may be used in subsequent court appearances. Therefore, the report should be confined to the facts.
- Whenever possible, objective and measurable evidence of the child's health and development should be presented.
- Where subjective views must be given, they should reflect balanced professional judgement.
- If the report is comprehensive and comprehensible, then the healthcare professional may not be called to give verbal evidence in person.
- Always keep a copy of your report.

Further Reading:
- *Legal Framework for Safeguarding Children in Individual Cases - from Greater Manchester SafeGuarding*

III. AGENCIES IN SAFEGUARDING CHILDREN

1. CHILDREN'S SOCIAL CARE (CSC)

- Commonly referred to as social services, take the lead in investigating and managing child protection cases. They will know whether or not a child and/ or family have been previously involved with children's social care.

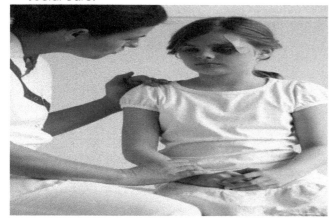

2. POLICE

- Safeguarding children is a fundamental part of the duties of all police officers.
- All forces have child abuse investigation units who undertake criminal investigations in cases of suspected child abuse.
- The child abuse investigation team will have knowledge of any previous criminal involvement of child/parents/carers.

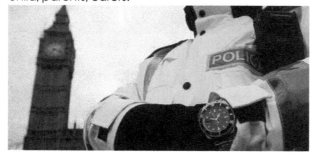

3. EDUCATION

- Schools have a statutory responsibility, like healthcare organisations, to safeguard children and young people.
- **School teachers** will have a good knowledge of a child's day to day demeanour and developmental/academic strengths and weaknesses.
- **The school nurse** will be aware of issues relating to health and development as well as other issues, if any, affecting the parents or other children in the family.

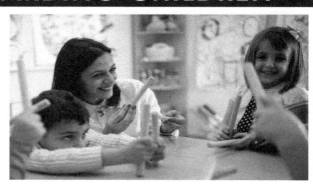

4. HEALTH

- All layers and elements of the health service have a statutory responsibility to safeguard children and young people.
- This includes **health visitors, GPs, staff in secondary and tertiary healthcare**, e.g. specialist hospitals, private hospitals, mental health services, genitourinary and family planning services, dentists and professions allied to medicine.

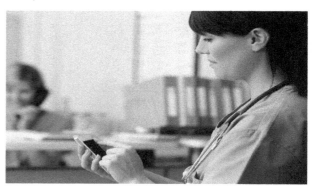

5. FAMILY JUSTICE SYSTEM

- **The Family Justice System** is a network of organizations including **family courts, the Children and Family Court Advisory and Support Service (CAFCASS), the Child Support Agency, and lawyers.**
- Safeguarding children's welfare is a key consideration for all professionals working in the Family Justice System.
- In all cases the child's welfare is the court's paramount consideration and the role of the court is to make decisions which are in the best interest of children based on the evidence before it and the law.

Further Reading:

- *Organisations responsible for dealing with child abuse - from CITIZEN ADVICE UK*

10. The Febrile Child

I. ASSESSMENT TOOL FOR THE FEBRILE CHILD

NICE TRAFFIC LIGHT SYSTEM [163]

TRAFFIC LIGHT ALERT FOR FEVERISH CHILDREN IN ED

	Green-low risk Check urine and **give** fever advice sheet	Amber – intermediate risk- admit	Red – high risk of life-threatening illness
Colour	• Normal colour of skin, lips and tongue	• Pallor reported by parent/carer	• Pale • Mottled • Ashen • Blue
Activity	• Responds normally to social cues • Content/smiles • Stays awake or awakens quickly • Strong normal cry/not crying	• Not responding normally to social cues • Wakes only with prolonged stimulation • Decreased activity • No smile	• No response to social cues • Appears ill to a healthcare professional • Does not wake or if roused does not stay awake • Weak, high-pitched or continuous cry
Respiratory		• Nasal flaring • RR > 50, age 6–12 mo. • RR > 40, age > 12 mo. • O_2 sat ≤ 95% in air • Crackles	• Grunting • RR > 60 /minute • Moderate or severe chest indrawing
Hydration	• Normal skin and eyes • Moist mucous membranes	• SBP >160 (<12 months), • SBP >150 (12-24 months) • SBP >140 (24-60 months) • Dry mucous membranes • Poor feeding in infants • CRT ≥ 3 seconds • Reduced urine output	• Reduced skin turgor
Other	• None of the amber or red symptoms or signs	• Fever for ≥ 5 days**	• Age 0–3 months, temperature ≥ 38 °C • Age 3–6 months, temperature ≥ 39 °C • Non-blanching rash • Bulging fontanelle • Neck stiffness • Status epilepticus • Focal neurological signs Focal seizures • Bile-stained vomiting

- *** Swelling of a limb, non-weight bearing, not using an extremity and a new lump >2cm**

- All febrile patients with green features should have a urine checked and be sent home with an advice sheet on fever.
- If any amber features and no diagnosis reached admit.
- If any red features refer child urgently to a paediatric registrar.
- All febrile babies under 6-months are red light. i.e. urgent

---

[163] National Institute for Health and Clinical Excellence. Feverish illness: assessment and initial management in children younger than 5 years.

London: NICE; https://www.nice.org.uk/guidance/ng143

CLINICAL ASSESSMENT TOOL FOR THE FEBRILE CHILD 0-5 YEARS

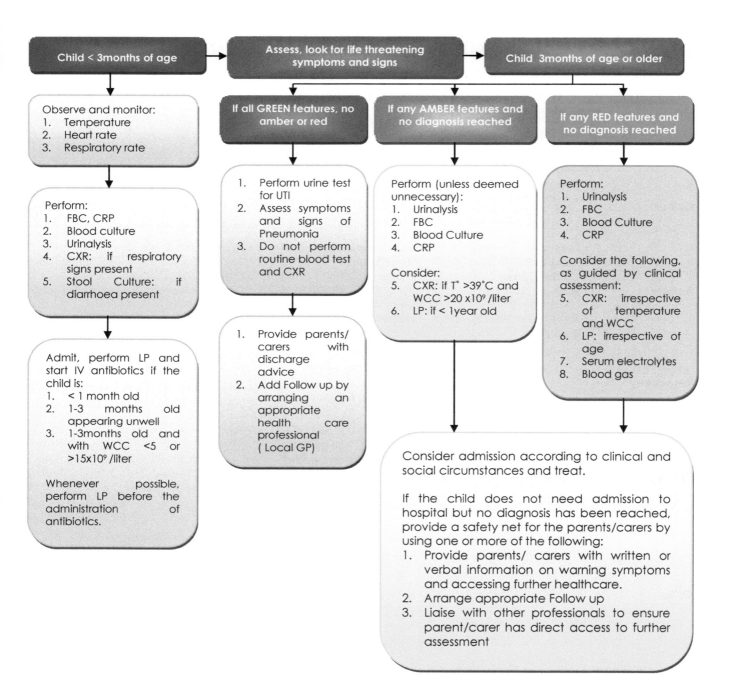

Child < 3months of age

Assess, look for life threatening symptoms and signs

Child 3months of age or older

If all GREEN features, no amber or red

If any AMBER features and no diagnosis reached

If any RED features and no diagnosis reached

Observe and monitor:
1. Temperature
2. Heart rate
3. Respiratory rate

Perform:
1. FBC, CRP
2. Blood culture
3. Urinalysis
4. CXR: if respiratory signs present
5. Stool Culture: if diarrhoea present

Admit, perform LP and start IV antibiotics if the child is:
1. < 1 month old
2. 1-3 months old appearing unwell
3. 1-3months old and with WCC <5 or >15x10⁹ /liter

Whenever possible, perform LP before the administration of antibiotics.

1. Perform urine test for UTI
2. Assess symptoms and signs of Pneumonia
3. Do not perform routine blood test and CXR

1. Provide parents/ carers with discharge advice
2. Add Follow up by arranging an appropriate health care professional (Local GP)

Perform (unless deemed unnecessary):
1. Urinalysis
2. FBC
3. Blood Culture
4. CRP

Consider:
5. CXR: if T° >39°C and WCC >20 x10⁹ /liter
6. LP: if < 1year old

Perform:
1. Urinalysis
2. FBC
3. Blood Culture
4. CRP

Consider the following, as guided by clinical assessment:
5. CXR: irrespective of temperature and WCC
6. LP: irrespective of age
7. Serum electrolytes
8. Blood gas

Consider admission according to clinical and social circumstances and treat.

If the child does not need admission to hospital but no diagnosis has been reached, provide a safety net for the parents/carers by using one or more of the following:
1. Provide parents/ carers with written or verbal information on warning symptoms and accessing further healthcare.
2. Arrange appropriate Follow up
3. Liaise with other professionals to ensure parent/carer has direct access to further assessment

II. APPROACH TO THE CHILD WITH PNEUMONIA

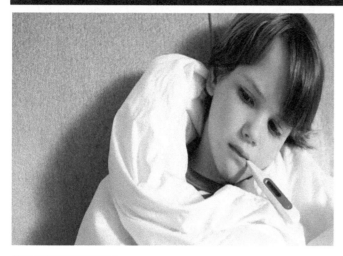

INTRODUCTION
- Pneumonia in childhood was responsible globally for 13% of deaths of children aged under 5 years in 2013 (WHO data).
- Infants, and children with congenital abnormalities or chronic illnesses, are at particular risk.
- A wide spectrum of pathogens causes pneumonia in childhood, and different organisms are important in different age groups.
- The incidence of viral infections decreases with increasing age, while the incidence of bacterial infections remains stable across all ages.
- Viral infections typically peak during the **autumn and winter season**, whereas bacterial pneumonia exhibits less marked seasonal fluctuation.
- **Organisms**
  - **In the newborn**: the most common pathogens are organisms from the mother's genital tract such as:
    - **Escherichia coli**
    - **Gram-negative bacilli**,
    - **Group B β-haemolytic Streptococcus**
    - **Chlamydia trachomatis.**
  - **In infancy**
    - **Respiratory viruses** are the most frequent cause,
    - **Streptococcus pneumoniae, Haemophilus** and, less commonly, **Staphylococcus aureus** are also important.
  - **In school-aged children**: Viruses become less frequent pathogens and bacterial infection, especially:
    - **Mycoplasma pneumoniae**,
    - **S. pneumoniae**
    - **Chlamydia pneumoniae**,

- **Bordetella pertussis** can present with pneumonia as well as with classic whooping cough, even in children who have been fully immunised. It can cause a severe pneumonitis, leading to respiratory failure in unimmunised infants.

CLINICAL PRESENTATION
- Fever, cough, breathlessness and chest recession in the younger child and lethargy are the usual presenting symptoms.
- The cough is often dry initially but then becomes loose. Older children may produce purulent sputum but in those below the age of 5 years it is usually swallowed.
- Pleuritic chest pain, neck stiffness and abdominal pain may be present if there is pleural inflammation.

INVESTIGATIONS & TREATMENT
- Classic signs of consolidation such as decreased percussion, decreased breath sounds and bronchial breathing are often absent, particularly in infants, and a **chest radiograph** is needed.
- This may show lobar consolidation, widespread bronchopneumonia or, rarely, cavitation of the lung.
- Pleural effusions may occur, particularly in bacterial pneumonia and this may organise to empyema.

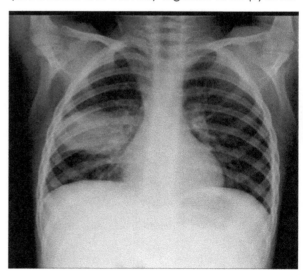

- **An ultrasound** of the chest will delineate the size and nature of pleural collection and if needed will guide placing of a chest drain.
- **Blood cultures, swabs** for viral isolation and an **FBC** should also be performed. It can be useful to save an acute serum for further microbiological diagnosis.

- All children diagnosed as having significant pneumonia should receive antibiotics.
- Oral antibiotics are sufficient in most cases, unless there is vomiting or severe respiratory distress.
- The initial choice of antibiotics depends on the age of the child and local policy:
- **Newborns and young infants:**
  o Should receive broad-spectrum IV antibiotics such as **cefotaxime or ceftriaxone.**

- **For older infants and preschool children:**
  o Oral **amoxicillin** is suitable.

- **For school-aged children:**
  o A macrolide such as **clarithromycin** is suitable.

- Antibiotics should be given for **7–10 days**, although complicated pneumonias, e.g. with empyema, may require several weeks' duration.
- In children with no respiratory difficulty, treatment will occur at home with a penicillin or macrolide.
- Infants, and children who look toxic, have definite dyspnoea, an SpO2 below 93%, grunting or signs of dehydration should be admitted and usually require IV treatment initially.
- **Oxygen** (if SpO2 < 93%) and an adequate **fluid intake** (70% maintenance, because of possible inappropriate ADH secretion) are also required.
- Mechanical ventilation is rarely required unless there is a serious underlying condition.

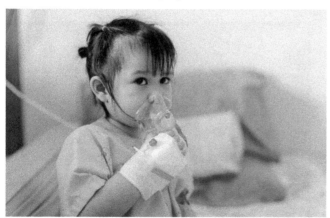

- Transfer to the PICU should be considered with the following:
  o An Fio2 >0.6 to keep the Spo2 at 94–98%,
  o Shock,
  o Exhaustion,
  o Rising CO2,
  o Apnoea or irregular breathing.

- If a child has recurrent or persistent pneumonia, they should be referred to a respiratory specialist so further investigation may be undertaken.

EMERGENCY TREATMENT OF PNEUMONIA

- Assess **ABC.**
- Provide a high concentration of oxygen via a face mask with reservoir bag.
- Attach a pulse oximeter; if a low flow maintains SpO2 at 94–98%, then nasal cannulae may be used with a flow <2 l/min.

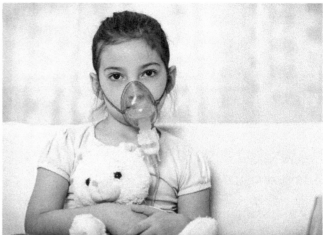

- It is not possible to differentiate reliably between bacterial and viral infection on clinical, haematological or radiological grounds, so children diagnosed as having significant pneumonia should receive antibiotics.

- The choice of antibiotic is usually according to local policy, but for infants and older children amoxicillin is effective against most bacteria.
- For young infants or if there is a septic component, **cefotaxime** would be considered.

- Other options include the use of:
  o **Flucloxacillin:** if Staphylococcus aureus is suspected, or
  o **Macrolide antibiotic:** if atypical pneumonia or pertussis (unimmunised infant) is suspected.

- **Maintain hydration:** extra fluid may be needed to compensate for loss from fever, and restriction may be needed because of inappropriate antidiuretic hormone (ADH) secretion.
- Fluid overload can contribute to worsening breathlessness.

- **Airway and breathing support** may especially be needed in children with neurodisability or neuromuscular weakness, who may have poor airway control and weak respiratory muscles even when well.

III. APPROACH TO THE FEBRILE CONVULSION

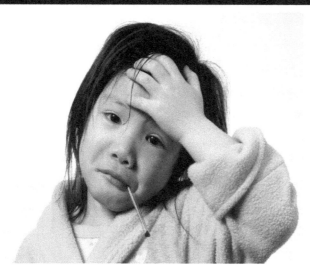

DEFINITIONS

- A seizure associated with fever occurring in a young child.
- Most occur between 18 months and 3 years of age.
- Febrile seizure is rare before **6 months and after 6 years.**
- **Simple febrile convulsion** is an Isolated, generalized tonic–clonic seizure lasting less than 15 minutes, which does not recur within 24 hours or within the same febrile illness.
- **Complex febrile seizures**, have one or more of the following features: a partial (focal) onset or focal feature during the seizure; duration of more than 15 minutes; recurrence within 24 hours, or within the same febrile illness; incomplete recovery within 1 hour.
- **Febrile status epilepticus** is a febrile seizure lasting longer than 30 minutes.
- Febrile convulsions arise most commonly from infection or inflammation outside the CNS in a child who is otherwise neurologically normal.
- Most febrile convulsions will have ceased by arrival in the ED.
- The child should initially be assessed in an ABCDE manner.
- The history and examination should aim to determine the cause of the fever (e.g. **viral upper respiratory tract infection, otitis media, urinary tract infection**, etc.).
- The above NICE traffic light system is helpful to identify the likelihood of serious underlying illness.
- If the child is still fitting on arrival in the ED, they should be managed using the status epilepticus guidance (See below).

DIAGNOSTIC APPROACH

- o **Resuscitation:** The priority is to stop the fit and to stabilise the patient following standard APLS guidelines.
- o **Don't ever forget Glucose (DEFG!)** - check BM in ALL.
- **History**
  - o **The state of health prior to the fit:** typically, the child is a little off colour or well prior to the fit.
  - o **Features of the fit:**
    - Obtain an accurate description of the fit if possible
    - Importantly - whether consciousness was lost.
    - The eyes may roll up, the limbs may stiffen, there may by cyanosis, there may be generalised movements of either upper and/or lower limbs.
  - o **Previous medical history:**
    - Particularly any previous history of fits.
    - Contact with infectious diseases.
    - Foreign travel.
  - o Family history of epilepsy or of febrile convulsions.
  - o Medication.
- **Assessment**
  - o The unconscious child should be assessed in accordance with APLS guidelines.
  - o Primary survey of ABCD, before a secondary survey general examination.
  - o Continuous pulse oxymetry.
  - o Investigation directed to the clinical findings, type of fit and age of the child.

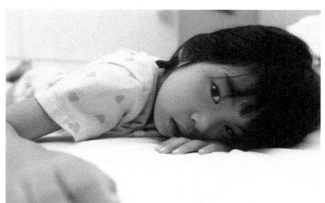

ED MANAGEMENT OF FEBRILE CONVULSION

1. CHILDREN LESS THAN 6 MONTHS OLD

- o Treat with caution any child under 6 months old with a high fever.
- o By definition this is not a febrile seizure (rare before 6 months and after 6-year-old)

o Assume is CNS infection until proven otherwise.
o All are treated as for **meningitis.**
o **Antibiotic therapy** must be commenced
o Urgent discussion with the ED Duty doctor and on call paediatrician
o Antibiotic treatment should not be delayed whilst the septic screen samples are collected.

2. AGE 6 - 18 MONTHS
o Treated with extreme caution
o Signs of serious infection are few
o If severely unwell a full septic screen should be carried out after appropriate resuscitative measures have been taken.
o Antibiotic therapy should not be delayed if obtaining these samples proves difficult.
o If mildly or moderately unwell, the child should be observed closely and the following investigations should be performed:

- **Laboratory:** Urine microscopy, Glucose, FBC, CRP, U&E, Calcium and Mg.
- Further investigation should be guided by continuing clinical review.

o A full septic screen should be considered if the child fails to show clinical improvement after appropriate healing measures, particularly if any of the following features are present:
- The child looks toxic or is irritable
- The child shows any sign of meningism
- The child shows signs of drowsiness or delayed recovery from the fit
- The fit is complex.
o Refer to the Paeds Doctor on duty

3. AGE OVER 18 MONTHS
o Older children are easier to assess clinically.
o If the child is severely unwell, investigations should be carried out as for the severely unwell child under 18 months of age.
o If mildly or moderately unwell, clinical assessment is of the greatest importance.
o Where there is an obvious source of infection, after thorough clinical assessment, no further investigations are required.
o Where the source of infection is not obvious or the fit was complex then proceed as per above investigations.

DISPOSAL
- Following a febrile fit, it may be reasonable to send the child home if the following criteria are met:
  o *Age > 1 year*
  o *The fit was simple*
  o *The child has fully recovered*

o *There is an obvious source of infection*
o *The child is not severely unwell*
o *The parents are not unduly anxious*
o *The child has had a previous febrile convulsion or there is a family history of febrile convulsions.*

- As a general rule, cases involving first febrile fits should be discussed with Senior ED staff or with the duty paediatrician.

- **Indications** for referral to the paediatric team after a febrile convulsion include:
  o *Children aged <18 months.*
  o *Signs of meningism.*
  o *Parental anxiety.*
  o *Complex or prolonged seizures*
  o *Systemically unwell.*
  o *Current or recent antibiotic use.*
  o *No clear focus of infection.*
  o *First febrile convulsion*
- All children presenting with a febrile convulsion who are less than 1 year of age should be admitted.
- Between 1 year and 18 months of age cases should be discussed with the duty admitting paediatrician.

DISCHARGE CHECKLIST
o If the child is to be discharged from the ED check:
- Appropriate treatment for the infection (if any)?
- Advice about keeping the child comfortable (remove clothing, Paracetamol 15mg per kg every 4-6 hours orally and/or Ibuprofen syrup 5mg per kg every 8 hours).
- An advice sheet should be given about febrile convulsions.
- Follow-up - should be arranged within 24-48 hours (normally with the General Practitioner but occasionally by return for ED senior review).

OUTCOME & PROGNOSIS
o The parents should be counselled fully (nearly all parents think that their child is dying during the first febrile fit).
o The recurrence risk is less than 30% (1 in 6 have 3 fits or more).
o Most recurrences occur within one year of the first convulsion.
o Often a strong family history, so siblings should be kept cool during illnesses.
o Simple febrile fits have no relationship to the development of epilepsy (if the convulsion was complex then outpatient follow-up with an EEG and/or CT scan is indicated).
o From a health prevention perspective, it is important to emphasise that the immunisation schedule should not be changed because of a simple febrile convulsion.

IV. THE CHILD WITH URINARY TRACT INFECTION

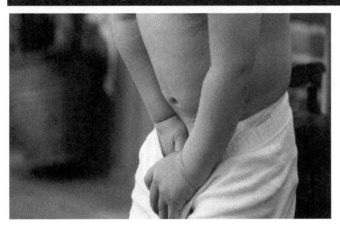

- The most common presentation of UTI in infants is an undiagnosed fever[164].
- Infants and children presenting with unexplained fever of 38°C or higher should have a urine sample tested after 24 hours at the latest.

COLLECTING THE URINE SAMPLE

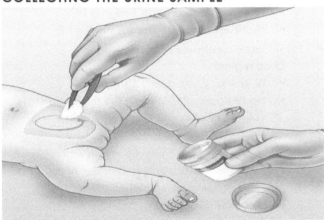

- A clean catch urine sample is the recommended method for urine collection.
- If a clean catch urine sample is not possible, use other non-invasive methods such as urine collection pads
- Do not use cotton wool balls, gauze or sanitary towels.
- If other non-invasive methods are not possible, use a catheter sample or suprapubic aspiration (SPA)
- Before SPA is attempted, ultrasound guidance should be used to demonstrate the presence of urine in the bladder.

DIAGNOSIS/ACUTE MANAGEMENT

- **Urine Microscopy result:** If Bacteriuria negative and Pyuria positive, antibiotic treatment should be started if clinically UTI.
- **Using dipstick test to diagnose UTI:**
  - If leukocyte esterase is negative and nitrite is positive, start antibiotic treatment if fresh sample was tested.
  - If leukocyte esterase is positive and nitrite is negative, only start antibiotic treatment if there is good clinical evidence of UTI.
- Treat with a different antibiotic, not a higher dose of the same antibiotic, if an infant or child is receiving prophylactic medication and develops an infection.

IMAGING TESTS

- Infants **younger than 6 months** should have **ultrasound** during the acute infection if they:
  - Do not respond well to treatment within 48 hours.
  - Have atypical UTI
  - Have recurrent UTI
- **In infants and children 6 months or older but younger than 3 years, MCUG** should not be performed routinely. It should be considered if the following features are present:
  - *Dilatation on ultrasound*
  - *Poor urine flow*
  - *Non-E. Coli-infection*
  - *Family history of VUR.*
- When a **Micturating Cystourethrogram (MCUG)** is performed, give oral prophylactic antibiotics for 3 days with MCUG taking place on the second day.

PROPHYLAXIS

- Antibiotic prophylaxis should not be routinely recommended in infants and children following first-time UTI (consider after recurrent UTI)

FOLLOW-UP

- Arrange follow up for infants and children with recurrent UTI, risk factors, atypical illness and abnormal imaging.
- Assessment of infants and children with renal parenchymal defects should include height, weight, blood pressure and routine testing for proteinuria.
- Infants and children with a minor, unilateral renal parenchymal defect do not need long-term follow-up unless they have recurrent UTI or family history or lifestyle risk factors for hypertension.

---

[164] *National Institute for Health and Clinical Excellence. Urinary tract infection in under 16s: diagnosis and management. Clinical guideline [CG54]Published date: August 2007 Last updated: October 2018. London: NICE; https://www.nice.org.uk/guidance/CG54*

11. The Convulsing Child

I. THE CHILD WITH STATUS EPILEPTICUS

INTRODUCTION

- Status epilepticus (SE) is a medical emergency associated with significant morbidity and mortality. SE is defined as a continuous seizure lasting more than 30 min, or two or more seizures without full recovery of consciousness between any of them.

- Based on recent understanding of the pathophysiology, it is now considered that any seizure that lasts more than 5 min probably needs to be treated as SE.

- There is a growing body of support for the definition to refer to seizures that persist for greater than 5 minutes without intervention. Status epilepticus (SE) is a common medical emergency associated with high morbidity, if not mortality. Mortality from SE varies from 3–50% in different studies. In elderly patients, refractory status epilepticus (RSE) may lead to death in over 76% cases[165].

- **Impending Status Epilepticus** has been advocated to describe continuous or intermittent seizures that persist **beyond 5 minutes** without neurological recovery.

- **Established SE** refers to clinical or electrographic seizures that persist for **30 minutes** or longer without full neurological recovery in between.

- **Refractory SE:** About 9–31% of patients with SE may fail to respond to standard treatment. This subgroup of RSE has greater morbidity and mortality. RSE is defined as continuous or repetitive seizures lasting longer than 60 min despite treatment with a benzodiazepine (lorazepam) and another standard anticonvulsant (usually phenytoin/fosphenytoin) in adequate loading dose[166].

- **Malignant SE** is a severe variant of RSE, in which the seizure fails to respond to aggressive treatment with even anesthetic agents. It typically occurs in young patients (18–50 years) in the setting of encephalitis.

- SE may be subdivided into convulsive and non-convulsive forms.

MANAGEMENT OF S.E. (See algorithm)[167]

- **Pre-hospital**
  - **ABC**: attention to airway, breathing and circulation, with the application of high flow oxygen where available.
  - **Blood glucose** should be checked and intravenous dextrose used to treat hypoglycaemia as indicated.
  - **Benzodiazepines**: **Diazepam** (rectal) or **Midazolam** (buccal or intranasal) may be used for this purpose.

- **On arrival in the ED**
  - Check **ABC**
  - Administer high-flow oxygen
  - Measure **blood glucose** and do **Pregnancy test**
  - **Drug regime**
    - **IV access**: Lorazepam **0.1 mg/kg IV**
    - **No IV access**: Diazepam **0.5 mg/kg PR**

- **10min later; continued seizure:**
  - **Drug regime**
    - **IV access**: Lorazepam **0.1 mg/kg IV**
    - **No IV access**: Paraldehyde **0.4 ml/kg (in same volume of olive oil) PR**

- **20min later; continued seizure:**
  - Request senior help, if not already present
  - Consider intraosseous access, consider IV cutdown if IV access not already established
  - **Drug regime**
    - Phenytoin **20 mg/kg IV** OR Phenobarbitone **20 mg/kg IV**
    - And Paraldehyde **0.4 ml/kg** (in same volume of olive oil) PR if not already given.

- **40 min later; continued seizure:**
  - Rapid sequence intubation
  - Transfer to intensive therapy unit (ITU)
  - **Drug regime:** Thiopental **4 mg/kg**

---

[165] *Logroscino G, Hesdorffer DC, Cascino GD, Annegers JF, Bagiella E, Hauser WA. Long-term mortality after a first episode of status epilepticus. Neurology. 2002;58:537–41.*

[166] *Shorvon S. Status epilepticus: Its clinical features and treatment in children and adults. Cambridge, England: Cambridge University Press; 1994. p. 201e.*

[167] *https://www.alsg.org/en/files/APLS/APLS_6e_Manual_updates.pdf*

STATUS EPILEPTICUS- APLS ALGORITHM

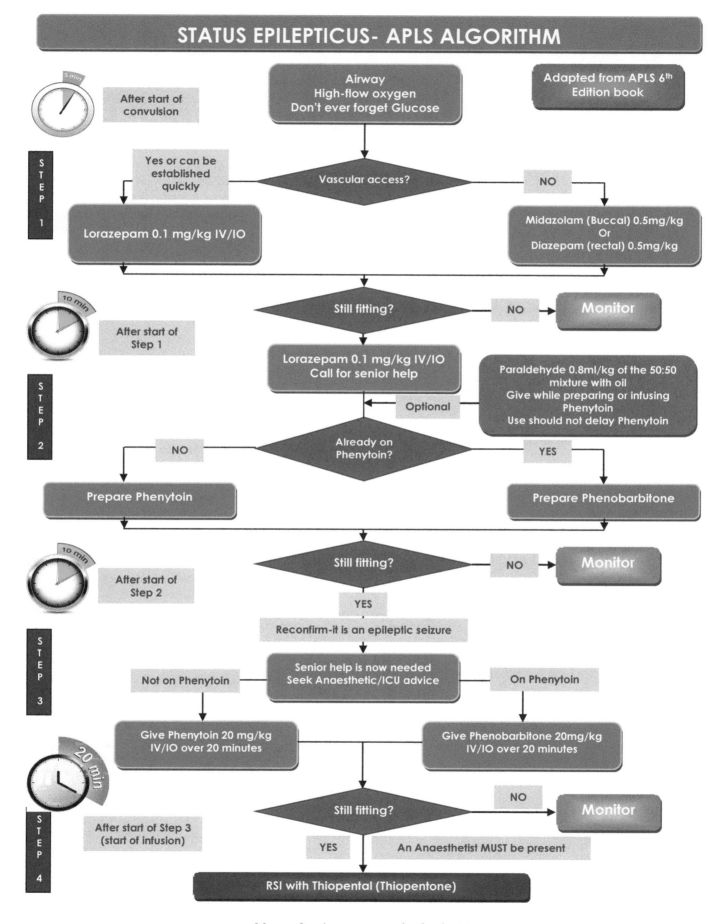

Airway
High-flow oxygen
Don't ever forget Glucose

Adapted from APLS 6th Edition book

After start of convulsion

STEP 1

Vascular access?

Yes or can be established quickly

NO

Lorazepam 0.1 mg/kg IV/IO

Midazolam (Buccal) 0.5mg/kg Or Diazepam (rectal) 0.5mg/kg

After start of Step 1

Still fitting? — **NO** → **Monitor**

STEP 2

Lorazepam 0.1 mg/kg IV/IO Call for senior help

Paraldehyde 0.8ml/kg of the 50:50 mixture with oil Give while preparing or infusing Phenytoin Use should not delay Phenytoin

Optional

Already on Phenytoin?

NO

YES

Prepare Phenytoin

Prepare Phenobarbitone

After start of Step 2

Still fitting? — **NO** → **Monitor**

YES

Reconfirm-it is an epileptic seizure

STEP 3

Senior help is now needed Seek Anaesthetic/ICU advice

Not on Phenytoin

On Phenytoin

Give Phenytoin 20 mg/kg IV/IO over 20 minutes

Give Phenobarbitone 20mg/kg IV/IO over 20 minutes

After start of Step 3 (start of infusion)

STEP 4

Still fitting? — **NO** → **Monitor**

YES

An Anaesthetist MUST be present

RSI with Thiopental (Thiopentone)

12. The Unwell Child

I. APLS APPROACH TO PRIMARY SURVEY

A & B. AIRWAY & BREATHING[168]

RECOGNITION OF POTENTIAL RESPIRATORY FAILURE

o The **Effort, Efficacy** and **Effect** of breathing need to be assessed bearing in mind the effects of respiratory inadequacy on other organs in the child's body.

o **Effort of breathing**
  - The degree of increase in the effort of breathing allows clinical assessment of the severity of respiratory disease.
  - It is important to assess the following:
    - Respiratory rate
    - Recession
    - Inspiratory or Expiratory noises: stridor, Wheezing
    - Grunting
    - Accessory muscle use
    - Flaring of the nostrils
    - Gasping

o **Efficacy of breathing:** Observations of the degree of chest expansion.

EFFECTS OF RESPIRATORY INADEQUACY ON OTHER ORGANS

1. Heart rate
  o Hypoxia produces tachycardia in the older infant and child.
  o Anxiety and a fever will also contribute to tachycardia, making this a non-specific sign.
  o **Severe or prolonged hypoxia leads to bradycardia>>> this is a pre-terminal sign.**

2. Skin colour
  o Hypoxia (via catecholamine release) produces vasoconstriction and skin pallor.
  o **Cyanosis is a late and pre-terminal sign of hypoxia** as it usually becomes apparent when SpO2 falls to <70%, and only in the absence of anaemia.
  o By the time central cyanosis is visible in acute respiratory disease, the patient is close to respiratory arrest.

o In the anaemic child, cyanosis may never be visible despite profound hypoxia.
o A few children will be cyanosed because of cyanotic heart disease, but may have adequate oxygen uptake within the lungs, and their cyanosis will be largely unchanged by oxygen therapy.

3. Mental status
  o The hypoxic or hypercapnic child will be agitated and/or drowsy.
  o Gradually drowsiness increases and eventually consciousness is lost.
  o These extremely useful and important signs are often more difficult to detect in small infants.
  o The parents may say that the infant is just 'not himself'.
  o The healthcare practitioner must assess the child's state of alertness by gaining eye contact and noting the response to voice and, if necessary, to painful stimuli.
  o A generalised muscular hypotonia also accompanies hypoxic cerebral depression.

C. CIRCULATION

1. RECOGNITION OF POTENTIAL CIRCULATORY FAILURE
  o The cardiovascular status needs to be assessed bearing in mind the effects of circulatory inadequacy on other organs.

2. CARDIOVASCULAR STATUS

Heart rate
  o The heart rate initially increases in shock due to catecholamine release and as compensation for decreased stroke volume.
  o The rate, particularly in small infants, may be extremely high (up to 220 beats per minute).
  o An abnormally slow pulse rate, or bradycardia, is defined as less than 60 beats per minute or a rapidly falling heart rate associated with poor systemic perfusion>>> This is a pre-terminal sign.

Pulse volume
  o Although blood pressure is maintained until shock is severe, an indication of perfusion can be gained by comparative palpation of both peripheral and central pulses.

---

[168] https://www.alsg.org/en/files/APLS/APLS_6e_Manual_updates.pdf

- o **Absent peripheral pulses and weak central pulses** are serious signs of advanced shock, and indicate that hypotension is already present.
- o **Bounding pulses** may be caused by an increased cardiac output (e.g. septicaemia), arteriovenous systemic shunt (e.g. patent arterial duct) or hypercapnia.

Capillary refill
- o Following cutaneous pressure on the **centre of the sternum** or on **a digit for 5 seconds**, capillary refill should occur within seconds.
- o A slower refill time than this can indicate poor skin perfusion, a sign which may be helpful in early septic shock, when the child may otherwise appear well, with warm peripheries.
- o The presence of fever does not affect the sensitivity of delayed capillary refill in children with hypovolaemia but a low ambient temperature reduces its specificity, so the sign should be used with caution in trauma patients who have been in a cold environment.
- o Poor capillary refill and differential pulse volumes are neither sensitive nor specific indicators of shock in infants and children, but are useful clinical signs when used in conjunction with the other signs described.
- o They should not be used as the only indicators of shock nor as quantitative measures of the response to treatment.
- o In children with pigmented skin, the sign is more difficult to assess.
- o In these cases, the **nail beds** are used and additionally **the sole of the feet** in young babies.

Blood pressure
- o In septic shock, target these normal values and respond to trends alongside the other indicators of shock.
- o Use of the correct cuff size is crucial if an accurate blood pressure measurement is to be obtained.
- o The width of the cuff should be more than 80% of the length of the upper arm and the bladder more than 40% of the arm's circumference.
- o If the blood pressure is less than the median systolic you should check for other signs of circulatory failure.
- o Hypotension (less than the 5th centile) is a late and pre-terminal sign of circulatory failure.
- o Once a child's blood pressure has fallen, cardiac arrest is imminent.
- o Hypertension can be the cause or result of coma and raised intracranial pressure.

3. EFFECTS OF CIRCULATORY INADEQUACY ON OTHER ORGANS

Respiratory system
- o A rapid respiration rate with an increased tidal volume, but without recession, may be caused by the metabolic acidosis resulting from circulatory failure.

Skin
- o Mottled, cold, pale skin peripherally indicates poor perfusion.
- o A line of coldness may be felt to move centrally as circulatory failure progresses.

Mental status
- o Agitation and then drowsiness leading to unconsciousness are characteristic of circulatory failure.
- o These signs are caused by poor cerebral perfusion.
- o In an infant, parents may say that he is 'not himself'.

Urinary output
- o A urine output of **less than 1 ml/kg/h in children and less than 2 ml/kg/h in infants** indicates inadequate renal perfusion during shock.
- o A history of reduced wet nappies or urine production should be sought.

Cardiac failure
- o The following features suggest a cardiac cause of respiratory inadequacy:
  - Cyanosis, not correcting with oxygen therapy
  - Tachycardia out of proportion to respiratory difficulty
  - Raised jugular venous pressure
  - Gallop rhythm/murmur
  - Enlarged liver
  - Absent femoral pulses

D. DISABILITY
RECOGNITION OF POTENTIAL CENTRAL NEUROLOGICAL FAILURE
- o Neurological assessment should only be performed after airway (A), breathing (B) and circulation (C) have been assessed and treated.
- o There are no neurological problems that take priority over ABC.
- o Both respiratory and circulatory failure will have central neurological effects.
- o Conversely, some conditions with direct central neurological effects (such as meningitis, raised intracranial pressure from trauma, and status epilepticus) may also have respiratory and circulatory consequences.

1. NEUROLOGICAL FUNCTION

Conscious level

o A rapid assessment of conscious level can be made by assigning the patient to one of these categories:

- **A: A**lert
- **V:** Responds to **V**oice
- **P:** Responds only to **P**ain
- **U: U**nresponsive to all stimuli

o If the child does not respond to voice, it is important that response to pain is then assessed.

o A painful central stimulus can be delivered by **sternal pressure**, by **supraorbital ridge pressure** or **squeezing the trapezius** or **Achilles tendon**.

o Commonly, a child who is unresponsive or who only responds to pain has a significant degree of coma, equivalent to 8 or less on the Glasgow Coma Scale (GCS).

o If the child responds to pain, it is best to note what the eyes and limbs did and what sounds or words were uttered, rather than simply categorising the child as 'P'. Simple descriptions that will form the basis of a subsequent formal GCS, such as 'opening eyes to pain' or 'localising to pain' are much more informative than 'P' alone.

- A child who does not open his eyes to pain, utters no sounds and extends his limbs has a GCS score of 4 and is likely to need prompt airway protection.
- A child who opens her eyes to pain, shouts recognisable words inappropriately and localises to the stimulus has a GCS of 10 and is at much less immediate risk.
- **Both are classified as 'P'.**

Posture

o Many children who are suffering from a serious illness in any system are hypotonic.

o Stiff posturing such as that shown by **decorticate** (flexed arms, extended legs) or **decerebrate** (extended arms, extended legs) children is a sign of serious brain dysfunction.

o These postures can be mistaken for the tonic phase of a convulsion. Alternatively, a painful stimulus may be necessary to elicit these postures.

o Severe extension of the neck due to upper airway obstruction can mimic the opisthotonos that occurs with meningeal irritation.

o A stiff neck and full fontanelle in infants are signs which suggest meningitis.

Pupils

o Many drugs and cerebral lesions have effects on pupil size and reactions.

o However, the most important pupillary signs to seek are **dilatation, unreactivity and inequality**, which indicate possible serious brain disorders.

2. RESPIRATORY EFFECTS OF CENTRAL NEUROLOGICAL FAILURE

o There are several recognisable breathing pattern abnormalities with raised intracranial pressure.

o However, they are often changeable and may vary from hyperventilation to **Cheyne–Stokes breathing** to apnoea.

o The presence of any abnormal respiratory pattern in a patient with coma suggests mid- or hind-brain dysfunction.

3. CIRCULATORY EFFECTS OF CENTRAL NEUROLOGICAL FAILURE

o Systemic hypertension with sinus bradycardia (Cushing's response) indicates compression of the medulla oblongata caused by herniation of the cerebellar tonsils through the foramen magnum.

o **This is a late and pre-terminal sign.**

E. EXPOSURE

Temperature

o A fever suggests an infection as the cause of the illness, but may also be the result of prolonged convulsions or shivering.

o In young infants, infection may present with a low body temperature.

Rash and bruising

o Examination is made for rashes, such as urticaria in allergic reactions, purpura, petechiae and bruising in septicaemia and child abuse, or maculopapular and erythematous rashes in allergic reactions and some forms of sepsis.

SUMMARY: THE RAPID CLINICAL ASSESSMENT OF AN INFANT OR CHILD

Airway and Breathing	Circulation	Disability	Exposure
Effort of breathing Respiratory rate/rhythm Stridor/wheeze Auscultation Skin colour	Heart rate Pulse volume Capillary refill Skin T°	Mental status Conscious level Posture Pupils	Fever Rash and bruising

II. APPROACH TO THE SERIOUSLY ILL CHILD

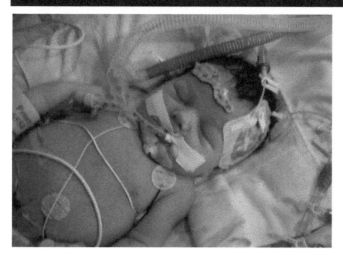

INTRODUCTION

o Treatment of a child in an emergency requires rapid assessment and urgent intervention.

o The structured approach includes:
  - Primary assessment
  - Resuscitation
  - Secondary assessment and looking for key features
  - Emergency treatment
  - Stabilisation and
  - Transfer to definitive care

1. PRIMARY ASSESSMENT & RESUSCITATION

o In a severely ill child, a rapid examination of vital functions is required.

o This primary assessment and any necessary resuscitation must be completed before the more detailed secondary assessment is performed.

AIRWAY

- **Primary assessment:** Assess patency by:
  - Looking for chest and/or abdominal movement
  - Listening for breath sounds
  - Feeling for expired air
  - Vocalisations, such as crying or talking, indicate ventilation and some degree of airway patency
  - If there is obvious spontaneous ventilation, note other signs that may suggest upper airway obstruction:
    - The presence of stridor
    - Evidence of recession
  - If there is no evidence of air movement then chin lift or jaw thrust manoeuvres must be carried out.

- Reassess the airway after any airway-opening manoeuvres. If there continues to be no evidence of air movement then airway patency can be assessed by performing an airway opening manoeuvre while giving rescue breaths.
- **Resuscitation:** If the airway is not patent, then this can be secured by:
  - A chin lift or jaw thrust
  - The use of an airway adjunct
  - Tracheal intubation

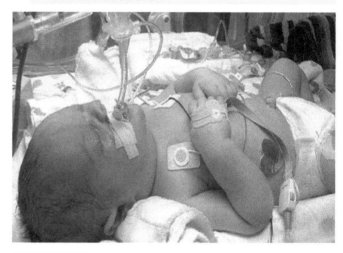

BREATHING

- **Primary assessment**
  - A patent airway does not ensure adequate ventilation.
  - The latter requires an intact respiratory centre and adequate pulmonary function augmented by coordinated movement of the diaphragm and chest wall.

- **Resuscitation**
  - **Give high-flow oxygen** (flow rate 15 l/min) through a mask with a reservoir bag to any child with respiratory difficulty or hypoxia.
  - In the child with inadequate respiratory effort, this should be supported either **with bag–valve–mask ventilation or intubation** and intermittent positive pressure ventilation.

CIRCULATION

- **Primary assessment**
  - It is more difficult to assess than breathing and individual measurements must not be used on their own to diagnose circulatory failure.

- **Resuscitation**
  - In every child with an inadequate circulation:

- **Give high-flow oxygen** through either a mask with a reservoir bag or an endotracheal tube if intubation has been necessary for airway control or inadequate breathing.
- **Venous or intraosseous access** should be gained and an immediate infusion of **crystalloid (20 ml/kg)** given.
- **Urgent blood samples, especially blood glucose**, may be taken at this point.

DISABILITY (NEUROLOGICAL EVALUATION)

- **Primary assessment**
  - Both hypoxia and shock can cause a decrease in conscious level.
  - Any problem with ABC must be addressed before assuming that a decrease in conscious level is due to a primary neurological problem.
  - In addition, any patient with a decreased conscious level or convulsions must have an **initial glucose stick test** performed.

- **Resuscitation**
  - Consider intubation to stabilise the airway in any child with a conscious level recorded as P or U (only responding to painful stimuli or unresponsive).
  - If hypoglycaemia has been found, treat hypoglycaemia with a **bolus of glucose (2 ml/kg of 10% glucose)** followed by an IV infusion of glucose, after taking blood for glucose measurement in the laboratory and a sample for further studies.
  - **Intravenous lorazepam, buccal midazolam or rectal diazepam** should be given for prolonged or recurrent fits).
  - Manage raised intracranial pressure if present.

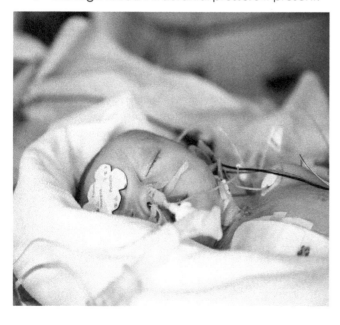

2. SECONDARY ASSESSMENT AND EMERGENCY TREATMENT

- The secondary assessment takes place once vital functions have been assessed and the treatment of life-threatening conditions has been instituted.
- It includes a medical history, a clinical examination and specific investigations.
- It differs from a standard medical history and examination in that it is designed to establish which emergency treatments are required to stabilise the child. At the end of secondary assessment, the practitioner should have a better understanding of the illness affecting the child and may have formulated a differential diagnosis.
- Emergency treatments will be appropriate at this stage – either to treat specific conditions (such as asthma) or processes (such as raised intracranial pressure). The establishment of a definite diagnosis is part of definitive care. The history often provides the vital clues that help the practitioner identify the disease process and hence be able to provide appropriate emergency care. In the case of children, the history is often obtained from an accompanying parent, although a history should be sought from the child if possible. Do not forget to ask pre-hospital staff about the child's initial condition and about treatments and response to treatments that have already been given. Some children will present with an acute exacerbation of a known condition such as asthma or epilepsy. Such information is helpful in focusing attention on the appropriate system but the practitioner should be wary of dismissing new pathologies in such patients. The structured approach prevents this problem. Unlike trauma (which is dealt with later), illness affects systems rather than anatomical areas.
- The secondary assessment must reflect this and the history of the complaint should be sought with special attention to the presenting system or systems involved. After the presenting system has been dealt with, all other systems should be assessed and any additional emergency treatments commenced as appropriate.
- The secondary assessment is not intended to complete the diagnostic process, but rather is intended to identify any problems that require emergency treatment. The following gives an outline of a structured approach in the first hour of emergency management. It is not exhaustive but addresses the majority of emergency conditions that are amenable to specific emergency treatments in this time period.

RESPIRATORY

- ## Secondary Assessment

Symptoms	Signs	Investigations
Breathlessness Coryza Cough Noisy breathing – grunting, stridor, wheeze Drooling and inability to drink Abdominal pain Chest pain Apnoea Feeding difficulties Hoarseness Acidotic breathing	Cyanosis Tachypnoea Recession Grunting Stridor Wheeze Chest wall crepitus Tracheal shift Abnormal percussion note Crepitations on auscultation	Oxygen saturation Peak flow if asthma suspected End-tidal/transcutaneous carbon dioxide if hypoventilation suspected Blood culture if infection suspected CXR (selective) ABG (selective)

EMERGENCY TREATMENT

If 'bubbly' noises are heard	The airway is full of secretions, which may require clearance by suction
If there is a harsh stridor associated with a barking cough	Croup should be suspected and the child given nebulised adrenaline (400 micrograms/kg or 0.4 ml/kg of 1:1000 (maximum 5 ml) nebulised in oxygen).
If there is a quiet stridor, drooling and a short history in a sick-looking child	Consider epiglottitis or tracheitis. Intubation is likely to be urgently required, preferably by a senior anaesthetist. Do not jeopardise the airway by any unpleasant or frightening interventions. Give IV cefotaxime or ceftriaxone once the airway is secure.
Sudden onset and significant history of inhalation	Consider a foreign body within the airway. If the 'choking child' procedure has been unsuccessful, the patient may require laryngoscopy. Do not jeopardise the airway by unpleasant or frightening interventions but contact a senior anaesthetist/ENT surgeon urgently
Stridor following ingestion/injection of a known allergen	Suggests anaphylaxis. Children in whom this is likely should receive IM adrenaline (10 mcg/kg or 150 mcg (<6 years), 300 mcg (6–12 yrs) or 500 mcg (>12 yrs)).

Children with a history of asthma or with wheeze and significant respiratory distress	Should receive oxygen therapy and inhaled β2-agonists
Infants with wheeze and respiratory distress	Have bronchiolitis and require only oxygen if hypoxic.
In acidotic breathing	Likely to take a blood sample for acid–base balance and blood sugar. Treat diabetic ketoacidosis with IV normal saline and insulin.

CARDIOVASCULAR (CIRCULATION)

- ## Secondary assessment

Symptoms	Signs	Investigations
Breathlessness Fever Palpitations Feeding difficulties Drowsiness Pallor Fluid loss Poor urine output	Tachy- or bradycardia Hypo- or hypertension Abnormal pulse volume or rhythm Abnormal skin perfusion or colour Cyanosis/pallor Hepatomegaly Crepitations on auscultation Cardiac murmur Peripheral oedema Absent femoral pulses Raised jugular venous pressure Hypotonia Purpuric rash	U&Es Full blood count ABG Coagulation studies Blood culture ECG CXR (selective)

EMERGENCY TREATMENT

- Further boluses of fluid should be given to shocked children who have not had a sustained improvement to the first bolus given at resuscitation.
- Consider inotropes, intubation and central venous pressure monitoring with the third bolus.
- Consider IV cefotaxime/ceftriaxone in shocked children with no obvious fluid loss, as sepsis is likely.
- If a patient has a cardiac arrhythmia the appropriate protocol should be followed.
- If anaphylaxis is suspected, give IM adrenaline (10 micrograms/kg or 150 micrograms (<6 years), 300 micrograms (6–12 years) or 500 micrograms (>12 years)), in addition to fluid boluses.

o Give **Prostin (alprostadil or dinoprostone)** if duct-dependent congenital heart disease is suspected, e.g. in neonates with unresponsive hypoxia or shock.

o Surgical advice and intervention may be needed for gastrointestinal emergencies.

o The following symptoms and signs may suggest this.

Symptoms	Signs
o Vomiting o Blood PR o Abdominal pain	o Abdominal tenderness o Abdominal mass o Abdominal distension

NEUROLOGICAL (DISABILITY)

- **Secondary assessment**

Symptoms	Signs	Investigations
Headache Convulsions Change in behaviour Change in conscious level Weakness Visual disturbance Fever	Altered conscious level Convulsions Altered pupil size and reactivity Abnormal posture Abnormal oculocephalic reflexes Meningism Papilloedema or retinal haemorrhage Altered deep tendon reflexes Hypertension Slow pulse Full and tense anterior fontanelle	U&E Blood sugar LFT Ammonia Blood culture ABG Coagulation studies Blood and urine toxicology including Carboxyhaemoglobin level CT Scan Brain

EMERGENCY TREATMENT

o For convulsions follow the status epilepticus protocol.

o If there is evidence of raised intracranial pressure (decreasing conscious level, asymmetrical pupils, abnormal posturing and/or abnormal ocular motor reflexes) then the child should undergo:

- Intubation and ventilation (to maintain a PCO2 of 4.5–5.0 kPa (34–38 mmHg).

- Nursing with head in-line and 20° head-up position (to help cerebral venous drainage).

- IV infusion with IV hypertonic (2.7) 3% saline 3 ml/kg, or mannitol 250–500 mg/kg (1.25–2.5 ml of mannitol 20%) over 15 minutes, and repeated if needed, provided serum osmolality remains below 325 mOsm/l.

- Consider dexamethasone (only for oedema surrounding a space-occupying lesion) 0.5 mg/kg 6-hourly.

o In a child with a depressed conscious level or convulsions, consider meningitis/encephalitis: Give cefotaxime/acyclovir.

o In drowsiness with sighing respirations, check blood sugar, acid–base balance and salicylate level.

o Treat diabetic ketoacidosis with IV normal saline and insulin.

o In unconscious children with pinpoint pupils, consider opiate poisoning: A trial of naloxone should be given.

EXTERNAL (EXPOSURE)

- **Secondary assessment**

Symptoms	Signs
o Rash o Swelling of lips/tongue o Fever	o Purpura o Urticaria o Angio-oedema

EMERGENCY TREATMENT

o In a child with circulatory or neurological symptoms and signs, a purpuric rash suggests septicaemia/meningitis.

o The patient should receive cefotaxime or ceftriaxone preceded by a blood culture.

o In a child with respiratory or circulatory difficulty, the presence of an urticarial rash or angio-oedema suggests anaphylaxis.

o Give IM adrenaline (10 micrograms/kg or 150 micrograms (<6 years), 300 micrograms (6–12 years) or 500 micrograms (>12 years)).

- **FURTHER HISTORY**
  - **Developmental and social history**
    - Particularly in a small child or infant, knowledge of the child's developmental progress and immunisation status may be useful.
    - The family circumstances may also be helpful – it may be worth prompting parents to remember other details of the family's medical history.

- **DRUGS AND ALLERGIES**
  - Any medication that the child is currently on or has been on should be recorded.
  - If poisoning is a possibility, it is important to document any medication in the home that the child might have had access to, as even relatively benign over-the-counter medications for adults may cause serious toxicity in small children.
  - A history of allergies should be sought.

13. Gastrointestinal Bleeding
I. APPROACH TO THE UPPER GI BLEEDING

- The upper GI tract is considered any location proximal to the Ligament of Treitz (distal duodenum). The common manifestations are **hematemesis or melena**, while very brisk UGI bleeding can present with hemodynamic changes (symptoms of dizziness, dyspnoea or shock) and/or haematochezia.
- The age of the paediatric patient is helpful when determining the differential diagnosis.

MOST COMMON ETIOLOGIES BY AGE	
Neonate	**3 Years - 5Years**
o Maternal blood o Haemorrhagic disease of the newborn o Coagulopathies: Liver failure, DIC o Gastritis: Stress, Sepsis, Protein Intolerance, Trauma (i.e. NG tube) o Necrotizing Enterocolitis	o Peptic Ulceration o Gastritis: Aspirin, NSAIDs o Varices o Epistaxis o Mallory-Weiss tear
1 Month - 1 Year	**5+ Year**
o Peptic ulcer, Reflux esophagitis, Gastritis o Foreign body o Medications: Aspirin, NSAIDs o Caustic Ingestion	o Peptic Ulceration o Varices o Coagulopathies: ITP, chemotherapy

HISTORY
- o Were there preceding complaints/signs of dyspepsia, dysphagia, abdominal pain, weight loss?
- o What drugs have the patient taken recently that may contribute to gastritis or coagulopathy?
- o Personal or family hx of easy bruising or bleeding?
- o Jaundice or change in stool color may signify underlying liver dysfunction.
- o A preceding choking bout may signify foreign body ingestion. Frequent epistaxis may indicate a nasopharyngeal source.

DIAGNOSIS
- o Is bleeding truly present? Red foods/liquids in the diet can resemble hematemesis.
- o Perform **Gastroccult/Hemoccult test** if unclear.
- o Consider naso/oropharyngeal or respiratory sources of bleeding. A careful exam of the nares and oral pharynx should be done.

- o The presence of **"coffee ground emesis"** represents blood altered by gastric contents and usually means that there has been slow bleeding from the region between the oesophagus and the duodenum.
- o **Perform NG tube aspirate** if significant blood loss estimated (more than teaspoon).
- o In addition to decreasing aspiration risk, this will aid in visualization via endoscope.
- o Other characteristics of upper GI bleeding are **elevated BUN** and **hyperactive bowel sounds**, although these findings are not sensitive.
- o **Endoscopy** is the preferred diagnostic modality, and 90% of cases can be diagnosed if endoscopy performed **within the first 24 hours.**
- o The most common causes have been identified as **gastritis, esophagitis, duodenal ulcers, and oesophageal varices.**
- o **Abdominal US** can assess portal HTN.
- o **Angiography** if endoscopy unsuccessful.

ASSESSMENT OF THE PATIENT
- o Hemodynamic stability is assessed by **vital signs,** which reflect the degree of blood loss.
- ▪ Age-adjusted increased heart rate is always the first compensatory mechanism, while increased capillary refill, orthostatic hypotension, weakness/dizziness, and syncope are also signs.
- o **Consider NG lavage** if bleeding is significant (>1 teaspoon)
- o Labs: **FBC, Coags, U&E, LFTs**
- o **Resuscitate** if hemodynamically unstable
- o **Refer to Paediatric/Surgery**

RESUSCITATION
- o **Typing and cross matching of blood** should be done to be prepared if necessary.
- o Fluid depletion should be corrected with **isotonic fluid** (IV/IO), as fast as necessary to reverse orthostatic hypotension. Hct is not a good measure of blood volume during acute hemorrhage.
- o If the bleeding is assessed to be severe, then the following should be considered: oxygenation, Foley catheterization of the bladder, central venous line, transfusion of whole blood or PRBC, use of pharmacologic agents, intubation and ventilator support.

II. THE LOWER GASTROINTESTINAL BLEEDING

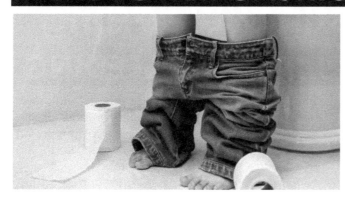

- Although gastrointestinal bleeding is worrisome for parents, unlike adult medicine, it is rarely associated with malignancies in paediatrics.

CONFIRMING THE PRESENCE OF BLOOD IN THE STOOL

- **Hemoccult or Hematest.** This test material contains a peroxide which interacts with peroxidates in hemoglobin and causes a visible color change.
  - **False negatives** can be caused by large amounts of ascorbic acid in the diet or if intestinal bacterial degrade hemoglobin to porphyrin.
  - **False positives** can be caused by large amounts of rare red meat and certain vegetables: broccoli, cauliflower, turnips, radishes, and cantaloupe.
  - **Foods and Medicines** that can make stool appear bloody include red licorice, red pop, koolaid, jello, beets, iron and Pepto Bismol.

UPPER VS. LOWER INTESTINAL TRACT BLEEDING

- An important part of the work-up of GI bleeding involves differentiating upper from lower GI tract bleeding.
  - If there is blood on the surface of the stool this is usually of anal-rectal origin
  - Bright red blood mixed in with stool usually is from below the ligament of Treitz but could be from above if bleed is brisk and large
  - Melena or tarry stools are usually above the ligament of Treitz

EVALUATION OF BLEEDING

- **HISTORY**
  - Amount of blood and appearance of stool (Bright red blood vs. tarry stools)
  - How long has there been bleeding?
  - Associated symptoms of fever, weight loss, diarrhoea, vomiting, constipation, pain
  - Change of appetite, Diet
  - Travel
  - Family History
  - Growth
- **PHYSICAL EXAM**
  - Pallor
  - Rashes, petechiae, purpura, hemangiomas, jaundice, telangiectasias
  - Mouth lesions
  - Abdominal exam for masses, tenderness
  - Rectal exam
  - Vital signs
  - Jaundice (hepatic failure) or cutaneous bruising

EVALUATION

- The evaluation of the infant or child with blood in their stools is dependent on the history, general condition of the child, growth and development, amount of blood in the stool, the condition of the child including heart rate, blood pressure, amount of discomfort, and degree of anaemia, if any.
- If necessary, the child should be stabilized.
- After a thorough history and physical exam, a **FBC, Reticulocyte count, smear, and Platelet count** should be performed.
- If the child is ill appearing, a **type and cross match** should be done.
- If the child is not ill and massive bleeding is not suspected, **an outpatient evaluation** may be performed.

MOST COMMON ETIOLOGIES BY AGE	
Neonate	**1 month – 1 Years**
o **NEC-** usually in preterm o **Hirschsprung's** disease associated with enterocolitis o Malrotation and associated **volvulus** o **Swallowed blood-** Do an **Apt test** to differentiate foetal from adult hemoglobin o **Coagulopathy**	o Anal or rectal **fissures** o **Formula intolerance** o **Meckel's diverticulum** o **Hirschsprung's** disease o **Intussusception-** most common in the ileocecal area o **Lymphonodular hyperplasia** o **Infectious diarrhoea/ HUS/ HSP**
1 Year – 5 Years	**5+ Year - Adolescence**
o **Polyps-** may have large amount of bleeding and often pass spontaneously o **Infectious diarrhoea-** either viral or bacterial	o Similar to younger with the addition of o **Inflammatory Bowel Disease**

14. The Child with Heart Conditions

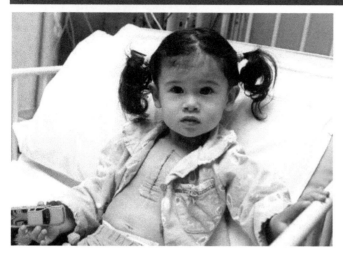

1. OVERVIEW

- In infancy, heart failure is usually secondary to structural heart disease, and medical management is directed at improving the clinical condition prior to definitive surgery.
- There are some complex congenital heart defects in which the presence of a **PDA** is essential to maintain pulmonary or systemic flow. The normal PDA closes functionally in the first 24 hours of life.
- Infants with duct-dependent right or left heart lesions present in the first few days of life as the ductus arteriosus starts closing in response to transition from foetal to postnatal life.
- With modern obstetric management, many infants are now diagnosed antenatally so that they may be delivered within cardiac units.
- Newborns also more commonly undergo newborn oximetry screening, which also allows earlier detection of cases. This has resulted in fewer infants with serious congenital heart disease, including those with duct-dependent disease, presenting to paediatric or emergency departments.
- In the older child, **myocarditis and cardiomyopathy** are the usual causes of the acute onset of heart failure and remain rare. Presenting features include fatigue, effort intolerance, anorexia, abdominal pain and cough. The presence of chest pain and arrhythmia should also be included as clues towards a diagnosis of myocarditis.

- On examination, a marked sinus tachycardia, hepatomegaly and raised jugular venous pressure are found with inspiratory crackles on auscultation.
- ECG and cardiac enzymes may be helpful in diagnosis.

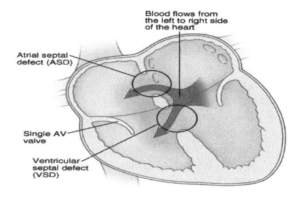

2. CAUSES OF HEART FAILURE THAT MAY PRESENT AS BREATHING DIFFICULTIES

LEFT VENTRICULAR VOLUME OVERLOAD OR EXCESSIVE PULMONARY BLOOD FLOW	LEFT HEART OBSTRUCTION
<ul><li>VSD</li><li>ASD</li><li>Common arterial trunk</li><li>Persistent arterial duct</li></ul>	<ul><li>Hypertrophic cardiomyopathy</li><li>Critical aortic stenosis</li><li>Aortic coarctation</li><li>Hypoplastic left heart syndrome</li></ul>
PRIMARY 'PUMP' FAILURE	**DYSRHYTHMIA**
<ul><li>Myocarditis</li><li>Cardiomyopathy</li></ul>	<ul><li>Supraventricular tachycardia</li><li>Complete heart block</li></ul>
CAUSES OF TACHYARRHYTHMIAS IN CHILDREN	
<ul><li>Re-entrant congenital conduction pathway abnormality (common)</li><li>Poisoning</li><li>Metabolic disturbance</li><li>After cardiac surgery</li><li>Cardiomyopathy</li><li>Long QT syndrome</li></ul>	

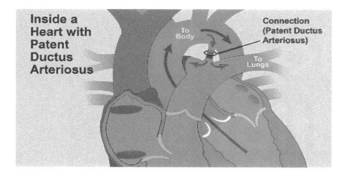

3. EMERGENCY TREATMENT OF PAEDIATRIC HEART FAILURE

- **Reassess ABC**
  - If there are signs of shock– treat the child for **cardiogenic shock.**
  - If circulation is adequate and oxygen saturation is normal or improves significantly with oxygen by face mask but there are signs of heart failure, then the breathing difficulty is due to pulmonary congestion secondary to a large left to right shunt.
    - The shunt may be through a ventricular septal defect (VSD), atrioventricular septal defect (AVSD), patent ductus arteriosus (PDA) or, more rarely, an aortopulmonary window or truncus arteriosus.
    - In many cases a heart murmur will be heard.
    - A chest X-ray will usually provide supportive evidence in the form of cardiomegaly and increased pulmonary vascular markings.
    - **Give high-flow oxygen by face mask with a reservoir, and diuretics should be commenced.**
    - In most cases, oral diuretics are adequate and a combination of loop diuretics **(frusemide)** with a potassium-sparing diuretic (**amiloride or spironolactone**) in twice or thrice daily doses should be commenced.
    - Electrolytes should be checked prior to commencing diuretics.
    - In severe cases, the first dose of frusemide may need to be given intravenously.
  - Babies in the first few days of life who present with breathlessness and increasing cyanosis largely unresponsive to oxygen supplementation are likely to have **duct-dependent congenital heart disease** such as **tricuspid or pulmonary atresia**.
  - Children of all ages who present with breathlessness from heart failure may have **myocarditis**. This is characterised by a marked sinus tachycardia and the absence of signs of structural abnormality.

- The patients should be treated with oxygen and diuretics.

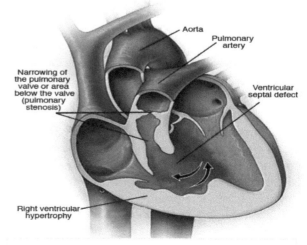

4. INVESTIGATIONS

  - FBC, U&E, Ca²⁺, Glucose, ABG
  - Blood Cultures: routine infection screen
  - CXR and ECG

5. MANAGEMENT

  - All patients suspected of having heart disease should be discussed with a paediatric cardiologist.
  - **Echocardiography** will establish the diagnosis in most cases.

Tetralogy of Fallot (ToF)

Tetralogy of Fallot, which is one of the most common congenital heart disorders, comprises:

1. Right ventricular (RV) outflow tract obstruction (RVOTO) (infundibular stenosis),
2. Ventricular septal defect (VSD),
3. Aorta dextroposition, and
4. RV hypertrophy (see the image below).

The mortality rate in untreated patients reaches 50% by age 6 years, but in the present era of cardiac surgery, children with simple forms of tetralogy of Fallot enjoy good long-term survival with an excellent quality of life.

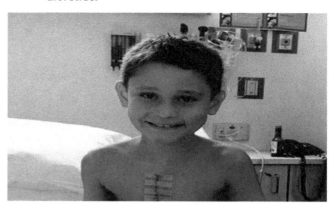

Tetralogy of Fallot

I. THE DUCT DEPENDENT HEART DISEASE

FEATURES SUGGESTING A CARDIAC CAUSE OF CIRCULATORY INADEQUACY
- *Cyanosis, not correcting with oxygen therapy*
- *Tachycardia out of proportion to respiratory difficulty*
- *Raised jugular venous pressure,*
- *Gallop rhythm/murmur*
- *Enlarged heart on chest X-ray,*
- *Enlarged liver*
- *Absent femoral pulses*

- The ductus arteriosus connects the systemic and pulmonary circulations in foetal life.
- Infants with duct-dependent right or left heart lesions present in the first few days of life as the ductus arteriosus starts closing in response to transition from foetal to postnatal life.

NEONATES WITH DUCT-DEPENDENT PULMONARY CIRCULATION
- **Pulmonary Atresia, Critical Pulmonary Stenosis, Tricuspid Atresia, Tetralogy of Fallot**
- Present in the first few days of life with increasing cyanosis unresponsive to supplemental oxygen and signs of severe hypoxaemia with little respiratory distress before collapsing with cardiogenic shock.
- A high index of suspicion is required to diagnose these conditions, as frequently there is no audible murmur. Patients may have **tachycardia, tachypnoea and an enlarged liver.**

NEONATES WITH DUCT-DEPENDENT SYSTEMIC CIRCULATION
- **Coarctation of the aorta, Critical Aortic Stenosis, Hypoplastic Left Heart Syndrome, Interrupted Aortic Arch**
- Usually present in the first few days of life with inability to feed, breathlessness, a grey appearance and collapse with poor peripheral circulation and cardiogenic shock.
- These infants are severely ill with signs of poor organ perfusion with severe metabolic acidosis, poor urine output and decreased conscious level.
- Pulses can be difficult to feel in these patients because of left-sided obstruction to cardiac output and a difference may be noticed in the upper and lower limb pulses and blood pressure depending on the site of the lesion.

CHILDREN WITH TRANSPOSITION OF THE GREAT ARTERIES
- They are duct dependent for both circulations (systemic and pulmonary).

- Having completed the primary assessment and resuscitation and identified by means of the key features that duct-dependent congenital heart disease is the most likely diagnosis, the child is reassessed.

INVESTIGATIONS
- Chest X-ray and ECG, FBC, U&E, Ca^{2+}, Glucose, ABG, Lactate, Blood cultures (since differential diagnosis with sepsis might be difficult).

EMERGENCY TREATMENT OF DUCT-DEPENDENT CONGENITAL HEART DISEASE
- **Reassess ABC**
- **Oxygen therapy** will often provide limited benefit.
- Since **it may accelerate duct closure**, use oxygen judiciously or discontinue if there is no effect.
- **Tracheal intubation and mechanical ventilation** in patients with cardiogenic shock. This decreases metabolic demands of the body and assists cardiac function.
- IV infusion of **Prostaglandin E2 (PGE2)**, this will usually reopen and keep the arterial duct patent, which will help in stabilising the patient before definitive surgical intervention.
  - **Cyanotic baby** or **one with poorly palpable pulses** who is otherwise well and non-acidotic: start at **10–15 nanograms/kg/min.**
  - **Acidotic or unwell baby** with suspected duct-dependent lesion: start at **20 nanograms/kg/min.**
  - If no response within first hour, increase to up to **50 nanograms/kg/min.**
- **In suspected left-sided obstruction:** aim for palpable pulses, normal pH and normal lactate.
- **In suspected right-sided obstruction:** aim for SpO2 75–85% and normal lactate.
- If there is suspected or known transposition of the great arteries or hypoplastic left or right heart syndrome with SpO2 <70% or worsening lactates liaise urgently with cardiology and/or intensive care as rapid assessment and atrial septostomy may be necessary.
- Prostaglandins can cause apnoea in some infants; frequent assessment is necessary to identify those who need ventilatory support.
- Prostaglandins can also cause vasodilatation and subsequent drop in blood pressure.
- Such patients may benefit from a fluid bolus to optimise preload.
- Frequent discussion with a paediatric cardiologist and intensivist is mandatory

II. THE CHILD WITH CARDIOMYOPATHY

- **Cardiomyopathy/Myocarditis** is uncommon, but may rarely be found in an infant or child presenting with shock, arrhythmias and signs of heart failure with no history of congenital heart disease.
- It may be difficult to differentiate these patients from septic patients and treatment is dictated by the management of shock.
- If such a patient were in the first few weeks of life, **a trial of prostaglandin (PGE1 or 2)** would be appropriate and would be beneficial for duct dependent circulations as discussed.

INVESTIGATIONS

- Chest X-ray and ECG, FBC, U&E, Ca^{2+},
- Glucose, ABG, Lactate
- Blood cultures

ED TREATMENT OF CARDIOMYOPATHY & MYOCARDITIS

- The management depends on whether the child presents with cardiac failure or shock.
  - Those presenting in heart failure need to be managed as per local guidance for heart failure, including use of **ACE inhibitors**.
  - In those presenting in shock and suspected to have myocarditis or cardiomyopathy, aggressive fluid resuscitation needs to be avoided and **inotropes need to be used** on advice of the intensive care team.
  - **Adrenaline** is usually the preferred inotrope and can be used both centrally and peripherally.
- **Reassess ABC**
- Give high-flow oxygen
- Give a **cautious fluid bolus of 5–10 ml/kg.**
- Children may be fluid depleted and have cardiac dysfunction, so judicious use of fluid would not be harmful.
- Aggressive fluid resuscitation needs to be avoided and inotropes (e.g. adrenaline and/or dobutamine) need to be used only on advice of the paediatric intensive care team or paediatric cardiologist.
- Treatment then needs to be titrated according to the clinical picture.
- Consider a **diuretic**, if the child is not shocked, to offload the heart, such as **IV Frusemide 0.5–1 mg/kg**

III. THE CHILD WITH BRADYCARDIA

- In Paediatric practice bradycardia is almost always a pre-terminal finding in patients with respiratory or circulatory insufficiency.
- Airway, breathing and circulation should always be assessed and treated if needed before pharmacological management of bradycardia.

CAUSES OF BRADYARRHYTHMIA IN CHILDREN:

- Pre-terminal event in hypoxia or shock
- Raised intracranial pressure
- Conduction pathway damage following cardiac surgery
- Congenital heart block (rare)
- Long QT syndrome

- Incidental bradycardia in a clinically well child may be seen in athletic and sporty children and does not require any treatment.

MANAGEMENT OF BRADYCARDIA IN CHILDREN:

- **Reassess ABC**
  - If there is hypoxia and shock, treat with:
    - High concentration Oxygen,
    - Bag–Mask Ventilation,
    - Intubation and
    - Intermittent Positive Pressure Ventilation.
  - Volume expansion: **20 ml/kg of crystalloid** repeated as recommended in the treatment of shock.
  - If the above is ineffective titrate slowly **Adrenaline 10 micrograms/kg IV.**
  - If the above is ineffective, **infuse adrenaline 0.05–2 micrograms/kg/min IV.**
  - If there has been vagal stimulation:
    - Treat with adequate ventilation.
    - Give **atropine 20 mcg/kg IV/IO** (min dose 100 micrograms; maximum dose 600 micrograms).
    - The dose may be repeated after 5 min (max total dose of 1mg in a child and 2mg in an adolescent).
  - If there has been poisoning, seek expert toxicology help.

IV. THE VENTRICULAR TACHYCARDIA (VT)

- Consider the following underlying causes:
  - Congenital heart disease and surgery.
  - Myocarditis or cardiomyopathy.
  - Poisoning with tricyclic antidepressants, procainamide or quinidine.
  - Renal disease or another cause of hyperkalaemia.
  - Channelopathies (long QT syndromes, catecholaminergic polymorphic VT).
  - Look for characteristics of the ECG indicative of torsade de pointes. This is seen in conditions characterised by a long QT interval or drug poisoning, such as with quinine, quinidine, disopyramide, amiodarone, tricyclic antidepressants or digoxin.
  - Check serum potassium, magnesium and calcium levels.

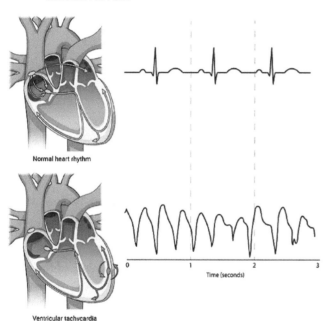

Normal heart rhythm

Ventricular tachycardia

MANAGEMENT OF TACHYCARDIA IN CHILDREN

- **Reassess ABC**
  - **In the haemodynamically unstable child**, the treatment is **synchronised DC cardioversion** starting at **2 J/kg.**
  - It can be repeated and the dose can be increased if needed.
  - **The treatment of the haemodynamically stable** child with VT should always include early consultation with a paediatric cardiologist.

- **They may suggest:**
  - **Amiodarone:** 5 mg/kg over 20 minutes; 30 minutes in neonates or
  - **IV Procainamide:** 15 mg/kg over 30–60 minutes; monitor ECG and blood pressure.
  - Both can cause hypotension, which should be treated with volume expansion.
  - Rare specific VT types may respond to IV verapamil.
  - In cases where the ventricular arrhythmia has been caused by **drug toxicity:**
    - Sedation/anaesthesia and DC shock may be the safest approach.
    - Use synchronous shocks initially, as these are less likely to produce ventricular fibrillation than an asynchronous shock.
    - If synchronous shocks are ineffectual, subsequent attempts will have to be asynchronous if the child is in shock.
  - **The treatment of torsade de pointes VT is:**
    - Emergency defibrillation followed by **Magnesium Sulphate** in a rapid IV infusion of 25–50 mg/kg (up to 2 g) and possibly lidocaine.
    - **IV β-blockers** may help calm the adrenergic storm.
- It is important not to delay a safe therapeutic intervention for longer than necessary in VT as the rhythm often deteriorates quite quickly into pulseless VT or VF.
- Sometimes **wide-complex tachycardia can be SVT with bundle branch block** and aberrant conduction:
  - This can be very difficult to differentiate from VT by a non-specialist.
  - A safer approach is to treat it as VT.
  - A dose of adenosine may help identify the underlying aetiology of the arrhythmia, but should be used with extreme caution in haemodynamically stable children with wide-complex tachycardia because acceleration of the tachycardia and significant hypotension are known risks and should not delay definitive treatment in children with shock.
  - Seek advice.

V. THE SUPRAVENTRICULAR TACHYCARDIA (SVT)

Supraventricular Tachycardia (SVT)

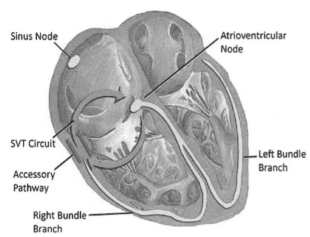

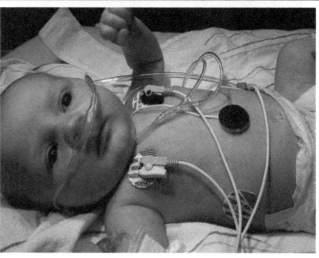

- Presenting complaints may range from tachycardia to poor feeding, irritability, heart failure, and shock.
- This is not usually a difficult diagnosis because the heart rate is sustained at **≥ 220 beats per minute with a QRS < 0.08 second**.
- ED management is dependent on the patient stability at presentation.

IN A STABLE PATIENT

- ○ **Vagal manoeuvers** at this age include icing the face, avoiding the nares.
- ○ If unsuccessful, IV access should be established, and adenosine **0.1 mg/kg IV push** followed immediately by flush should be administered (maximum of 6 mg/kg).
- ○ If SVT persists then a second dose of adenosine **0.2 mg/kg IV** (maximum of 12 mg/kg).
- ○ After a further two minutes, another dose of **0.3 mg/kg adenosine** should be given
- ○ If the child remains in stable SVT despite these measures then the guidelines recommend that following be considered:
  - ▪ **Adenosine 0.4-0.5 mg/kg**
  - ▪ **Synchronous DC shock**
  - ▪ **Amiodarone**

AN UNSTABLE PATIENT

- ○ Without IV access should be treated with **synchronized cardioversion** (1 - 2 J/kg).
- ○ If there is established IV access and adenosine is readily available, then the initial cardioversion may be attempted pharmacologically.
- ○ If the SVT is unresponsive to adenosine or synchronized cardioversion or if a wide QRS is suspected, then **amiodarone 5 mg/kg IV over 20-60 minutes** may be administered.
- ○ Alternatively, **Procainamide 15 mg/kg IV over 30-60 minutes** may be administered.
- ○ Amiodarone and Procainamide should not be administered together because the combination can lead to **hypotension and widening of the QRS complex.**
- ○ **Lidocaine 1 mg/kg IV** is a final option for a wide QRS and should only be used in consultation with a paediatric cardiologist.
- ○ A 12-lead ECG should be obtained prior to and after conversion from SVT to normal sinus rhythm.

- This is a useful diagnostic tool for the cardiologists to help determine further management.
- A Paediatric Cardiologist should be consulted for further evaluation.

15. Pain Management
I. ASSESSMENT OF ACUTE PAIN IN CHILDREN

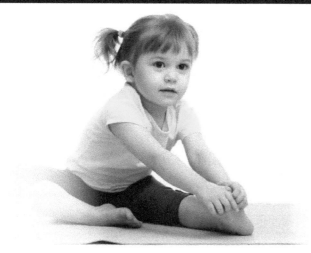

PAIN MEASUREMENT SCALE

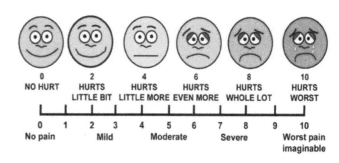

OVERVIEW

o Acute pain is one of the most common adverse stimuli experienced by children, occurring as a result of injury, illness and necessary medical procedures. It is associated with increased anxiety, avoidance, somatic symptoms and increased parent distress[169].

o Pain is commonly under-recognised, under-treated and treatment may be delayed.

o For moral, ethical, humanitarian and physiological reasons, pain should be anticipated and safely and effectively prevented and controlled in all age groups[170].

- **Assessment of acute pain in children in the ED**
  o **Children < 5 years:** FLACC
  o **Children 5-7 years:** Wong Baker FACES
  o **Children >7 years:** Use VAS (scale 0-10 [10 worse pain ever])

Wong-Baker FACES® Pain Rating Scale

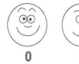

0	2	4	6	8	10
No Hurt	Hurts Little Bit	Hurts Little More	Hurts Even More	Hurts Whole Lot	Hurts Worst

HOW TO TREAT PAIN

1. Non-Pharmacological
  o **Psychological strategies:** involving parents, cuddles, child-friendly environment, and explanation with reassurance all help build trust.
  o Also, distraction with toys, blowing bubbles, reading, or story-telling using superhero or magical imagery to make the pain go away.
  o Non-pharmacological adjuncts such as limb immobilisation, dressings for burns[171].

2. Pharmacological
- **Pain management - Meds**
  o Pharmacological agents, via a variety of routes: see below descriptions.
  o Use **TAC** in preference to EMLA for topical anaesthesia.
  o For superficial wounds, topical anaesthesia should be used in preference to Lignocaine infiltration.
  o Also, local or regional anaesthesia are useful (e.g. femoral and auricular blocks).
  o For procedures, departments may consider conscious sedation using Ketamine (IV / IM) (more on Ketamine sedation).
  o PO/IV/IN options include, Non-opioid, Opioid (including intra-nasally delivered Fentanyl) and inhaled (N_2O).

[169] American Academy of Paediatrics, American Pain Society. The Assessment and Management of Acute Pain in Infants, Children and Adolescents. Paediatrics 2001; 108(3):793-797.

[170] Morton NS. Prevention and control of pain in children. Br J Anaesthesia 1999; 83; 118-229.

[171] RCEM Management of Pain in Children, Simon Smith FRCP, FCEM. Consultant in Emergency Medicine, John Radcliffe Hospital, Oxford. July 2017

II. ORAL AND PARENTERAL ANALGESIA

A. LOCAL ANAESTHETICS

1. AMETOP GEL (This contains tetracaine (amethocaine) base 4%.)

o It is used under an occlusive dressing, Analgesia is achieved after 30–45 minutes;
o Anaesthesia remains for 4–6 hours after removal of the gel
o Slight erythema, itching and oedema may occur at the site
o Not to be applied on broken skin, mucous membranes, eyes or ears
o Can cause sensitisation on repeated exposure.
o Not recommended for a patient under 1 month of age

2. EMLA

o A mixture of **lidocaine 2.5% and prilocaine 2.5%** can be used in a similar fashion where sensitivity to Ametop occurs.
o EMLA, however, takes around 60 minutes to work effectively and tends to cause vasoconstriction rather than vasodilatation.

3. ETHYL CHLORIDE SPRAY: This works immediately

4. LIGNOCAINE 1%

o 1% lidocaine is used for rapid and intense sensory nerve block. It is often used with adrenaline to prolong the duration of sensory blockade and to limit toxicity by reducing absorption (adrenaline concentration 5 micrograms/ml).
o Adrenaline-containing local anaesthetic should not be used in areas served by an end artery, such as a digit.
   - Onset of action: within **2 minutes**
   - Duration of action: up to **2 hours**
   - The maximum body dose is **3 mg/kg for plain** solutions and **7 mg/kg for solutions that contain adrenaline.**

5. BUPIVACAINE

o This local anaesthetic is used – at a concentration of 0.25% or 0.5% – when longer lasting local anaesthesia is required, such as in femoral nerve blocks.
o **L-Bupivacaine** used in the same dose is associated with less toxicity.
   - Onset of action: up to **15 minutes**
   - Duration of action: up to **8 hours.**
   - Maximum body dosage is **2 mg/kg.**
o Local anaesthetics are manufactured to a pH of 5 (to improve shelf-life) and are painful for this reason.

o Overdose or inadvertent injection of local anaesthetics into an artery or vein may result in cardiac arrhythmias and convulsions.
o Resuscitative facilities and skills must therefore be available wherever and whenever these drugs are injected.

6. ADRENALINE & COCAINE GEL

o 1ml of gel per 1cm of wound, to max 4mls
o Not on mucous membranes or abrasions
o Controlled drug

B. NON-OPIOID ANALGESICS

- These drugs exhibit varying degrees of analgesic, antipyretic and anti-inflammatory activity.

1. PARACETAMOL

o Paracetamol is probably the most widely used analgesic in paediatric practice.
o It may be administered by the oral, rectal and intravenous routes.
o It is thought to work through inhibiting cyclo-oxygenase in the central nervous system but not in other tissues, so that it produces analgesia without any anti-inflammatory effect.
o It does not cause respiratory depression.
o It is very safe when administered at the recommended dose although overdosage in a large single dose or too frequent smaller doses may cause hepatotoxicity.
o Higher loading doses have been shown to improve pain control.

2. NONSTEROIDAL ANTI-INFLAMMATORY DRUGS

o These are anti-inflammatory and antipyretic drugs with moderate analgesic properties.
o They are less well tolerated than paracetamol, causing **gastric irritation, platelet disorders, bronchospasm and renal impairment.**
o They should therefore be avoided in children with a history of gastric ulceration, platelet abnormalities and dehydration or renal problems.
o Their advantage is that they are especially useful for post-traumatic pain because of the additional anti-inflammatory effect.
o Ibuprofen is given by mouth, and if rectal administration is necessary then diclofenac can be used.

C. OPIATE ANALGESICS

1. MORPHINE

o Administered intravenously, Morphine produces a rapid onset of excellent analgesia and remains the treatment of choice in many situations.

o It may be titrated to effect and reversed if necessary.

o Side effects include:

- Respiratory depression,
- Nausea and vomiting.
- Cardiovascular effects include peripheral vasodilatation and venous pooling, but in single doses it has minimal haemodynamic effect in a supine patient with normal circulating volume.
- In hypovolaemic patients it will contribute to hypotension but this is not a contraindication to its use and merely an indication for cardiovascular monitoring and action as appropriate.
- Opioids produce a dose-dependent depression of ventilation primarily by reducing the sensitivity of brain-stem respiratory centres to hypercarbia and hypoxia.

o This means that a patient who has received a dose of an opioid requires observation and/or monitoring and should not be discharged home until it is clear that the effects of the opiate are significantly reduced.

o The nausea and vomiting produced in adults by morphine seems to be less common in children.

o The intranasal route for the administration of opiates such as **Diamorphine and Fentanyl** has been shown to be a safe and effective route and is becoming increasingly popular for children.

o It also has the advantage of being quick and easy, avoiding the trauma of an intravenous cannula.

D. OPIATE ANTAGONISTS

2. NALOXONE

o Naloxone is a potent opioid antagonist. It antagonises the sedative, respiratory-depressive and analgesic effects of opioids.

o It is rapidly metabolised and is given parenterally because of its rapid first-pass extraction through the liver following oral administration.

o Following intravenous administration, Naloxone reverses the effects of opiates virtually immediately.

o Its duration of action, however, is much shorter than the opiate agonist.

o Therefore, repeated doses or an infusion may be required if continued opiate antagonism is wanted.

E. INHALATIONAL ANALGESIA

1. ENTONOX

o Nitrous oxide is a colourless, odourless gas that provides analgesia in subanaesthetic concentrations.

o It is supplied in premixed cylinders at a 50% concentration with oxygen or at a concentration of up to 70% with oxygen via a blender.

o Delivery devices either act on a demand principle, i.e. the gas is only delivered when the patient inhales and applies a negative pressure, or via a free-flowing circuit. The latter delivery system requires a scavenger circuit. Generally during nitrous oxide therapy, the patient has to be awake and cooperative to be able to inhale the gas; this is an obvious safeguard with the technique.

o Because nitrous oxide is inhaled and has a low solubility in blood, its onset of effect is very rapid.

o It takes 2–3 minutes to achieve its peak effect.

o For the same reason, the drug wears off over several minutes, enabling patients to recover considerably quicker than if they received narcotics or sedatives. Laryngeal protective reflexes do not always remain intact.

o Nitrous oxide is therefore most suitable for procedures where short-lived intense analgesia is required, e.g. dressing changes, suturing, needle procedures such as venous cannulation, lumbar punctures and for pain relief during splinting or transport.

o It is also of benefit for immediate pain relief on presentation until definitive analgesia is effective.

o Using a free flow circuit, nitrous oxide **can be used by children as young as 2 years of age**, although children will need to be 4 or 5 years of age before they can trigger the demand valve of a premixed cylinder. Nitrous oxide may cause nausea, vomiting, euphoria and disinhibition.

o Prolonged exposure to high concentrations can cause bone marrow depression and neuronal degeneration. Nitrous oxide is contraindicated in children with possible intracranial or intrathoracic air because gas diffusion into the confined space may increase pressure.

F. SEDATIVE DRUGS

- In addition to analgesics, psychotropic drugs may also be useful when undertaking lengthy or repeated procedures.

- Sedatives relieve anxiety but not pain and may reduce the child's ability to communicate discomfort and therefore should not be given in isolation.

- The problems associated with the use of sedatives are those of side effects (usually hyperexcitability) and the time required for the child to be awake enough to be allowed home if admission is not necessary.

1. MIDAZOLAM

o This is an amnesic and sedative drug. It can be given intravenously, intramuscularly, orally or intranasally (although this is unpleasant).

o It has an onset time of action of 15 minutes after an oral administration and recovery occurs after about an hour. t may cause respiratory depression, necessitating monitoring of respiratory function and pulse oximetry.

o A few children become hyperexcitable with this drug.

o Whilst its action can be reversed by **Flumazenil**, intravenously this is rarely necessary and can precipitate seizures.

2. KETAMINE

o Ketamine is a potent anaesthetic agent that has an established place in paediatric procedural pain relief in many emergency settings. It causes a dissociative anaesthesia, which is **amnesic and analgesic**, but has **little effect on breathing and maintaining protective airway reflexes**. Side effects include hypersalivation, tachycardia and hypertension, but previous concerns with regard to increasing intracranial pressure are no longer valid.

o Laryngospasm is a rare complication that may be precipitated by instrumentation of the upper airway.

o Ketamine should be considered as an anaesthetic agent and used with all the precautions generally associated with anaesthesia. Emergence phenomenon can be treated with midazolam if necessary but are much less common in paediatric than in adult practice.

o **CONTRA-INDICATIONS**
  o Prior adverse reaction to ketamine
  o Age less than 12 months
  o Active upper or lower respiratory tract infection
  o Active asthma
  o Unstable or abnormal airway: Tracheal surgery or stenosis.
  o Proposed procedure within the mouth or pharynx
  o Patients with severe psychological problems such as cognitive or motor delay or severe behavioural problems
  o Previous psychotic illness/ Uncontrolled epilepsy/ Intra-ocular pathology

o Significant cardiac disease
o Recent significant head injury or reduced level of consciousness
o Intracranial hypertension with CSF obstruction
o Hyperthyroidism or thyroid medication
o Porphyria
o A relative contra-indication that might result in a child receiving in-patient general anaesthesia is commonly **a lack of adequate ED resources:** typically, because of excess departmental workload.

o **CONSENT**
o Seek informed consent from the parent/guardian and older child, including in your discussion potential risks vs benefits, adverse events and alternative options.

o **Dosage**
  - **IV route: Ketamine IV 1 mg/kg slowly** (no less than a minute) so as to avoid apnoea.
  - Within 60 seconds you should sense that the child becomes vacant, demonstrating occasional nystagmus.
  - Supplemental (slow) **IV doses of 0.5 mg/kg** may be required should you deem the level of sedation inadequate, or if the procedure is prolonged.
  - **IM route:** An alternative strategy is **2.5 mg/kg IM injection in the lateral aspect of a thigh** (prepared with topical local anaesthetic if time allows).
  - Expect to wait 5 – 8 minutes for clinical effect.
  - Use top-up doses of **1 mg/kg IM** as required.

o **POST-PROCEDURE**
o **College of Emergency Medicine post-procedure advice:**
  - The child should recover in a quiet, observed and monitored area under the continuous observation of a trained member of staff.
  - Recovery should be complete between **60 and 120 minutes**, depending on the dose and route used.
  - The child can be safely discharged once they are able to ambulate and vocalise/converse at pre-sedation levels.
  - An advice sheet should be given to the parent or guardian advising rest, quiet and supervised activity for the remainder of that day.
  - The child should not eat or drink for two hours after discharge because of the risk of nausea and vomiting.

16. The Limping Child

I. DIFFERENTIAL DIAGNOSIS

COMMON CAUSES OF LIMPING IN CHILDREN

a. All ages

- Trauma (fracture, haemarthrosis, soft tissue)
- Infection (septic arthritis, osteomyelitis, discitis)
- Secondary to various viral illnesses
- Tumor
- Sickle cell disease
- Serum sickness

b. Toddler (1-3 years)	c. Child (4-10 years)	d. Adolescent (11-16 years)
• Transient synovitis	• Transient synovitis	• Slipped upper femoral epiphysis
• Toddler's fracture	• Juvenile arthritis	• Spondylosis
• Child abuse (NAI)	• Perthes disease	• Osgood-Schlatter
• Developmental dysplasia of the hip	• Rheumatic fever	• Chondromalacia
• Juvenile arthritis	• Haemophilia	• Overuse syndromes
• Neuromuscular disease	• Henoch-Schönlein purpura	• Osteochondritis dissecans
• Haemophilia	• Kohler's Disease	
• Henoch-Schönlein purpura	• Rickets	
• Rickets		
• Cerebral palsy		

II. THE CHILD WITH SEPTIC ARTHRITIS

- Septic arthritis in children is an orthopaedic emergency that has serious consequences if not diagnosed promptly and treated effectively.
- The presenting symptoms include pain, non-weight bearing and fever. Inflammatory markers are raised and ultra-sonography demonstrates a joint effusion.
- Diagnosis is by exclusion.
- **Kocher's criteria for child with painful hip: "NEW T"**
  - o **N**on-weight bearing on the affected side
  - o **E**SR >40
  - o **W**CC > 12
  - o **T**emperature > 38.5
- Remember that not all of the features may be present and that the younger the child, the more subtle the presentation can be!
- Staphylococcus aureus is the most common pathogen[172].
- Other causative organisms include group A *Streptococcus* and *Enterobacter* species.

- *Haemophilus influenzae* septic arthritis may occur in children who have not been vaccinated.
- The incidence of Kingella kingae septic arthritis is almost certainly significant but underreported because of its fastidious nature in culture.

INVESTIGATIONS

- o **FBC, ESR, and CRP: negative results** do not rule the disease out.
- o **Blood cultures:** useful in identifying the organism but do not help confirm or exclude the diagnosis in the ED.
- o **X-ray:** used as useful baseline, can be initially normal.
- o **Lateral X-rays** may show bone destruction.
- o **Joint aspiration** and **synovial fluid analysis:** (most important diagnostic test): Fluid should be sent **for gram stain, cultures, crystal examination**, and **cell count**.

MANAGEMENT

- o IV Antibiotics: **Flucloxacillin and benzylpenicillin.**
- o **Analgesia:** consider splintage in addition to pharmacological treatment.
- o **Urgent orthopaedic referral:** for joint irrigation/drainage.

---

[172] Kang SN, Sanghera T, Mangwani J, Paterson JM, Ramachandran M. The management of septic arthritis in children: systematic review of the English language literature. J Bone Joint Surg Br 2009;91:1127–33.

III. THE CHILD TRANSIENT SYNOVITIS

- Transient synovitis is a benign, self-limiting condition that involves synovial inflammation and effusion formation. The condition is poorly understood but a viral aetiology is suspected.
- Although transient synovitis is more common than septic arthritis, given the serious nature of the latter condition, any child presenting with joint irritability should be considered to have septic arthritis until proven otherwise. It is a relatively common problem, especially in children between the ages of **3 and 6 years** old which is usually self-limiting within approximately one week.
- There is a higher incidence in boys than girls.
- Rapid onset of hip pain and limping in an otherwise well child. +/- history of **preceding viral illness**
- Hip held in flexion and abduction, limitation of internal rotation.
- Only mild reduction of hip movements.

IV. THE CHILD WITH PERTHE'S DISEASE

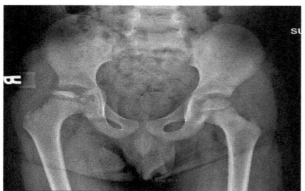

Perthes Disease- From orthokids.org

- Legg-Calve-Perthes disease (LCPD) is idiopathic osteonecrosis or idiopathic avascular necrosis of the capital femoral epiphysis of the femoral head.
- This process is also known as coxa plana, Legg-Perthes, Legg Calve or Perthes disease[173].
- The cause of Legg-Calve-Perthes disease is not known. It may be idiopathic or due to other etiology that would disrupt blood flow to the femoral epiphysis such as trauma (macro or repetitive microtrauma), coagulopathy, and steroid use.
- Thrombophilia is present in approximately 50% of patients and some form of coagulopathy is present in up to 75% [174].

- Age range **2-12 years** (majority **4-8yrs**)
- Boys: Girls = **4 :1, 15%** may be bilateral

CLINICAL:

- **History May Uncover:**
  - Limp of acute or insidious onset, often painless (1 to 3 months)
  - If pain is present, it can be localized to the hip, or refer to the knee, thigh, or abdomen
  - With progression, pain typically worsens with activity
  - No systemic symptoms should be found

- **Physical Examination May Reveal:**
  - Decreased internal rotation and abduction of the hip
  - Pain on rotation referred to the anteromedial thigh and/or knee
  - Atrophy of thighs & buttocks (from pain leading to disuse)
  - Afebrile
  - Leg length discrepancy
  - Gait Evaluation
  - Antalgic Gait (acute): Short-stance phase secondary to pain in the weight-bearing leg
  - Trendelenburg gait (chronic): Downward pelvic tilt away from affected hip during the swing phase

IMAGING:

- The abnormalities are best seen on a **frog-leg lateral view**.
- Perthe's disease **may be bilateral,** so it is important to look specifically for flattening and sclerosis of the femoral head & epiphyseal widening, not simply to compare the two sides. If the diagnosis is in doubt **MRI** is the investigation of choice

COMPLICATIONS

- The most common are coxa magna (widening of the femoral head) and coxa plana (flattening).
- If the femoral head is damaged, it can result in premature physeal arrest which can lead to leg length discrepancy.
- A poorly formed femoral head can also lead to acetabular dysplasia and resultant hip incongruency. This can lead to altered mechanics and subsequent labral tears.
- Lateral hip subluxation or extrusion is a complication associated with a poor outcome and can lead to lifelong problems for the patient.
- A late complication of this childhood disease is hip arthritis.

[173] Leroux J, Abu Amara S, Lechevallier J. Legg-Calvé-Perthes disease. Orthop Traumatol Surg Res. 2018 Feb;104(1S):S107-S112.

[174] Vosmaer A, Pereira RR, Koenderman JS, Rosendaal FR, Cannegieter SC. Coagulation abnormalities in Legg-Calvé-Perthes disease. J Bone Joint Surg Am. 2010 Jan;92(1):121-8.

PROGNOSTIC FACTORS

- **Child's age:** Younger children (age 6 and below) have a greater potential for developing new, healthy bone.
- **The degree of damage to the femoral head:** If more than 50% of the femoral head has been affected by necrosis, the potential for regrowth without deformity is lower. Fifty percent of patients almost fully recover, with no long-term sequelae [175].
- **The stage of disease at the time the child is diagnosed:** How far along the child is in the disease process affects which treatment options to recommend.

V. THE CHILD WITH OSTEOMYELITIS

- Approximately 50% of cases occur in preschool-aged children. Young children primarily experience acute hematogenous osteomyelitis due to the rich vascular supply in their growing bones and therefore most commonly affects **the long bone metaphysis** as these are rapidly growing and highly vascular. It may spread to involve an adjacent joint.
- Symptoms are: **pain, redness, swelling & reduced use of the affected area** (which may be the only sign in infants).
- *Staphylococcus aureus* is the most common pathogen, followed by *Streptococcus pneumoniae and Streptococcus pyogenes.*
- Gram-negative bacteria and group B streptococci are frequently seen in newborns.
- *Pseudomonas aeruginosa* is often associated with osteomyelitis and osteochondritis following penetrating wounds of the foot through a tennis shoe.
- Children who are immunocompromised are prone to infection with various fungi and bacteria, in addition to common pathogens.
- Bony lesions due to *Bartonella henselae* (cause of catscratch disease) have also been reported.
- *Salmonella* is an important cause of osteomyelitis in children with sickle cell disease and other hemoglobinopathies.
- *Kingella kingae,* a fastidious gram-negative rod, is increasingly recognized as a cause of osteoarticular infections, particularly in the first 2 years of life and following a respiratory tract infection.

- Anaerobes such as *Bacteroides, Fusobacterium, Clostridium,* and *Peptostreptococcus* rarely cause osteomyelitis.
- The diagnosis is easily missed in the early stages, so a high index of suspicion and close follow up is required.
- Optimal antibiotic selection, adequate dosing, and a sufficiently prolonged antibiotic course with monitoring for clinical response and for the toxicity of therapy are essential.

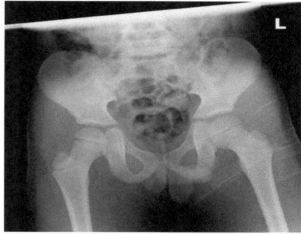

Pelvic Osteomyelitis – From Journal of Orthopaedic Case Reports

INVESTIGATIONS

- o **FBC, ESR, CRP and Blood cultures.**
- o Microbiological diagnosis should be obtained from **blood, joint aspirate or bone aspirate** with Gram stain & culture.
- o **Bone biopsy** can be performed if other diagnoses are suspected, e.g. tumour.
- o **MRI** is the gold standard investigation to confirm the diagnosis.
- o **Plain radiographs** are initially normal but will show bone destruction once this develops, **usually 10-15 days** after the start of infection.

VI. AVULSION FRACTURES OF THE APOPHYSES

- Apophyseal avulsion fractures of the pelvis are rare injuries typically affecting young athletes with not yet ossified cartilaginous growth plates[176].
- Avulsion fractures of the apophyses of the growing pelvis and hip are typically seen in **adolescent athletes (age range 14-25 years)** and are caused by forceful contraction of the muscle avulsing its bony attachment through the physis (growth plate).

---

[175] *Heesakkers N, van Kempen R, Feith R, Hendriks J, Schreurs W. The long-term prognosis of Legg-Calvé-Perthes disease: a historical prospective study with a median follow-up of forty one years. Int Orthop. 2015 May;39(5):859-63. .*

[176] *Fractures of the apophyses in adolescent athletes.*

Howard fm, piha rj jama. 1965 jun 7; 192:842-4.

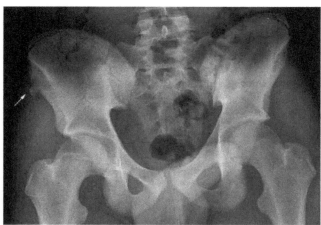

Traumatic avulsion of the anterior superior iliac spine (ASIS) - Image courtesy researchgate.net

MANAGEMENT

o Initially non-operative with **rest, ice, analgesia, passive and active mobilisation after 1 week,** and then a **gradual return to sporting activity.**

o Occasionally delayed surgical fixation may be required for marked displacement & painful non-union.

VII. THE TODDLER'S FRACTURE

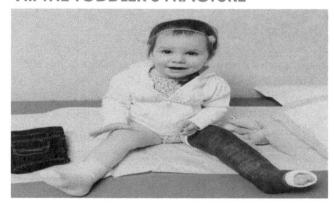

- Toddler's fracture, also called *childhood accidental spiral tibial fracture* or *CAST fracture*, is a fracture unique to ambulatory infants and young children.
- It is caused by a twisting injury while tripping, stumbling, or falling.
- Children usually present limping or refusing to walk. Tenderness at the fracture site is common but is at times hard to elicit in young children.
- Toddler's fracture is diagnosed clinically and frequently can be documented with radiographs.
- They are typically seen in children aged **9 months-3 years.** Usually they are seen in the mid-shaft, but may occur in the upper or lower tibia
- Toddler's fracture may present without specific history of trauma (although usually it does; 92% in one study)

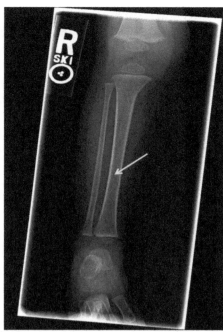

Toddler Fracture | Image courtesy Radiologypics.com

- Radiologic evidence of a broken bone helps confirm fracture, but in the case of TF it is frequently difficult to see a line of fracture on initial x-ray films.
- Presumptive diagnosis helps secure timely treatment, and a repeated x-ray scan after 10 to 14 days helps confirm a diagnosis if a fracture line can be seen[177]. There are no clinical features that can reliably differentiate toddler's fracture from other causes of limp.
- **ED ultrasound** diagnosis of TF in the emergency department was proposed by Lewis and Logan after plain radiographs failed to confirm the diagnosis, and they used the fracture hematoma for guidance[178].

MANAGEMENT OF TODDLER'S FRACTURE SHOULD INCLUDE:

o Treatment is supportive.
o A backslab can be applied.
o An above-knee walking cast for 4 weeks is optional
o Consider NAI* as appropriate
o Analgesia
o Above knee back slab.
o Fracture clinic in 2 weeks with x-ray
o Weight bear as able
o Advice to parents to return if condition worsens or if there are any ongoing concerns
- *NAI: Non-Accidental Injury

---

[177] Toddler's fracture. Clancy J, Pieterse J, Robertson P, McGrath D, Beattie TF J Accid Emerg Med. 1996 Sep; 13(5):366-7.

[178] Lewis D, Logan P. Sonographic diagnosis of toddler's fracture in the emergency department. J Clin Ultrasound. 2006;34(4):190–4.

VIII. THE SLIPPED UPPER FEMORAL EPIPHYSIS

- Slipped Upper Femoral Epiphysis (SUFE) or Slipped Capital Femoral Epiphysis (SCFE) is the most common hip disorder in the adolescent age group.
- It occurs when weakness in the proximal femoral growth plate allows displacement of the capital femoral epiphysis. SCFE is a misnomer; it is the metaphysis that displaces anteriorly and superiorly, leading to the slipped state[179].
- Klein lines are drawn along the superior cortex of the femoral neck. A normal Klein line will intersect the epiphysis. An abnormal Klein line does not intersect the epiphysis, as the femoral neck has moved proximally and anteriorly relative to the epiphysis
- Late childhood/early adolescence, tends to occur in **10 – 15-year olds.** Weight often > 90th centile.
- Boys: Girls = **2:1, 25%** may be bilateral

CLINICAL

o Presents with pain in hip or knee and associated limp.
o The hip appears externally rotated and shortened.
o There is decreased hip movement - especially internal rotation.
- **Risk Factors**: Obesity, Male sex, Immature skeleton, Family history of SUFE
- **Imaging:** AP views alone may miss subtle changes therefore **bilateral 'frog view'** is required

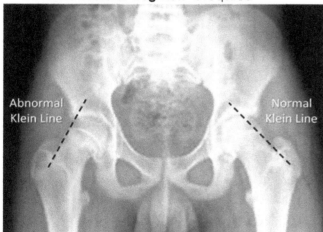

Right SUFE- Image courtesy of John M. Flynn, MD

COMPLICATIONS

- *Long term degenerative osteoarthritis: ~90%*
- *Avascular necrosis of the femoral head (10-15%): increased incidence with the number of attempted reductions and with multiple screws for pinning*
- *Chondrolysis (7-10%): acute cartilage necrosis*

- *Deformity*
- *Limb length discrepancy*

MANAGEMENT

- Refer to Ortho

IX. THE CHILD WITH SARCOMAS

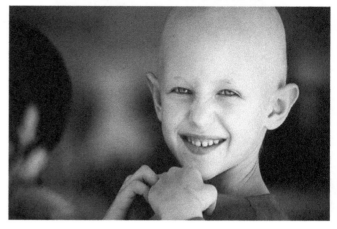

- Soft tissue sarcomas in children are relatively rare.
- Paediatric sarcomas are a heterogenous group of tumours that arise from primitive mesenchymal tissue.
- They can develop from smooth muscle, connective tissue, nerve or muscle at any site in the body and at any age from infancy onwards.
- Rhabdomyosarcoma (RMS) is the most common soft tissue sarcoma among children less than 15 years old, with an incidence of 4.6 per million per year[180].
- Patients may present with a **painless mass** or with symptoms from adjacent tissues, e.g. pain, muscle weakness/reduced use of a limb, abnormal neurology, erythema, urinary retention, pathological fracture, back pain etc.
- They may also present with systemic symptoms such as **fever or weight loss**, particularly when metastases are present.
- Examination of a child with a suspected sarcoma must therefore be comprehensive, including:
  o Careful inspection and palpation of painful sites
  o Neurological examination for asymmetrical weakness or numbness
  o Respiratory examination for signs of metastases Skin examination for purpura (thrombocytopaenia due to bone metastases.

---

[179] *Loder RT, Aronsson DD, Dobbs MB, et al. Instructional course lecture: slipped capital femoral epiphysis. J Bone Joint Surg Am. 2000 Aug;82-A(8):1170-88.*

[180] *Gurney J, Young JL, Jr, Roffers SD, et al. Cancer incidence and survival among children and adolescents: United States SEER Program 1975–1995. Bethesda (MD): National Cancer Institute; SEER Program; 1999. Vol NIH Pub 99-4649.*

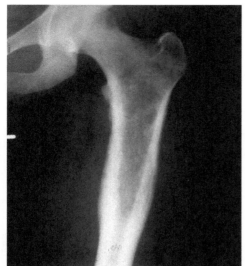

Ewing's sarcoma - Proximal femur - From Tumor Library

ED INVESTIGATION:

o **Plain x-ray:** Initially to look for soft tissue mass and signs of bone involvement such as erosion or pathological fracture.

o **MRI:** is required to determine the extent of the disease, and should be done emergently if there is neurological involvement such as suspected spinal cord compression.

X. THE CHILD WITH OSGOOD-SCHLATTER DISEASE

- Osgood-Schlatter disease is a common cause of knee pain in growing adolescents. **It is an inflammation** of the area just below the knee where the patella tendon attaches to the tibial tuberosity

- **Risk factors for OSD include the following:**
  o Age: female 8-12 years & male between 12-15 years
  o Male sex (3:1)
  o Rapid skeletal growth
  o Repetitive sprinting and jumping sports
- Osgood Schlatter in adults can occur, especially if it has not been looked after during teenage years but is more unusual.
- **Activity -** As the young athlete's bones grow quickly, it can take some time for the muscles and tendons to catch up.
- These changes result in a pulling force from the patella tendon, on to the tibial tuberosity at the top of the shin.
- **This area then becomes inflamed, painful and swollen.**
- This is frequent in younger people because their bones are still soft and are not yet fully grown.

- It is seen more often in children involved with **running and jumping activities** which put a much greater strain on the patella tendon.

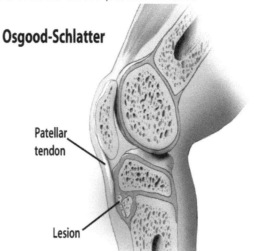

SYMPTOMS

- Symptoms of Osgood Schlatter's disease typically consist of pain at the **tibial tuberosity or bony bit at the top of the shin.**
- The tibial tuberosity may become swollen or inflamed and may even become more prominent than normal.
- Tenderness and pain are worse during and after exercise but usually improves with rest.
- The athlete is likely to experience pain when contracting the quadriceps muscles or performing squat type exercises.

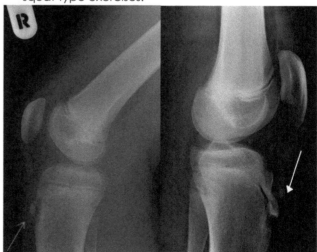

TREATMENT

- **PRICE** principles
  o **P**rotection of the knee from further injury.
  o **R**est
  o **I**ce
  o **C**ompression
  o **E**levation

17. Rashes in Children

INTRODUCTION

o Because childhood rashes may be difficult to differentiate by appearance alone, it is important to consider the entire clinical presentation to help make the appropriate diagnosis[181].

o Considerations include the appearance and location of the rash; the clinical course; and associated symptoms, such as pruritus or fever.

o A fever is likely to occur with roseola, erythema infectiosum (fifth disease), and scarlet fever.

• Pruritus sometimes occurs with atopic dermatitis, pityriasis rosea, erythema infectiosum, molluscum contagiosum, and tinea infection.

• Originally six classical exanthems were described, however vaccination coverage has resulted in a fall in many of these illnesses and more recently newer exanthems such as **Gianotti Crosti Syndrome** have been described.

DEFINITIONS

o **An exanthem** is an eruptive skin rash associated with a fever or other constitutional symptoms.

o Exanthems may arise from an infectious disease or may be drug related.

o **Enanthema** is an eruptive lesion on the mucous membranes occurring as a symptom of disease.

THE ORIGINAL SIX CLASSICAL CHILDHOOD EXANTHEMS

N°	OTHER NAMES	AETIOLOGY (IES)
1. First disease	Rubeola, Measles	**Paramyxovirus**
2. Second disease	Scarlet Fever or Scarlatina	**Streptococcus**
3. Third disease	Rubella, German measles, 3-day measles	**Rubella virus**
5. Fifth disease	Erythema infectiosum	**Parvovirus B19**
6. Sixth disease	Exanthem subitum, Roseola infantum,	**Human Herpes Virus 6B** **Human Herpes Virus 7**

[181] AMANDA ALLMON, MD; KRISTEN DEANE, MD; and KARI L. MARTIN, MD, University of Missouri–Columbia School of Medicine, Columbia, Missouri. Am Fam Physician. 2015 Aug 1;92(3):211-216.

HISTORY AND PHYSICAL EXAMINATION

o The initial approach to a child with a rash begins with the history, which should include the duration of the rash, the initial appearance and how it has evolved, the location, and any treatments that have been used. Parents should also be asked if other household members have a similar rash and if there have been any new medication, product, or environmental exposures. The presence or absence of associated symptoms can help clinicians develop a differential diagnosis. A fever is likely with roseola, erythema infectiosum, and scarlet fever. Pruritus sometimes occurs with atopic dermatitis, pityriasis rosea, erythema infectiosum, molluscum contagiosum, and tinea infection.

o On physical examination, certain clinical findings may be useful in determining a diagnosis. It is important to determine the type of lesions, such as macules, papules, vesicles, plaques, or pustules. Other important characteristics include location and distribution, arrangement, shape, color, and presence or absence of scale.

MACULOPAPULAR ERUPTIONS

o Measles (rubeola)
o Rubella
o Erythema infectiosum (fifths disease)
o Exanthum subitum (roseola)
o Lyme's disease
o Drug related eruptions
o Steven Johnsons Syndrome
o Erythema Multiforme
o Meningiococcaemia

DIFFUSE ERYTHEMA WITH DESQUAMATION

o Scarlet fever
o Toxic shock syndrome
o Scalded skin syndrome
o Kawasaki disease

VESICOBULLOUS/ PUSTULAR ERUPTIONS

o (Diffuse) Varicella zoster
o (Diffuse) disseminated Gonnococaemia
o (Local) hand foot and mouth
o (Local) Herpes zoster
o Staphylococcal bacteraemia
o Rickettsia

SEVEN BROAD TYPES HAVE BEEN IDENTIFIED:

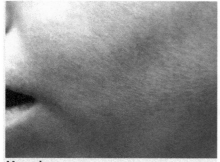

Macule

A macule is a circumscribed area of change in normal skin colour, with no skin elevation or depression. It may be any size.

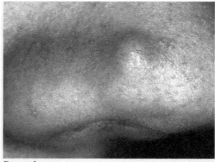

Papule

A papule is a solid raised lesion up to 0.5 cm in greatest diameter.

Note, however, that some text definitions use 1.0 cm as a cut-off limit instead of 0.5 cm.

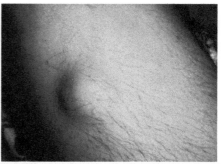

Nodule

A nodule is similar to a papule but is located deeper in the dermis or subcutaneous tissue.

Nodules are differentiated from papules by palpability and depth, rather than size

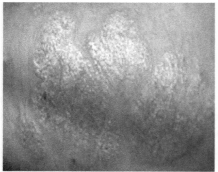

Plaque

A plaque is an elevation of skin occupying a relatively large area in relation to its height.

It can often be formed by a confluence of papules.

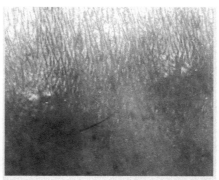

Pustule

A pustule is a circumscribed elevation of skin containing purulent fluid of variable character. The fluid may be white, yellow, greenish or haemorrhagic.

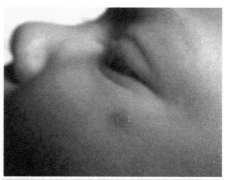

Vesicle

A vesicle is a circumscribed, elevated, fluid-containing lesion less than 0.5 cm in its greatest diameter. It may be intra-epidermal or sub-epidermal in origin.

Note, however, that some text definitions use 1.0 cm as a cut-off limit instead of 0.5 cm.

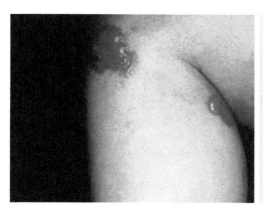

Bulla

A bulla is similar to a vesicle, except the lesion is more than 0.5 cm in its greatest diameter.

Note, however, that some text definitions use 1.0 cm as a cut-off limit to replace 0.5 cm

I. THE CHILD WITH MEASLES

OVERVIEW

- Measles is one of the most contagious infectious diseases, with at least a 90% secondary infection rate in susceptible domestic contacts.
- Despite being considered primarily a childhood illness, measles can affect people of all ages. See the image below. It is caused by a **paramyxovirus** and is still a leading cause of morbidity and mortality in developing countries.
- Measles has been a notifiable illness since the 1940s.
- MMR vaccinations are administered at **12-15 months** of age and **3 to 5 years of age.**

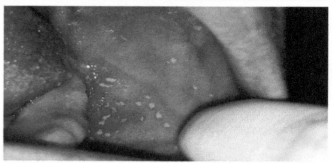

Koplik spots- image source aafp.org

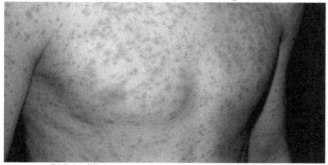

Child with Measles- Image source Echolive.ie

CLINICAL ASSESSMENT/ RISKS

- The patient history is notable for exposure to the virus. The incubation period from exposure to onset of measles symptoms ranges from 7 to 14 days (average, 10-12 days).
- Measles occurs in epidemics in winter and spring, the infection is **spread by droplet spread or less commonly by aerosol spread.**
- The primary site of infection is the nasopharynx.
- The first sign of measles is usually a high fever (often >40° C) that typically lasts 4-7 days.
- This prodromal phase is marked by malaise, fever, anorexia, and the classic triad of conjunctivitis (see the image below), cough, and coryza (the "3 Cs").
- Other possible associated symptoms include photophobia, periorbital edema, and myalgias.
- The characteristic enanthem generally appears 2-4 days after the onset of the prodrome and lasts 3-5 days. Small spots (**Koplik spots**) can be seen inside the cheeks during this early stage
- **Associated signs** described in measles are:
  - **Pin point elevations of the soft palate**, which coalesce to cause a reddened pharynx.
  - **Kolpik spots:** These are blue white area sounded by erythema and occur on the buccal mucosa opposite the second molar. They last around 1-2 days and are pathognomonic of measles.

COMPLICATIONS

- **ENT:** Otitis media, Tonsillitis, Laryngotracheobronchitis
- **Respiratory:** Bronchopneumonia
- **GIT:** Diarrhoea
- **CNS:** Acute encephalitis, Sub acute sclerosing panencephalitis

INVESTIGATIONS

- The investigation is performed using **oral fluid or serum sampling** for measles **IgM antibody.**
- In acute cases measles can be detected using **throat swabs or in the urine.**

MANAGEMENT OF MEASLES

- Treatment is largely symptomatic.
- **Prophylactic antibiotics** to children with measles in geographical areas with a high case fatality rate or with a high incidence of post- measles pneumonia. Antibiotics have been shown to reduce the incidence of complications of pneumonia, otitis media and tonsillitis.
- **Human Normal Immunoglobulin (HNIG)**
  - HNIG may be used to prevent or reduce the severity of an attack if used **within 72 hours** of contact in the following groups:
    - Immunocompromised
    - Pregnant women
    - Infants under the age of 12 months
- **MMR vaccine (13 months and 3.5 years)**
  - Is indicated in the healthy unimmunised or partially immunised within 72 hours of exposure to measles.
- **Vitamin A therapy**
  - Vitamin A deficiency can be a risk factor for severe measles.
- **Notification:** this disease should be notified based on clinical suspicion.
- Children should be kept off school until 5 days after the appearance of the rash.

II. THE CHILD WITH SCARLET FEVER

OVERVIEW

- Scarlet fever is diagnosed in 10% of children presenting with streptococcal tonsillopharyngitis[182].
- It is caused by certain strains of group A beta-hemolytic streptococci that release a streptococcal pyrogenic exotoxin (erythrogenic toxin). Patients who have a hypersensitivity to the toxin may develop the characteristic rash associated with scarlet fever.
- Most children have a fever and sore throat one to two days before the rash develops on the upper trunk. The rash spreads throughout the body, sparing the palms and soles, with characteristic circumoral pallor. This differs from some viral exanthems that develop more slowly.

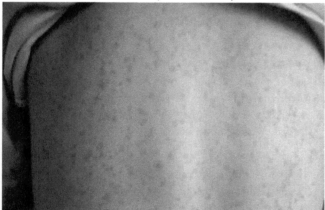

Scarlet Fever – image Source Healthline

- The rash is characterized by confluent, erythematous, blanching, fine macules, resembling a sunburn, and sandpaper-like papules.
- In skinfolds, such as the axilla, antecubital fossa, and buttock creases, an erythematous, nonblanching linear eruption (Pastia lines) may develop. Petechiae on the palate may occur, as well as erythematous, swollen papillae with a white coating on the tongue (white strawberry tongue). Red strawberry tongue occurs after desquamation of the white coating.
- After several weeks, the rash fades and is followed by desquamation of the skin, especially on the face, in skin-folds, and on the hands and feet, potentially lasting four to six weeks[183].

CLINICAL ASSESSMENT

---

[182] Ferri FF. Scarlet fever. In: Ferri's Clinical Advisor. Philadelphia, Pa.: Elsevier; 2014.

[183] Festekjian A, Pierson SB, Zlotkin D. Index of suspicion. Pediatr Rev. 2006;27(5):189–194.

- Scarlet fever is more common in childhood.
- The illness usually begins with a sore throat, headache, fever, tender cervical lymphadenopathy, malaise and also abdominal pain may occur in children. This is followed by a confluent **erythematous rash with a sandpaper like quality.**
- **Other features associated with Scarlet fever:**
  - o **Pastias lines** in the flexural folds such as axilla, neck (due to linear petechiae formations.)
  - o **Circumoral pallor**
  - o **Pharyngitis**
  - o **Desquamation of hands, feet and groin** areas at 7-10 days
  - o **Red strawberry tongue**

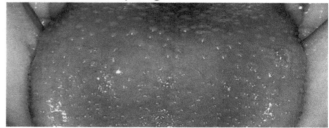

Strawberry tongue- Image source

COMPLICATIONS OF SCARLET FEVER

- o **ENT:** Sinusitis, Mastoiditis, Peritonsillar Abscess
- o **Respiratory:** Pneumonia,
- o **CVS:** Meningitis, Cerebral Abscess.
- o **Systemic infections:** Septicaemia, Osteomyelitis, Septic Arthritis, Myocarditis and toxic shock like syndrome.
- o **Renal:** Glomerulonephritis
- o **Rheumatological:** Acute Rheumatic Fever

INVESTIGATION

- o **Throat swab culture** (Gold standard test) can be performed, but a good quality specimen is required, results can take 24 to 48 hours to become available.
- o **Streptococcal antibody tests (ASOT)** are not indicated during acute illness

MANAGEMENT

- o Antibiotic treatment is indicated (**Penicillin V or Erythromycin or Cephalosporin) for 10 days.**
- o Notification
- o Patients diagnosed with this should have 5 days off from school or work following the commencement of antibiotics.

III. THE CHILD WITH RUBELLA

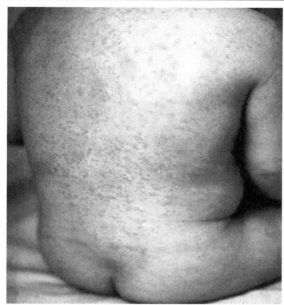

Rubella – Image source cdc.gov

DEFINITION

o Rubella is a viral illness that causes a mild fever and a skin rash. It's also called **German measles**, but is not caused by the same virus that causes measles (rubeola). Rubella is spread through contact with fluid from the nose and throat. It can be prevented with a vaccine.

o It spreads by **airborne transmission** or **droplet** spread from 7 days before to around 7 days after the onset of the rash.

o The incubation period is around **2 weeks** after which a prodrome of headaches, fever and lymphadenopathy occur.

o Immunisation programmes have had a major impact on this illness in developed countries and the incidence of rubella has been markedly reduced in the UK.

CLINICAL ASSESSMENT

o Rubella is associated with a characteristic macular rash, which starts on the face, passing down through the body to the feet and is associated with a fever, tender occipital and posterior auricular lymphadenopathy, arthralgia and respiratory involvement.

o The clinical signs of Rubella may be difficult to distinguish from other viral illnesses such as Parvovirus B19, measles, dengue, Human herpes virus 6. Therefore, laboratory diagnosis is required.

o This vital in especially during pregnancy due to consequences to the foetus

COMPLICATIONS

o Encephalitis, hepatitis, pericarditis,
o Neuritis
o Conjunctivitis
o Orchitis
o Arthralgia
o Arthritis is more common in postmenopausal women.
o Haemolytic anaemia
o Thrombocytopenia

CONGENITAL RUBELLA SYNDROME

• The occurrence of congenital defects is the highest (85%) if the mother develops the rash in the first 12 weeks of pregnancy.

COMPLICATIONS:

o **Ophthalmogical:**
  ▪ Cataracts, Microopthalmos and Congenital glaucoma
o **Cardiac:**
  ▪ Patent ductus arteriosus (PDA) and Peripheral pulmonary artery stenosis
o **Auditory:**
  ▪ Sensory neural hearing impairment
o **Neurological:**
  ▪ Meningoencephalitis

INVESTIGATION STRATEGIES

o **IgG and IgM assays are used.**
o The clinical diagnosis of rubella is unreliable and therefore laboratory confirmation and follow up of this disease is important.
o This is vital especially during pregnancy due to the consequences to the foetus.

MANAGEMENT

o **Children or adults with Rubella should remain of school for at least 5 days after the onset of the rash.**
o This is a notifiable disease.
o Women should avoid pregnancy until 3 months after immunisation
o **MMR vaccine (13 months and 3.5 years)**

IV. THE CHILD WITH PARVOVIRUS B19

- Erythema infectiosum, or fifth disease, is caused by parvovirus B19. It is a common childhood infection characterized by a prodrome of low-grade fever, malaise, sore throat, headache, and nausea followed several days later by an erythematous "slapped cheek" facial rash.
- After two to four days, the facial rash fades. In the second stage of the disease process, pink patches and macules may develop in a lacy, reticular pattern, most often on the extremities.
- After one to six weeks, the rash resolves but may reappear with sun exposure, heat, or stress. Arthralgias occur in approximately 8% of young children with the disease but are much more common in teens and young adults.
- Patients are no longer considered infectious once the rash appears. Treatment is symptomatic and includes nonsteroidal anti-inflammatory drugs for arthralgias and antihistamines for pruritus[184].

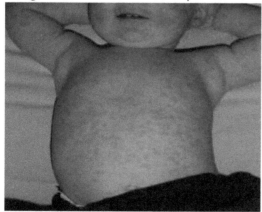

Parvovirus B19 – Source Wikipaedia.org

CLINICAL ASSESSMENT

o Fever and nonspecific symptoms occur early and this is followed approximately 2 to 3 weeks later by a rash and arthropathy. The classical rash **(stage 1)** has been described as a **slapped cheek appearance**, which lasts for up to 4 days.

o The rash is a confluent erythematous, oedematous rash with patches or plaques on cheeks with sparing of nasal bridge and periorbital areas

o This is followed by **(stage 2)** a **maculopapular rash to the trunk and limbs.**

o This rash can vary in intensity and duration. As the rash begins to fade it can take on a lacy appearance.

o Arthropathy can occur in around 5% of the paediatric population and up to 60% of the adult population. Children tend to follow a milder course whereas in adults a symmetrical arthropathy affecting hands, wrists and feet can be more severe.

- **Clinical spectrum** of illness associated with Parvovirus B19:
  o Arthropathy, Henoch Schönlein purpura, Autoimmune disorders
  o Myocarditis, Hepatitis, Papular purpuric glove and socks syndrome
  o Meningitis and encephalitis
  o Fibromyalgia and chronic fatigue syndrome
- Chronic infection in patients with immunodeficiency

COMPLICATIONS

- Complications of parvovirus infections are seen in the following groups:
  o Haemoglobinopathies: **aplastic crises**
  o Immunocompromised
- Pregnant women: **hydrops fetalis** Transient aplastic crises can occur in those with and without underlying chronic haemolytic illness.
- Approximately 60% of women are immune to this virus. Viral transmission in pregnancy is more likely to occur during the first and second trimester.
- **Foetal hydrops** is more likely to occur in the second trimester.

INVESTIGATION STRATEGIES

o **IgM antibodies** appear around 10 days' post infection and remain detectable for up to 2-3 months.

o **IgG antibodies** appear at about 14 days' post infection and remain for life.

o Pregnant women in contact with Parvovirus B19 or with suspected parvovirus B19 should have serological testing and referral to the obstetricians for regular monitoring and follow up.

MANAGEMENT

o For the majority of patients Erythema infectiosum is **self-limiting.**

o **Analgesia** may be needed for joint pains.

o **Transfusion** may be indicated for patients with aplastic crises.

o **Intravenous immunoglobulin,** which contains pooled neutralising anti B19 antibody has been used to treat immunocompromised patients

o Children in high risk groups should be **referred.**

---

[184] Servey JT, Reamy BV, Hodge J. Clinical presentations of parvovirus B19 infection. Am Fam Physician. 2007;75(3):373–376.

V. THE CHILD WITH ROSEOLA INFANTUM

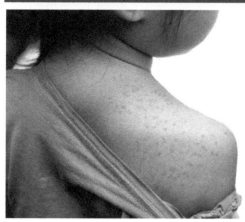

Roseola Infantum – From Steward Health care

- Roseola is most commonly caused by human herpesvirus 6 and affects infants and children younger than three years[185].
- It is characterized by the abrupt onset of high fever lasting one to five days. During this period, children often appear well with no focal clinical signs except possible mild cough, rhinorrhea, or mild diarrhea.
- Once the fever resolves, an erythematous macular to maculopapular rash usually appears, starting on the trunk and spreading peripherally.
- This rash is similar in appearance to that of rubeola (measles).
- In contrast with roseola, the rash associated with measles starts on the face (usually behind the ear) or mouth (Koplik spots) and moves downward[186].
- Children with roseola usually appear well, whereas those with measles are typically more ill-appearing. Roseola is a self-limited illness requiring no treatment, and the diagnosis is clinical[187].

CLINICAL ASSESSMENT

o The illness is associated with a mild respiratory illness, 3-5 days of a high fever of 39-40ºC and cervical lymphadenopathy (30%).
o The fever disappears coinciding with a rash.
o Around 10% of US infants are reported to develop the characteristic rash **commencing behind the ears i.e. discrete blanching macules and papules which are surrounded by halos.**
o The rash lasts around 1-2 days.

---

185 *Yamanishi K, Okuno T, Shiraki K, et al. Identification of human herpes-virus-6 as a causal agent for exanthem subitum. Lancet. 1988;1(8594):1065–1067.*

186 *Lampell MS. Childhood rashes that present to the ED part I: viral and bacterial issues. Pediatr Emerg Med Pract. 2007;4(3):1–24.*

187 *Okada K, Ueda K, Kusuhara K, et al. Exanthema subitum and human herpesvirus 6 infection. Pediatr Infect Dis J. 1993;12(3):204–208.*

o Palpebral oedema has been observed before the onset of the rash in the absence of ocular pathology.

SYMPTOMS AND SIGNS SEEN IN EXANTHEM SUBITUM

o Palpebral oedema in 30%
o Uvulopalatal junction ulcers.
o Erythematous papules on the soft palate also known as **Nagayama's spots** (65%)
o Diarrhoea (68%)
o Cough (50%)
o Prenatal and perinatal infections are uncommon due to maternal antibodies.

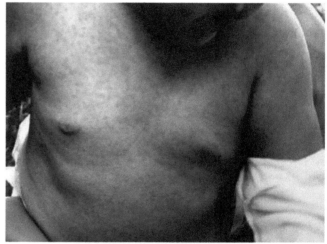

Roseola Infantum – From Medscape

INVESTIGATION STRATEGIES

o For the majority of cases serological testing is not necessary.

COMPLICATIONS ASSOCIATED WITH EXANTHEM SUBITUM:

o Meningoencephalitis
o Encephalitis
o Hemiplegia

MANAGEMENT

o HHV6 causes a benign illness and in the majority of cases antiviral therapy is not needed.
o Reactivation of this virus can occur in transplant recipients.
o The rash is often misdiagnosed as measles.

VI. THE CHILD WITH CHICKEN POX

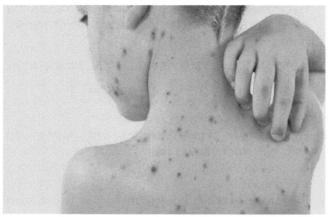

Varicella-zoster virus - From Yahoo News

- Varicella-zoster virus (VZV) is a human neurotropic alphaherpesvirus that causes a primary infection commonly known as chickenpox (varicella) [188].
- Chicken pox (varicella) is a common worldwide highly infectious illness and primarily a disease of childhood.
- The period of infectivity is from the time when symptoms first appear until all lesions have crusted over. This is usually around 5-6 days after the onset of the illness. This disease is usually mild and resolves spontaneously.
- Incubation is from **10 to 21 days.**
- This highly contagious virus is transmitted by directly touching the blisters, saliva, or mucus of an infected person. It is also transmitted through the air by coughing and sneezing.
- VZV initiates primary infection by inoculating the respiratory mucosa. It then establishes a lifelong presence in the sensory ganglionic neurons and, thus, can reactivate later in life causing herpes zoster (shingles), which can affect cranial, thoracic, and lumbosacral dermatomes.
- Acute or chronic neurologic disorders, including cranial nerve palsies, zoster paresis, vasculopathy, meningoencephalitis, and multiple ocular disorders, have been reported after VZV reactivation resulting in herpes-zoster.

PRESENTATION

- With varicella, an extremely pruritic rash follows a brief prodromal stage consisting of a low-grade fever, upper respiratory tract symptoms, tiredness, and fatigue.

[188] *Kennedy PG, Rovnak J, Badani H, et al. A comparison of herpes simplex virus type 1 and varicella-zoster virus latency and reactivation. J Gen Virol. 2015;96(Pt 7):1581-1602.*

- This exanthem develops rapidly, often beginning on the chest, trunk, or scalp and then spreading to the arms and legs.
- Varicella also affects mucosal areas of the body, such as the conjunctiva, mouth, rectum, and vagina.
- It is possible to be infected with no symptoms.
- Fever tends to resolve by day 4.
- Prolonged fever > 4 days should prompt the suspicion of complications of Varicella such as secondary bacterial sepsis.

COMPLICATIONS

o Most children have a mild illness with no complications.
o The risks to the mother are the highest in the third trimester and the risks to the foetus are the greatest in the first and second trimester.
o Groups which may be at a risk of greater severity of illness with chicken pox:
- Neonates
- Immunocompromised
- Pregnant women
- Patients with chronic steroid use.

COMPLICATIONS OF CHICKEN POX

o Pneumonia
o Bacterial superinfection of skin
o Bacteraemia/ toxic shock syndrome
o Encephalitis
o Acute cerebellar ataxia
o Necrotising fasciitis
o Purpura fulminans/ disseminated zoster
o Thrombocytopenia
o Glomerulonephritis
o Arthritis/ Hepatitis

CONGENITAL COMPLICATIONS

o Shortened limbs
o Skin scarring
o Cataracts
o Growth retardation.
o There is currently no routine immunisation against Varicella in the UK.
- Since 2003 vaccination is recommended to non-immune health care workers.

MANAGEMENT

o **Oral acyclovir** reduces the total number of lesions and the duration of fever when used within 24 hours of the onset of rash in immunocompetent children.

o It has not been shown to reduce the incidence of VZV pneumonia or complications when compared to placebo. The results do not support the widespread use of acyclovir in the immunocompetent child.

o **Varicella zoster immunoglobulin** should be given to neonates whose mothers develop the rash 7 days before or 7 days after the delivery, to reduce the risk of **severe neonatal Varicella.**

o Neonates presenting with a chickenpox rash **should be admitted for acyclovir 10mg/Kg.**

o In the majority of cases simple treatment advice can be given and the child can be managed at home.

o Children should be kept off school until all the lesions have crusted over and no new crops have occurred, this is usually **around 5-6 days.**

o Patients with chickenpox should **avoid contact** with pregnant women, neonates and the immunocompromised.

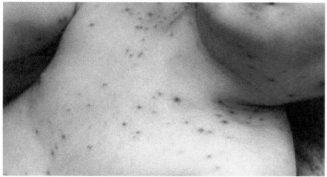

Varicella-zoster virus - From urdupoint.com

VARICELLA ZOSTER AND PREGNANCY

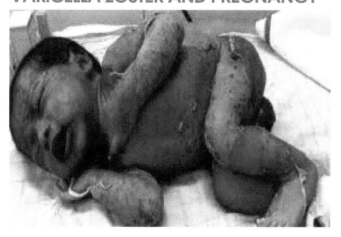

• Any pregnant woman who has not had chickenpox or who is found to be seronegative for **VZV IgG** should be advised to minimize any contact with chickenpox and shingles and to seek medical help immediately if exposed.

• If a pregnant woman is exposed, the first course of action is to perform a blood test and check for **VZV immunity**.

• If she is not immune and the history of the exposure is significant, she should be given **VZV immunoglobulin** as soon as possible.

• It is effective **up to 10 days after being exposed.**

• A pregnant woman that develops chickenpox should seek medical help urgently.

• There is an increased maternal risk of **Pneumonia, Encephalitis** and **Hepatitis** as well as the 1% risk of developing **FVS.**

• **Acyclovir** should be used with caution before 20 weeks gestation, but is recommended after 20 weeks if the woman presents within 24 hours of the onset of the rash.

SUMMARY OF CHILDHOOD EXANTHEMS		
Diseases	**Aetiology**	**Description**
Measles	Paramyxovirus	An erythematous maculopapular rash beginning on the head
Scarlet fever	Group A beta-haemolytic streptococci	A confluent erythematous rash with a sandpaper-like quality
Rubella	Rubella virus	Macular in form, starting on the face then passing down the body to the feet
Erythema infectiosum	Parvovirus B19	Resembling a slapped cheek and lasting up to 4 days
Exanthem subitum	Human herpesvirus 6 or Human herpesvirus 7	Discrete blanching macules and papules surrounded by halos
Chicken pox	Varicella virus	Fluid-filled vesicles which progress over the trunk
Gianotti-Crosti syndrome	A range of different viruses and bacteria	Papular or papulovesicular in form and distributed symmetrically on the face, buttocks and extremities

VII. THE CHILD WITH KAWASAKI'S DISEASE

BACKGROUND

o Kawasaki's is a disease of exclusion and the diagnosis and treatment of possible cases must be discussed with senior medical staff.

DIAGNOSIS

o There is no diagnostic test and diagnosis is based on clinical criteria and the exclusion of other diseases.

o Infection must be considered and often in practice children are treated with antibiotics for 24-48 hours.

o The criteria may present sequentially such that an 'incomplete' case can evolve with time to become 'complete'.

o This makes the definite exclusion of Kawasaki's difficult and **the disease should be considered in any irritable child with a fever for 5 or more days.**

DIAGNOSTIC CRITERIA

o Fever more than 5 days plus 4 of the following:
  - Conjunctivitis
  - Lymphadenopathy
  - Rash
  - Changes to lips or oral mucosal (strawberry tongue)
  - Changes of extremities

Signs & Symptoms of Kawasaki Disease

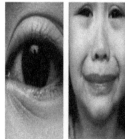
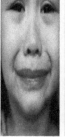
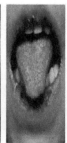
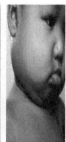
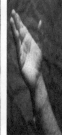
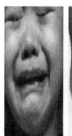
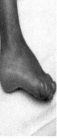
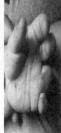
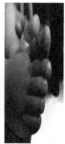

Kawasaki disease - From Tribun Jatim

DIFFERENTIAL DIAGNOSIS

- Toxic Shock Syndrome
- Scalded skin syndrome
- Scarlet fever
- EBV,
- CMV,
- Mycoplasma
- Polyarteritis nodosa
- Juvenile idiopathic arthritis
- Malignancy (lymphoma)

INITIAL INVESTIGATIONS

o K.D. is associated with many non-specific laboratory findings.
  - Acute phase proteins raised Neutrophilia, ESR raised
  - Thrombocytosis towards the end of the second week and therefore is not useful diagnostically
  - LFTs may be deranged
  - Pyuria,
  - CSF pleocytosis

OTHER INVESTIGATIONS:

- FBC and Film, ESR, CRP, Renal profile, LFT, Coagulation
- Autoimmune profile
- ASOT, anti-DNase Serology: mycoplasma, enterovirus, adenovirus, measles, parvovirus, EBV, CMV
- Blood Cultures, Urine MC&S
- ECG and echocardiogram
- Consider CXR

TREATMENT

o **Aspirin:** Given during the acute phase of the illness at high dose **(30mg/kg/day)** and then reduced to **5mg/kg/day** when the inflammatory markers have returned to normal.

o **Immunoglobulin:** Early recognition and treatment with IVIG has been shown to reduce the occurrence of coronary artery aneurysms.

o For maximum benefit it should be given before day 10 of the illness but should not be withheld if diagnosed after this time.

o If you suspect KD then it should be treated regardless of what the echo shows.

o Recommended dose is **2g/Kg over 12 hours** except where there is cardiac compromise when a smaller volume in divided doses may be preferable.

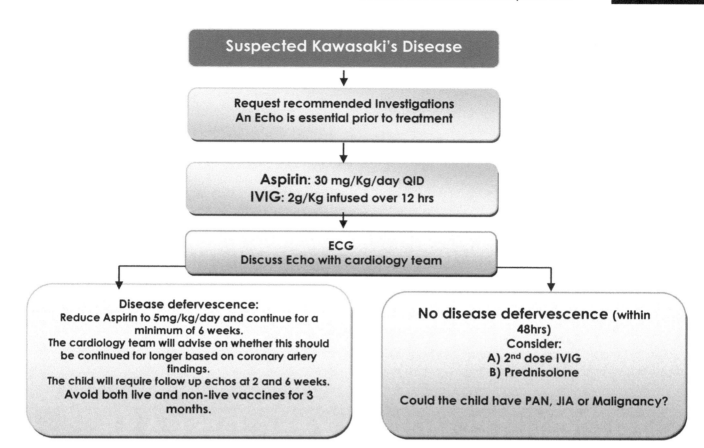

Suspected Kawasaki's Disease

↓

Request recommended Investigations
An Echo is essential prior to treatment

↓

Aspirin: 30 mg/Kg/day QID
IVIG: 2g/Kg infused over 12 hrs

↓

ECG
Discuss Echo with cardiology team

Disease defervescence:
Reduce Aspirin to 5mg/kg/day and continue for a minimum of 6 weeks.
The cardiology team will advise on whether this should be continued for longer based on coronary artery findings.
The child will require follow up echos at 2 and 6 weeks.
Avoid both live and non-live vaccines for 3 months.

No disease defervescence (within 48hrs)
Consider:
A) 2nd dose IVIG
B) Prednisolone

Could the child have PAN, JIA or Malignancy?

VIII. THE CHILD WITH PEMPHIGOID

BACKGROUND
o Commonest autoimmune sub-epidermal blistering disorder.
o Auto-antibodies target "adhesion complexes" in the skin's basement membrane=blister formation.
o High relapse rate.

CLINICAL
o Itchy +++, tense fluid filled blisters skin and/or mucous membranes.
o Usually limbs, groin, and abdomen.
o Older patients.
o Beware septicaemia (especially if immunocompromised).

DIFFERENTIAL DX
o Bullous pemphigoid.
o Linear IgA disease.
o Epidermolysis bullosa acquisita.
o Bullous drug reaction.

INVESTIGATIONS
o Clinical diagnosis.
o Confirmatory biopsy +/- immunofluorescence.
o ↑CRP & ↑ESR.

MANAGEMENT
o **Potent topical steroids** (clobetasol propionate).
o **Oral steroids or Dapsone** (esp. for mucous membrane disease).
o **Tetracyclines +/- nicotinamide** in milder cases.
o **Immunosuppressants (**MTX / Azathioprine) in severe cases.
o **Regular skin antiseptic soaks.** And protective non-adherent dressings.

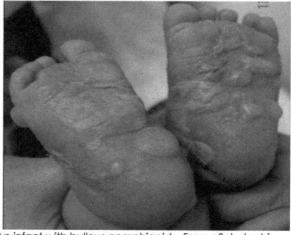

An infant with bullous pemphigoid – From eScholarship.org

IX. THE HAND, FOOT AND MOUTH DISEASE

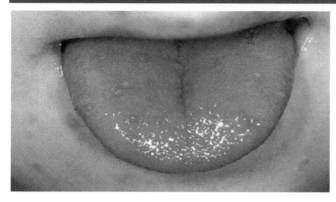

CLINICAL

- **Coxsackie virus** (more serious Enterovirus clusters in Asia)
- Person to person spread.
- Max children **1 - 4 years** (common up to 10 years).
- Sores in mouth, rashes on hands & feet and buttocks.

- "Textbook" vesicles occur at junction of hard and soft skin (palm, sole/ankle area).
- Commonest cause of mouth sores (painful, small yellow sores, red halo) children.
- Painful eating then hand rash.
- May have low fever, anorexia, sore throat, abdominal pain for 7 days.
- Usually mild but beware dehydration and occasional arthropathy.

CLINICAL DIAGNOSIS

- Rarely progress to encephalitis / transverse myelitis (flaccid - so do neuro exam).
- Hydration, analgesia (mouth ulcers), control pyrexia.
- Keep from school only if ill (may attend school if rash alone)

X. THE CHILD WITH LYME DISEASE

BACKGROUND

- **Spirochete Borrelia burgdorferi** infection via **tick bite**

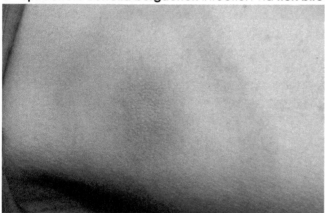

Tick Bite – From daily Express

CLINICAL

- **Erythema migrans** - macular erythematous rash with central clearing
- Starts at bite site (3-21 days later) and spreads (spirochetes migrate from wound site)
- Rash disappears after 1 month or may never be noticed
- May have associated '"flu" like fatigue, fever etc.
- **Late symptoms seen in 2/3 if untreated:**

- **Neuroborreliosis:** Mononeuritis Multiplex (e.g. Bell's) or Meningitis
- **Oligoarthralgia:** (knees) - Synovial ↑WCC and PCR + Positive for spirochetes
- **Pancarditis:** AV Block, or Myocarditis

COMPLICATIONS

- Bell's palsy
- Carditis and heart block
- Mononeuritis multiplex
- Arthritis

INVESTIGATIONS

- **Serology testing** to confirm suspicious cases.

MANAGEMENT

- If erythema migrans or strong suspicion for Lyme disease - treat with **Doxycycline**, then ask for serology testing.
- If neuroborrelliosis - admit neurology
- If oligoarthritis get (sterile procedure) synovial aspirate
- If cardiac, beware heart block (atropine ±pacing) and admit cardiology
- Please contact microbiology for antibiotic advice

XI. THE CHILD WITH ATOPIC ECZEMA

1. INTRODUCTION

- Atopic dermatitis is the most common childhood skin disorder in developed countries[189].
- This chronic, pruritic skin disease is relapsing in nature. Atopic dermatitis typically presents in infancy and early childhood and may persist into adulthood.
- Children may present with a variety of skin changes, including erythematous plaques and papules, excoriations, severely dry skin, scaling, and vesicular lesions.

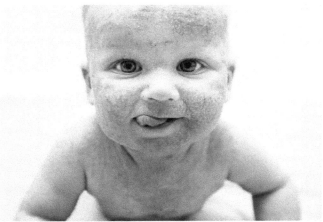

Atopic dermatitis - MIMS Malaysia

- Clinical findings of atopic dermatitis are variable but can be categorized into three groups of diagnostic features: essential, important, and associated[190]. Atopic dermatitis is common in flexural areas and on the cheeks and buttocks.
- The distribution of atopic dermatitis lesions can vary based on the age of the child. Infants and younger children often have lesions on the extensor surfaces of extremities, cheeks, and scalp. Older children and adults often present with patches and plaques on the flexor surfaces (antecubital and popliteal fossa).
- Hands and feet are also commonly affected.
- Thickened plaques with a lichenified appearance may be seen in more severe cases.
- Children with atopic dermatitis often have dry, flaky skin and are at risk of secondary cutaneous infections.

- The treatment is aimed at controlling, not curing, the disease with parent counseling on good skin care (e.g., liberal use of emollients and avoidance of triggers, such as cold weather, frequent hot baths, fragrant products, and harsh detergents).
- Despite good skin care practices, topical corticosteroids are usually needed during flare-ups.
- Atopic lesions that do not respond to traditional therapies should be biopsied or cultured if there is concern for infection. Atopic eczema (atopic dermatitis) is a chronic inflammatory skin condition.
- It is common in childhood affecting about 10% of school-aged children. Moderately severe eczema is miserable for the whole family. Itch and sleep deprivation are the main complaints.
- Topical treatment is messy and time consuming.
- Many parents who end up bringing their child to the ED will be exhausted and fed up.
- It is important that they get consistent, clear messages about treatment.
- Flares are common, and sometimes there will be a treatable exacerbating factor such as infection.

ANTIBIOTICS

- Most patients with atopic dermatitis have *Staphylococcus aureus* infection[191].
- The relationship between *S. aureus* infection and atopic dermatitis flare-ups has been debated but remains unclear.
- The use of antiseptic baths and washes also should be avoided.

SYSTEMIC THERAPY

- Rarely, systemic therapy is indicated for severe, resistant disease.
- Systemic corticosteroids are effective at acutely controlling atopic dermatitis in adults, but their use should be restricted to the short term.
- Rebound flare-ups and diminishing effectiveness severely limit use[192].

OTHER THERAPIES

- Ultraviolet (UV) phototherapy using UVB, narrowband UVB, UVA, or psoralen plus UVA may be beneficial for the treatment of severe disease if it is used appropriately, depending on the patient's age.

[189] Williams H, Robertson C, Stewart A, Ait-Khaled N, Anabwani G, Anderson R, et al. Worldwide variations in the prevalence of symptoms of atopic eczema in the International Study of Asthma and Allergies in Childhood. J Allergy Clin Immunol. 1999;103(1 pt 1):125–38....

[190] Eichenfield LF, Hanifin JM, Luger TA, Stevens SR, Pride HB. Consensus conference on pediatric atopic dermatitis. J Am Acad Dermatol. 2003;49:1088–95.

[191] Gambichler T. Narrowband UVB phototherapy in skin conditions beyond psoriasis. J Am Acad Dermatol. 2005;52:660–70.

[192] Sidbury R, Hanifin JM. Systemic therapy of atopic dermatitis. Clin Exp Dermatol. 2000;25:559–66.

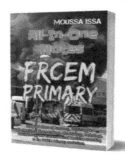
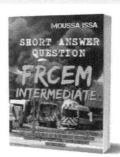
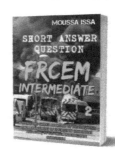
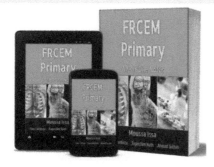
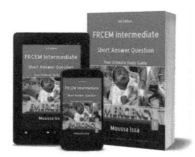
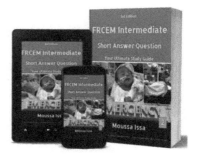
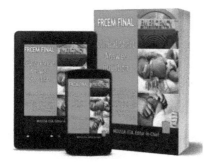
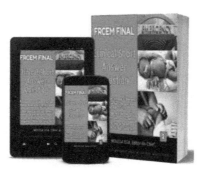
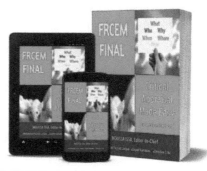
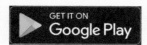
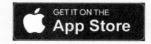

Section V. Anaesthetic Competences

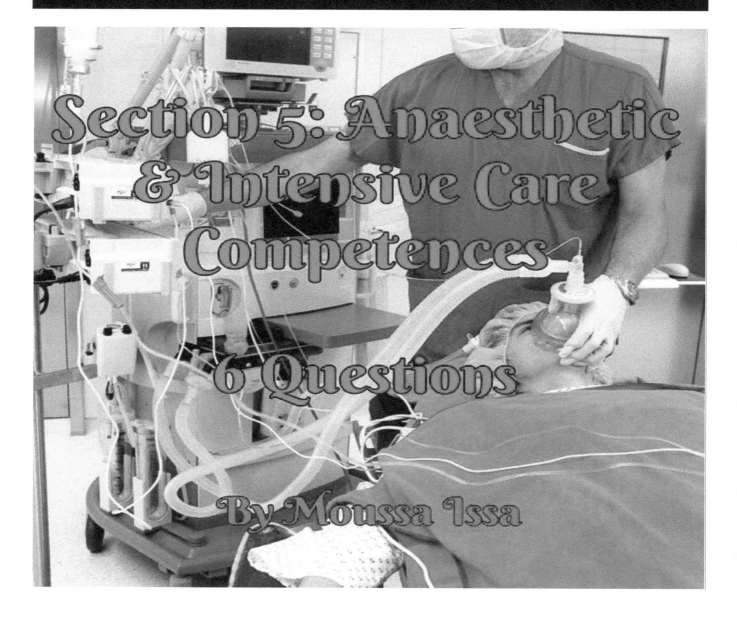

Section 5: Anaesthetic
& Intensive Care
Competences

6 Questions

By Moussa Issa

Ebook for only £3/month!

Get our Reading App for your Android smartphone or tablet to start enjoying the Moussa Issa eBookstore discovery and digital reading experience.

Download our APP on your Smart device Now.

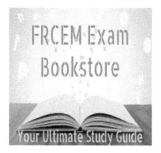

FRCEM Exam eBookstore

FRCEM Exam Bookstore   Books & Reference

PEGI 3

Offers in-app purchases

This app is compatible with all of your devices.

Installed

A static eBook with little interactivity cannot draw your attention any more. Thus it is essential to engage readers with interactive reading experience.
Moussa Issa eBookstore proves to be on top of the interactive eBook game, enabling readers to watch integrated videos related to the subject directly on the page.
The additional flipping effect makes the eBook fully interactive and dynamic.

Customize your experience with multiple font and page styles and social sharing tools.

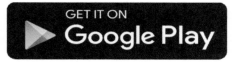

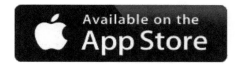

Distributed by Moussa Issa Bookstore Ltd

Website: www.moussaissabooks.com

Email: info@moussaissabooks.com

eBook subscription: www.moussaissabooks.com/read-ebook-online

1. Preoperative Assessment

I. PRE-OPERATIVE HISTORY & EXAMINATION

- The **pre-operative assessment** is an opportunity to identify co-morbidities that may lead to patient **complications during the anaesthetic, surgical, or post-operative period**. Patients scheduled for elective procedures will generally attend a pre-operative assessment 2-4 weeks before their date of surgery. The pre-operative history follows the same structure as typical history taking, with the addition of some anaesthetic and surgery specific topics.

- **History of the Presenting Complaint** - A brief history of why the patient first attended and what procedure they have subsequently been scheduled for. One should also confirm the side on which the procedure will be performed (if applicable).

- **Past Medical History** - A full PMH is required, with the following specifically asked about:
  - **Cardiovascular disease** (including hypertension and exercise tolerance).
    - The risk of an acute cardiac event is increased during anaesthesia.
  - **Respiratory disease**, as adequate planned oxygenation is essential in reducing the risk of acute ischaemic events in the peri-operative period.
  - **Renal disease**, as many features of renal disease (such as anaemia, coagulopathy, biochemical disturbances) can increase the incidence of surgical complications.
    - Blood loss or IV contrast given during some procedures can cause significant renal dysfunction, so extra care may be taken
  - **Endocrine disease**, specifically diabetes mellitus and thyroid disease
    - Many medications often require specific changes to be made in the peri-operative period

Other specific questions: it may be useful to ask themselves the following questions:
- Female of reproductive age – could they be pregnant?
- African or Afro-Caribbean descent – could they have undiagnosed sickle cell disease?

- **Past Surgical History** - Has the patient had any **previous operations**? If so, what, when, and why?
- **Past Anaesthetic History** - Has the patient **had anaesthesia before**? If so, were there any issues? Were they well post-operatively? Has the patient experienced to any previous post-operative nausea and vomiting?
- **Drug History** - A **full drug history** is required, as some medications require stopping or altering prior to surgery. Ask about any known **drug allergies**.
- **Family History** - An important condition to ask about is malignant hyperthermia, yet any other adverse reactions in surgery of immediate family members should also be documented.
- **Social History** - Ensure to ask the patient about **smoking history and alcohol intake** and their exercise tolerance

II. PRE-OPERATIVE EXAMINATION

- In the pre-operative examination, two distinct examinations are performed; the **general examination** (to identify any underlying pathology) and the **airway examination** (to predict the difficulty of intubation).
- If appropriate, the area relevant to the operation can also be examined. Perform a full general examination, looking closely for any obvious cardiovascular, respiratory, or abdominal signs.
- An anaesthetic exam, including an airway assessment, will also be performed by the anaesthetist prior to any surgery.

ASA CLASSIFICATION[193]

ASA	Health status of patient
I	A normal healthy patient
II	A patient with mild systemic disease
III	A patient with severe systemic disease
IV	A patient with severe systemic disease that is a constant threat to life
V	A moribund patient who is not expected to survive without the operation
VI	A declared brain-dead patient whose organs are being removed for donor purposes

193 *Published in British Journal of anaesthesia 2014 Reliability of the American Society of Anesthesiologists physical status scale in clinical practice Ashwin Sankar, Simon R Johnson, William Scott Beattie, Gordon Tait, D N Wijeysundera*

II. PRE-OPERATIVE INVESTIGATIONS

The nature of the exact investigations required depends on a number of factors, including co-morbidities, age and the seriousness of the procedure. Each specific hospital is likely to provide local guidelines; however, it is useful to understand the tests than could be done pre-operatively and have an appreciation as to why each may be requested. NICE produce a colour traffic light table which can further guide your investigative decisions.

BLOOD TESTS
- **Full Blood Count** (FBC)
  - Most patients will get a full blood count, predominantly used to assess if there is **undiagnosed anaemia or thrombocytopenia**, as this requires correction pre-operatively to reduce the risk of cardiovascular events.
- **Urea & Electrolytes** (U&Es)
  - To assess the **baseline renal function** of the kidneys, which will indicate potential co-morbid status and help inform any potential IV fluid management intra-operatively.
- **Liver Function Tests** (LFTs)
  - Important in the assessing **liver metabolism and synthesising function**, useful for peri-operative management; if there is suspicion of liver impairment, LFTs may help direct medication choice and dosing.
- **Clotting Screen**
  - Any indication of **deranged coagulation**, such as iatrogenic causes (e.g. warfarin), inherited coagulopathies (e.g. haemophilia A/B), or liver or renal impairment, will need identifying and correcting before surgery

GROUP AND SAVE VERSUS CROSS-MATCH
Group and Save (G&S) and Cross-Match (X-match) are two tests often cause a great deal of confusion:
- **A G&S** determines the patient's blood group (ABO and RhD) and screens the blood for any atypical antibodies. The process takes around 40 minutes and no blood is issued. A G&S is recommended if blood loss is not anticipated, but blood may be required should there be greater blood loss than expected.
- **A X-match** involves physically mixing the patient's blood with the donor's blood, in order to see if any immune reaction takes places. If it does not, the donor blood is issued and can be transfused in to the patient, otherwise alternative blood is trialled.

This process also takes ~40 minutes (in addition to the 40 minutes required to G&S the blood, which must be done first). A X-match is done if blood loss is anticipated.

IMAGING
ECG: is often performed in individuals with a history of cardiovascular disease or for those undergoing major surgery. It can indicate any underlying cardiac pathology and provide a baseline if there are post-operative signs of cardiac ischaemia.
*N.B.: **An echocardiogram (ECHO)** can be considered if the person has (1) a heart murmur (2) cardiac symptom(s) (3) signs or symptoms of heart failure.*

Chest X-ray: should be used only when absolutely necessary and should not be performed routinely. Local guidelines should be available to aid decision-making and indications may include:
- *Respiratory illness who have not had a CXR within 12 months*
- *New cardiorespiratory symptoms*
- *Recent travel from areas with endemic tuberculosis*
- *Significant smoking history*

If a patient has a chronic lung condition, **spirometry** may be of use in assessing current baseline and predicting post-operative pulmonary complications in these patients.

OTHER TESTS
- **Pregnancy Testing:** Consider in women of reproductive age; carry out a pregnancy test with the woman's consent if there is any doubt about whether she could be pregnant.
- **Sickle Cell Test:** Do not routinely offer testing for sickle cell disease or sickle cell trait before surgery. If the person has any member of their family with sickle cell disease, or is Africa or Afro-Caribbean descent, strongly consider performing a sickle cell test.
- **MRSA Swabs:** All patients will have swabs taken from the nostril ± perineum ± other sites for MRSA colonisation. If this is isolated, antiseptic hair and body wash, along with topical ointment applied to the nostrils, will be given; in some hospitals, this is given for all elective patients pre-operatively, even if this means the operation is delayed.
- **Urinalysis:** is performed if any evidence or suspicion of ongoing glycosuria or urinary tract infection, yet should not be done routinely pre-operatively.

III. INFORMING THE PATIENT & CONSENT

WHAT IS CONSENT?

It is an agreement by the patient to undergo a specific procedure. Only the patient can make the decision to undergo the procedure, even though the doctor will advise on what is required. Although the need for consent is usually thought of in terms of surgery, in fact it is required for any breach of a patient's personal integrity, including examination, performing investigations and administering an anaesthetic.

A patient can refuse treatment or choose a less than optimal option from a range offered (providing an appropriate explanation has been given — see below), but he or she cannot insist on treatment that is not on offer.

WHAT ABOUT AN UNCONSCIOUS PATIENT?

This usually arises in the emergency situation, for example a patient with a severe head injury.

Asking a relative or other individual to sign a consent form for surgery on the patient's behalf is not appropriate, **as no one can give consent on behalf of another adult.** Under these circumstances medical staffs are required to act **'in the patient's best interests.**

This will mean taking into account not only the benefits of the proposed treatment, but also any views previously expressed by the patient (e.g. refusal of blood transfusion by a Jehovah's Witness).

This will often require discussion with the relatives, and this opportunity should be used to inform them of the proposed treatment and the rationale for it.

All decisions and discussions must be clearly documented in the patient's notes.

WHAT CONSTITUTES EVIDENCE OF CONSENT?

Most patients will be asked to sign a consent form before undergoing a procedure. However, there is no legal requirement for such before anaesthesia or surgery (or anything else); the form **simply shows evidence of consent at the time it was signed.**

Consent may be given verbally and this is often the case in anaesthesia.

It is recommended that a written record of the content of the conversation be made in the patient's case notes.

WHAT DO I HAVE TO TELL THE PATIENT?

In obtaining consent it is essential the patient is given an adequate amount of information in a form that they can understand.

This will vary depending on the procedure, but may include:

- **The environment of the anaesthetic room and who they will meet**, particularly if medical students or other healthcare professionals in training will be present.
- Establishing **intravenous access and IV infusion**.
- The need for, and type of, any **invasive monitoring**.
- What to **expect during the establishment of a regional technique**.
- Being conscious throughout surgery if a regional technique alone is used, and **what they may hear**.
- **Preoxygenation**
- **Induction of anaesthesia:** although most commonly intravenous, occasionally it may be by inhalation.
- Where they will **'wake up'**: This is usually the recovery unit, but after some surgery it may be the ICU or HDU. In these circumstances the patient should be given the opportunity to visit the unit a few days before and meet some of the staff.
- **Numbness and loss of movement** after regional anaesthesia.
- The possibility of **drains, catheters and drips:** their presence may be misinterpreted by the patient as indicating unexpected problems.
- The possibility of a need for **blood transfusion**.
- **Postoperative pain control**, particularly if it requires their co-operation; for example, a patient-controlled analgesia device.
- Information on **any substantial risks** with serious adverse consequences associated with the anaesthetic technique planned.

Although the anaesthetist will be the best judge of the type of anaesthetic for each individual, patients should be given an explanation of the choices, along with the associated benefits and risks in terms they can understand. Most patients will have an understanding of general anaesthesia — the injection of a drug, followed by loss of consciousness and lack of awareness throughout the surgical procedure.

If regional anaesthesia is proposed, it is essential that the patient understands and accepts that remaining conscious throughout is to be expected, unless some form of sedation is to be used. Most patients will want to know when they can last eat and drink before surgery, if they are to take normal medications and how they will manage without a drink.

Some will expect or request a premed and in these circumstances the approximate timing, route of administration and likely effects should be discussed.

Finally, before leaving ask if the patient has any questions or wants anything clarified further.

2. Premedication

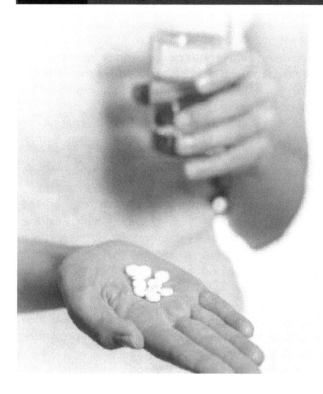

THE "6 AS" OF PREMEDICATION

1. Anxiolysis
2. Amnesia
3. Antiemetic
4. Antacid
5. Anti-autonomic
6. Analgesia

1. ANXIOLYSIS

- The most commonly prescribed drugs are the **benzodiazepines.**
- They produce a degree of **sedation and amnesia**, are well absorbed from the gastrointestinal tract and are usually given orally, **45– 90mins preoperatively.**
- Those most commonly used include **Temazepam 20–30mg, Diazepam 10–20mg and Lorazepam 2–4mg.** In patients who suffer from excessive somatic manifestations of anxiety, for example tachycardia, **beta blockers** may be given.
- A preoperative visit and explanation is often as effective as drugs at alleviating anxiety, and sedation does not always mean lack of anxiety.

2. AMNESIA

- Some patients specifically request that they not have any recall of the events leading up to anaesthesia and surgery. This may be accomplished by the administration of **Lorazepam** (as above) to provide anterograde amnesia.

3. ANTIEMETIC

- Reduction of nausea and vomiting
- Nausea and vomiting may follow the administration of opioids, either pre- or intraoperatively.
- Certain types of surgery are associated with a higher incidence of postoperative nausea and vomiting (PONV), for example gynaecology.
- Unfortunately, none of the currently used drugs can be relied on to prevent or treat established PONV.

4. ANTACID

- To modify pH and volume of gastric contents.
- Patients are starved preoperatively to reduce the risk of regurgitation and aspiration of gastric acid at the induction of anaesthesia (see below).

INTRODUCTION

- The main indication for premedication remains anxiety, for which a benzodiazepine is usually prescribed, sometimes with metoclopramide to promote absorption.
- Premedication serves several purposes: anxiolysis, smoother induction of anaesthesia, reduced requirement for intravenous induction agents, and possibly reduced likelihood of awareness.
- Intramuscular opioids are now rarely prescribed as premedication.
- The prevention of aspiration pneumonitis in patients with reflux requires premedication with an H2 antagonist, the evening before and morning of surgery, and sodium citrate administration immediately prior to induction of anaesthesia.
- Topical local anaesthetic cream over two potential sites for venous cannulation is usually prescribed for children.
- Anticholinergic agents may be prescribed to dry secretions or to prevent bradycardia, e.g. during squint surgery.
- Usual medication should be continued up to the time of anaesthesia.

o This may not be possible or effective in some patients:
  - Those who require emergency surgery;
  - Those who have received opiates or are in pain will show a significant delay in gastric emptying;
  - Those with a hiatus hernia, who are at an increased risk of regurgitation.
o A variety of drug are used to try and increase the pH and reduce the volume.
  - **Oral sodium citrate (0.3M):** 30mL orally immediately preinduction, to chemically neutralize residual acid.
  - **Ranitidine** (H₂ antagonist): 150mg orally 12 hourly and 2 hourly preoperatively.
  - **Metoclopramide:** 10mg orally preoperatively. Increases both gastric emptying and lower oesophageal sphincter tone. Often given in conjunction with ranitidine.
  - **Omeprazole** (Proton Pump Inhibitor): 40mg 3–4 hourly preoperatively.
o If a naso- or orogastric tube is in place, this can be used to aspirate gastric contents.

COMMONLY USED ANTI-EMETIC DRUGS, DOSE AND ROUTE OF ADMINISTRATION

Type of drug	Example	Usual dose
Dopamine antagonists	Metoclopramide	10 mg orally or IV
5-hydroxytryptamine antagonists	Ondansetron	4–8 mg orally or IV
Antihistamines	Cyclizine	50 mg IM or IV
Anticholinergics	Hyoscine	1 mg transdermal patch

5. ANTIAUTONOMIC
o Reduce salivation (antisialogogue), for example during fibreoptic intubation, surgery or instrumentation of the oral cavity or ketamine anaesthesia.

Anticholinergic
o Reduce the vagolytic effects on the heart, for example before the use of suxamethonium (particularly in children), during surgery on the extra ocular muscles (squint correction), or during elevation of a fractured zygoma.

Antisympathomimetic effects
o **Atropine and hyoscine** have now largely been replaced pre- operatively by **Glycopyrrolate 0.2–0.4mg IM.**
o Many anaesthetists would consider an IV dose given at induction more effective.

o Increased sympathetic activity can be seen at intubation, causing tachycardia and hypertension.
o This is undesirable in certain patients, for example those with ischaemic heart disease or raised intracranial pressure. These responses can be attenuated by the use of beta blockers given preoperatively (e.g. atenolol, 25–50mg orally) or intravenously at induction (e.g. Esmolol).
o Peri-operative beta blockade may also decrease the incidence of adverse coronary events in high risk patients having major surgery.
o An alternative is to give a potent analgesic at induction of anaesthesia, for example fentanyl, alfentanil or remifentanil.

6. ANALGESIA
o Although the oldest form of premedication, analgesic drugs are now generally reserved for patients who are in pain preoperatively.
o The most commonly used are **Morphine, Pethidine** and **Fentanyl.**
o Morphine was widely used for its sedative effects but is relatively poor as an anxiolytic and has largely been replaced by the benzodiazepines.
o Opiates have a range of unwanted side-effects, including **nausea, vomiting, respiratory depression and delayed gastric emptying.**

7. MISCELLANEOUS
A variety of other drugs are commonly given prophylactically before anaesthesia and surgery; for example:
o **Steroids:** to patients on long-term treatment or who have received them within the past 3 months;
o **Antibiotics:** to patients with prosthetic or diseased heart valves, or undergoing joint replacement;
o **Anticoagulants:** as prophylaxis against deep venous thrombosis;
o **Transdermal glyceryl trinitrate (GTN):** as patches in patients with ischaemic heart disease to reduce the risk of coronary ischaemia;
o **Eutectic mixture of local anaesthetics (EMLA):** a topically applied local anaesthetic cream to reduce the pain of inserting an IV cannula

COMMON HOME MEDICATIONS WHICH AFFECT ANAESTHESIA

Drug	Effect
ETOH	Tolerance to anaesthesia
B-blockers	Bronchospasm
Antibiotics	Prolongation of NMJ blockade
Benzodiazepines	Tolerance to anaesthesia
Diuretics	Hypovolemia, Hypokalaemia

3. Anaesthetic Agents

I. SEDATION AGENTS

1. MIDAZOLAM

- A short acting water-soluble benzodiazepine which at higher doses causes intense **sedation** (anaesthesia) and **retrograde amnesia.**
- The initial dose is **0.02-0.1mg/Kg** in adults older than 60 and the chronically ill or debilitated
- Onset of action: **30-60 sec** with Peak action at **12min.**
- Half-life: **2hrs**; Risk: May cause **hypotension.**
- Antidote: **Flumazenil** (caution!!! must be taken as it may have a shorter duration of action than the sedative agent, resulting in re-sedation.)

2. PROPOFOL

- Propofol is now used for procedural sedation in many EDs worldwide. **Has no analgesic property**
- Its mechanism of action is unclear but is thought to act by potentiating the inhibitory neurotransmitters GABA and glycine, which enhances spinal inhibition during anaesthesia.
- Although initially introduced for anesthetic induction and maintenance, propofol's pharmacodynamic profile including a rapid onset, rapid recovery time, and lack of active metabolites has accounted for its popularity in the arena of procedural sedation[194].

DOSAGE:

- For induction of anaesthesia **is 1 mg/kg initially then 0.5mg/kg every 1-2min.**
- For maintenance of anaesthesia is **4-12 mg/kg/hour.**
- Following intravenous injection propofol acts within **30 seconds** and its duration of action is **5-10 minutes.**

SIDE EFFECTS OF PROPOFOL

- Pain on injection (in up to 30%)
- Hypotension, Hyperventilation
- Transient apnoea
- Headache, Coughing and hiccup
- Thrombosis and phlebitis

CONTRAINDICATIONS

- **Absolute**
  - Known hypersensitivity to propofol or any of its components
  - Allergies to egg, egg products, soybeans or soy products (not Milk allergy)
  - Disorders of fat metabolism
- **Relative:**
  - Known case of epilepsy
  - Untreated HTN
  - Compromises left ventricular function
  - Hepatic or Renal impairment
  - Pregnant and lacting mother
  - Paediatric age <3 yrs

3. KETAMINE

- Ketamine is the only anaesthetic agent available that has **analgesic, hypnotic, and amnesic properties**. When used correctly it is a very useful and versatile drug. Ketamine acts by non-competitive antagonism of the NMDA receptor Ca^{2+} channel pore and also inhibits NMDA receptor activity by interaction with the phenylcyclidine binding site.
- Ketamine has also been shown to be a valuable agent for procedural sedation in combative patients, mentally disabled patients or autistic patients[195].

DOSAGE AND ROUTES:

- Ketamine can be used intravenously and intramuscularly.
- **10 mg/kg IM:** when used by this route it acts within **2-8 minutes** and has a duration of action of **10-20 minutes**.
- **1.5-2 mg/kg IVI:** administered over a period of 60 seconds. When used intravenously it acts within **30 seconds** and has a duration of action of **5-10 minutes** Ketamine is also effective when administered orally, rectally, and nasally.
- Baroreceptor function is well maintained and arrhythmias are uncommon

---

194 *Propofol anesthesia for invasive procedures in ambulatory and hospitalized children: experience in the pediatric intensive care unit. Hertzog JH, Campbell JK, Dalton HJ, Hauser GJPediatrics. 1999 Mar; 103(3):E30.*

195 *Combination of oral ketamine and midazolam as a premedication for a severely autistic and combative patient. Shah S, Shah S, Apuya J, Gopalakrishnan S, Martin T J Anesth. 2009; 23(1):126-8.*

SIDE EFFECTS OF KETAMINE

- Tachycardia, Nausea and vomiting
- Increase BP, CVP, Cardiac Output
- Nystagmus, Diplopia, Rash
- *Ketamine 1 – 2 mg/kg IV is the ideal induction agent in asthmatic patients due to its bronchodilatory effects.*
- **Rocuronium and suxamethonium** are commonly used as paralytic agents. Rocuronium has the added advantage of providing a longer period of paralysis, which avoids ventilator asynchrony in the early stages of management.

4. ENTONOX

- Entonox is a **50/50 mix of oxygen and nitrous oxide**.
- Its main actions are **analgesia and depression of the central nervous system.**
- It is not known for certain how it works but it is postulated that it acts via the modulation of enkephalins and endorphins within the central nervous system.
- It takes approximately **30 seconds** to act and continues for approximately **60 seconds** after inhalation has ceased.
- Entonox is stored in **white or blue cylinders with blue and white shoulders.**

INDICATIONS OF ENTONOX

- As an adjuvant to general anaesthesia
- As an analgesic during labour
- As an analgesic during painful procedures

SIDE EFFECTS OF ENTONOX

- Nausea and vomiting (15% of patients)
- Dizziness, Euphoria
- Inhibition of vitamin B12 synthesis
- Potential respiratory and hemodynamic effects of nitrous oxide include a dose-dependent negative depressant effect on myocardial contractility and increases in pulmonary artery pressure. Nitrous oxide also causes dose-dependent respiratory depression, resulting in an elevation of the resting $PaCO_2$ level and blunting of the central respiratory response to hypercarbia and hypoxemia[196].

CONTRAINDICATIONS OF ENTONOX

- **Entonox should be avoided in patients with:**
  - *Head injuries, Chest injuries,*
  - *Suspected bowel obstruction,*
  - *Middle Ear disease,*
  - *Early pregnancy and B12 or folate deficiency.*

5. METHOXYFLURANE (PENTHROX)

- The Penthrox inhaler is a hand-held **inhaler** used for **self-administration** of **methoxyflurane** for **pain relief.**

INDICATIONS

- The Penthrox inhaler is indicated for use by children and adults for the self-administration of methoxyflurane for analgesia in emergency and remote settings.
- A non-**opioid** alternative to **morphine**, this device is also easier to use than **nitrous oxide**.

CONTRAINDICATIONS

- Due to the risk of organ (especially **kidney**) **toxicity**, methoxyflurane is **contraindicated** in patients with pre-existing **kidney disease** or **diabetes mellitus**, and is not recommended to be administered in conjunction with **tetracyclines** or other potentially **nephrotoxic** or **enzyme-inducing** drugs.

DOSING

- The maximum recommended dose is **6 milliliters per day** or **15 milliliters per week** because of the risk of cumulative dose-related nephrotoxicity, and the inhaler should not be used on consecutive days.

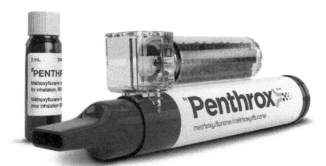

DELIVERY

- This portable, disposable, single-use inhaler device, along with a single 3 milliliter brown glass vial of methoxyflurane is provided in doctor's kits that allow conscious **hemodynamically** stable patients (including children over the age of 5 years) to self-administer the drug, under supervision.
- Each 3 milliliter dose lasts approximately 30 min.

ADVERSE EFFECTS

- Despite the potential for renal impairment when used at anesthetic doses, no significant adverse effects have been reported in the literature when it is used at the lower doses (up to 6 milliliters) used for producing analgesia and sedation.

196 *Levels of consciousness and ventilatory parameters in young children during sedation with oral midazolam and nitrous oxide. Litman RS, Berkowitz RJ, Ward DS Arch Pediatr Adolesc Med. 1996 Jul; 150(7):671-5.*

II. INHALATION ANAESTHETICS

COMMON FEATURES OF INHALED ANAESTHETICS

- Modern inhalation anesthetics are **nonflammable, nonexplosive agents**.
- Decrease cerebrovascular resistance, resulting in **increased perfusion of the brain**,
- **Cause bronchodilation**, and decrease both spontaneous ventilation and hypoxic pulmonary vasoconstriction (increased pulmonary vascular resistance in poorly aerated regions of the lungs, redirecting blood flow to more oxygenated regions).

MAC (POTENCY)

- The minimum alveolar concentration (MAC) is a measure of anaesthetic potency.
- MAC is defined as the minimum alveolar concentration at steady state of inhaled anaesthetic at 1 atm pressure that prevents movement (e.g. withdrawal) in response to a standard surgical midline incision in 50% of a test population.
- It reflects the actions of an inhalation agent on spinal cord-mediated reflexes by measuring somatic responses and is not necessarily a surrogate for lack of awareness[197].
- The anaesthetic requirement for preventing consciousness is better estimated by the MAC-awake, that is, the end-tidal concentration of inhaled anaesthetics that prevents appropriate voluntary responses to spoken commands in 50% of a test population. This endpoint measures perceptive awareness rather than memory.
- MAC-awake is typically half the value of MAC but are more difficult to define as the endpoint of unconsciousness and are less clearly defined than movement. By performing anaesthetic washout experiments, it has been concluded that MAC awake is approximately one-third of MAC for isoflurane, sevoflurane, and desflurane.

Factors that can increase MAC (make the patient less sensitive) include:

- Hyperthermia,
- Drugs that increase CNS catecholamines,
- Chronic ethanol abuse.

Factors that can decrease MAC (make the patient more sensitive) include:

- Increased age,
- Hypothermia,
- Pregnancy,
- Sepsis,
- Acute intoxication,
- Concurrent IV anesthetics,
- a2 -adrenergic receptor agonists (for example, clonidine, dexmedetomidine).

1. HALOTHANE

PHYSICAL PROPERTIES

- Halothane is a halogenated alkane .
- The carbon–fluoride bonds are responsible for its nonflammable and nonexplosive nature.
- Thymol preservative and amber-colored bottles retard spontaneous oxidative decomposition.

ADVANTAGES:

- Potent anesthetic,
- Rapid induction & recovery
- Neither flammable nor explosive,
- Sweet smell, non-irritant
- Does not augment bronchial and salivary secretions.
- Low incidence of post-operative nausea and vomiting.
- Relaxes both skeletal and uterine muscle, and can be used in obstetrics when uterine relaxation is indicated.
- Not hepatotoxic in pediatric patient, and combined with its pleasant odor, this makes it suitable in children for inhalation induction.

DISADVANTAGES:

- **Weak analgesic** (thus is usually coadministerd with N2O, opioids)
- Is a strong **respiratory depressant**
- Is a strong **cardiovascular depressant**; halothane is vagomimetic and cause atropine-sensitive bradycardia.
- **Cardiac arrhythmias**: serious if hypercapnia develops due to hypoventilation and an increase in the plasma concentration of catecholamines)
- **Hypotensive effect** (phenylephrine recommended)
- **Hepatotoxic**: is oxidatively metabolized in the liver to tissue toxic hydrocarbons (e.g., trifluroethanol and bromide ion).
- **Malignant hyperthermia**

---

[197] *Khurram Saleem Khan, Ivan Hayes, Donal J Buggy, Pharmacology of anaesthetic agents II: inhalation anaesthetic agents,* Continuing Education in Anaesthesia Critical Care & Pain, *Volume 14, Issue 3, June 2014, Pages 106–111, https://doi.org/10.1093/bjaceaccp/mkt038*

CONTRAINDICATIONS

- It is prudent to withhold halothane from patients with unexplained liver dysfunction following previous anaesthetic exposure.
- Halothane, like all inhalational anaesthetics, should be used with care in patients with intracranial mass lesions because of the **possibility of intracranial hypertension** secondary to increased cerebral blood volume and blood flow.
- Hypovolemic patients and some patients with severe reductions in left ventricular function may not tolerate halothane's negative inotropic effects.
- Sensitization of the heart to catecholamines limits the usefulness of halothane when exogenous epinephrine is administered or in patients with pheochromocytoma.

DRUG INTERACTIONS

- The myocardial depression seen with halothane is exacerbated by **β-adrenergic-blocking agents** and **calcium channel-blocking agents.**
- **Tricyclic antidepressants** and **Monoamine Oxidase Inhibitors** have been associated with fluctuations in blood pressure and arrhythmias, although neither represents an absolute contraindication.
- The combination of **halothane and aminophylline** has resulted in serious ventricular arrhythmias.

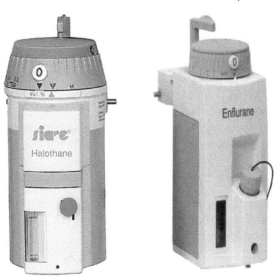

2. ENFLURANE

ADVANTAGES:

- Less potent than halothane, but produces rapid induction and recovery
- ~2% metabolized to fluoride ion, which is excreted by the kidney
- Has some analgesic activity

- **Differences from halothane:**
  o Fewer arrhythmias,
  o Less sensitisation of the heart to catecholamines,
  o Greater potentiation of muscle relaxant due to more potent **"curare-like"** effect.

DISADVANTAGES:

- CNS excitation at twice the MAC,
- Can induce seizure

3. ISOFLURANE

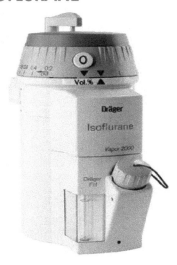

ADVANTAGES:

- A very stable molecule that undergoes little metabolism
- Not tissue toxic
- Does not induce cardiac arrhythmias
- Does not sensitise the heart to the action of catecholamines
- Produces concentration-dependent hypotension due to peripheral vasodilation
- It also dilates the coronary vasculature, increasing coronary blood flow and oxygen consumption by the myocardium, this property may make it beneficial in patients with IHD.

CONTRAINDICATIONS

- Isoflurane presents **no unique contraindications.**
- Patients with severe hypovolemia may not tolerate its vasodilating effects.
- It can trigger malignant hyperthermia.

DRUG INTERACTIONS

- Epinephrine can be safely administered in doses up to 4.5 mcg/kg.
- Nondepolarizing NMBAs are potentiated by isoflurane.

4. DESFLURANE

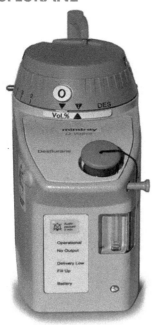

ADVANTAGES
- Rapidity of induction and recovery: outpatient surgery
- Like isoflurane, it decreases vascular resistance and perfuse all major tissues very well.

DISADVANTAGES
- Less volatility (must be delivered using a special vaporiser
- Irritating cause apnea, laryngospasm, coughing, and excessive secretions

CONTRAINDICATIONS
- Severe hypovolemia,
- Malignant hyperthermia,
- Intracranial hypertension.

DRUG INTERACTIONS
- Desflurane potentiates nondepolarizing neuromuscular blocking agents to the same extent as isoflurane.
- Epinephrine can be safely administered in doses up to 4.5 mcg/kg as desflurane does not sensitize the myocardium to the arrhythmogenic effects of epinephrine.
- Switching from isoflurane to desflurane toward the end of anaesthesia does not significantly accelerate recovery, nor does faster emergence translate into faster discharge times from the postanesthesia care unit. Desflurane emergence has been associated with delirium in some paediatric patients.

5. SEVOFLURANE

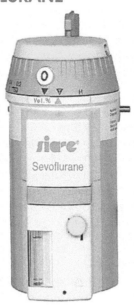

- Has low pungency,
- Not irritating the airway during induction; making it suitable for induction in children
- Rapid onset and recovery
- Metabolized by liver, releasing fluoride ions; thus, like enflurane, it may prove to be **nephrotoxic.**

CONTRAINDICATIONS
- Severe hypovolemia,
- Susceptibility to malignant hyperthermia,
- Intracranial hypertension.

DRUG INTERACTIONS
- sevoflurane potentiates NMBAs.
- It does not sensitize the heart to catecholamine-induced arrhythmias.

6. METHOXYFLURANE
- The most potent and the best analgesic anesthetic available for clinical use.
- **Nephrotoxic** and thus seldom used.

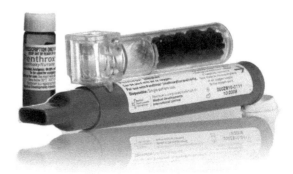

III. INTRAVENOUS INDUCTION AGENTS

1. PROPOFOL

- Propofol, Phenol derivative, it is an IV sedative-hypnotic used in the induction and or maintenance of anesthesia.
- Onset is smooth and rapid (40 seconds)
- It is occasionally accompanied by excitatory phenomena, such as muscle twitching, spontaneous movement, or hiccups.
- Propofol can cause pain during injection which may be attenuated by co-administration of lidocaine or by formulation in medium chain, rather than long-chain triglycerides.
- It has a short initial distribution half-life (2–8 min).
- Propofol is rapidly metabolized in the liver by conjugation to glucuronide and sulphate, producing water-soluble compounds which are excreted mainly by the kidneys[198].
- **Poor analgesia.**

PHARMACODYNAMIC EFFECTS

- **Cardiovascular**
  o Propofol reduces systemic vascular resistance, cardiac contractility, and preload.

- **Respiratory**
  o Like thiopental, propofol causes profound respiratory depression.

- **Cerebral**
  o Propofol decreases cerebral oxygen requirements, cerebral blood flow, and intracranial pressure.
  o It also has useful antiemetic effects.
  o Although during induction, it may cause spontaneous movements, muscle twitching, or hiccups, it has predominantly anticonvulsant properties at high infusion doses and causes burst suppression on EEG.
  o It has been used successfully to terminate status epilepticus.

- **Potential toxicity**
  o Long-term infusions of high doses of propofol cause **'propofol infusion syndrome'** characterized by severe metabolic acidosis, rhabdomyolysis, renal failure, lipaemia, and cardiac failure in association with critical illness.

2. KETAMINE

- Ketamine (phencyclidine derivative) a short-acting, anesthetic, **induces a dissociated state** in which the patient is unconscious (but may appear to be awake) and does not feel pain.
- Ketamine is used mainly in children and elderly adults for short procedures.

PHARMACODYNAMICS

- **Cardiovascular**
  o Ketamine, in contrast to other i.v. anaesthetics, increases arterial pressure, heart rate, and cardiac output due to central stimulation of the sympathetic nervous system.
  o It increases the pulmonary arterial pressure and myocardial work.
  o It is relatively contraindicated in patients with coronary artery disease and poorly controlled hypertension.
  o It is often used as an i.v. anaesthetic agent in patients with acute hypovolaemic shock[199].

- **Respiratory**
  o Ketamine has minimal effects on ventilatory drive. It is a potent bronchodilator and preserves upper airway reflexes, but patients with increased risk of aspiration may require airway protection.

- **Cerebral**
  o Ketamine increases cerebral blood flow, intracranial pressure, and cerebral oxygen requirements.
  o It induces a state of *dissociative anaesthesia* which results in the patient appearing conscious (e.g. eye opening, swallowing, muscle contraction) but unresponsive to pain.
  o Unpleasant dreams, hallucinations, and delirium may follow its use, but these adverse effects can be minimized by co-administration with benzodiazepines.
  o It has analgesic and opioid-sparing properties.

- **Potential toxicity**
  o Numerous animal studies in rodents indicate that NMDA receptor antagonists, including ketamine, induce neurodegeneration in the developing brain.

[198] *Khurram Saleem Khan, Ivan Hayes, Donal J Buggy, Pharmacology of anaesthetic agents I: intravenous anaesthetic agents,* Continuing Education in Anaesthesia Critical Care & Pain, *Volume 14, Issue 3, June 2014, Pages 100–105, https://doi.org/10.1093/bjaceaccp/mkt039*

[199] *Khurram Saleem Khan, Ivan Hayes, Donal J Buggy, Pharmacology of anaesthetic agents I: intravenous anaesthetic agents,* Continuing Education in Anaesthesia Critical Care & Pain, *Volume 14, Issue 3, June 2014, Pages 100–105, https://doi.org/10.1093/bjaceaccp/mkt039*

o There is also evidence that other general anaesthetics, such as isoflurane, can induce neuronal cell death (apoptosis) in neonatal animal models during key neurodevelopmental periods, which may be exacerbated by concurrent administration of midazolam or nitrous oxide.

o Concern has recently arisen regarding the safety of anaesthesia in infants and children.

1. THIOPENTONE

- Thiopental sodium is a very short acting barbiturate that is primarily used for the induction of anaesthesia.
- Barbiturates are thought to act primarily at synapses by depressing post-synaptic sensitivity to neurotransmitters and by impairing pre-synaptic neurotransmitter release.
- The dose for **induction of anaesthesia** is **2-7 mg/kg.**
- Following intravenous injection thiopental sodium rapidly reaches the brain and causes unconsciousness within **30-45 seconds** and the effects last **5-15 minutes.**
- Its effects are cumulative with repeated administration.

PHARMACODYNAMICS

- **Cardiovascular**
  o Thiopental causes direct myocardial depression, with decreased mean arterial pressure (MAP) due to inhibition of medullary vasomotor centre and reduced sympathetic outflow, resulting in dilatation of capacitance vessels.
  o It results in an elevation in heart rate due to baroreceptor-mediated sympathetic reflex stimulation of the heart in response to decrease in cardiac output and arterial pressure.
  o The effects are more pronounced in hypovolaemia, β-blockade, pericardial tamponade, and valvular heart disease[200].

- **Respiratory**
  o Thiopental causes depression of the medullary ventilatory centre and decreases the response to hypercapnoea and hypoxia.
  o It does not completely depress noxious airway reflexes and may predispose to laryngospasm and bronchospasm.
  o It also has antanalgesic effects.

- **Cerebral**
  o Thiopental decreases cerebral metabolic oxygen consumption rate ($CMRO_2$), the cerebral blood flow, and intracranial pressure.
  o Large doses cause electrical silence (burst suppression) on EEG, which may protect the brain from episodes of focal ischaemia.

- **Potential toxicity**
  o Owing to slow metabolism and prolonged elimination kinetics, thiopental is rarely used as a continuous infusion.
  o No specific toxicity has been associated with it, other than extension of its known side-effects

2. ETOMIDATE

- It is an intravenous induction agent associated with a **rapid recovery.**
- The dose for induction of anaesthesia is **0.3 mg/kg.**
- Following intravenous injection etomidate acts in **10-65 seconds** and its duration of action is **6-8 minutes**.
- Etomidate is notable for its relative **cardiovascular stability.** Its effects are non-cumulative with repeated administration.

PHARMACODYNAMICS

- **Cardiovascular**
  o Etomidate is known for its cardiovascular stability in comparison with propofol and thiopental. At induction dose of 0.3 mg kg^{-1}, etomidate has no effect on systemic vascular resistance, myocardial contractility, and heart rate.

- **Respiratory**
  o Etomidate has minimal effect on ventilation and does not cause apnoea at appropriate clinical doses.

- **Cerebral**
  o Etomidate decreases cerebral metabolic rate, blood flow, and intracranial pressure to the same extent as thiopental. Because of minimal cardiovascular effects, cerebral perfusion pressure is well maintained.

- **Potential toxicity**
  o Etomidate binds to the P450 enzyme 11-β-hydroxylase, which is important for steroidogenesis. This effect is due to binding of a nitrogen atom in etomidate's imidazole ring to the Fe^{2+} within the haem ring on the 11-β-hydroxylase enzyme resulting in the inhibition of steroid formation.
  o Long-term infusions of etomidate cause adrenocortical suppression. This led to abandonment of etomidate's use as a sedative in intensive care units.

---

[200] *Khurram Saleem Khan, Ivan Hayes, Donal J Buggy, Pharmacology of anaesthetic agents I: intravenous anaesthetic agents,* Continuing Education in Anaesthesia Critical Care & Pain, *Volume 14, Issue 3, June 2014, Pages 100–105,* https://doi.org/10.1093/bjaceaccp/mkt039

Drug	Induction and recovery	Main unwanted effects	Notes
Thiopental	Fast onset (accumulation occurs, Giving slow recovery), Hangover	CVS and Resp depression Decreased urine output	Used as induction agent declining. ↓CBF and O2 consumption Injection pain
Etomidate	Fast onset Fairly fast recovery	Excitatory effects during induction Adrenocortical suppression	Less CVS and resp depression than Thiopenthal. Injection pain
Propofol	Fast onset Fast recovery	CVS and Resp depression Pain at injection site	Most common induction agent Rapidly metabolized Possible to use as continuous infusion Injection pain Antiemetic
Ketamine	Slow onset, After effects common during recovery	Psychotomimetic effects following recovery, Postop Nausea-vomiting	Produces good analgesia and amnaesia No injection site pain
Midazolam	Slower onset than other agents	Minimal CVS and resp depression	Little Resp and CVS depressions, No pain, good amnaesia

ADJUNCTS TO ANAESTHESIA

1. FENTANYL
- A potent synthetic opiate with a rapid onset of action and short half-life.
- **Used to blunt sympathetic reflexes to laryngoscopy** and **the rise in ICP** associated with intubation.
- Dosage intravenously of **0.05-1mcg/kg.**
- May cause significant **respiratory depression, rigid chest syndrome** if given too rapidly and **hypotension.**

2. ATROPINE
- A competitive muscarinic antagonist, which causes vagal inhibition at the SA and AV nodes resulting in increased heart rate.
- Used **to counter reflex bradycardia** in children under 10 yrs or after repeat dose suxamethonium.
- Dosage intravenously of <u>**0.02mg/kg**</u> **3 minutes before** administration of Suxamethonium.

IV. MUSCLE RELAXANTS

- If intubation is required, it may be necessary to paralyse the patient using:
  - **Depolarizing muscle relaxants:** Suxamethonium
  - **Non-depolarizing muscle relaxants**
    - Rocuronium, Cistracurium,
    - Vecuronium, Atracurium.

1. SUXAMETHONIUM

- Suxamethonium is a short acting muscle relaxant. The main uses in anaesthesia are to allow intubation of the trachea or to maintain relaxation for short surgical procedures[201]. Binds to the postsynaptic acetylcholine receptors, resulting in transient receptor agonism and muscle contraction followed by a refractory period of muscle relaxation within **30–60 seconds** lasting several minutes.
- Its relatively short-lived effects are the result of its metabolism by **Plasma Cholinesterase.**
- Dosage intravenously is **0.5-2 mg/kg.** If second dose required – **consider atropine pre-treatment.**
- Onset of action **45-60 seconds** usually preceded by fasciculation within 15 seconds. Initial return of muscle activity occurs within **3-5 minutes** and adequate spontaneous ventilation within **8-10 minutes**. May cause hypotension and bradycardia (after second dose, in younger children (atropine pre-treatment), in the presence of hypoxia).

SIDE EFFECTS OF SUXAMETHONIUM
- Hyperkalemia
- Malignant hyperthermia
- Muscle pain
- Cardiac arrhythmias
- Rapid increase in intraocular pressure

CONTRAINDICATIONS
- **Recent burns** but can be given in the first 24 hours following the burn.
- **Spinal cord trauma** causing paraplegia. It can be given immediately after the injury but should be avoided from approximately day-10 to day-100 after the injury.
- Other contraindications to the use of suxamethonium include:
  - Severe muscle trauma
  - Hyperkalaemia
  - History of malignant hyperthermia

2. ATRACURIUM

- Atracurium is a highly selective, competitive or non-depolarising neuromuscular blocking agent.
- It is used as an adjunct to general anaesthesia or sedation in the intensive care unit (ICU), to relax skeletal muscles, and to facilitate tracheal intubation and mechanical ventilation[202].
- Atracurium competes with acetylcholine for nicotinic (N2) receptor binding sites at the post-synaptic membrane of the neuromuscular junction.
- This prevents acetylcholine from stimulating the receptors. Because the blockade is competitive muscle paralysis occurs gradually.
- In order to enhance neuromuscular recovery post nondepolarizing relaxation at the end of surgery, the amount of acetylcholine in the synapse is increased by inhibiting the **acetylcholinesterase enzyme** using a reversal agent such as **Neostigmine.** The 'intubating' dose of atracurium is **0.3-0.6 mg/kg** and subsequent doses are one-third of this amount. Satisfactory intubating conditions are produced within **90 seconds** of administration.
- **The duration of action of atracurium is prolonged by the following factors:**
  - Hypocalcaemia, Hypokalaemia
  - Hypoproteinaemia, Hypercapnia
  - Hypermagnesaemia
- Dehydration, Acidosis and **Histamine release** may occur if doses > 600 µg/kg are used. This can result in cutaneous flushing, hypotension and bronchospasm. Bradycardia has also been reported.

Drug	Dose	Precautions
Morphine	0.05-0.20mg/Kg	Resp depression Histamine release with hypotension, N&V, itching, bronchospasm,
Ketofol 10mg/ml sol	IV 1:1 ratio; 1-3ml every 2 min until desired effect achieved	
Naloxone	1-2mg IV. Additional every 2-3min to a total 10mg	Clinical duration shorter than longer acting opioids
Flumazenil	0.02mg/kg -2mg over 15 secs Additional 0.2mg doses at 1min interval until desired state of consciousness achieved	Contraindicated in patients taking benzodiazepines for an extended amount of time, Underlying seizure disorder In Patients on TCA

---

[201] *Suxamethonium Dr I. Kestin, Consultant Anaesthetist, Derriford Hospital, Plymouth*

[202] *https://www.medicines.org.uk/emc/product/4433/smpc*

V. REVERSAL OF MUSCLE RELAXANTS

1. ANTICHOLINESTERASE AGENTS

- **Neostigmine, Edrophonium, and Pyridostigmine** are used to reverse neuromuscular blockade.
- **Edrophonium** has a rapid onset, but is not as effective as neostigmine for deep blocks.
- **Pyridostigmine** has a slow onset, which makes it ill-suited to the reversal of intermediate-acting neuromuscular agents.

1. NEOSTIGMINE

- Remains the most commonly used anticholinesterase agent, although many principles can also apply to edrophonium and pyridostigmine. Reduces the intensity of neuromuscular blockade in a dose-dependent manner up to **0.04-0.05 mg/kg**, but higher doses have little if any additional benefit.
- The agent must be injected only when sufficient spontaneous recovery is observed.
- It is recommended to wait until there are four visible twitches following train-of-four (TOF) stimulation before administering neostigmine.
- If no fade is visible, significant residual blockade is possible, but adequate reversal requires only **0.02-0.03 mg/kg of neostigmine**.
- If three or fewer twitches are visible, it is preferable to maintain anesthesia until there are four visible twitches and then give neostigmine at the usual **0.04-0.05 mg/kg doses.** When the reversal agent is administered too early, recovery might be incomplete, and residual paralysis difficult to diagnose, as human senses cannot detect fade when the TOF ratio is 0.4 or greater.
- Neostigmine is typically administered along with an antimuscarinic agent like glycopyrrolate or atropine to attenuate the parasympathomimetic activity at other non-muscular acetylcholine receptor sites[203].

2. SUGAMMADEX

- BRIDION (sugammadex) is indicated for the reversal of neuromuscular blockade induced by rocuronium bromide and vecuronium bromide in adults undergoing surgery[204]. As a result, Sugammadex inactivates rocuronium molecules and indirectly decreases the intensity of neuromuscular blockade.
- Once bound, the kidney excretes the Sugammadex-rocuronium complex.

- To a lesser extent, Sugammadex also shows an affinity for **Vecuronium and Pancuronium**; however, it has no affinity for other neuromuscular blockers such as Succinylcholine, Atracurium, Cistracurium, and Doxacurium. The recovery time following Sugammadex administration is exceptionally fast, i.e., approximately **2 minutes**.

DOSAGE
Routine reversal:
- A dose of **4 mg/kg** sugammadex is recommended if recovery has reached at least 1-2 post-tetanic counts (PTC) following rocuronium or vecuronium induced blockade. Median time to recovery of the T_4/T_1 ratio to 0.9 is around 3 minutes.
- A dose of 2 mg/kg sugammadex is recommended, if spontaneous recovery has occurred up to at least the reappearance of T_2 following rocuronium or vecuronium induced blockade. Median time to recovery of the T_4/T_1 ratio to 0.9 is around 2 minutes.
- Using the recommended doses for routine reversal will result in a slightly faster median time to recovery of the T_4/T_1 ratio to 0.9 of rocuronium when compared to vecuronium induced neuromuscular blockade.

Immediate reversal of rocuronium-induced blockade:
- If there is a clinical need for immediate reversal following administration of rocuronium a dose of 16 mg/kg sugammadex is recommended. When 16 mg/kg sugammadex is administered 3 minutes after a bolus dose of 1.2 mg/kg rocuronium bromide, a median time to recovery of the T_4/T_1 ratio to 0.9 of approximately 1.5 minutes can be expected.
- There is no data to recommend the use of sugammadex for immediate reversal following vecuronium induced blockade.

Re-administration of sugammadex:
- In the exceptional situation of recurrence of neuromuscular blockade post-operatively (see section 4.4) after an initial dose of 2 mg/kg or 4 mg/kg sugammadex, a repeat dose of 4 mg/kg sugammadex is recommended.
- Following a second dose of sugammadex, the patient should be closely monitored to ascertain sustained return of neuromuscular function.

Re-administration of rocuronium or vecuronium after sugammadex:
- For waiting times for re-administration of rocuronium or vecuronium after reversal with sugammadex.

---

[203] Adeyinka A, Kondamudi NP. StatPearls [Internet]. StatPearls Publishing; Treasure Island (FL): Mar 24, 2019. Cholinergic Crisis.

[204] https://www.merckconnect.com/bridion/mechanism-of-action/

4. Airway Assessment & Management

I. BASIC AIRWAY MANAGEMENT

OVERVIEW

- The role of airway assessment is to identify potential problems with the maintenance of oxygenation and ventilation during airway management.
- Indications for the use of airway management are:
  (1) failure to oxygenate;
  (2) failure to ventilate;
  (3) failure to maintain a patent airway.
- The modality of airway management primarily depends on the cause and severity of the patient condition, but is also subject to factors such as environment and clinician skill.
- Airway management is performed through the utilization of both noninvasive and invasive techniques:
  - Noninvasive airway management includes passive oxygenation, bag-valve-mask ventilation, supraglottic airways, and noninvasive positive-pressure ventilation.
  - Invasive airway management comprises advanced skills such as endotracheal intubation, cricothyroidotomy, and tracheostomy[205].

CAUSES OF AIRWAY OBSTRUCTION

- Infection, including:
  - Retropharyngeal abscess
  - Peritonsillar abscess,
  - Tonsillitis,
  - Epiglottitis
- Trauma to larynx (blunt and penetrating)
- Tumour
- Anaphylaxis
- Foreign body
- Blood
- Angioedema Vomit
- Secretions
- Penetrating neck injury

A. SIMPLE AIRWAY MANOEUVRES

1. SUCTION

- Suctioning may be required to clear the airway of secretion and debris through the use of a Yankauer suction tip. The patient should have been oxygenated for several minutes prior to suctioning. Obviously, this will not be possible in the patient with an obstructed airway[206].
- Suction should be applied for less than 10-15 seconds in the adult; less than 5 seconds in the pediatric patient. If repeat suctioning is required, ensure the patient remains adequately oxygenated. All suctioning should be done under direct vision and should be as atraumatic as possible. The Yankauer catheter is a rigid tube used to clear secretions and other foreign material from the oropharynx. It is inserted into the oral cavity under direct visualization and slowly withdrawn while the suction is activated.

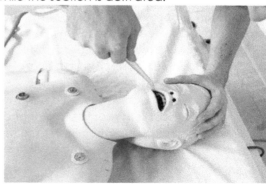

2. THE CHIN-LIFT MANOEUVRE

- This maneuver should only be used if the physician is confident there is no risk of injury to the c-spine. Standing on the patient's right hand side, the physicians left hand is used to apply pressure to the forehead to extend the neck[207].

[205] Webb MP, Helander EM, Meyn AR, Flynn T, Urman RD, Kaye AD. Preoperative Assessment of the Pregnant Patient Undergoing Nonobstetric Surgery. Anesthesiol Clin. 2018 Dec;36(4):627-637.

[206] https://handbook.bcehs.ca/treatment-guidelines/clinical-procedures/airway-management-and-oxygenation/basic-airway-management/

[207]elentra.healthsci.queensu.ca/assets/modules/basic-airway-management/simple_airway_maneuvers.html

o The volar surfaces of the tips of the index and middle finger are used to elevate the mandible which will lift the tongue from the posterior pharynx.

o The pillow effectively flexes the neck in relation to the torso; the chin-lift manoeuvre extends the head in relation to the neck.

o The so called **'sniffing position'** is achieved.

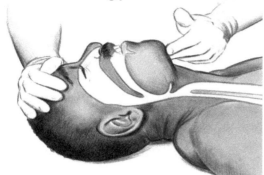

3. THE JAW THRUST

• Where there is risk of c-spine injury, such as a patient who is unconscious as a result of a head injury, the airway should be opened using a maneuver that does not require neck movement. The jaw thrust is performed by having the physician stand at the head of the patient looking down at the patient[208].

• The middle finger of the right hand is placed at the angle of the patient's jaw on the right.

• The middle finger of the left hand is similarly placed at the angle of the jaw on the left. An upward pressure is applied to elevate the mandible which will lift the tongue from the posterior pharynx.

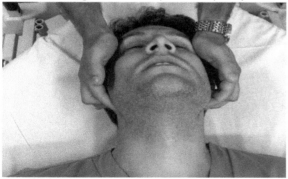

o **The chin-lift** is suitable for those patients who, with an open airway, are breathing adequately. **A high flow oxygen mask** can be applied.

o **A jaw thrust** is more suitable for patients who require **bag-mask ventilation**, since it is difficult to apply a mask and a chin-lift simultaneously.

o **In trauma patients** (suspected cervical spine injury), apply the **jaw thrust** not the chin-lift manoeuvre.

B. SIMPLE AIRWAY ADJUNCTS

1. OROPHARYNGEAL AIRWAY

• The OPA is designed to prevent the tongue and other soft tissues from obstructing the glottis. It is indicated for unresponsive patients who do not have an intact gag reflex[209].

o Ensure the correct size is employed. Measure the OPA from the angle of the jaw to the midline of the mouth.

o Ensure the mouth has been cleared of secretions or debris.

o The traditional method is to insert the OPA upside down or at a 90-degree angle to avoid catching the tongue, and then rotating it into proper position after passing the crest of the tongue.

o The OPA may also be inserted using a tongue depressor to displace the tongue while the device is inserted with the bevel posteriorly over the crest of the tongue.

o If an oropharyngeal airway becomes plugged with emesis, blood or other secretions change out the airway.

o Utilization of the OPA does not remove the requirement for manual maneuvers previously described including jaw thrust, positioning the patient and suctioning.

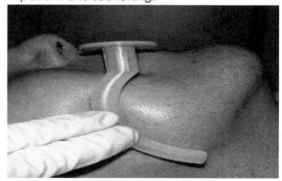

2. NASOPHARYNGEAL AIRWAY

o The nasopharyngeal airway is a soft rubber or plastic hollow tube that is passed through the nose into the posterior pharynx. The tubes come in sizes based on the internal diameter(i.d.) of the tube.

o The larger the internal diameter the longer the tube. An 8.0 – 9.0 i.d. is used for a large adult, a 7.0 – 8.0 i.d. for a medium adult and a 6.0 – 7.0 i.d. for a small adult.

o These tubes can be used when the use of an oropharyngeal airway is difficult, such as when a patient is clenching their jaw.

---

[208]elentra.healthsci.queensu.ca/assets/modules/basic-airway-management/simple_airway_maneuvers.html

[209]https://elentra.healthsci.queensu.ca/assets/modules/basic-airway-management/airway_adjuncts.html

o   As well, the nasopharyngeal airway is generally better tolerated than the oropharyngeal airway in a semiconscious patient[210].

o   To insert, the nasopharyngeal airway is lubricated with water soluble lubricant or anesthetic jelly along the floor of the nostril into posterior pharynx behind the tongue.

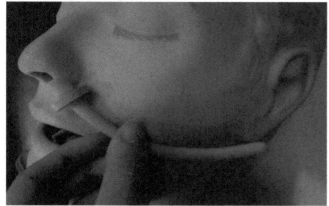

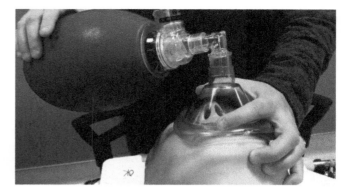

- More resistance in the bag then you might anticipate suggests a problem.
- Recognise your limitations as a single-handed airway practitioner.
- If you sense a problem ask someone to squeeze the bag as per your instructions, whilst you attempt to provide better airway patency and mask seal using your right hand opposite your left.

C. BAG VALVE MASK VENTILATION

- Most patient can be successfully oxygenated and if need be ventilated using good Bag Valve Mask (BVM) technique and adapting a staged approach for the Difficult Bag Valve Mask (DBVM) patient.
- Good, one person BVM technique starts with a well fitting mask, and a properly executed "EC" grip where the index finger and thumb encircle the base of the mask and the middle, ring and small fingers hook the mandible.
- Key to a successful mask seal is to lift the face into the mask with the EC grip as opposed to pushing the mask onto the face. This is action is the "lift and squeeze technique"
- Adequate ventilation can be confirmed by:
  o   Looking for chest wall rise and fall,
  o   Improvement in oxygen saturation.

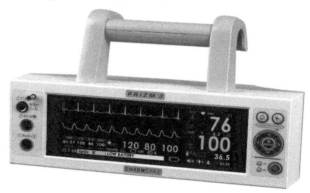

DIFFICULTY IN VENTILATION

- The difficult airway should be defined in terms of the key components of airway management:
  1. Bag-mask ventilation
  2. Supraglottic airway insertion
  3. Tracheal intubation
  4. Infraglottic airway insertion

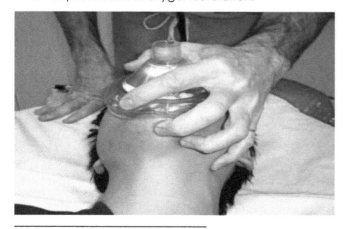

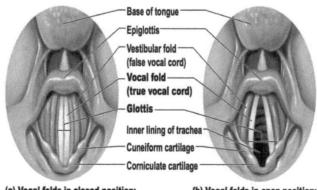

- Base of tongue
- Epiglottis
- Vestibular fold (false vocal cord)
- Vocal fold (true vocal cord)
- Glottis
- Inner lining of trachea
- Cuneiform cartilage
- Corniculate cartilage

(a) Vocal folds in closed position; closed glottis

(b) Vocal folds in open position; open glottis

[210]https://elentra.healthsci.queensu.ca/assets/modules/basic-airway-management/airway_adjuncts.html

II. DIFFICULT AIRWAY MANAGEMENT

INTRODUCTION

o A difficult airway is defined as the clinical situation in which a conventionally trained anesthesiologist experiences difficulty with facemask ventilation of the upper airway, difficulty with tracheal intubation, or both. The difficult airway represents a complex interaction between patient factors, the clinical setting, and the skills of the practitioner[211].

o **Difficult facemask or supraglottic airway (SGA) ventilation (e.g., laryngeal mask airway [LMA], intubating LMA [ILMA], laryngeal tube):** It is not possible for the anesthesiologist to provide adequate ventilation because of one or more of the following problems: inadequate mask or SGA seal, excessive gas leak, or excessive resistance to the ingress or egress of gas. Signs of inadequate ventilation include (but are not limited to) absent or inadequate chest movement, absent or inadequate breath sounds, auscultatory signs of severe obstruction, cyanosis, gastric air entry or dilatation, decreasing or inadequate oxygen saturation (SpO2), absent or inadequate exhaled carbon dioxide, absent or inadequate spirometric measures of exhaled gas flow, and hemodynamic changes associated with hypoxemia or hypercarbia (e.g., hypertension, tachycardia, arrhythmia).

o **Difficult SGA placement:** SGA placement requires multiple attempts, in the presence or absence of tracheal pathology.

o **Difficult laryngoscopy:** It is not possible to visualize any portion of the vocal cords after multiple attempts at conventional laryngoscopy.

o **Difficult tracheal intubation:** Tracheal intubation requires multiple attempts, in the presence or absence of tracheal pathology.

o **Failed intubation:** Placement of the endotracheal tube fails after multiple attempts.

• **CAN'T INTUBATE, CAN'T VENTILATE (CICV)** is when a failed intubation is compounded by an inability to maintain adequate oxygen saturation with BVM.

CAUSES OF DIFFICULT AIRWAY:

o Poor Preparation
o Inadequate positioning
o Poor availability of equipment
o Lack of suitable personnel
o Inadequate training

---

[211] https://anesthesiology.pubs.asahq.org/article.aspx?articleid=1918684

MALLAMPATI SCORE[212]

o Seated patient
o Open their mouth as far as they can.
o Using a tongue depressor or laryngoscope blade if necessary.
o If only the base of the uvula, or less, can be visualised, intubation may be more challenging.
o It is difficult to assess in the immobilised or obtunded patient.

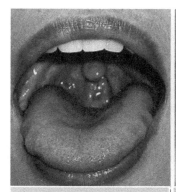

Class I: Full visibility of tonsils, uvula and soft palate

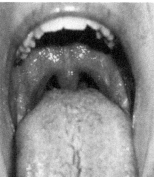

Class II: Visibility of hard and soft palate, upper portion tonsils and uvula

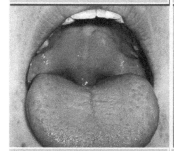

Class III: Soft and hard palate and base of the uvula are visible

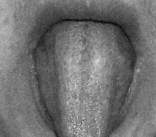

Class IV: Only hard palate visible

3-3-2 Rule

A normal patient should be able to accomodate:

A. **3** finger breadths between incisors
B. **3** fingers from the tip of the chin to the neck
C. **2** fingers from the chin / neck junction to the thyroid cartilage

• The presence of indicators of possible difficulty does not mean an airway will be difficult; more importantly, their absence does not mean it will be easy.

---

[212] Mallampati, SR; Gatt, SP; Gugino, LD; Desai, SP; Waraksa, B; Freiberger, D; Liu, PL (Jul 1985). "A clinical sign to predict difficult tracheal intubation: a prospective study". Canadian Anaesthetists' Society Journal. **32** (4): 429–34.

- It is also vital to remember that pathology compromising the airway might progress rapidly. The difficulty of an airway is not a static concept.
- Pathological processes, which can compromise an airway, might develop rapidly.

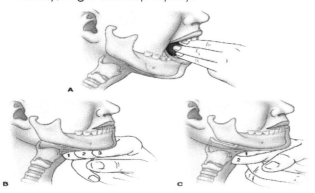

- For example: **Upper airway burns; a mildly hoarse voice** may quickly progress to airway obstruction and the need for an emergency surgical airway.
- Penetrating injuries to the neck; can cause a **rapidly expanding haematoma** which may compress the airway.

Difficulty Endotracheal Intubation= LEMON	Difficult Bag-Mask-Valve (BMV)= MOANS
- **L**ook externally - **E**valuate 3-3-2 - **M**allampati - **O**bstruction/Obesity - **N**eck Mobility	- **M**ask seal (Beard, Blood...) - **O**bstructed/Obese - **A**ge > 55 - **N**o teeth/Neck Stiffness / Neck Mass - **S**tridor / Snores/ Stiff Lungs
Difficult Laryngeal Mask Airway (LMA)=RODS	Difficult Cricothyrotomy = SHORT
- **R**estricted Mouth Opening - **O**bstruction - **D**istorted airway anatomy - **S**tiff Lungs / Neck	- **S**urgery - **H**ematoma, Have Infection (Abscess) - **O**besity - **R**adiation - **T**rauma, Tumor

CORMACK-LEHANE VIEWS

- A variety of clinical tests and models have been described to predict difficult laryngoscopy and difficult intubation.
- Most prediction models describe difficult laryngoscopy based on Cormack-Lehane laryngoscopic views, in which 4 grades are classified based on the view obtained at laryngoscopy:
  - **Grade I,** the glottis is completely visible.
  - **Grade II,** only the posterior commissure or posterior portion of the laryngeal aperture is visible.
  - **Grade III,** only the epiglottis is visible.
  - **Grade IV,** no glottic structures are visible, only the soft palate.

- Higher **Cormack-Lehane** views (grades III and IV) are associated with difficult intubation.
- Whereas difficult tracheal intubation is uncommon (incidence of 1–3%, based on varying definitions used in the literature), the inability to view the larynx during direct laryngoscopy may be as high as 6% in adult patients.

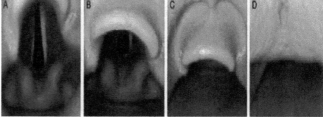

Laryngoscopic view grading system as initially developed by Cormack and Lehane.

MANAGEMENT OF DIFFICULT AIRWAY

- Call for help, if not already done
- Re-position patient (neck flexed 35° onto chest and 15° face extension)
- Reduce cricoid force
- Attempt **'BURP'** manoeuvre (see below)
- Use gum elastic bougie
- Try alternative laryngoscopy blade: If successful >>> Tracheal Intubation
- If there is still no improvement, try a laryngeal mask airway

DISCHARGE STATUS

- Patients should be formally assessed for discharge suitability from the clinical area where sedation has taken place. Discharge criteria are as follows:
  - The patient has returned to their baseline level of consciousness.
  - Vital signs are within normal limits for that patient.
  - Respiratory status is not compromised.
  - Pain and discomfort have been addressed.

- If there is a requirement to discharge the patient prior to meeting these criteria they should be transferred to an appropriate clinical environment, usually level 2 care with continuation of periprocedure monitoring standards.
- Patients meeting discharge criteria following sedation who go on to be discharged home from the ED should be discharged into the care of a responsible third party.
- Verbal and written instructions should be given

5. Rapid Sequence Intubation

I. DEMONSTRATE RSI

1. CLINICAL INDICATIONS FOR RSI

o **Isolated head injury:** Hypoxic, GCS 5, facial injury, blood in the pharynx, masseter spasm
o **Chest injury:** requiring urgent ventilation (for example, bilateral flail segments; pulmonary contusion; drained haemopneumothoraces with hypoxia despite adequate drainage and supplemental oxygen)
o **Asthma:** Exhausted asthmatic on maximal therapy
o **Status epilepticus:** unresponsive to other therapy
o **Patient who has taken an overdose:** comatose, cardiovascularly stable and maintaining a patent airway. Protection of the airway is desirable but not required immediately

2. CONTRAINDICATIONS OF RSI

o Spontaneous breathing with adequate ventilation
o Operator concern that both intubation and BVM may not be successful
o Major laryngeal trauma
o Distorted facial/ airway anatomy

3. COMPLICATIONS OF RSI

o Failure to intubate
o Hypoxia
o Unrecognised oesophageal intubation
o Aspiration of stomach contents
o Hypotension
o Awareness
o Arrhythmias, Cardiac arrest

• Aspiration of gastric content – the risk is higher if:
o There has been recent ingestion
o Gastric emptying is delayed secondary to trauma, pain, diabetes or opioids
o The lower oesophageal sphincter is incompetent owing to obesity, pregnancy or hiatus hernia
o The patient has been manually ventilated for a long time before performing the RSI, since this inflates the stomach

o The appropriate cricoid pressure has not been applied
• Inability to intubate, exacerbated by trauma from repeated attempted intubations.
• Intubation of the oesophagus.
• Dislodgement of the tube.
• **Bronchial intubation:** commonly a tube inserted too far will occlude the right upper main bronchus, resulting in collapse of the lung section. If placed further, the entire left main bronchus may not be ventilated, leading to collapse of the lung and a higher risk of pneumothorax.
• **Tracheal stenosis:** prolonged intubation, especially with an inflated cuff, and more common in children who have soft, more easily damaged tracheas.
• Severe hypoxia if prolonged attempts are undertaken.
• Chipping, loosening or dislodgement of teeth.

4. EQUIPMENT

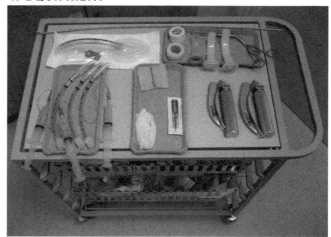

• Size 3 or 4 Macintosh laryngoscope (curved blade)
• Cuffed endotracheal tubes (sizes 7 and 8)
• Wide-bore suction and tilting bed
• 10 mL syringe for inflating the cuff
• Gum elastic bougie and stylet

- Aqueous gel lubricant, Pillow
- Magill's forceps, Ribbon or tape to secure the endotracheal (ET) tube
- Colorimetric end-tidal CO2 monitor
- Anaesthetic drugs
- Emergency drugs (adrenaline and atropine)
- Difficult-airway set

> ↓ Before you commence intubation, you should already have a back-up plan (plan B) in the event that you cannot
> ↓ Intubate and cannot ventilate the patient.

It is crucial that your team members be aware of this plan and so can prepare accordingly.

The three major situations encountered in the emergency department are:

1. A rapid sequence induction (RSI) where the patient is awake and unstarved (a full stomach). Measures are made to reduce the risk of aspiration, with a minimum delay between the patient being awake and asleep with cuffed tube in trachea.
2. Intubation where the patient is obtunded or is suspended. In these circumstances, the patient will not need to be sedated or paralysed.
3. Failed intubation where the patient cannot be ventilated or intubated.

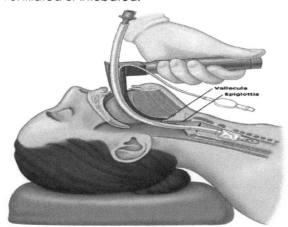

5. DRUG DOSAGES FOR RSI

- IBW = ideal body weight, TBW = total body weight
  - o **INDUCTION AGENTS**
    - Ketamine 1.5-2 mg/kg IBW
    - Etomidate 0.3-0.4 mg/kg TBW
    - Fentanyl 2-10 mcg/kg TBW
    - Midazolam 0.1-0.3 mg/kg TBW
    - Propofol 1-2.5 mg/kg IBW + (0.4 x TBW) (others simply use 1.5 mg/kg x TBW as the general guide)
    - Thiopental 2-7 mg/kg TBW

- o **NEUROMUSCULAR BLOCKERS:**
  - Suxamethonium 1-2 mg/kg TBW
  - Rocuronium 0.6-1.2 mg/kg IBW
  - Vecuronium 0.15-0.25 mg/kg IBW

6. ESSENTIAL FEATURES OF RAPID SEQUENCE INDUCTION

- o Pre-oxygenation with 100% oxygen
- o Predetermined induction doses of drugs
- o Cricoid pressure
- o Cuffed endotracheal tube
- o Equipment and strategy to manage failed intubation

7. SUGGESTED APPROACH

- The situation that you are presented with – a patient with a GCS of 6 who is being oxygenated with a bag–valve mask and has undetectable saturations on 15 L of O2 – is suggestive of imminent full respiratory arrest.
- You should identify this and call for help (invariably in the examination, the anaesthetist will be unavailable).
- Ask the nurse to apply monitoring.
- Do not assume that the airway is patent because there is an oropharyngeal airway already in situ and ongoing bag–valve ventilation.
- Assess the airway for obstruction, confirm that the oropharyngeal airway is the appropriate size, and confirm successful ventilation with bag–valve ventilation (a two-person technique may be needed).
- The use of an LMA is an option. In this scenario, the bag–valve mask continues to be inadequate and intubation should be considered.
- Ventilation should continue, since some degree of oxygenation may be occurring while you prepare for intubation, but you should be aware of gastric insufflation.

THE EMERGENCY INTUBATION

It is worth being aware of the '10 Ps' of ET intubation before you plan your procedure:

1. *Preparation*
2. *Plan for failure*
3. *Positioning the head*
4. *Pre-oxygenation*
5. *Pre-treatment*
6. *Protection from aspiration (cricoid pressure)*
7. *Paralysis with induction*
8. *Placement of the ET tube*
9. *Proof of correct ET tube placement*
10. *Post-intubation placement*

1. PREPARATION

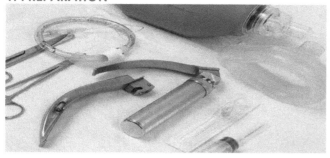

It is essential that you have the right equipment and staff for the planned procedure.
You should:

- Have a back-up plan if you run into difficulties.
- Have the patient on full monitoring (ECG/BP/pulse oximetry).
- Check all of the equipment (suction, laryngoscope, ET tube cuff).
- Ensure that there is IV access and the cannula is patent.
- Ensure that the emergency drugs are drawn up and labelled.
- Ensure that you have a trained assistant.

2. PLAN FOR FAILURE

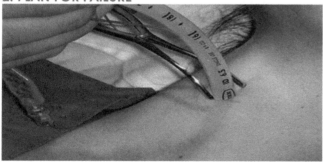

- The importance of having a back-up plan in the event that you cannot intubate the patient cannot be overstressed.
- If you are not comfortable in executing your back-up plans B, C or even D then you should really question whether you are the right person to be intubating the patient.

3. POSITIONING THE HEAD

- The goal of positioning the head is to have the oral, pharyngeal and laryngeal inlets positioned in a straight line facilitating direct laryngoscopy.
- The ideal position is achieved by placing a pillow under the patient's head and extending the head on the neck in a **'sniffing the morning air' position.**
- This is the optimum position for intubation; however, a neutral position and in-line immobilization must be maintained when you suspect a C-spine injury.

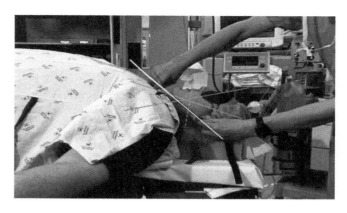

4. PRE-OXYGENATION

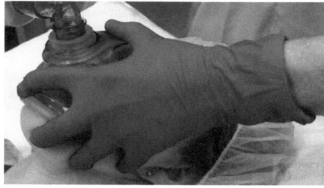

- Pre-oxygenation is performed with the patient breathing 100% oxygen through a tight-fitting non-rebreathing facemask **for 3 minutes.**
- This allows replacement of nitrogen-containing air with oxygen, and acts as an oxygen reservoir delaying the onset of hypoxia in cases of prolonged apnoea or difficult intubation.
- After each failed attempt at intubation, the patient should be pre-oxygenated.

5. PRE-TREATMENT

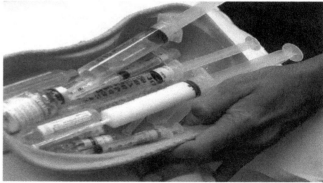

Some situations require medications to attenuate the hypertensive response to larygnoscopy:

- **Lidocaine**
- **Opioids (e.g. Fentanyl or alfentanil)**
- These are not normally given in a crash induction, where the priority is securing the airway quickly and safely.

6. PROTECTION OF THE AIRWAY

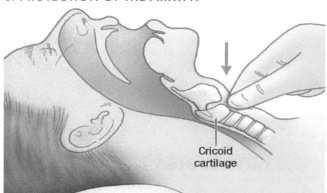

Cricoid cartilage

- Protection of the airway from aspiration of gastric contents is only achieved when a tube is positioned within the trachea, with no leakage of air around the cuff.
- However, before the tube can be placed within the trachea, **cricoid pressure** must be applied to reduce the occurrence of passive regurgitation.
- Cricoid pressure (**Sellick's manoeuvre**, Figure above) should be applied by a trained assistant using anteroposterior pressure on the cricoid cartilage at the onset of induction.
- The full 44 newtons of force should be applied when neuromuscular blocking agents are administered or when the patient is obtunded.
- The complete circumferential ring of the cricoid compresses the lumen of the oesophagus against the sixth cervical vertebra.
- **It does not prevent active vomiting**, and continued application in such circumstances can result in oesophageal rupture. This is the only situation in which it should be released prematurely, and **the bed tilted head down with the patient on the left lateral position** to reduce aspiration.
- Otherwise, the cricoid should only be released after confirmed correct tube placement and adequate cuff inflation.

7. PARALYSIS WITH INDUCTION

- Only those trained in RSI and who routinely perform these techniques should administer muscle relaxants and anaesthetic agents, owing to contraindications and adverse complications associated with their use in the emergency setting.
- Give an appropriate intravenous induction agent: **thiopental or propofol.** These both cause hypnosis and amnesia.
- To ease laryngeal intubation, high-speed muscle relaxation is important. The drug of choice in most circumstances is **suxamethonium**, although you should be aware of its contraindications.

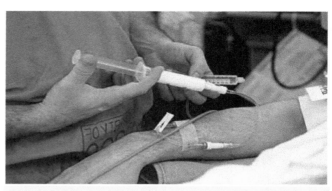

- Suxamethonium is a depolarizing muscle relaxant and causes muscle fasciculation before muscle relaxation.

8. PLACEMENT OF THE ET TUBE

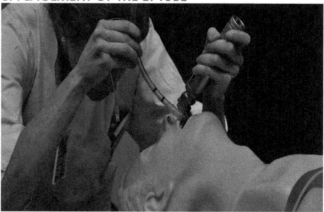

You will be asked to demonstrate this on the manikin.

- Stand behind the patient.
- Hold the laryngoscope with your **left hand** and insert it into the mouth over the **right side** of the tongue.
- Sweep the tongue **from right to left** and push it upwards so that the tip of the epiglottis comes into view. Make sure that you do not use the teeth as a fulcrum and that the lower lip does not get caught between the blade of the laryngoscope and the teeth.
- Advance the tip of the laryngoscope into the valecula between the epiglottis and the tongue.
- To visualize the vocal cords, lift the contents of the oropharynx by moving the laryngoscope along the central axis of the handle.
- If you have a good view of the cords, you should insert the ET tube with your right hand so that it passes between the vocal cords into the trachea, ensuring that the cuff has passed beyond the vocal cords.
- In most adults, the tube will usually lie between **22 and 24 cm** at the level of the incisors.

- Stabilize the tube until it is taped or tied in place.
- Connect the tube via a catheter mount and ventilate the patient with 12–15 L of oxygen.
- The cuff should be inflated until no audible leak of ventilation gases is heard to pass around the cuff.

9. PROOF OF CORRECT ET TUBE PLACEMENT

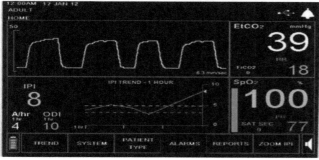

It is imperative that you ensure that the ET tube is in the correct place and at the correct depth, by (in chronological order):

1. Direct visualisation of the tube passing through the cords
2. Compliance of the reservoir bag on manual ventilation and fogging of the tube
3. Symmetrical expansion of the chest wall
4. Auscultation of the chest bilaterally for breath sounds and auscultation over the epigastrium to exclude oesophageal intubation
5. Attachment of an end-tidal CO2 monitor (capnograph or calometric)
6. Obtaining a chest X-ray to ensure placement of the tube above the carina and below the level of the cords

10. POST TUBE PLACEMENT

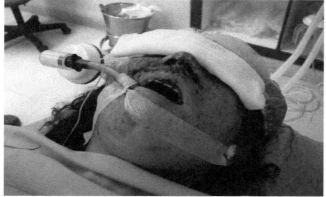

- The tube should be secured and the level at the central incisors noted in case of tube migration.
- The patient should be carefully monitored, and, once they have been stabilized, **a portable chest X-ray** should be performed to ensure that the main bronchus has not been inadvertently intubated.

THE SELLICK MANOEUVRE[213]

- It is cricoid pressure applied during endotracheal intubation. It is used to reduce the risk of regurgitation of gastric contents and works by virtue of the cricoid pressure occluding the oesophagus, which passes directly behind it.

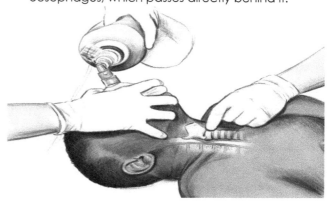

BURP MANOEUVRE[214]

- It is used to improve the view of the glottis during laryngoscopy (not to prevent regurgitation like The Sellick Manoeuvre). The 'BURP' manoeuvre requires an assistant to apply pressure of the thyroid cartilage posteriorly (1), then upwards (2), and finally laterally towards the patients right (3).

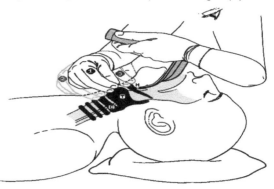

AIRWAY/VENTILATION PROBLEMS ASSOCIATED WITH SERIOUS ILLNESS AND INJURY

- Pre-oxygenation may be impossible or ineffective
- Positioning for intubation may be difficult if the cervical spine is immobilised
- The airway may be partially obstructed by trauma, blood, vomitus or secretions
- The patient may be uncooperative
- They patient may already be hypoxic or haemodynamically compromised
- It may be impossible to predict whether the patient is likely to represent a difficult intubation.

---

213 Sellick BA. Cricoid pressure to control regurgitation of stomach contents during induction of anaesthesia. Lancet 1961;2:404–6

214 Takahata O, Kubota M, Mamiya K, et al. The efficacy of the "BURP" maneuver during a difficult laryngoscopy. Anesth Analg. 1997;84:419-421.

II. PROCEDURAL SEDATION

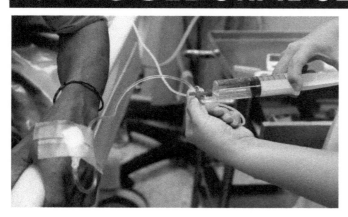

DEFINITION

- Procedural sedation involves the use of short-acting analgesic and sedative medications to enable clinicians to perform procedures effectively, while monitoring the patient closely for potential adverse effects. This process was previously (and inappropriately) termed "conscious sedation," but because effective sedation often alters consciousness, the preferred term is now "procedural sedation and analgesia" (PSA)[215].

INDICATIONS

o There are no absolute indications for the performance of procedural sedation and analgesia (PSA). PSA may be used for any procedure in which a patient's pain or anxiety may be excessive and may impede performance.

o PSA is often useful for procedures where deep relaxation facilitates performance (eg, closed reduction of a dislocated joint).

o Common procedures in which PSA may be beneficial include electrical cardioversion, closed joint reduction, complicated laceration repair, abscess incision and drainage, and lumbar puncture.

CONTRA-INDICATIONS

o Allergy or hypersensitivity to the relevant medications

o Lack of appropriately trained personnel to perform the sedation

o Patients have an ASA IV and above

o Lack of appropriate monitoring and resuscitation equipment (for Potential G.A.)

o High risk of aspiration, e.g. acute alcohol intoxication

DEPTH OF SEDATION AND DEFINITIONS

- Sedation is a continuum which extends from normal alert consciousness to complete unresponsiveness.

- Sedation and recovery move patients along this scale, but it is difficult to accurately assess the precise degree of sedation at any one time, and even harder to maintain a patient at a pre-defined target level. The American Society of Anesthesiologists (ASA) uses the following useful definitions for sedation[216]:

- **Minimal Sedation (Anxiolysis)** is a drug-induced state during which patients respond normally to verbal commands. Although cognitive function and coordination may be impaired, ventilatory and cardiovascular functions are unaffected. In the Emergency Department this is most often achieved using inhaled Entonox (50% NO & 50% oxygen).

- **Moderate Sedation/Analgesia** ('Conscious Sedation') is a drug-induced depression of consciousness during which patients respond purposefully to verbal commands, either alone or accompanied by light tactile stimulation. No interventions are required to maintain a patent airway, and spontaneous ventilation is adequate. Cardiovascular function is usually maintained. In the Emergency Department this is most often achieved using a combination of opioids and benzodiazepines.

- **Deep Sedation/Analgesia** is a drug-induced depression of consciousness during which patients cannot be easily aroused but respond purposefully following repeated or painful stimulation. The ability to independently maintain ventilatory function may be impaired. Patients may require assistance in maintaining a patent airway, and spontaneous ventilation may be inadequate. Cardiovascular function is usually maintained.

- **General Anaesthesia** is a drug-induced loss of consciousness during which patients are not rousable, even by painful stimulation. The ability to independently maintain ventilatory function is often impaired. Patients often require assistance in maintaining a patent airway, and positive pressure ventilation may be required because of depressed spontaneous ventilation or drug-induced depression of neuromuscular function. Cardiovascular function may also be impaired.

---

[215] Green SM, Krauss B. Procedural sedation terminology: moving beyond "conscious sedation". Ann Emerg Med 2002; 39:433.

[216] RCEM Safe Sedation in the Emergency Department - Report and Recommendations.pdf, November 201. Available at RCEM PDF

PERFORMING PROCEDURAL SEDATION

- **Informed consent** — Before performing procedural sedation and analgesia (PSA), the clinician must discuss the risks, benefits, and alternatives of the procedure and the planned sedation with the patient and answer any questions. A printed informed consent form may be used. Implied consent is acceptable in some cases where the patient is unable to provide explicit consent due to severe pain or altered mental status[217].
- **Prerequisites and personnel** — Although previously the domain of anesthesia practitioners, PSA is performed safely by other clinicians, including emergency and critical care physicians and nurse specialists[218]. Clinicians providing PSA should have in-depth knowledge of the relevant drugs, including their mechanism of action, doses, side effects, and reversal agents. Such clinicians must also be well versed in advanced cardiovascular life support, including airway management.
- **Equipment** — All equipment necessary to perform the procedure and manage the airway should be available at the bedside during the performance of PSA. Such equipment includes suction to manage vomiting or oral secretions, airway adjuncts, such as a bag-valve mask and oral and nasal airways, and equipment to perform endotracheal intubation. Intravenous access should be established. Resuscitation medications, including advanced cardiac life support medications and reversal agents (ie, naloxone and flumazenil) should be available. Appropriate monitors should be in place.
- **Monitoring and preoxygenation** — Proper monitoring of patients during the performance of PSA is crucial. The patient's blood pressure, heart rate, and respiratory rate should be measured at frequent, regular intervals; the oxygen saturation (SpO_2), end-tidal carbon dioxide ($EtCO_2$) level, and cardiac rhythm should be monitored continuously[219].
- **AMPLE system**: This assessment should include a past medical history, drug history and focussed clinical examination to identify any existing medical illnesses, particularly cardiovascular or respiratory disease and allergy.

AIRWAY ASSESSMENT

- Airway Evaluation is performed in anticipation of possible intubation. The patient's airway should be assessed; this includes identifying features associated with increased risk of difficult intubation and/or ventilation. Using the **LEMON** Mnemonic: highlights patients who may be **difficult to intubate:**
  - o **L:** Look externally (facial trauma, beard, large incisors, large tongue)
  - o **E:** Evaluate the 3-3-2 rule
  - o **M:** Mallampati score
  - o **O:** Obesity/obstruction (stridor in particular is worrying)
  - o **N:** Neck mobility

LEVEL OF SEDATION

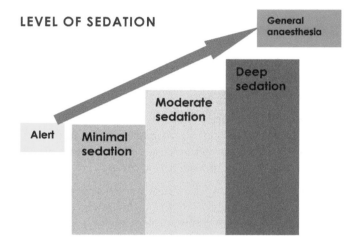

FASTING

- Aspiration is a rare complication of procedural sedation.
- There is a paucity of evidence to make an absolute recommendation regarding minimum fasting times prior to procedural sedation; however, the following principles should be borne in mind:
  - o Protective airway reflexes are more likely to be impaired with deep sedation, making aspiration more likely in the event of regurgitation.
  - o In circumstances where life or limb are not threatened, a procedure may be delayed to ensure safer sedation without altering the clinical outcome.
  - o There is a paucity of evidence to suggest a minimum pre-sedation fasting time, however the practitioner should consider the urgency of any procedure when managing an unfasted patient.

---

[217] Godwin SA, Caro DA, Wolf SJ, et al. Clinical policy: procedural sedation and analgesia in the emergency department. Ann Emerg Med 2005; 45:177.

[218] Harrington L. Nurse-administered propofol sedation: a review of current evidence. Gastroenterol Nurs 2006; 29:371.

[219] Miner JR, Burton JH. Clinical practice advisory: Emergency department procedural sedation with propofol. Ann Emerg Med 2007; 50:182.

PHARMACEUTICAL AGENTS

- **Intravenous Analgesic/Sedative drugs should be given slowly** – over 30 – 60 seconds **and in small, incremental doses that are titrated to the desired end-point of analgesia and sedation**
- It is best to regard procedural sedation as a 2 step process - analgesia then sedation
- Most importantly the team should choose an agent with which they are familiar.

Choice of agents:

- **Level 1:** We suggest nitrous oxide and or an Opiate and anxiolytic doses of a Benzodiazepine. The analgesic is given first in appropriate dose and then a bolus of Benzodiazepine. Fentanyl is the opioids and Midazolam is the Benzodiazepine of choice, anxiolytic doses are 1 – 2 mg. Elderly patients might be deeply sedated on very small doses of Midazolam, hence we suggest in the over 65 years old patients Midazolam is considered as a level 3 sedation drug

- **Level 2:** The agents used for Level2 sedation should preserve cardio respiratory function and protective airway reflexes but alter consciousness state. The drug of choice is Ketamine

- **Level 3:** The drugs used for this level of sedation may impair protective airway reflexes and depress respiratory function. These drugs include Propofol, Etomidate and higher doses of Benzodiazepines. A combination of Propofol and ketamine (0.5mg/kg of each) is an acceptable alternative

- All syringes must be labelled with dose and concentration and time
- All drug doses agreed and are called out in ml and mg prior to delivery and upon delivery
- Drugs should be drawn up by the team member who will use them and correctly labelled
  - All Analgesics in 10 ml syringes
  - All Sedatives including Midazolam in 20 ml syringes

DISSOCIATIVE SEDATION

- A separate sedation category, **'dissociative sedation'**, has therefore been introduced[220].
- **Dissociative sedation** is defined as 'a trance like cataleptic state characterized by profound analgesia and amnesia, with retention of protective airway reflexes, spontaneous respirations, and cardiopulmonary stability.'

- **Ketamine** is a unique drug in sedation practice because it causes a dissociative state that does not fit the standard definitions of sedation listed above.
- We recognise that an important boundary exists between moderate or 'conscious' sedation, where the patient responds purposefully to verbal commands, and deeper levels of sedation where the patient responds only to painful stimuli, or not at all. Once verbal contact with the patient is lost it becomes difficult to determine the level of unconsciousness, and over-sedation with an associated risk of airway and cardio-respiratory complications is possible.
- Deeper levels of sedation are, to all intents and purposes, indistinguishable from general anaesthesia and should therefore be treated as such. Because sedation is a continuum, it is not always possible to predict how the individual patient will respond.
- Patients in whom conscious sedation is intended have the potential to become more deeply sedated. Practitioners intending to produce a given level of sedation must therefore be able to 'rescue' patients from a deeper level of sedation than intended.
- A clinician intending to achieve 'deep sedation' should therefore have the knowledge and skills to manage and rescue a patient from general anaesthesia.

RECOMMENDATIONS FOR SAFE SEDATION IN THE ED[221]

- Immediate Life Support comprises the essential knowledge and skills to enable recognition of the acutely ill patient and treatment of a patient in cardiac arrest while awaiting the arrival of a resuscitation team.
- Competencies within the domain of ILS include: delivery of high-quality chest compressions, basic airway management, safe defibrillation using either manual or automated external defibrillators (AEDs), and being a cardiac arrest team member.

- **OXYGEN**
  - Oxygen should be given to sedated patients, who may experience a fall in oxygen saturation from the baseline level measured on room air.
  - Oxygen should be given from the start of sedative administration until the patient is ready for discharge from the recovery area.

---

220 RCEM Safe Sedation in the Emergency Department - Report and Recommendations.pdf, November 201. Available at RCEM PDF

221 RCEM Safe Sedation in the Emergency Department - Report and Recommendations.pdf, November 201. Available at RCEM PDF

- **CAPNOGRAPHY**
  - The use of continuous capnography is mandatory wherever deep sedation, dissociative sedation, general anaesthesia or RSI occurs, except in rare cases where it would substantially interfere with surgical access.
  - Capnography is also recommended at lighter levels of sedation; this is an emerging area of practice, and the use of capnography is expected to become routine.

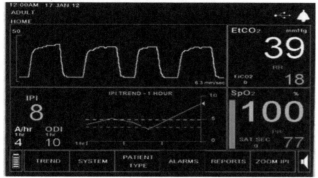

- **DOCUMENTATION**
  - Standard forms should be routinely used for patient pre-assessment, patient information, consent, monitoring, discharge information and clinical audit.
  - Past medical history, medications, allergies and physical examination of vital signs, airway and cardiopulmonary status should all be recorded prior to the procedure.
  - Good practice guidelines, issued by the Department of Health, include standard consent forms for patients undergoing procedures including sedation and general anaesthesia, but national agreement has not been established in the other documentation areas, and the development of appropriate forms would be welcomed.

- **POST-PROCEDURE MONITORING**
  - All patients who have received sedation should continue to be managed in a clinical area that provides the same level of facilities and monitoring as those required during the procedure, until the level of consciousness and other vital signs have returned to pre-procedure baseline levels.
  - This includes the presence of a clinician who has been trained in the core skills required of recovery nurses, as described in guidelines issued by the Association of Anaesthetists of Great Britain and Ireland.

  - These skills include **the monitoring and measurement of vital signs** and **overall patient status**, including **respiratory rate, blood pressure, heart rate, Glasgow Coma Score and basic life support training.**

- **DISCHARGE STATUS**
  - Patients should be formally assessed for discharge suitability from the clinical area where sedation has taken place.
  - **Discharge criteria are as follows:**
    - The patient has returned to their baseline level of consciousness.
    - Vital signs are within normal limits for that patient.
    - Respiratory status is not compromised.
    - Pain and discomfort have been addressed.

- **ACTING ON INCREASED ASPIRATION RISK**[222]
  - Where the risk of aspiration is significantly increased steps should be taken to mitigate this risk.
  - Suggested approaches include:
    - **Delaying the procedure**, if clinically appropriate.
    - **Adopting an alternative technique**: Rapid sequence induction of anaesthesia and tracheal intubation is considered the 'gold standard' where there is an increased aspiration risk, but pulmonary aspiration may still occur. In addition, RSI introduces other risks, such as inability to intubate or ventilate the patient and the risk of adverse reaction to induction and neuromuscular blocking drugs.
    - **Regional anaesthetic techniques** may allow the required procedure to be performed with no or minimal sedation.
    - **Reducing the depth and duration of sedation**: This increases the risk of procedural failure, but may be appropriate in some instances.
    - **Promote gastric emptying:** administration of **Ranitidine or PPIs, Metoclopramide and Sodium Citrate is appropriate** to neutralise gastric acid and promote gastric emptying.
    - In all cases of increased aspiration risk the advice of an expert sedationist should be sought. However, there is no consensus on this subject, even among experts.

---

[222] *RCEM Safe Sedation in the Emergency Department - Report and Recommendations.pdf, November 201. Available at* RCEM PDF

6. Postoperative Analgesia

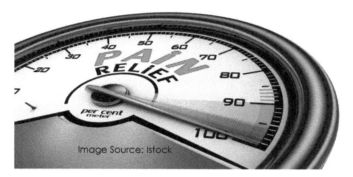

Image Source: Istock

INTRODUCTION

- The provision of effective pain relief during the postoperative period is dependent on anaesthetic technique, type and extent of surgery and patient factors such as age and personality. In practice, a combination of opioid, non-steroidal anti-inflammatory drugs (NSAIDs) and local anaesthetic techniques is often used.

- Preoperative patient evaluation and planning is vital to successful postoperative pain management. Recommended preoperative evaluation includes a directed pain history, a directed physical exam and a pain control plan; however, the literature is insufficient in regards to efficacy[223].

- Likewise patient preparation should include adjustments of preoperative medications to avoid withdrawals effect, treatment to reduce preoperative pain/anxiety, and preoperative initiation of treatment as part of a multimodal pain management plan. There is some support that preoperative pain levels may predict levels of postsurgical pain[224].

- Certain preoperative variables such as age, anxiety levels, and depression may have an effect on levels of postoperative pain.[Z] Higher postoperative pain levels can be associated with lower quality of care.

- Although preoperative patient and family education are recommended, the literature is equivocal regarding its impact on postoperative pain, anxiety, and time to discharge[225].

PAIN ASSESSMENT

- Pain, by definition, is a subjective sensation and is difficult for an observer to accurately assess. The provision of a reliable and valid means of assessing pain is important because it allows the degree of improvement, after an analgesic intervention, to be documented in a reproducible way.

- There are a number of specific pain assessment scales that are used in the postoperative setting to ensure that a history of the patient's pain is recorded in a useful form so as to inform treatment decisions.

- These include:
  o *Verbal rating scale (VRS)*
  o *Numerical rating scale (NRS)*
  o *Visual analogue scale (VAS)*

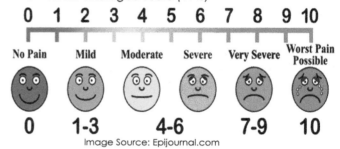

Image Source: Epijournal.com

- In very young children, physiological and behavioural indicators are used. Older children may choose from ranked facial expressions on a chart.

- **The verbal rating scale** is simple and easy to use. The patient is asked to rate the pain as 'none', 'mild', 'moderate', or 'severe' when at rest and on movement.

- **The numerical rating scale** consists of a numerical scale representing the pain from 0 = 'no pain' to 10 (or 5) ='the worst imaginable pain'.

- **The visual analogue scale** consists of a 10 cm long line which represents a spectrum of pain intensity from 'no pain at all' on the extreme left through to 'the worst pain imaginable' on the extreme right.

- The patient is asked to mark the point on this line that corresponds to the severity of the pain. The VAS is primarily a research tool and, performed correctly, is arguably too complex for routine postoperative use.

- There is no obvious advantage of the more detailed methods in terms of practical patient management.

---

[223] *Practice guidelines for acute pain management in the perioperative setting: an updated report by the American Society of Anesthesiologists Task Force on Acute Pain Management. American Society of Anesthesiologists Task Force on Acute Pain Management.Anesthesiology. 2012 Feb; 116(2):248-73.*

[224] *Preoperative prediction of severe postoperative pain. Kalkman CJ, Visser K, Moen J, Bonsel GJ, Grobbee DE, Moons KG Pain. 2003 Oct; 105(3):415-23.*

[225] *What is the effect of preoperative information on patient satisfaction? Walker JA Br J Nurs. 2007 Jan 11-24; 16(1):27-32.*

ACUTE PAIN SERVICE

- The importance of effective postoperative pain relief, and the increased complexity of analgesic techniques such as PCA and continuous epidural infusions, has resulted in the formation of acute pain services in many hospitals. They provide a multidisciplinary approach to postoperative pain control with the involvement of anaesthetists, specialist nurses and clinical pharmacists.
- An acute pain service carries out regular patient assessment and provides backup forward staff.
- It is also involved in 'in-house' training of medical and nursing staff to improve understanding of analgesic methods and pain assessment.

ADVERSE EFFECTS OF POSTOPERATIVE PAIN

- **Cardiovascular**
  - Tachycardia
  - Hypertension
  - Increased myocardial oxygen demand
- **Respiratory**
  - Decreased vital capacity
  - Decreased functional residual capacity
  - Decreased tidal volume
  - Chest infections
  - Basal atelectasis
- **Gastrointestinal**
  - Nausea and vomiting
  - Ileus
- **Other effects**
  - Urinary retention
  - Deep venous thrombosis
  - Pulmonary embolus

TREATMENT OF PAIN

1. OPIOIDS

- Opioids may be given via the following routes: intramuscular, subcutaneous, intravenous, oral, intrathecal or extradural.
- The dose of opioid required in the postoperative period shows marked interpatient variability.
- This is due to both pharmacokinetic and pharmacodynamic factors with up to a fivefold difference in plasma concentrations after identical doses of intramuscular opioid.
- There are also differences in opioid receptor sensitivity between patients.
- The conventional regime of on-demand intramuscular opioid often fails to provide adequate pain relief as delays in administration, lack of patient awareness of availability and time taken for onset of action result in plasma levels falling below that required to produce analgesia.

- Usual dosage is **10–15 mg every 2–4 hours**. There may be slow absorption in patients with poor peripheral perfusion.
- Subcutaneous opioid administration via indwelling cannulae is associated with similar limitations but avoids repeated needle insertion.
- All opioids have significant side effects that limit their use. The most important side effect is respiratory depression that could result in hypoxia and respiratory arrest. Hence, regular monitoring of respiration and oxygen saturation is essential in patients on opioids postoperatively. In addition, nausea, vomiting, pruritus, and reduction in bowel motility leading to ileus and constipation are also common side effects of these medications[226].
- Longer-term use of opioids can lead to dependence and addiction. Once the patient is able to tolerate oral intake, oral opioids can be initiated and continued after discharge from the hospital. With the development of enhanced recovery protocols, particularly in colorectal surgery, primarily opioid-based regimens are being challenged by other agents and approaches to postoperative pain management[227].

A. INTRAVENOUS OPIOIDS

- **Patient-controlled analgesia (PCA)** was developed to further improve opioid analgesia by accounting for the variation in opioid requirement from patient to patient and the reduction in opioid required with time. The theoretical advantage of this technique is that the patient should maintain a plasma concentration at around the minimum effective analgesic plasma concentration, with resultant good pain control and reduced side effects.
- It is safer than intravenous infusion techniques as the associated sedation when the patients are pain-free results in reduced usage. In practice, patients may not alleviate their pain completely with this technique because of their worries about addiction and side effects.
- The success of PCA is dependent on patient education during the preoperative visit, adequate pain control in the recovery room and regular review by nursing and anaesthetic staff. **Morphine** is the most commonly used opioid, although other drugs such as **Alfentanil** and **Pethidine** have been used with good effect.

---

[226] *Influence of intravenous opioid dose on postoperative ileus. Barletta JF, Asgeirsson T, Senagore AJ Ann Pharmacother. 2011 Jul; 45(7-8):916-23.*

[227] *The evolution of analgesia in an 'accelerated' recovery programme for resectional laparoscopic colorectal surgery with anastomosis.Zafar N, Davies R, Greenslade GL, Dixon AR Colorectal Dis. 2010 Feb; 12(2):119-24.*

- A demand dose of **Morphine 1 mg** is used with a lock-out period of 5 minutes.
- The main side effects associated with parenteral opioid administration are **nausea and vomiting, and cardiorespiratory depression.**
- The risk of this is increased in patients receiving background opioid infusions or other sedative drugs. The elderly and patients with pre-existing sleep apnoea also have an increased risk of respiratory depression.

B. ORAL OPIOIDS

- Patients who are able to tolerate oral intake may benefit from opioids given by this route. It is a particularly useful technique in children as it avoids needle or cannula insertion. A dose of **morphine 0.2 mg/kg** is adequate in most instances.

C. SPINAL OPIOIDS

- Opioid administration via the intrathecal or extradural route can provide excellent postoperative pain control. The commonest side effects associated with this technique are **nausea, pruritus, sedation and urinary retention.**
- Respiratory depression is an infrequent complication, but it can occur up to 24 hours after administration of **intrathecal opioids**, and therefore patients must be observed in the high dependency unit for a 24-hour period to monitor their respiratory status. Patients receiving **extradural opioids** are at a lower risk of developing respiratory depression but they must also be managed on a ward where this potentially fatal complication can be recognised and treated.
- **Intravenous Naloxone** given in titrated doses is effective at reversing the opioid induced respiratory depression without reducing the analgesic effect.

2. NON-STEROIDAL ANTI-INFLAMMATORY DRUGS

- This group of drugs have both analgesic and anti-inflammatory properties.
- They are effective for treatment of mild to moderate postoperative pain and, after the first 24–36 hours, may be used as the sole analgesic in major surgical patients.
- Nonsteroidal anti-inflammatory agents (NSAIDS) are useful in reducing the amount of opiates requested and administered to the patient thus reducing opioid side effects[228].

- NSAIDs have several advantages over opioid analgesics:
  - Their use is not associated with respiratory depression or gastric stasis
  - They are not controlled drugs, they are readily available.
- The use of NSAIDs is associated with **potentially serious side effects:**
  - Gastrointestinal haemorrhage,
  - Gastric ulceration,
  - Renal impairment
  - Increased risk of postoperative bleeding due to impairment of platelet function.
- There is a risk of bleeding with these agents, so use of NSAIDs is dependent on the individual patient's risk factors. Nonselective agents such as ibuprofen do have an increased side effect profile (bleeding, antiplatelet effect); however, general consensus in the literature is that COX-1 inhibitors are preferred over selective COX-2 inhibitors such as celecoxib, given the recent evidence of cardiovascular risks associated with COX-2 agents[229].
- **NSAIDs are contraindicated in patients with:**
  - History of peptic ulcer disease,
  - Gastrointestinal bleeding,
  - Renal impairment,
  - Previous hypersensitivity reactions to aspirin or NSAIDs,
  - Asthma,
  - Bleeding diathesis.
- They should be avoided in the dehydrated or hypovolaemic patient and care should be taken when using NSAIDs in the elderly.
- The salicylates are absolutely contraindicated in children less than 12 years of age - **Reye's syndrome**, an acute encephalopathy with fatty infiltration of the liver, is associated with administration of these drugs in this age group.

3. LOCAL ANAESTHETICS

- Local infiltration, peripheral nerve blocks and epidural analgesia are often used to produce postoperative pain relief, both alone and in conjunction with other analgesic methods.
- The advantage of local anaesthetic techniques is that profound analgesia can be produced without respiratory depression or nausea and vomiting. However, local anaesthetic toxicity may occur as a result of inadvertent intravenous administration or after large doses.

---

[228] A randomized, controlled trial to compare ketorolac tromethamine versus placebo after cesarean section to reduce pain and narcotic usage. Lowder JL, Shackelford DP, Holbert D, Beste TM Am J Obstet Gynecol. 2003 Dec; 189(6):1559-62; discussion 1562

[229] Cardiovascular and gastrointestinal toxicity of selective cyclo-oxygenase-2 inhibitors in man. Dajani EZ, Islam K J Physiol Pharmacol. 2008 Aug; 59 Suppl 2():117-33.

7. Postoperative Nausea & Vomiting

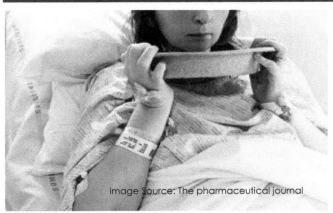

Image Source: The pharmaceutical journal

DEFINITIONS

- **Nausea** is the subjective sensation of the need to vomit.
- **Vomiting** is the forced expulsion of GI contents through the mouth.
- Postoperative nausea and vomiting (PONV) is a patient-important outcome; patients often rate PONV as worse than postoperative pain[230].
- PONV usually resolves or is treated without sequelae, but may require unanticipated hospital admission and delay recovery room discharge[231].

INCIDENCE

- ~30% overall after GA.
- Up to 80% in high-risk patients.

ASSOCIATED MORBIDITY

- Decreased patient satisfaction,
- Delayed hospital discharge,
- Unexpected hospital admission.
- Wound dehiscence,
- Bleeding,
- Pulmonary aspiration,
- Oesophageal rupture.
- Fluid and electrolyte disturbances.

RISK FACTORS ASSOCIATED WITH PONV

Patient factors
- Female gender
- Age***
- Non-smoker
- Anxiety
- History of motion sickness[232]
- Previous PONV
- Delayed gastric emptying
- Obesity

Anaesthetic factors
- **Drugs**
  o Opioids
  o Intravenous induction agents
  o Nitrous oxide
  o Neostigmine
- **Technique**
  o Gastric insufflation
  o Subarachnoid block

Surgical factors
- Emergency procedure
- Day-case surgery
- ENT surgery
- Strabismus correction
- Gynaecological procedures
- Gastrointestinal surgery
- Postoperative pain
- Ileus, gastric distension

*** In adults, the incidence of PONV decreases as patients age; for paediatric patients, age increases the risk, such that children older than 3yr have an increased risk of PONV, compared with children younger than 3yr.

In children, young age appears to be protective. POV rarely occurs in children <3 years of age, and increases in frequency with age >3, decreasing again with puberty[233]

---

[230] Macario A, Weinger M, Carney S, Kim A. Which clinical anesthesia outcomes are important to avoid? The perspective of patients. Anesth Analg 1999; 89:652.

[231] Hill RP, Lubarsky DA, Phillips-Bute B, et al. Cost-effectiveness of prophylactic antiemetic therapy with ondansetron, droperidol, or placebo. Anesthesiology 2000; 92:958.

[232] Koivuranta M, Läärä E, Snåre L, Alahuhta S. A survey of postoperative nausea and vomiting. Anaesthesia 1997; 52:443.

[233] Eberhart LH, Geldner G, Kranke P, et al. The development and validation of a risk score to predict the probability of postoperative vomiting in pediatric patients. Anesth Analg 2004; 99:1630.

RISK SCORES FOR PREDICTING PONV

- Currently, there are two simplified PONV risk scores for adults, and one simplified PONV risk score for children.
- **Koivuranta's PONV risk score**[234] features five risk factors:
  - Female gender,
  - Non-smoking status,
  - History of PONV,
  - History of motion sickness, and
  - Duration of surgery >60 min.

Number of risk factor	Incidence of PONV (%)
0	17
1	18
2	43
3	54
4	74
5	87

- **Apfel et al.**[235] developed a simplified risk score that reduced the number of risk factors in the model from five to four.
- The Apfel simplified score includes:
  - Female gender,
  - History of PONV and/or motion sickness,
  - Non-smoking status, and
  - Post-operative use of opioids.

Number of risk factor	Incidence of PONV (%)
0	10
1	20
2	40
3	60
4	80

- **The POVOC score** is the simplified risk score for predicting PONV in children. The four independent risk factors are:
  - Duration of surgery ≥30min,
  - Age ≥3yr,
  - Strabismus surgery,
  - History of PONV in the child or of PONV in his/her relatives.

Number of risk factor	Incidence of PONV (%)
0	9
1	10
2	30
3	55
4	70

---

[234] Koivuranta M, Läärä E, Snåre L, Alahuhta S. A survey of postoperative nausea and vomiting. Anaesthesia 1997; 52:443.

[235] Apfel CC, Läärä E, Koivuranta M, et al. A simplified risk score for predicting postoperative nausea and vomiting: conclusions from cross-validations between two centers. Anesthesiology 1999; 91:693.

MANAGEMENT OF PONV

- PONV is multifactorial; therefore, a multimodal approach is most effective.

1. PHARMACOLOGICAL METHODS

- Prophylaxis versus treatment remains controversial.
- **First line therapy:**
  - **Serotonin antagonists:** Ondansetron, Palonosetron,
  - **Corticosteroids:** Dexamethasone,
  - **Dopamine antagonists:** Droperidol
- They all have a similar efficacy against PONV, with a relative risk reduction of about 25%. Each drug results in similar relative risk reduction, giving an additive, but declining, absolute effect.
- **Second line therapy:**
  - **Metoclopramide** (D2 antagonist), but associated with extrapyramidal and sedative side effects.
  - **Cyclizine** is an antihistamine and is effective, but associated with a significant rate of side effects such as sedation, dry mouth, visual disturbance, and urinary retention.
  - **Transdermal scopolamine** is a cholinergic antagonist that reduces the risk of PONV by 40% when applied prior to surgery but carries a 3-fold increased risk of visual disturbance, compared with placebo.

2. NON-PHARMACOLOGICAL METHODS

- **Acupuncture**—pericardium (P6) point on the palmar aspect of the wrist. As effective as standard antiemetics, but no side effects (number needed to treat, NNT = 5).
- Others include:
  - Ginger root extract,
  - Hypnosis, Suggestion,
  - Homeopathy.

THE VOMITING PATIENT

- Reassurance.
- Correct vital signs appropriately.
- Ensure adequate analgesia and hydration.
- Look for a surgical cause (e.g. distended abdomen—insert or aspirate via NGT).
- **Antiemetics:**
  - Check if a prophylactic antiemetic was given.
  - **Ondansetron** is no more effective than placebo for rescue treatment if the patient received a 5-HT3 receptor antagonist intra-operatively as prophylaxis.
  - Antiemetics administered as rescue treatment should be of a different class than the drug administered as prophylaxis.

8. Postoperative Oxygen Therapy

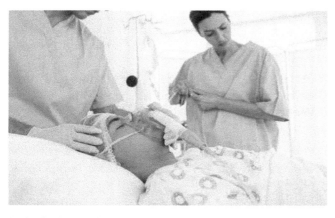

INDICATIONS

- Supplemental oxygen should be administered for at least 10 minutes to all patients during emergence from anaesthesia to prevent the development of tissue hypoxia.
- Any patient who is at risk of developing tissue hypoxia or is already hypoxaemic should be given supplemental oxygen.
- Gift et al. [236] state that the rational cost-effective use of supplemental oxygen in the early postoperative period in patients that have undergone peripheral surgery can be adjusted according to the level of oxygen saturation upon admission to the postanesthesia care unit (PACU). From this point of view, a safe level of oxygen saturation might indicate that routine oxygen administration is unnecessary[237].

INDICATIONS FOR OXYGEN THERAPY IN THE POSTOPERATIVE PERIOD

- **Patient factors**
  - Cardiorespiratory disease
  - Obesity
  - Elderly
  - Shivering

- **Surgical factors**
  - Upper abdominal procedures
  - Thoracic surgery
- **Physiological factors**
  - Hypovolaemia
  - Hypotension
  - Anaemia
- **Postoperative analgesic technique**
  - Patient-controlled analgesia
  - IV opioid infusion
  - Epidural infusion (both local anaesthetic agents and opioids).

TECHNIQUES OF ADMINISTRATION

- They may be subdivided into variable or fixed performance devices.
- **Variable-performance devices** are so called because the inspired oxygen concentration (FiO2) and degree of rebreathing vary from patient to patient and at different times in the same patient.
- This is dependent on the respiratory rate, inspiratory flow rate and length of expiratory pause. This type of device is most commonly used, as an accurate FiO2 is not required in the majority of patients.
- **The Hudson mask** is a clear plastic facemask that is placed over the nose and mouth and, at a flow rate of 4 litres per minute, provides an FiO2 of approximately **0.4**. Addition of a reservoir bag to these masks increases the maximum obtainable FiO2 to approximately **98%.**
- Patient compliance is poor due to a claustrophobic feeling and the need to remove it during eating and drinking and for routine mouth care.
- **Nasal cannulae** provide a more comfortable and continuous method of oxygen delivery. At a flow rate of **2–4 litres per minute**, these devices provide an FiO2 comparable with the face mask.

- **The fixed-performance devices** provide an accurate FiO2 and avoid rebreathing. They may be further subdivided into **high airflow oxygen enrichment (HAFOE) devices**, e.g. Venturi masks, or **lower flow devices such as anaesthetic breathing systems.**

---

[236] Gift AG, Stanik J, Karpenick J, et al. Oxygen saturation in postoperative patients at low risk for hypoxemia: is oxygen therapy needed? Anesth Analg 1995;80:368-72.

[237] DiBenedetto RJ, Graves SA, Gravenstein N, Konicek C. Pulse oximetry can change routine oxygen supplementation practices in the postanesthesia care unit. Anesth Analg 1994;78:365-8.

- **Venturi masks** use injectors of different sizes to deliver set oxygen concentrations varying from 24% to 60% by entraining air in oxygen using the Venturi principle.
- The appropriate oxygen flow rate for each mask is printed on the injector, which is also colour coded.
- For example, a 24% oxygen valve requires an oxygen flow of 2 litres per minute and entrains 38 litres of air per minute.

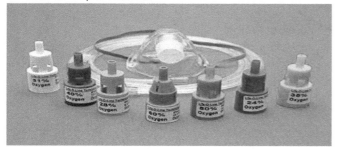

- Patients who require these masks include those at risk of respiratory failure if given high oxygen concentrations, i.e. those who are reliant on a hypoxic drive for ventilation.

OXYGEN DELIVERY SYSTEMS IN THE POSTOPERATIVE PERIOD

Variable performance

- Hudson mask
- MC mask
- Nasal cannulae
- Nasal catheter (nasopharyngeal catheter)

Fixed performance

- Venturi masks
- Anaesthetic breathing circuits

- In patients who are taken to recovery with a laryngeal mask in situ, supplemental oxygen may be provided by a T-piece connected to it as an alternative to a Mapleson C. This may be run as simply an open-ended tube or as a fixed-performance device.
- The use of anaesthetic breathing systems is reserved for the immediate postoperative period, when 100% oxygen may need to be delivered via a tight-fitting mask, for example when there is airway obstruction or laryngeal spasm.

HUMIDIFICATION

- Humidification is only required when oxygen is delivered at high flow rates or when the upper airway humidification processes are bypassed, as occurs after tracheostomy orduring prolonged tracheal intubation. It is therefore rarely required during the postoperative period.

DURATION

- There is no consensus on how long supplemental oxygen therapy should be given. However, the incidence of hypoxaemia is greatest on the second or third postoperative night after major surgery and the PaO_2 may not return to preoperative levels until the fifth night. Supplemental oxygen should therefore be given, where indicated, for at least three days postoperatively.

COMPLICATIONS

- Supplemental oxygen administration is a safe technique. However, problems may occur when inappropriate methods
- are used. Two common problems are the occurrence of **barotrauma** and the **risk of interference with hypoxic drive** in certain patients.

1. BAROTRAUMA

- Barotauma occurs when oxygen is directly delivered to the lower airway without free outflow of any excess gas.
- The practice of placing a variable-performance face mask over the open end of a tracheal tube or laryngeal mask should be avoided as there have been reports of the oxygen inlet part of the face mask impacting on the male connector of the tracheal tube.
- This resulted in delivery of oxygen at a flow rate of 4 litres per minute and a pressure of 400 kPa, with fatal consequences.
- The use of a T-piece system, where excess gas is vented to the atmosphere, is a much safer alternative.

2. LOSS OF HYPOXIC VENTILATORY DRIVE

- Approximately 10% of patients with chronic respiratory failure depend on hypoxic ventilatory drive to maintain an adequate $PaCO_2$.
- In this group of patients administration of a high FiO_2 will cause hypoventilation, with subsequent CO_2 retention and respiratory acidosis. However, the fear of causing CO_2 retention must not prevent the provision of appropriate oxygen therapy.
- A PaO_2 of 7–8 kPa must be attained. At this level of PaO_2 a slight increase will have a marked effect on oxygen content as this equates to the steepest part of the oxygen–haemoglobin dissociation curve.
- In practice, 24–28% oxygen should be given in the first instance followed by blood gas analysis to assess clinical response.
- A higher FiO_2 should be administered if the PaO_2 is too low and, if required, ventilatory support should be instituted to control the $PaCO_2$.

9. Critically Ill Patient
I. THE ICU PATIENT GOING TO THEATRE

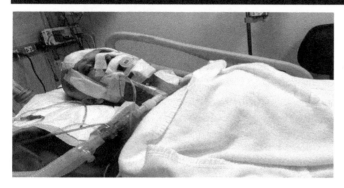

The planning, transfer, and monitoring of a critically ill patient on the ICU needing surgery can be challenging.

Physiological instability should be anticipated, detected, and acted upon promptly and effectively. Senior anaesthetists and surgeons must be involved.

CONSENT

Informed consent is often impossible, as the patient may be sedated or comatose. While the family is not able to give consent in law, the reasons for surgery and risks should be discussed with them, whenever possible.

PREOPERATIVE ASSESSMENT

- Routine aspects of the preoperative assessment (e.g. history of previous anaesthetics, chronic medical conditions, allergies) are just as relevant to the critically ill patient as they are to the elective case.
- Assess the patient's current condition from discussion with the critical care team and from information on the observation and drug charts.
- Note the current fluid requirements and rate/concentration of inotrope infusions; ensure that there is an adequate supply of inotrope prepared for theatre; consider which vasopressors may be required.
- Note the patient's O2 requirement, lung compliance, minute volume, PEEP, etc. to enable prediction of the ventilator settings that will be necessary in theatre. In the absence of a suitable ventilator in the operating room, it will be necessary to use a ventilator from the ICU.
- Check IV access, and consider if any additional cannulae may be required.

- Many ICU patients have had all peripheral access removed. Check which antibiotics the patient is receiving and whether any doses will be due in theatre. Check the most recent FBC, U&Es, and ABG, and ensure that blood is available.
- If the patient is being transferred to a more remote facility, such as the X-ray department, ensure adequate anaesthetic assistance. If the patient's lungs have poor compliance and are requiring high PEEP, it may be necessary to use an ICU ventilator.
- On occasions, it may be necessary to undertake an MRI scan on a critically ill patient—the inability to take ferrometallic objects into the scan room is problematic.

TRANSFER TO THE OPERATING ROOM

- Familiarize yourself with the transport equipment, and ensure it is functioning before leaving the ICU.
- If the patient is already ventilated, establish on the transfer ventilator before leaving the ICU to ensure adequate ventilation can be maintained.
- Modern transfer ventilators provide many of the functions of an ICU ventilator.
- Consider increasing the patient's sedation for the transfer. If the patient is not already sedated and ventilated, decide whether to induce in the ICU, the anaesthetic room, or theatre; factors influencing the decision will be safety, available assistance, haemodynamic instability, and patient comfort.
- Monitor the patient fully en route.
- Disentangle all lines; re-establish full monitoring, and check IV access before the start of surgery.

TRANSFER BACK TO THE INTENSIVE CARE UNIT

- Inform the ICU staff when surgery is about to finish; this enables them to prepare to receive the patient, and possibly to assist in the transfer.
- Ensure that a full verbal and written handover is given to the ICU medical and nursing staff, and communicate the post-operative requirements.

II. TRANSFERRING THE CRITICALLY ILL

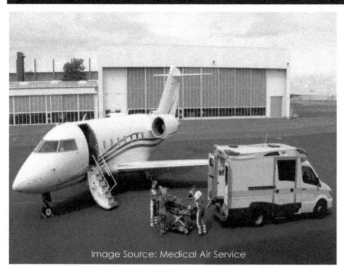

Image Source: Medical Air Service

- Safe transfer demands experienced staff and careful preparation. Several studies have demonstrated that patients are often inadequately resuscitated and monitored during transfer.
- All acute hospitals must have systems and resources in place to resuscitate and stabilize critically ill patients and carry out time-critical transfers when required[238]. In the UK, the majority of primary transfers are conducted by the ambulance service.
- Secondary transfer duties usually fall to anaesthetic/critical care doctors, accompanied by a member of the nursing staff and a paramedic crew.

DANGERS OF TRANSFER

- **Deranged physiology,** worsened by movement (acceleration/ deceleration leads to CVS instability)—15% of patients develop avoidable hypoxia and hypotension.
- **Cramped conditions, isolation, and temperature and pressure changes**.
- **Vehicular crashes.**
- Principles of safe transfer Staff experienced in intensive care and transfer—specialist transport teams may improve outcome but may cause delay.
- Use of appropriate equipment and vehicle, extensive monitoring, careful stabilization, continuing reassessment, direct handover, documentation, and audit.

[238] Whiteley, S., Macartney, I., Mark, J., Barratt, H., and Binks, R. **Guidelines for the transport of the critically ill adult.** The Intensive Care Society, ; 2011

THE TRANSFER VEHICLE

- UK inter-hospital transfers are typically via land ambulance. Factors influencing the decision to transfer by air include urgency of care, geography, platform availability, weather, and access to airports/helipads.
- Fixed and rotary wing transfer follow the same basic principles, but have additional considerations which are beyond the scope of this article.
- The equipment and constraints of air-transfer vary depending on platform and provider; only clinicians confident and competent in aeromedical transfer should undertake such missions.
- Regardless of the platform, the clinical team should position themselves safely to enable observation and access to the patient and any ancillary equipment (e.g. monitoring, ventilator, syringe drivers, etc.). If clinical actions are required, a decision must be taken between the transfer team and ambulance crew weather to stop the vehicle to allow safe intervention.
- Consider air if over 150 miles (remember decreasing PaO2 at altitude, expanding air spaces requiring NGT/orogastric tube, temperature, noise, and vibration).
- Decreased barometric pressure leads to **expansion of gas-filled cavities** (patients should have NGTs and may need chest drains).
- Pressurizing the cabin pressure to sea level can decrease these problems but increases fuel costs!
- **Air in the ETT cuff should be replaced by saline.**

PROBLEMS DURING TRANSFER

- Vibration leads to failure and inaccuracy of NIBP monitoring.
- Invasive monitoring should be used, if at all possible.
- Access to the patient may be limited.
- Acceleration/deceleration may lead to CVS instability.
- Hypothermia, particularly during transfer between vehicles.

SPECIFIC CONSIDERATIONS FOR CHILDREN

- Hypothermia is a greater risk, particularly in the infant.
- Monitor the central temperature, and use warming mats, 'bubble wrap', hats, etc. to maintain temperature.
- A secure IV access is paramount before departure.

CALCULATING OXYGEN RESERVES

- Anticipate your length of journey, and ensure you have plenty of spare O2 available for unanticipated delays.

- When transferring a patient, it is important to have an understanding of both oxygen requirements and cylinder sizes. One of the key principals of safe transfer practice is ensuring that there is an adequate amount of oxygen available, particularly in mechanically ventilated patients.

- The predicted transfer time should be estimated and to ensure that there is a reasonable margin for error and to allow for unexpected delays it is convention to allow for twice the expected transfer time. The flow rate required to deliver the desired percentage of oxygen should also be determined.

- Table below gives the approximate operating times for different O2 cylinders venting at different rates.

Operation time (in min) for different minute volumes at FiO2 1.0

Size of O2 cylinder (volume, L)	Minute volume 5L/min	Minute volume 7L/min	Minute volume 10L/min
D (340)	56	42	30
E (680)	113	85	61
F (1360)	226	170	123

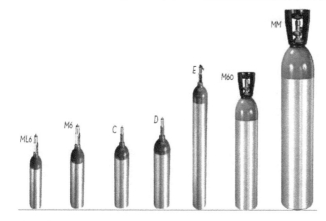

1. CALCULATE OXYGEN REQUIRED

- In mechanically ventilated patients it is important to remember that the ventilator itself requires an **additional 1 L of oxygen per minute to operate**.

- From these estimations it is possible to derive the following formula:

> **Oxygen required = 2 x (oxygen required by patient + ventilator) x transfer time**

- The amount of oxygen required to oxygenate the patient can be calculated by the product of the fractional inspired O2 (FiO2) and the minute volume (MV).

- The minute volume being the product of the respiratory rate and the tidal volume.

- Therefore, the total oxygen requirement for any given transfer can be calculated by:

> **Oxygen required = ([FiO2 x MV] + O2 required by ventilator] x (2 x transfer time)**

2. CALCULATE NUMBER OF CYLINDERS REQUIRED

Calculate the amount of oxygen required (Number of Cylinders) for the journey using the following:

> **Number of Cylinders = 2 x duration of journey x Flow (l/min) / Cylinder Capacity (Liters)**

3. CALCULATE ESTIMATED REMAINING TIME

Estimate the remaining time that oxygen can be delivered at a given flow rate for the journey using the following:

> **Approx. Remaining time (hours) = Oxygen Cylinder (psig) /200 x Oxygen Flow Rate (l/min)**

- **Example 1,** if oxygen is provided at **10 l/min** for a journey intended to take 120 minutes,
  No Cylinder=2 x120 x10/600= 4

- This would need **4 size E cylinders**, each containing 600 litres. This allows for at least twice as much oxygen as the estimated journey time requires. Always take more than one cylinder in case of leakage or failure.

- **Example 2,** an E-cylinder of oxygen with a pressure of 1,000 psig, used at an oxygen flow rate of 5 L/min would be depleted in **[1,000/(200x5) ≈ 1 hour**

- *An E-cylinder has an internal volume of 4.8 L and when "full" is pressurized to 2,000 psig.*

- *Since psig is the pressure measured in excess of atmospheric pressure (14.7 psia, **p**ounds per **s**quare **i**nch **a**bsolute pressure), the cylinder pressure is 2,014.7 psia.*

- *Applying Boyle's Law:* **2,014.7X4.8=14.7XV2**

- *Therefore, V2, the volume of oxygen in a "full" E-cylinder at 1 atm is* **(2,014.7X4.8)/14.7=658L**

PREPARATION

- Ensure meticulous stabilization prior to transfer.

- Take a full history, and make a thorough examination.

- Full monitoring, including invasive BP and CVP where indicated.

- Blood tests, radiographs, and CT prior to transfer.

- Explain the procedure to the patient and family.

- Use the checklist in Table below.

- It is sensible to have a transfer pack already prepared with the things you are most likely to need.

LIST OF RECOMMENDED ITEMS TO CONSIDER

Checklist for preparation to transfer a patient

A: airway
- Is the airway safe?
- If in doubt, intubate.
- Cervical spine control

B: breathing
- Portable ventilator settings.
- Check ABG before departure after 15min on the portable ventilator.
- Self-inflating bag–valve device in the event of a ventilator/O2 failure.
- Suction.
- Adequate sedation, analgesia, and relaxation.
- Adequate O2 reserves.
- Insert a chest drain if there is a possibility of a pneumothorax (e.g. fractured ribs).

C: circulation
- Stable circulation with good access.
- Controlled external bleeding.
- Invasive BP and CVP, when indicated.
- Inotropes—if in doubt, have them prepared and ready to run.
- Pumps and batteries.
- Insert a urinary catheter, and monitor output.

D: disability
- GCS (mannitol, IPPV),
- Pupillary signs.
- NGT/orogastric tube.

E: exposure
- Temperature loss.
- Splint long bones.

F: forgotten?
- All notes, referral letter, results, radiographs (including CT scans), and blood products.
- Inform the receiving unit that you are leaving the base hospital.
- Inform relatives.
- Take contact numbers.
- Take warm clothing, mobile phone, food, and credit card/money for the team!
- Plan for the return journey.
- Medical indemnity and insurance for death or disability of transfer staff.

Equipment and drug box guidelines

Airway and Breathing
- Suction equipment, Tracheal tubes, connectors, ties
- Stethoscope, Tracheostomy tubes (if appropriate)
- Face masks, airways, self-inflating bag with reservoir
- Laryngoscopes, spare batteries
- Gum elastic bougie

Circulation
- Cannulae plus IV dressings and tape
- IV fluids and giving set
- Syringes and needles
- Mini-sharps receptacle

Resuscitation drugs
- Adrenaline,
- Adenosine
- Noradrenaline
- Hydrocortisone
- Lorazepam
- Salbutamol nebulizers
- Lidocaine
- Glucose
- Amiodarone, Metoprolol
- Sodium bicarbonate
- Furosemide
- Atropine
- Saline ampoules
- Naloxone
- GTN spray
- Calcium chloride
- Plain drug labels

Sedation/muscle relaxants
- Propofol, Midazolam
- Atracurium or Rocuronium
- Suxamethonium
- Paediatric equipment—extras
- Paediatric O2 mask with reservoir bag

Tracheal tubes
- Small cannulae Paediatric drug doses
- Appropriate self-inflating bag with reservoir
- Laryngoscope and stylets
- Intraosseous needle Magill forceps and suction catheters
- Masks and airways 10% glucose for infusion

10. Safe use of Vasoactive Drugs and Electrolytes

I. INOTROPES AND VASODILATORS

A. ADRENORECEPTORS

Adrenoreceptors		
α1	• Vasoconstriction • Increased Peripheral Resistance • Increased BP • Mydriasis • Increased closure of internal sphincter of bladder	
α2	**Inhibition of:** • Norepinephrine release • Ach release • Insulin release	
β1	• Increased heart rate. • Increased myocardia contractility • Increased release of renin • Increased lipolysis • Increased platelet aggregation	
β2	• Vasodilation • Bronchodilation • Slightly decreased Peripheral resistance • Increased muscles and liver glycogenolysis • Increased release glucagon • Relax uterine smooth muscles	
β3	• Lipolysis	

B. VASOACTIVE AGENTS

- **INOTROPES:**
  - Agents that increase myocardial contractility or inotropy (β1 effect)
  - e.g. **Dobutamine**, Adrenaline, Isoprenaline, Ephedrine

- **VASOPRESSORS:**
  - Agents that cause vasoconstriction leading to increased systemic and/or pulmonary vascular resistance (↑SVR, PVR/ α1 effect)
  - e.g. **Noradrenaline**, Vasopressin, Metaraminol, Methylene blue

- **INODILATORS:**
  - Agents with inotropic effects that also cause vasodilation leading to **decreased** systemic and/or pulmonary vascular resistance (↓SVR, PVR)
  - e.g. **Milrinone**, Levosimendan

1. INOTROPES AND INODILATORS

MECHANISM OF ACTION

- The main mechanism of action for most inotropes involves increasing intracellular calcium, either by increasing influx to the cell during the action potential or increasing release from the sarcoplasmic reticulum.
- Choice of inotrope will depend on factors such as the patient's underlying disease state and the clinician's preference. There is limited evidence to suggest that one particular inotrope is better than another[239].

CATECHOLAMINES

- The most commonly used inotropes are the catecholamines; these can be endogenous (eg, adrenaline, noradrenaline) or synthetic (eg, dobutamine, isoprenaline).
- These medicines act on the sympathetic nervous system. Most commonly their cardiac effects are attributed to stimulation of alpha and beta adrenergic receptors (specifically α_1, β_1, and β_2). However, this is a simplification: there are several subtypes of α_1 receptors as well as α_2, β_3, and various dopaminergic receptors that are involved.
- The main receptor in the cardiac muscle that affects the rate and force of contraction is the β_1 receptor.

---

[239] Packer M, Carver JR, Rodeheffer RJ, et al. *Effect of oral milrinone on mortality in severe chronic heart failure. New England Journal of Medicine* 1991;325:1468–75.

- Binding to ß1 receptors results in increased calcium entry into the cell via the opening of L-type calcium channels and release of intracellular calcium from the sarcoplasmic reticulum. More calcium is available to bind with troponin-C, thereby enhancing myocardial contractility.
- Most catecholamines have a short half-life (about two minutes) and steady-state blood concentrations are reached within 10 minutes.
- They are therefore usually given by continuous infusion.

DOBUTAMINE

- Dobutamine is predominantly a ß1 agonist and therefore increases cardiac contractility and heart rate. It also acts at ß2 receptors causing vasodilation and decreasing afterload.
- Because of this vasodilation, and to ensure adequate MAP is achieved, it may be necessary to administer dobutamine in combination with a vasopressor (eg, noradrenaline).
- The main side effects of dobutamine are increased heart rate, arrhythmias and raised myocardial oxygen demand.
- These can cause myocardial ischaemia.

ISOPRENALINE

- Isoprenaline has a similar profile to dobutamine but tends to cause more tachycardia.
- It is sometimes used for bradycardic patients requiring inotropic support.

NORADRENALINE

- Because noradrenaline acts primarily via a1 receptors, it is usually used as a vasopressor (increasing SVR to maintain MAP) rather than an inotrope.
- It is often used with other inotropes, such as dobutamine, to maintain adequate perfusion, as discussed above.

ADRENALINE

- Adrenaline has activity at all adrenergic receptors (predominantly acting as a ß agonist in low doses and an a agonist at higher doses); other more specific inotropes are often preferred over adrenaline.
- Adrenaline is used mainly during resuscitation after cardiac arrest (in this case it is given as a bolus).
- It is not recommended for use in cardiogenic shock because of metabolic side effects, including hyperlactataemia and hyperglycaemia[240].

DOPAMINE

- Dopamine is a complicated inotrope because it has dose-dependent pharmacological effects.
- Low-dose dopamine (2–5µg/kg/min) exerts mainly dopaminergic effects, at medium doses (5–10µg/kg/min) the ß1 inotropic effects predominate and at high doses (10–20µg/kg/min) a1 vasoconstriction predominates.

PHOSPHODIESTERASE-3 INHIBITORS

- Phosphodiesterase-3 (PDE3) is an enzyme found in cardiac and smooth muscle cells.
- Inhibition of PDE3 increases intracellular calcium causing vasodilation and increased myocardial contractility.
- The mechanism of action is independent of adrenergic receptors and therefore PDE3 inhibitors are particularly useful if these receptors have become down-regulated (eg, in patients with chronic heart failure).
- **Milrinone** is the most commonly used PDE3 inhibitor. It has a relatively long half-life (two hours) and can accumulate in patients with renal failure.

LEVOSIMENDAN

- Levosimendan is a novel inotrope that sensitises troponin-C to calcium, thereby increasing the force of contraction.
- It also acts on potassium channels in smooth muscle to cause vasodilation.
- Levosimendan increases CO without increasing myocardial oxygen consumption[241].
- Levosimendan is administered as a continuous infusion (with or without an initial bolus dose) over 24 hours.
- It has a half-life of about one hour, but active metabolites mean that the inotropic effect can continue for up to five days after the infusion has finished.[242]
- Despite levosimendan's potentially favourable pharmacological profile, the evidence supporting its use remains controversial and it is expensive and unlicensed.

MONITORING

- Inotropes are usually only used in clinical areas where patients' haemodynamics can be monitored adequately. Continuous monitoring of MAP, CO and CVP allows haemodynamic changes to be detected and addressed rapidly.

[240] Dickstein K, Cohen-Solal A, Filippatos G, et al. ESC guidelines for the diagnosis and treatment of acute and chronic heart failure 2008. European Heart Journal 2008;29:2388–442.

[241] Ukkonen H, Saraste M, Akkila J, et al. Myocardial efficiency during levosimendan infusion in congestive heart failure. Clinical Pharmacology and Therapeutics 2000;68:522–31.

[242] Kivikko M, Lehtonen L, Colucci WS. Sustained hemodynamic effects of intravenous levosimendan. Circulation 2003;107:81–6.

- It is essential that pharmacists in critical care understand the pharmacology of inotropes and the haemodynamic monitoring required to ensure safe practice.
- Pharmacists can help to identify medicines that might need to be stopped when these therapies are started (eg, beta-blockers).

2. VASOPRESSORS

1) NOREPINEPHRINE

- Norepinephrine (Levophed) acts on both alpha-1 and beta-1 adrenergic receptors, thus producing potent vasoconstriction as well as a modest increase in cardiac output.
- A reflex bradycardia usually occurs in response to the increased mean arterial pressure (MAP), such that the mild chronotropic effect is canceled out and the heart rate remains unchanged or even decreases slightly.
- Norepinephrine is the preferred vasopressor for the treatment of septic shock.

2) PHENYLEPHRINE

- Phenylephrine (Neo-Synephrine) has purely alpha-adrenergic agonist activity and therefore results in vasoconstriction with minimal cardiac inotropy or chronotropy.
- MAP is augmented by raising systemic vascular resistance (SVR).
- A potential disadvantage of phenylephrine is that it may **decrease stroke volume**, so it is reserved for patients in whom norepinephrine is contraindicated due to arrhythmias or who have failed other therapies.
- Although SVR elevation increases cardiac afterload, most studies document that cardiac output (CO) is either maintained or actually increased among patients without pre-existing cardiac dysfunction.

3) VASOPRESSIN AND ANALOGS

- Vasopressin (antidiuretic hormone) is used in the management of diabetes insipidus and esophageal variceal bleeding; however, it may also be helpful in the management of vasodilatory shock.
- Although its precise role in vasodilatory shock remains to be defined, it is primarily used as a second-line agent in refractory vasodilatory shock, particularly septic shock or anaphylaxis that is unresponsive to epinephrine. It is also used occasionally to reduce the dose of the first-line agent.

- **Terlipressin**, a vasopressin analog, has been assessed in patients with vasodilatory shock.
- The effects of vasopressin may be dose dependent.
- The higher dose was more effective at increasing the blood pressure without increasing the frequency of adverse effects in these patients.
- Doses of vasopressin above 0.03 units/min have been associated with coronary and mesenteric ischemia and skin necrosis in some studies, although some of these studies were in animals and necrosis in humans may also have been due to coexisting conditions (e.g., disseminated intravascular coagulation).
- Doses higher than the therapeutic range (0.04 units/min) are generally avoided for this reason unless an adequate mean arterial pressure (MAP) cannot be attained with other vasopressor agents.
- **Rebound hypotension** appears to be common following withdrawal of vasopressin. To avoid rebound hypotension, the dose is slowly tapered by **0.01 units/min every 30 minutes**.
- Other potential adverse effects of vasopressin include **hyponatremia and pulmonary vasoconstriction**.
- Terlipressin appears to have a similar side effect profile to vasopressin.

II. ELECTROLYTE DISTURBANCES

- Electrolyte homeostasis is essential: at a cellular level it is important for maintaining membrane potentials and stability.
- This affects all organs but is particularly important for cardiovascular, renal, and neurological function.
- Many cellular processes depend upon specific electrolyte concentrations as cofactors in chemical reactions. On a broader scale, electrolyte disturbances can cause significant fluid imbalance between different compartments.

1. SODIUM

Definition	Serum [Na+] (mmol/l)
Hyponatraemia	< 135
Normal	135 - 145
Mild Hypernatremia	146 - 149
Moderate Hypernatraemia	150 - 169
Severe Hypernatraemia	≥ 170

- Sodium is the main extracellular cation and so the major determinant of osmolarity and ECF volume.
- The normal plasma value is **135–145mmol/L.**
- Sodium is actively pumped out of the cells against its concentration gradient by the Na^+-K^+ ATPase to help maintain the resting membrane potential of cells.
- Sodium is absorbed from the intestine, and is filtered and actively reabsorbed by the kidney.
- Levels of sodium are regulated by the hypothalamus (via osmoreceptors) and the renin–angiotensin system. Atrial natriuretic peptide also has a role via fluid volume changes.
- Abnormalities of sodium balance are the result of excessive or insufficient sodium intake and/or changes in extracellular water volume. Imbalance will affect ICF volume, hypernatraemia reducing it and hyponatraemia increasing it, through osmosis.

A. HYPONATRAEMIA (serum Na <135mmol/L)
- This is a common condition, seen in 15–30% of hospitalized patients and is caused by **either increased sodium loss** or **excessive water intake.**
- Symptoms of hyponatraemia range from lethargy, irritability, nausea, and vomiting to confusion, drowsiness, seizures, and coma.
- **Rapid correction of hyponatraemia** should be avoided as this can lead to **central pontine myelinolysis.**

- Na+ levels should generally be corrected at **<0.5mmol/L/h.**
- Causes of hyponatraemia are given in Table below according to the volaemic status of the patient.
- Treatment should primarily be directed at the cause of the hyponatraemia.

CAUSES OF HYPONATRAEMIA

Hypovolaemic	Normovolaemic	Hypervolaemic
Cerebral salt wasting syndrome	SIADH	SIADH
Diuretic therapy	Thiazide diuretics	CCF
Diarrhoea/vomiting	Adrenal insufficiency	Nephrotic syndrome
Sweating	Hypothyroidism	Cirrhosis
Adrenal insufficiency	Iatrogenic	Renal failure
Blood loss		Iatrogenic (excessive fluid administration)
		'TUR' syndrome

SIADH
- Excess ADH results in inappropriate water retention by the kidneys leading to hyponatraemia.
- The diagnosis requires:
  - **Hyponatraemia + Low Serum Osmolality:** Less than 275mosm/Kg
  - **High urine osmolality/Concentrated urine:** Sodium >20 mmol/L and osmolality >300 mosm/kg
  - Absence of hypovolaemia, oedema, or diuretics.

1. CAUSES OF SIADH
  - **CNS:** Meningitis, Encephalitis, Abscess, Stoke, Subarachnoid Haemorrhage, Subdural Haemorrhage, Head Injury.
  - **Malignancy:** Small Cell Lung Cancer, Pancreatic Cancer, Prostate Cancer, Lymphoma.
  - **Respiratory:** Pneumonia, Aspergillosis.
  - **Metabolic:** Porphyria.
  - **Drugs:** Diuretics, Antidepressants, ACE Inhibitors, Antipsychotics, COX2 Inhibitors, PPI.
  - **Trauma.**

2. ED MANAGEMENT OF SIADH
  - Treat the underlying cause
  - Cessation of offending drug.
  - Fluid restriction to less than 1l/day.
  - **Demeclocycline:** if persistent SIADH.
  - Urgent review by a renal consultant

B. HYPERNATRAEMIA (Serum Na >145mmol/L)

- Hypernatraemia is less common than hyponatraemia and can be caused by **decreased water intake**, **excess water loss**, or **excess salt intake**.
- Neurological symptoms such as weakness, lethargy, and seizures can occur when it is severe.
- The most common cause is fluid loss or 'dehydration'.
- **Diabetes insipidus (DI)** is relatively common following brain injury, particularly in patients selected for organ donation in whom brain stem death has been diagnosed.
- DI results from decreased secretion of ADH leading to decreased water reabsorption by the kidney and a diuresis. **Nephrogenic DI** exists where the kidney does not respond to ADH. In DI **plasma osmolarity is high (>305mosm/L)** and the patient produces large volumes of dilute urine (osmolarity <350mosm/L).
- A simple test is to use a urine dipstick to measure specific gravity: **dilute urine will be < 1.005.**
- Treatment of hypernatraemia should be directed at the cause but may also involve the administration of water either enterally or intravenously as 5% dextrose.
- Excessively rapid correction of hypernatraemia can lead to **cerebral oedema.**

1. CAUSES OF HYPERNATRAEMIA

Excessive Water losses	Decreased Fluid Intake
Renal:	o Neurologic impairment
▪ Central/Nephrogenic Diabetes insipidus	o Hypothalamic disorder
▪ Diuretics	o Restricted access to fluid
▪ Tubulopathies	o Fluid restriction
▪ Hyperglycaemia	o Ineffective breastfeeding
Insensible:	**Excess Na⁺ administration**
▪ Fever or High ambient temperature	o Hypertonic NaCl
▪ Exercise	o Sodium hydrochloride
▪ Burns	o Normal saline, blood products
▪ Respiratory illnesses	o Na⁺ ingestion
Gastrointestinal	
▪ Gastroenteritis	
▪ Osmotic Diarrhoea	
▪ Colostomy/Ileostomy	
▪ Malabsorption	
▪ Vomiting	

2. POTASSIUM

- Potassium is the main intracellular cation. The normal plasma concentration is **3.5–5.0mmol/L.**
- Potassium's most important action is in the maintenance of the cell membrane potential and action potentials.
- Potassium is absorbed from the intestine and excreted via the kidney.
- Abnormalities of potassium homeostasis are generally due to excessive or insufficient intake or excretion, or movement into or out of cells.

A. HYPOKALAEMIA (SERUM K <3.5MMOL/L)

- This common electrolyte abnormality is frequently asymptomatic but can lead to weakness and malaise.
- Severe adverse effects are unlikely until the level is <2.5mmol/L when muscle weakness and cardiac arrhythmias can occur.
- **ECG changes include:**
  - o Prolongation of the PR interval,
  - o ST depression,
  - o Prolonged QT interval,
  - o T wave inversion and
  - o Prominent U waves.
- Treatment is by potassium replacement, but high concentrations of potassium given quickly IV can cause cardiac arrest: maximum recommended infusion rates are **10–20mmol/h.**

CAUSES OF HYPOKALAEMIA

Reduced intake	• IV fluids without K • Low potassium diet (rare)
Increased loss	**Renal:** • Diuretics • Hyperaldosteronism **Gastrointestinal:** • Vomiting • Diarrhoea • Fistulae
Shift into cells	• Metabolic alkalosis • Insulin • Catecholamines (β agonists)

B. HYPERKALAEMIA (serum K >5.0mmol/L)

- Severe hyperkalaemia is a life-threatening condition and requires immediate treatment.
- ECG changes are progressive:
  - o Tall tented T waves,
  - o Diminished P waves, ultimately leading to a sinusoidal trace and asystole.
- Muscle weakness is reported when hyperkalaemia is severe.

CAUSES OF HYPERKALAEMIA

Increased intake	• Potassium replacement • Blood transfusion • Potassium containing drugs

Decreased excretion	• Renal failure
	• Potassium-sparing diuretics
	• Hypoaldosteronism
	• **Drugs:**
	  o ACE inhibitors
	  o a2 blockers
	  o NSAIDs

Shift from inside cells	• **Drugs:**
	  o Suxamethonium
	  o Metabolic acidosis
	  o Tissue necrosis

- Management is initially directed at driving potassium into the cells with insulin and dextrose (e.g. 15 units fast-acting insulin and 50mL 50% glucose) and β-agonists (nebulized salbutamol).
- Calcium gluconate should also be given to protect from cardiac arrhythmias (10mL of 10% calcium gluconate).
- However, these are only temporizing measures and ultimately the excess potassium needs to be removed from the body. This may require renal replacement therapy, although potassium exchange resins (e.g. calcium resonium) can be used if renal replacement is not possible, or delayed.

3. CALCIUM

- The majority of the body's calcium is stored within bone.
- The normal plasma level is **2.12–2.65mmol/L**, a significant proportion of which is bound to proteins, mostly albumin. It is therefore important that the reported value is corrected for the albumin level.
- Free ionized calcium is approximately 1.2mmol/L. Free calcium is important for cardiac and skeletal muscle contraction: it acts as a second messenger and neurotransmitter, and it is an important cofactor for some enzymatic reactions, notably in coagulation.
- Calcium homeostasis is regulated by the actions of vitamin D, parathyroid hormone, and calcitonin.
- **Parathyroid hormone** is secreted from the parathyroid gland in response to **hypocalcaemia and hypomagnesaemia** and it acts to increase absorption from the intestine, kidney, and bone, and increases conversion of vitamin D to the active form.

- Vitamin D is formed in the skin or absorbed in the gut.
- The active metabolite 1,25-dihydroxycholecalciferol is formed in two stages by the liver and then the kidney.
- It also acts to increase reabsorption of calcium.
- **Calcitonin** is secreted by the parafollicular cells of the thyroid gland in response to hypercalcaemia.
- It acts to inhibit calcium resorption from bone and increases renal excretion of calcium and phosphate.

A. HYPOCALCAEMIA (serum Ca <2.12mmol/L)
Hypocalcaemia is associated with reduced parathyroid hormone or vitamin D activity, renal failure, pancreatitis, and alkalosis. It is particularly important to check for hypocalcaemia following thyroidectomy.
Features include:
- Neuromuscular excitability: paraesthesia (or convulsions in severe cases), +ve Chvostek's and Trousseau's signs
- Cardiac manifestations: low cardiac output state + ECG changes (prolonged QT interval)
- Torsade's de pointes may occur, but is much less common than with hypokalaemia or hypomagnesaemia.
- Treatment is directed at the predisposing cause together with calcium replacement (**10mL 10% calcium chloride or gluconate** administered slowly intravenously).

B. HYPERCALCAEMIA (serum Ca >2.65mmol/L)
- Common causes of hypercalcaemia are **hyperparathyroidism and malignancy** (both primary and bony metastases).
- The clinical features are classically memorized as **bones** (bone pain), **stones** (renal stones), **groans** (abdominal pain), and **moans** (psychiatric disorders).
- Treatment is to administer **normal saline by IV infusion** to dilute the plasma level, sometimes combined with diuretics to promote excretion of calcium.
- Bisphosphonates also have a role some cases.

COMPLICATION OF HYPERCALCAEMIA
o **Cardiac Arrhythmia**
o **ECG changes**
  ▪ QT shortening
  ▪ Prolonged PR
  ▪ Widened QRS
  ▪ Notched QRS with increased voltage
  ▪ AV block

Electrolyte imbalance

CAUSES OF HYPERCALCAEMIA

Malignancy	Endocrine
• Breast, Lung, Thyroid, Kidney, Prostate cancers • Myeloma, • Leukaemia • Lymphoma: Hodgkin's and non-Hodgkin's	• Primary and Tertiary Hyperparathyroidism • Addison's • Pheochromocytomas • Hyperthyroidism

Drugs	
• Thiazides diuretics • Lithium • Theophylline toxicity • Hypervitaminose A • Hypervitaminose D	

Other Causes	Fictitious
• Rhabdomyolysis • Respiratory: Sarcoidosis, TB • Dehydration • Immobilisation • Milk-Alkali syndrome • Familial hypocalciuric hypercalcaemia	• Not corrected level for albumin • Prolonged cuff time • Paget's (non-malignant increased bone turnover)

INVESTIGATIONS
o **Blood:** Ca^{2+} adjusted for albumin, Phosphate, PTH, U&E
o **ECG**
o **High Ca^{2+} and High PTH**= Primary and Tertiary hyperparathyroidism
o **High Ca^{2+} and Low PTH**= Malignancy and other rarer causes

ED MANAGEMENT OF HYPERCALCAEMIA
- **Rehydration**
  o **IV Normal saline 0.9%** 4-6 liters in 24hrs
  o Consider **Haemodialysis** if severe Renal failure
  o Must monitor or replace K and Mg as these will be lost in the urine along with the calcium
  o **Do not give THIAZIDES**, they will worsen condition
  o Treatment with FRUSEMIDE is controversial as it promotes Calcium bone reuptake.

- **After rehydration:**
  o **IV Biphosphonates:**
    ▪ Zoledronic acid 4mg over 15min or
    ▪ Pamidronate 30-90mg at 20mg/hr or Ibandronic acid 2-4mg

- **Second line treatment**
  o **Prednisolone 40mg** daily (indicated in Lymphoma, other granulomatous diseases or 25-OHD poisoning)
  o **Calcitonin 4-8IU SC/IM BD** (if poor response to Biphosphonates)
  o **Calcimetics 30mg po BD** (indicated for primary hyperthyroidism, Parathyroid carcinoma or renal failure)
  o **Parathyroidectomy**: if poor response to other measures

4. MAGNESIUM
- Magnesium is mostly found in the ICF. The normal plasma level is **0.7–1.05 mmol/L.**
- Whilst an oversimplification, magnesium can be thought of as an antagonist to calcium in its actions. It is a cofactor in many reactions including ATP and nucleic acid production.
- In anaesthesia it is used for the treatment of bronchospasm in asthma, as an anticonvulsant in pre-eclampsia and eclampsia, and as an antiarrhythmic. It has also been used as an adjuvant to postoperative analgesia.
- Magnesium decreases acetylcholine release at the neuromuscular junction and can increase the action of non-depolarizing muscle relaxants.

A. HYPOMAGNESAEMIA (serum Mg <0.7mmol/L)
- Hypomagnesaemia can be treated with an IV infusion (10–20mmol) of magnesium sulphate (note that 1g is equivalent to 4mmol of MgSO4). It is common in critical care to aim for plasma levels of >1.0mmol/L.

B. HYPERMAGNESAEMIA
- It is treated by stopping magnesium supplementation and inducing a diuresis.
- In severe cases **IV calcium** should be given.

III. ACID–BASE ABNORMALITIES

A. NORMAL ABG VALUES

- Blood gas analysis is a commonly used diagnostic tool to evaluate the partial pressures of gas in blood as well as acid-base content.
- Understanding and use of blood gas analysis enables providers to interpret respiratory, circulatory and metabolic disorders[243].
- On inspired room air :

pH	7.350-7.450	
	kPa	mm Hg
pCO₂	4.67-6.00	35-45
pO₂	10.67-13.33	80-100
Bicarbonate		23-28 mmol/L
Base excess		-2 to +2 mmol/L

- **No compensation:**
  - pH remains abnormal, and the 'other' value (where the problem isn't occurring, i.e. CO2 or HCO3-) will remain normal or has made no attempt to help normalise the pH.
  - For example: in uncompensated metabolic acidosis: pH ↓7.23, HCO3- ↓15mmol/L, and the CO2 will be normal at 40mmHg.
- **Partial compensation:**
  - pH is still abnormal, and the 'other' value is abnormal in an attempt to help normalise the pH.
  - For example: in partially compensated respiratory alkolosis: pH ↑7.62, CO2 ↓27 and the HCO3- will be abnormal at ↓17mmol/L
- **Full compensation:**
  - The pH is normal, as the 'other' value is abnormal and has been successful in normalising the pH.
  - For example: Fully compensated metabolic acidosis pH 7.38, HCO3- ↓15mmol/L and the CO2 ↓30mmHG

BASE EXCESS / BASE DEFICIT
- Calculation of the base excess or deficit is a way of quantifying HCO3-.
- Base excess is the quantity of base (HCO3-, in mEq/L) that is above or below the normal range of buffer base in the body (22 -28 mEq/L).
- This cannot be calculated from PCO₂ and pH as the haemoglobin also contributes to the buffer base.

- One can use the **Siggaard-Andersen Nomogram** to estimate base excess or deficit.
- **Severe metabolic acidosis** is associated with a base deficit of -10 mEq/L
- **A positive number** is called a **base excess** and indicates a **metabolic alkalosis.**
- **A negative number** is called a **base deficit** and indicates a **metabolic acidosis.**

Acid-Base disturbances can be of either:
- **Respiratory origin** where the disturbance is primarily of CO₂ exchange.
- **Metabolic origin** where the disturbance is due to bicarbonate
- If the pH moves towards normal, this is termed **compensation.**
- **Correction** is when normal pH is restored.
- The next compensatory change in pH occurs by **altering respiratory rate** and therefore blood pCO₂.
- The following equilibrium equation is crucial to understanding acid-base balance:

$$H2O + CO2 \leftrightarrow H2CO3 \leftrightarrow HCO3^- + H+$$

- This equation shows that carbon dioxide (CO2) in blood dissolves to form carbonic acid (H2CO3), which dissociates to form acidic H+ (which can then combine with physiological bicarbonate to push the equation back to the left).

- The final compensatory change is renal handling (i.e. excretion) of acid (and subsequent reabsorption of HCO3-).

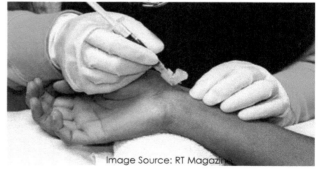
Image Source: RT Magazine

Look for additional electrolyte disturbances, such as:
- Raised glucose (with ketones and acidosis: diabetic ketoacidosis, DKA)
- Raised anion gap (metabolic acidosis)
- Hypokalaemia and hypochloraemia (metabolic alkalosis)
- Hyperchloraemia (normal-anion-gap acidosis)
- Acidosis with raised urea and creatinine (may suggest hypovolaemia or renal failure)

---

[243] Gattinoni L, Pesenti A, Matthay M. Understanding blood gas analysis. Intensive Care Med. 2018 Jan;44(1):91-93.

ANION GAP
This is defined as follows:

$$AG = (Na^+ + K^+) - (Cl^- + HCO3^-)$$

- The Anion Gap (AG) is a derived variable primarily used for the evaluation of metabolic acidosis to determine the presence of unmeasured anions
- The normal anion gap depends on serum phosphate and serum albumin concentrations
- An elevated anion gap strongly suggests the presence of a metabolic acidosis
- The normal anion gap varies with different assays, but is typically **4 to 12mmol/L** (if measured by ion selective electrode; **8 to 16** if measured by older technique of flame photometry)
  - o If AG > 30 mmol/L then metabolic acidosis invariably present
  - o If AG 20-29mmol/L then 1/3 will not have a metabolic acidosis
  - o K can be added to Na+, but in practice offers little advantage

Actual and expected values for PaCO2 and HCO3⁻
These calculations are useful for determining whether the disturbance is acute or chronic and what the degree of compensation is:

Corrected HCO3⁻ = Measured HCO3⁻ + (anion gap−18)

Expected PaCO2 = (0.2 × serum HCO3⁻) + 1
(Winters' formula)

- o Expect HCO3⁻ to rise 1.5 mmol/L per 1 kPa rise in PaCO2 acutely.
- o Expect HCO3⁻ to rise 3.0 mmol/L per 1 kPa rise in PaCO2 chronically.

ESTIMATION OF FIO2
When uncontrolled oxygen is being given to a patient (i.e. via a nasal cannula, a Hudson mask or a non-rebreathing reservoir mask), you will need to estimate FiO2 from the following formula:

FiO2=[L/min 100% O2+(MV−L/min 100% O2)× 0.21]/MV

where MV is the minute volume, given by respiratory rate (RR) × tidal volume (TV).

PACO2
Assume that the alveolar partial pressure of CO2 (PACO2) is equal to the measured PaCO2.

Alveolar (A) – arterial (a) gradient
This is defined as follows:

Aa gradient = PAO2 − PaO2

where PaO2 is measured and PAO2 is calculated as follows: **PAO2 = FiO2 × 95 − (PaCO2/0.8)**

- The Aa gradient increases with the patient's age from less than 2 kPa in the young to up to 5 kPa in the elderly.
- It is useful in distinguishing whether hypoxia is due to a ventilation/perfusion (V/Q) mismatch or to shunting (perfusion without ventilation).
- It is particularly useful when you suspect a pulmonary embolism.

B. UNCOMPENSATED ACID-BASE DISORDERS
1. METABOLIC ACIDOSIS
↓pH, ↓HCO3⁻

- Classification of a metabolic acidosis depends on the anion gap – the difference between the major plasma cations (Na+ and K+) and anions (Cl- and HCO3-): **Anion gap = (Na+ + K+) − (Cl- + HCO3-)**
- A normal anion gap is in the range **9-14 mmol/l.**
- Calculating the anion gap often helps **identify the cause of the acidosis**.
- o **HAGMA:**
  - By contrast to a low serum anion gap, an elevated serum anion gap is a relatively common occurrence, particularly among hospitalized patients[244]. High Anion Gap Metabolic Acidosis. A raised anion gap can be due to excess acid production or ingestion contributing extra H+: **CAT MUDPILERS**

METABOLIC ACIDOSIS AND ANION GAP			
HAGMA		**NAGMA**	
C	CO Cyanide	P	K+ sparing diuretics (Spironolactone)
A	Alcohol Aminoglycosides	A	Acetazolamide
T	Toluene	R	Rhabdomyolysis, RTA
		A	Alimentation feeding
M	Methanol	M	Mineral Acids
U	Urea	E	Enterostomy
D	DKA (and AKA)	D	Diarrhoea
P	Paracetamol Paraldehyde Phenformin	I	Intestinal fistula
I	Iron Isoniazid	C	Cholestyramine
L	Lactic acidosis	Or **ABCD:**	
E	Ethanol Ethylene glycol	**A**ddison crisis, **B**icarbonate loss: GIT, Renal, RTA	
S	Salicylate OD Solvents Starvation	**C**hloride excess **D**rugs: Acids, Spironolactone, Acetazolamide, Cholestyramine	

244 Lolekha PH, Vanavanan S, Lolekha S: Update on value of the anion gap in clinical diagnosis and laboratory evaluation. Clin Chim Acta**307** :33– 36,200

o **NAGMA:**
  - Normal Anion Gap Metabolic Acidosis.
  - In a normal anion gap acidosis, bicarbonate is lost from the gut or the kidneys and there is a raised chloride, which compensates for the extra cations, thus keeping the gap normal.
  - This occurs as a result of reabsorption of sodium chloride via the kidneys: **PARAMEDIC**

2. RESPIRATORY ACIDOSIS $\downarrow$pH, $\uparrow$pCO2

CAUSES OF RESPIRATORY ACIDOSIS[245]:
o Airway obstruction
  - Upper
  - Lower
    o COPD
    o Asthma
    o other obstructive lung disease
o CNS depression
o Sleep disordered breathing (OSA or OHS)
o Neuromuscular impairment
o Ventilatory restriction
o Increased CO_2 production: shivering, rigors, seizures, malignant hyperthermia, hypermetabolism, increased intake of carbohydrates
o Incorrect mechanical ventilation settings

3. METABOLIC ALKALOSIS $\uparrow$pH, $\uparrow$HCO$_3^-$

CAUSES OF METABOLIC ALKALOSIS:
- **Hypovolemia with Cl- depletion**
  o GI loss of H+
    - Vomiting, gastric suction, villous adenoma, diarrhea with chloride-rich fluid
  o **Renal loss H+**
    - Loop and thiazide diuretics, post-hypercapnia (especially after institution of mechanical ventilation)
- **Hypervolemia, Cl- expansion**
  o Renal loss of H+: edematous states (heart failure, cirrhosis, nephrotic syndrome), hyperaldosteronism, hypercortisolism, excess ACTH, exogenous steroids, hyperreninemia, severe hypokalemia, renal artery stenosis, bicarbonate administration

4. RESPIRATORY ALKALOSIS $\uparrow$pH, $\downarrow$pCO2

- **In respiratory alkalosis,** there is low pCO$_2$ and a consequent high pH as a result of the equation **moving to the left** and lowering H+.

CAUSES OF RESPIRATORY ALKALOSIS[246]:

o CNS stimulation: fever, pain, fear, anxiety, CVA, cerebral edema, brain trauma, brain tumor, CNS infection
o Hypoxemia or hypoxia: lung disease, profound anemia, low FiO2
o Stimulation of chest receptors: pulmonary edema, pleural effusion, pneumonia, pneumothorax, pulmonary embolus
o Drugs, hormones: salicylates, catecholamines, medroxyprogesterone, progestins
o Pregnancy, liver disease, sepsis, hyperthyroidism
o Incorrect mechanical ventilation settings

C. COMPENSATION OF ACID-BASE DISORDERS

- Compensatory mechanisms restore pH towards normal by altering pCO$_2$ and HCO$_3^-$.

1. COMPENSATION OF METABOLIC ACIDOSIS
o The lowered pH acts on peripheral chemoreceptors to stimulate the ventilation.
o Respiratory rate increases and pCO2 falls: $\uparrow$**RR,** $\downarrow$**Pco2**
$$\downarrow CO_2 + H_2O \leftarrow H_2CO_3 \leftarrow H^+ + HCO_3^-$$
o [H+] therefore falls, as does [HCO$_3^-$].
o There is also increased reabsorption of HCO$_3^-$ and increased excretion of H+ from the kidneys but this is not instant.

2. COMPENSATION OF METABOLIC ALKALOSIS
o Conversely, in metabolic alkalosis, the higher pH acts on the chemoreceptors to reduce ventilation and increase pCO$_2$: $\downarrow$**RR,** $\uparrow$**Pco2**
$$\uparrow CO_2 + H_2O \leftarrow H_2CO_3 \leftarrow H^+ + HCO_3^-$$
o The renal response is then to decrease HCO$_3^-$ reabsorption and decrease H+ excretion.
o This usually occurs fairly quickly, but if the alkalosis is caused by vomiting, resulting in dehydration, the overriding renal response is to increase Na+ and HCO$_3^-$ reabsorption.
o Therefore, effective rehydration will help to more rapidly correct the alkalosis.

3. COMPENSATION OF RESPIRATORY ACIDOSIS
o The problem here is within the ventilatory system, with the kidneys acting to compensate which can take a significant length of time **(up to two days).**
o The [H+] is raised, thus the rate of H+ secretion is also increased.

---

[245] *Interpretation of Arterial Blood Gases (ABGs) David A. Kaufman, MD Chief, Section of Pulmonary, Critical Care & Sleep Medicine, Bridgeport Hospital-Yale New Haven Health*

[246] *Interpretation of Arterial Blood Gases (ABGs) David A. Kaufman, MD Chief, Section of Pulmonary, Critical Care & Sleep Medicine, Bridgeport Hospital-Yale New Haven Health*

o This results in **increased HCO3- reabsorption**, despite HCO3- already being higher as a result of the equation shifting to the right:

$$\uparrow CO_2 + H_2O \rightarrow H_2CO_3 \rightarrow \uparrow H^+ + \uparrow HCO_3^-$$

o Although the secretion of H+ brings the pH closer to normal, the pH will not be restored to normal without correction of the underlying respiratory disorder.

4. COMPENSATION OF RESPIRATORY ALKALOSIS

o In respiratory alkalosis, the [H+] decreases due to a primary reduction in pCO2.

o There is therefore less H+ in the renal tubules and reduced H+ secretion.

o As a consequence, **less HCO3- is reabsorbed causing a further fall in [HCO3-]**.

o To restore pCO2 and HCO3- completely to normal, the primary ventilatory problem must be corrected (i.e. The respiratory rate must reduce).

D. MIXED ACID-BASE PICTURE

Disorder	Characteristics	Selected situations
Respiratory acidosis with metabolic acidosis	↓in pH ↓ in HCO3 ↑ in PaCO2	• Cardiac arrest • Intoxications • Multi-organ failure
Respiratory alkalosis with metabolic alkalosis	↑in pH ↑ in HCO3- ↓ in PaCO2	• Cirrhosis with diuretics • Pregnancy with vomiting • Over ventilation of COPD
Respiratory acidosis with metabolic alkalosis	pH in normal range ↑ in PaCO2, ↑ in HCO3-	• COPD with diuretics, vomiting, NG suction • Severe hypokalemia
Respiratory alkalosis with metabolic acidosis	pH in normal range ↓ in PaCO2 ↓ in HCO3	• Sepsis • Salicylate toxicity • Renal failure with CHF or pneumonia • Advanced liver disease
Metabolic acidosis with metabolic alkalosis	pH in normal range HCO3- normal	• Uremia or ketoacidosis with vomiting, NG suction, diuretics,

• A mixed acid-base disturbance is where there is **more than one primary disorder at a time**.

• This often occurs in acutely unwell patients.

• **NB**: *it is impossible to have more than one respiratory disorder in a mixed picture. i.e. a metabolic acidosis and alkalosis can co-exist, but not a respiratory acidosis and alkalosis.*

• When considering all mixed disturbances, the clinical picture will usually indicate the underlying problem – the blood gas results should always be put in a clinical context.

E. OTHER RESULTS ON THE ABG

• Other results are detailed below.

o **Potassium**: when low, this indicates a possible **Metabolic Alkalosis**.

o **Chloride**: this also has a bearing on metabolic acid-base disorders and is required for calculating the anion gap.

o **Lactate**: immensely important in the diagnosis of **Sepsis** and **global hypoperfusion**.

  ▪ **A lactate >4 mmol/l** in the presence of suggested infection would initiate Early Goal Directed Therapy.

  ▪ Remember, ↑lactate in the presence of abdominal pain suggests **Ischaemic bowel**.

o **Glucose**: remember raised glucose with acidosis can indicate **ketoacidosis**. Glucose is also an important target in the Surviving Sepsis Campaign: it should be maintained above the lower limit of normal, **but less than 8.3 mmol/l.**

o **Haemoglobin**: if the Hb is low, there is less O2 carrying capacity within the blood.

o **Carboxyhaemoglobin**: CO binds to Hb to form carboxyhaemoglobin (COHb);

  ▪ It binds **230-270 times more strongly than O2** and causes a leftward shift in the oxyhaemoglobin dissociation curve, so less oxygen is available to hypoxic tissues.

  ▪ The main early symptom is headache which occurs when levels reach around **10%**.

  ▪ But when levels reach **50-70%**, seizures and death can result.

  ▪ When breathing air, CO has a **half-life of 3-4 hours**, but only **30-90 minutes** when breathing 100% O2.

  ▪ Hyperbaric oxygen reduces this further.

Disorder	pH	Primary problem	Compensation

Metabolic acidosis	↓	↓ in HCO₃-	↓ in PaCO₂
Metabolic alkalosis	↑	↑ in HCO₃-	↑ in PaCO₂
Respiratory acidosis	↓	↑ in PaCO₂	↑ in [HCO₃-]
Respiratory alkalosis	↑	↓ in PaCO₂	↓ in [HCO₃-]

OXYHAEMOGLOBIN DISSOCATION CURVE (ODC)

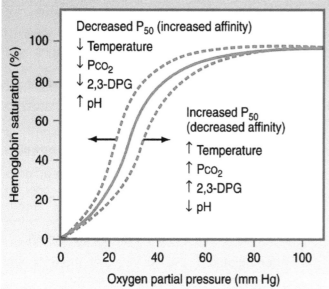

LIRD affinity: **L**eft **I**ncreases and **R**ight **D**ecreases affinity
CO Poisoning, Fetal Hb and Myoglobin have higher affinity to O2 (left shift)

- The ODC looks at the relationship between oxygen tension (pressure) and oxygen saturation.
- It helps us better understand how our blood interacts with oxygen, i.e. how and why it picks up and lets oxygen go.
- The S shape tells us that after an amount of oxygen has accumulated in the blood, there isn't room for any more, no matter how much oxygen you throw at the haemoglobin molecule, it wont change.
- Affinity basically means how much we (or blood) are attracted to someone (oxygen).
- The ODC shows us what changes the affinity of blood for oxygen.
  - **RIGHT SHIFT (ACIDOSIS)**
    - Shift of the curve to right decreases affinity - meaning that the Hb isn't very attracted to

oxygen, and when it does pick up oxygen, it lets it go very quickly.
  - Increased temperature and CO2 help this right shift.
  - **LEFT SHIFT (ALKALOSIS)**
    - Shift of the curve to the left increases affinity - meaning that the Hb is very attracted (oh la la) to oxygen and when oxygen is picked up, the Hb has a hard time letting it go at the cellular level.
    - Decreased temperature and CO2 help the curve move to the left[247].

---

[247] Dickson, S. 1995 Understanding the Oxyhemoglobin Dissociation Curve. Critical care Nurse 15, 10, 54-58.

11. Local & Regional Anaesthesia

I. LOCAL ANAESTHETIC TOXICITY

SYSTEMIC TOXICITY

- Systemic effects usually occur when blood concentrations of local anaesthetic increase to toxic levels.
- Adding a vasoconstrictor (e.g. adrenaline) can reduce the systemic absorption of an anaesthetic, thus increasing the maximum safe dosage. For lidocaine, the maximum safe dose is 3 mg per kg of body weight; 7 mg/kg can be used if the solution has adrenaline added.

Dose of lignocaine mcg/ml	Presenting symptoms
5	• Light-headedness • Circumoral paraesthesia • Slurred speech • Tinnitus
10	• Convulsions • Loss of consciousness
15	• Coma • Myocardial depression
20	• Respiratory arrest • Cardiac arrhythmia
>25	• Cardiac arrest

- There are few reports of local anaesthetic toxicity in infants and children. However, seizures, arrhythmias, cardiac arrest, and transient neuropathic symptoms have been reported[248].
- Lidocaine toxicity has been reported after subcutaneous administration, oral administration, and intravascular injection[249].
- The progression of lidocaine toxicity correlates well with ascending serum levels, with initial benign symptoms developing at 5 µg/mL, deteriorating into life-threatening cardiac arrest at levels above 25 µg/mL. Therefore, the development of tinnitus, light-headedness, circumoral numbness, diplopia and a metallic taste in the mouth indicate the onset of toxicity and possible impending development of severe symptoms.
- Cardiovascular toxicity usually manifests itself as tachycardia and hypertension but with increasing toxicity bradycardia and hypotension occur. Ventricular arrythmias and cardiac arrest are also known side effects[250].

COMPLICATIONS OF LOCAL ANAESTHESIA

Technique-related
- Direct nerve trauma
- Bleeding
- Haematoma
- Infection
- Intravascular injection
- Damage to surrounding structures (tendons, pneumothorax)

Drug-related
- Anaphylactoid
- Methaemoglobinuria (prilocaine)
- Toxicity by intravascular injection
- Toxicity by overdose and systemic absorption

MANAGEMENT OF SEVERE LOCAL ANAESTHETIC TOXICITY[251]

1. Recognition

- **Signs of severe toxicity:**
  o Sudden alteration in mental state, severe agitation or loss of consciousness, with or without tonic-clonic convulsions
  o Cardiovascular collapse: sinus bradycardia, conduction blocks, asystole and ventricular tachyarrhythmias may occur

[248] **Gunter JB**. Benefit and risk of local anesthetics in infants and children. Paediatr Drugs2002;**4**:649–72.

[249] **Smith M**, Wolfram W, Rose R. Toxicity seizures in an infant caused by (or related to) oral viscous lidocaine use. J Emerg Med1992;**10**:587–90

[250] **Brown DL**, Skiendzielewski JJ. Lidocaine toxicity. Ann Emerg Med1980;**9**:627–9.

[251] Association of Anaesthetists of Great Britain and Ireland and available for download at: www.aagbi.org/publications/guidelines/docs/la_toxicity_2010.pdf

o Local anaesthetic (LA) toxicity may occur some time after an initial injectionConsider the use of **Intralipid** in local-anaesthetic-induced cardiac arrest or circulatory failure that is unresponsive to standard therapy.

2. Immediate management

- Stop injecting the LA
- Call for help
- Maintain the airway and, if necessary, secure it with a tracheal tube
- Give 100% oxygen and ensure adequate lung ventilation (hyperventilation may help by increasing plasma pH in the presence of metabolic acidosis)
- Confirm or establish intravenous access
- Control seizures: give a benzodiazepine, thiopental or propofol in small incremental doses
- Consider drawing blood for analysis, but do not delay definitive treatment to do this

3. Treatment

IN CIRCULATORY ARREST

- Start cardiopulmonary resuscitation (CPR) using standard protocols
- Manage arrhythmias using the same protocols, recognising that arrhythmias may be very refractory to treatment
- Consider the use of cardiopulmonary bypass if available
- **GIVE INTRAVENOUS LIPID EMULSION** (following the regimen overleaf)
  o Continue CPR throughout treatment with lipid emulsion
  o Recovery from LA-induced cardiac arrest may take >1h
  o Propofol is not a suitable substitute for lipid emulsion
  o Lidocaine should not be used as an anti-arrhythmic therapy

WITHOUT CIRCULATORY ARREST

- Use conventional therapist to treat:
  o Hypotension,
  o Bradycardia,
  o Tachyarrhythmia
- **CONSIDER INTRAVENOUS LIPID EMULSION** (following the regimen overleaf)
  o Propofol is not suitable substitute for lipid emulsion
  o Lidocaine should not be used as an antiarrhythmic therapy

4. Follow-up

- Arrange safe transfer to a clinical area with appropriate equipment and suitable staff until sustained recovery is achieved
- Exclude pancreatitis by regular clinical review, including daily amylase or lipase assays for two days
- Report cases as follows: in the United Kingdom to the National Patient Safety Agency (via www.npsa.nhs.uk).
- In the republic of Ireland to the Irish Medicines Board (via www.imb.ie).
- If Lipid has been given, please also report its use to the international registry at www.lipidregistry.org.

AAGBI Safety Guidelines Management of Severe Local Anaesthetic Toxicity[252]

INTRALIP EMULSION

Immediately		
Give an initial intravenous bolus injection of 20% lipid emulsion 1.5ml/kg/ over 1 min	**and**	Start an intravenous infusion of 20% lipid emulsion at 15ml/kg/h

After 5 mins		
Give a maximum of two repeat boluses (same dose) if: • Cardiovascular stability has not been restored or • An adequate circulation deteriorates Leave 5 min between boluses A maximum of three boluses can be given (including the initial bolus)	**and**	Continue infusion at same rate, but : Double the rate to 30 ml.kg-1.h-1 at any time after 5 min, if: • Cardiovascular stability has not been restored or • An adequate circulation deteriorates Continue infusion until stable and adequate circulation restored or maximum does of lipid emulsion given

Do not exceed a maximum cumulative dose of 12 ml/kg

---

[252] *Association of Anaesthetists of Great Britain and Ireland and available for download at: www.aagbi.org/publications/guidelines/docs/la_toxicity_2010.pdf*

II. REGIONAL NERVE BLOCK

1. SUPRATROCHLEAR NERVE BLOCK

ANATOMY
- To anesthetize the forehead from the orbital ridge to the vertex of the scalp.
- **The supratrochlear nerve** also is a branch of the ophthalmic division of the trigeminal nerve and exits through the superior medial aspect of the orbit.

INDICATIONS
- Relief from neuropathy[253]
- Analgesia for wound closure or debridement
- Analgesia for local excision or biopsy

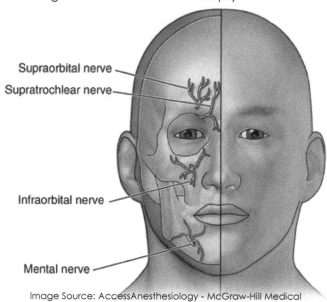

Supraorbital nerve
Supratrochlear nerve
Infraorbital nerve
Mental nerve

Image Source: AccessAnesthesiology - McGraw-Hill Medical

CONTRAINDICATIONS
- Patient refusal or inability to obtain consent
- Allergy to available local anesthetics
- Inability of patient to cooperate with or tolerate procedure
- Infection at injection site
- Distortion of surface or bony anatomy

PROCEDURE
1. Inject local anaesthetic solution over the midline of the forehead at eyebrow level.
2. Inject a 25- or 27-gauge needle through skin wheal aimed laterally while injecting 3–5 mL local anaesthetic subcutaneously.
3. Stop infiltrating when the needle reaches the midline of the orbit.

2. SUPRAORBITAL NERVE BLOCK

ANATOMY
- **The supraorbital nerve** emerges from the supraorbital foramen/notch and is a branch of the ophthalmic division of the trigeminal nerve.

INDICATIONS
- Wound closure[254]
- Pain relief
- Anesthesia for debridement
- Contraindication to general anesthesia

CONTRAINDICATIONS
- Any allergy or sensitivity to the anesthetic agent
- Evidence of infection at the injection site
- Distortion of anatomical landmarks
- Uncooperative patient

ANAESTHESIA
- A supraorbital nerve block requires 1-3 mL of the chosen anesthetic agent.
- Lidocaine (Xylocaine) is the most commonly used agent.
  - The onset of action for lidocaine is approximately 4-6 minutes.
  - The duration of effect is approximately 75 minutes.
- Bupivacaine (Marcaine) is another frequently used anesthetic agent.
  - The onset of action of bupivacaine is slower than that of lidocaine.
  - The duration of anesthesia of bupivacaine is about 4-8 times longer than that of lidocaine.
- The dose of anesthetic used in typical volumes for this procedure is not toxic.

3. INFRAORBITAL NERVE BLOCK

ANATOMY
- **The infraorbital nerve** emerges from the infraorbital foramen and is a branch of the maxillary division of the trigeminal nerve.
- Anaesthesia to the infraorbital nerve will also provide anaesthesia to its terminus, **the superior alveolar nerves**.

INDICATIONS
- Wound closure
- Pain relief

---

253 https://emedicine.medscape.com/article/1826449-overview

254 https://emedicine.medscape.com/article/82641-overview#a1

- Anesthesia for debridement
- Contraindication to general anesthesia

CONTRAINDICATIONS

- Any allergy or sensitivity to the anesthetic agent[255]
- Evidence of infection at the injection site
- Distortion of anatomical landmarks
- Uncooperative patient

PROCEDURE: EXTRAORAL APPROACH

1. Palpate the inferior orbital foramen in its midline position. The infraorbital nerve is often tender on palpation as it exits the foramen.
2. Inject a 25- or 27-gauge needle just above the infraorbital foramen injecting 1–2 mL of local anaesthetic.
3. Take care not to inject into the foramen because there is an increased risk of intraneural injection.
4. Hold a finger on the inferior orbital rim to avoid ballooning of the lower eyelid with injection.
5. Intraoral approach is possible and preferred because it is less painful.

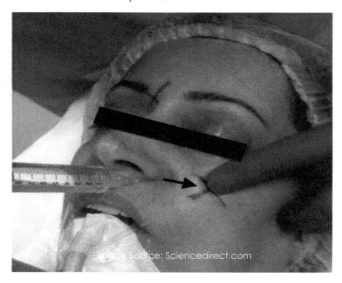

Image Source: Sciencedirect.com

PROCEDURE: INTRAORAL APPROACH

1. Apply topical benzocaine or lidocaine gel to the point of insertion, which is the height of the mucobuccal fold over the first premolar, which is the site of insertion. Wipe off after 1–3 min.
2. Palpate with the finger of the noninjecting hand over the inferior border of the inferior orbital rim.
3. Retract the lip with the noninjecting hand.
4. Using a long 25- to 27-gauge needle, with the bevel toward the bone, advance the needle at the insertion site toward the infraorbital foramen.
5. Once the target is reached, aspirate and inject 1 mL of local anaesthetic.

6. Exert pressure on the foramen for 1 min after injection to force the anaesthetic through the infraorbital foramen.
7. If the needle is difficult to advance and the patient experiences pain on insertion, redirect the needle laterally and advance.
8. If analgesia is attained for the lip but not the eyelid, the analgesia was placed inferior to foramen, and if analgesia is attained for the eyelid but not the lip, placement was superior to the foramen.

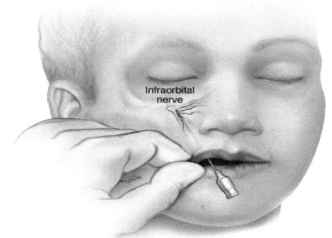

Image Source: Sciencedirect.com

4. MENTAL NERVE BLOCK

ANATOMY

- **The mental nerve** emerges from the mental foramen and is a branch of the mandibular division of the trigeminal nerve. Mental foramen lies in the vertical plane with the midpoint of the pupil and sits in the middle of the body of the mandible.

INDICATIONS

- Lacerations of the lower lip, especially if the vermillion border is involved[256]
- Lacerations to the soft tissue of the chin that extends from the lip anteriorly to the alveolar process and caudally to the mid-body of the mandible
- Surgical removal of facial tumors/lesions
- Relief from postherpetic neuralgia

CONTRAINDICATIONS

- Noncooperative patient
- Overlying infection
- Allergic reaction to local anesthetic
- Patient refusal
- Distorted anatomy

---

[255] https://emedicine.medscape.com/article/82660-overview#a7

[256] https://emedicine.medscape.com/article/82603-overview#a3

PROCEDURE: EXTRAORAL APPROACH

1. Inject local anaesthetic solution over the identified location of the mental foramen, creating a skin wheal.
2. Advance a 25- or 27-gauge needle through the skin wheal until the mandible is contacted, injecting 1–2 mL of local anaesthetic.
3. Intraoral approach is possible and preferred because it is less painful.

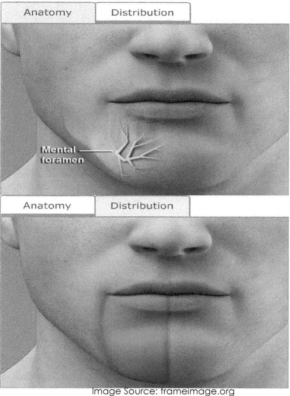

Image Source: frameimage.org

PROCEDURE: INTRAORAL APPROACH

1. Apply topical benzocaine or lidocaine gel to the point of insertion, which is the mucobuccal fold between the apices of the first and the second premolars. Wipe off after 1–3 min.
2. Insert a 25- to 27-gauge needle, with the bevel toward the mandible, aimed toward the mental foramen.
3. After advancing one-third the depth of the mandible and contacting the mandible, inject 1–2 mL of local anaesthetic.
4. By pressing firmly on the mental foramen for 2–3 min after the mental foramen has been blocked, **an incisive nerve block is also created**.
5. This is useful if anaesthesia to the lower anterior teeth is also desired.

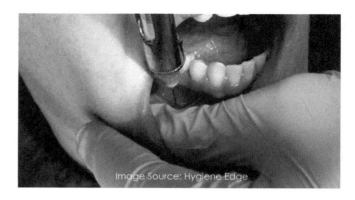

Image Source: Hygiene Edge

5. EXTERNAL EAR BLOCK

INDICATIONS

- In the emergency department, a nerve block of the external ear is most suitable for, but not limited to the following situations[257]:
  - o Analgesia to allow for a more thorough exam and repair of the external ear in trauma
  - o Patients with contraindications to general anesthesia and procedural sedation
  - o Incision and drainage, followed by packing of an auricular hematoma
  - o Incision and drainage of abscesses and cysts
  - o Laceration repair
  - o Foreign body removal
  - o Red ear syndrome
  - o Great auricular neuralgia

Auricular ring block technique

Auricular block anesthetizes four nerves that innervate the auricle:
1. Lesser occipital nerve,
2. Greater auricular nerve,
3. Auricular branch of vagus nerve,
4. Auriculotemporal nerve

---

[257] Jeon Y, Kim S. Treatment of great auricular neuralgia with real-time ultrasound-guided great auricular nerve block: A case report and review of the literature. Medicine (Baltimore). 2017 Mar;96(12):e6325.

CONTRAINDICATIONS

- Known anesthetic agent allergy
- Uncooperative patient
- Cellulitis or erythema overlying the injection site (relative contraindication due to the theoretical risk of spreading the infection)
- Coagulopathy

PROCEDURE: AURICULAR RING BLOCK

1. Using a 25- to 27-gauge needle, insert the needle just inferior to the earlobe directing it toward the tragus.
2. Aspirate and advance the needle superiorly subcutaneously injecting 3–4 mL of local anaesthetic.
3. Withdraw the needle without fully removing it and redirect it posterosuperiorly along the inferior posterior auricular sulcus, aspirating and injecting as before.

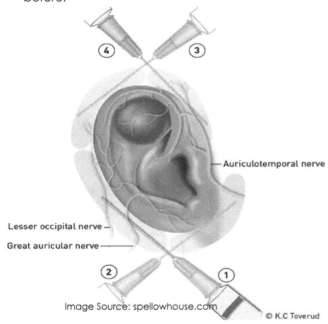

Image Source: spellowhouse.com

© K.C Toverud

4. Remove the needle and insert it just superior to the point of helix insertion into the scalp.
5. Advance the needle and aspirate and inject in the direction of the tragus. Inject into the subcutaneous tissue while avoiding the ear cartilage.
6. Withdraw and redirect the needle posteriorly and inferiorly toward the skin behind the ear, injecting as before.
7. Beware of inadvertent cannulation of the **superficial temporal artery**, which crosses the zygomatic arch and crosses medial to the ear.
8. If the artery is violated, it requires 20–30 min application of firm pressure.

6. WRIST BLOCK

INDICATIONS

- To anesthetize the hand in preparation for laceration repair, fracture or dislocation reduction, or pain relief.

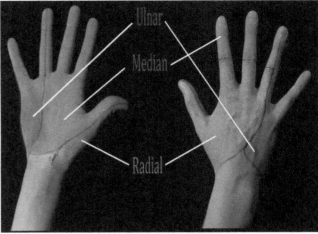

Nerve distribution in the hand

1. WRIST BLOCK: MEDIAN NERVE
PROCEDURE[258]

- Advance the needle at 45° to the skin towards the wrist. The median nerve runs 1–1.5 cm deep; 3–5 ml of LA is injected.
- Paraesthesia of the thumb or index finger warrants withdrawal of the needle by 1–2 mm.
- In order to block the palmar cutaneous branch of the median nerve, the needle is advanced subcutaneously towards the flexor retinaculum and a further 3–5 ml of LA is injected as the needle is withdrawn.
- Note that in patients with carpal tunnel syndrome, block of the median nerve at the wrist could cause pressure-induced neuropraxia in the tight carpal tunnel.

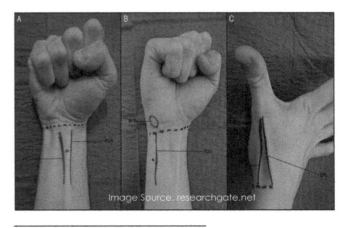

Image Source: researchgate.net

[258] *RA McCahon, NM Bedforth, Peripheral nerve block at the elbow and wrist*, Continuing Education in Anaesthesia Critical Care & Pain, *Volume 7, Issue 2, April 2007, Pages 42–44,*

2. WRIST BLOCK: RADIAL NERVE
PROCEDURE
- At the wrist, the radial nerve is separated into numerous terminal branches.
- LA is injected subcutaneously between the radial styloid and the midpoint of the dorsum of the wrist.

This should be confluent with the LA infiltration of the dorsal cutaneous branch of the ulnar nerve[259].

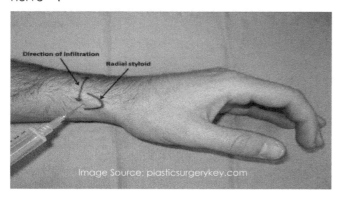

Image Source: plasticsurgerykey.com

3. WRIST BLOCK: ULNAR NERVE
PROCEDURE
- To block the ulnar nerve, the same needle can be advanced beneath the tendon of FCU towards the radial border of the forearm, to a depth of 1–1.5 cm. The needle is redirected subcutaneously around the ulnar aspect of the wrist in order to block the dorsal cutaneous branch of the ulnar nerve. This medial approach to the ulnar nerve reduces the risk of intra-arterial needle placement.
- The alternative is to make an anterior approach, medial to the ulnar artery and lateral to the tendon of FCU. This approach may require a second injection around the ulnar border of the wrist.
- Using either method, 3–5 ml of LA is injected at each site[260].

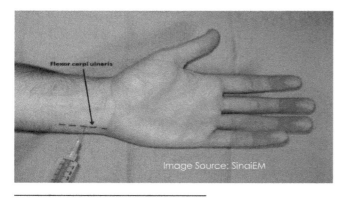

Image Source: SinaiEM

[259] RA McCahon, NM Bedforth, Peripheral nerve block at the elbow and wrist, Continuing Education in Anaesthesia Critical Care & Pain, Volume 7, Issue 2, April 2007, Pages 42–44,

[260] RA McCahon, NM Bedforth, Peripheral nerve block at the elbow and wrist, Continuing Education in Anaesthesia Critical Care & Pain, Volume 7, Issue 2, April 2007, Pages 42–44,

7. DIGITAL NERVE BLOCKS: RING, WEB SPACE, AND TENDON SHEATH
INDICATIONS
- To anesthetize the digits in preparation for laceration repair, nail bed repair, joint reduction, or pain relief.

1. RING BLOCK
PROCEDURE
1. Insert a 25-gauge needle on the dorsal surface of the proximal phalanx of the digit to be anesthetized. Inject 1 mL along the dorsal surface and withdraw the needle.
2. Reinsert the needle again perpendicular to the last injection and running on the lateral surface of the phalanx. Inject 1–1.5 mL of local anaesthetic to just past the phalanx base
3. Repeat the injection in the same fashion on the medial aspect of the phalanx.
4. Do not inject more than 5 mL into a digit.
5. Toe blocks are similar to finger ring blocks, except that the great toe requires plantar surface injection as well, owing to its unique nerve supply.

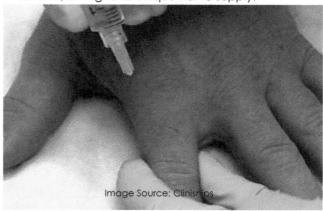

Image Source: Clinisrips

2. WEB SPACE DIGITAL BLOCK
PROCEDURE
1. Have the patient abduct the fingers.
2. Palpate the metacarpophalangeal joint and then insert a 25- to 27-gauge needle into the lateral web space subcutaneously, directing it dorsally. Aspirate then inject 1 mL of local anaesthetic.
3. Withdraw the needle but before the exiting skin, redirect toward the palmar aspect until the tip is next to the metacarpophalangeal joint, and inject 1 mL of local anaesthetic.
4. Repeat the procedure on the medial web space of the digit.
5. Each digit blocked requires injection on both the lateral and the medial web spaces.

ac

3. INTRATHECAL DIGITAL BLOCK: FLEXOR TENDON SHEATH

PROCEDURE

1. Inject anaesthetic directly into the flexor tendon sheath. Palpate on the palmar surface over and proximal to the metacarpophalangeal joint. Gentle flexion of digit may better reveal the sheath. Have the patient abduct the fingers.

2. Insert a 25-gauge needle at a 45° angle to the skin and along the long axis of the digit directly into the flexor tendon sheath at the level of the distal skin crease.

3. Inject 2 mL of local anaesthetic. The anaesthetic should flow freely if it is in the sheath. If it does not, it is likely in the tendon and should be withdrawn slightly.

4. Contraindications to intrathecal block are **local infection** and **preexisting flexor tendon injury**.

5. Risk of tenosynovitis; sterilize the skin before introducing the needle.

6. If laceration has involved the tendon, anaesthetic may leak from the wound.

8. INTERCOSTAL BLOCK

- **Indications:** thoracic or upper abdominal surgery, rib fractures[261], breast surgery.
- **Landmarks:** angle of the rib (6-8 cm lateral to the spinous process)
- **Needle insertion:** Under the rib with approximately 20-30° cephalad angulation
- **Target:** needle insertion 0.5 cm past the inferior border of the rib
- **Local anaesthetic: 3-5 mL** per intercostal level.

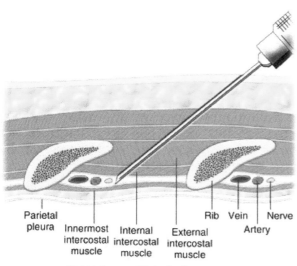

Parietal pleura   Innermost intercostal muscle   Internal intercostal muscle   External intercostal muscle   Rib   Vein   Artery   Nerve

Image Source: Clinicalgate.com

9. FEMORAL NERVE BLOCK/ FASCIA ILIACA BLOCK

OVERVIEW

o Historically, the technique was sometimes termed the **"3 in 1 block"** because it was thought a single injection could block the **femoral, lateral femoral cutaneous and obturator nerves**. Femoral (3 in 1) block should be performed under **ultrasound guidance**

o Used for **fractured shaft of femur** or **fractures of the patella.**

o If possible, obtain IV access before performing this technique

o There is a low but definite risk of local anaesthetic toxicity

o **Max dose of local anaesthetic Bupivacaine 2 mg/kg (= 0.4 ml/kg of 0.5% bupivacaine)**

o You can use a mixture of lignocaine and Bupivacaine. If mixture used, then maximum dose should be **2mg/kg in TOTAL.**

INDICATIONS

- The femoral nerve block (FNB) is indicated for surgery on the anterior aspect of the thigh. It may also be combined with a sciatic nerve block to provide complete lower extremity coverage below the knee, and additionally with an obturator block to provide complete lower extremity anesthesia.

- Both single injection and continuous infusions provide pain relief following total knee replacement[262].

- Femoral nerve block is also useful for analgesia in femoral neck fractures, femur fractures, and patellar injuries. Femoral nerve block may be utilized alone or as part of a multi-modal pain management plan[263].

CONTRAINDICATIONS

- Absolute contraindications include patient refusal, inability to cooperate, and severe allergy to local anesthetic agents.

- Relative contraindications include current infection at the site of local injection, patients on anticoagulation and antithrombotic medications, and patients with bleeding disorders.

[262] Ilfeld BM, Le LT, Meyer RS, Mariano ER, Vandenborne K, Duncan PW, Sessler DI, Enneking FK, Shuster JJ, Theriaque DW, Berry LF, Spadoni EH, Gearen PF. Ambulatory continuous femoral nerve blocks decrease time to discharge readiness after tricompartment total knee arthroplasty: a randomized, triple-masked, placebo-controlled study. Anesthesiology. 2008 Apr;108(4):703-13.

[263] Chan EY, Fransen M, Parker DA, Assam PN, Chua N. Femoral nerve blocks for acute postoperative pain after knee replacement surgery. Cochrane Database Syst Rev. 2014 May 13;(5):CD009941.

[261] Hwang EG, Lee Y. Effectiveness of intercostal nerve block for management of pain in rib fracture patients. J Exerc Rehabil. 2014 Aug;10(4):241-4.

- The Emergency Physician should discuss the possibility of further nerve damage in patients with pre-existing nerve damage or those who may be susceptible to nerve injury (such as severe diabetes, trauma to nerves, etc.) [264]

LANDMARKS AND SURROUNDING STRUCTURES

o *Important landmarks include the femoral crease, ASIS, pubic tubercle, femoral artery (palpable) and veins (not palpable), both located medially.*

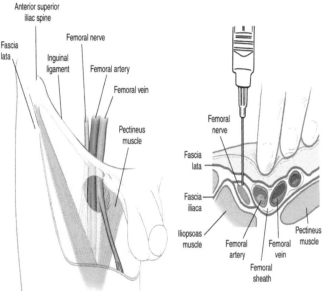

Image Source: Access Emergency Medicine -McGraw-Hill Medical

- **TRADITIONAL FEMORAL BLOCK**
  o **A line is drawn from the ASIS to the pubic tubercle**, in order to outline the inguinal ligament. The femoral artery is marked.
  o A 4 cm 22 ga. needle is inserted just **lateral to the femoral artery**.
  o The femoral nerve is often found within a triangular hyperechoic region, **lateral to the femoral artery and superficial to the iliopsoas muscle**.

FASCIA ILIACA COMPARTMENT BLOCK
INDICATIONS[265]

- The aim is to reduce the requirement for systemic analgesics such as opioids and non-steroidal anti-inflammatories, along with their side-effects.
- This is particularly important in elderly patients, who form by far the largest group admitted with neck of femur fractures.

- Pre-operative analgesia for patients with neck of femur or femoral shaft fractures
- Analgesia for the application of plaster in children with femoral fractures (following discussion with a senior clinician).

CONTRA-INDICATIONS[266]

- Patient refusal
- Known true allergy or previous anaphylactic reaction to local anaesthetic.
- Inflammation or infection over the site.
- Previous femoral-bypass surgery, or near a graft site.
- Anticoagulation – INR >1.5 o Consider recent clopidogrel/high dose aspirin/low molecular weight heparin. o Use clinical judgement and discuss with a senior clinician.

GENERAL PREPARATION

- Confirm the indication and correct patient, rule out contra-indications, obtain informed (verbal) consent, and ensure that you have the right assistance, monitoring and equipment.
- Specific equipment required:
  o Fascia iliaca block pack (kept in 'theatre' in the Emergency Department).
  o Skin antiseptic solution (0.5% chlorhexidine spray or ChloraPrep® sponges). 30-40mls of long acting local anaesthetic. We advise 0.25% (2.5mg/ml) chirocaine/levobupivacaine, 30mls if patient weighs 50kg. 1-2mls of 1% lignocaine for skin infiltration if necessary.

LANDMARK PROCEDURE[267]

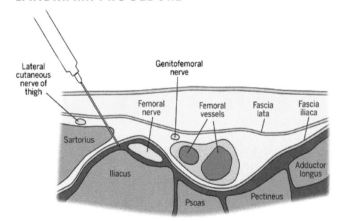

Image Source: Link.springer.com

- The landmarks for the procedure are the anterior superior iliac spine (ASIS) and the ipsilateral pubic tubercle.

---

[264] Kasibhatla RD, Russon K. Femoral nerve blocks. J Perioper Pract. 2009 Feb;19(2):65-9.

[265] Fascia Iliaca Compartment Block: Landmark Approach Guidelines For Use In The Emergency Department, June 2016- RCEM.PDF

[266] Fascia Iliaca Compartment Block: Landmark Approach Guidelines For Use In The Emergency Department, June 2016- RCEM.PDF

[267] Fascia Iliaca Compartment Block: Landmark Approach Guidelines For Use In The Emergency Department, June 2016- RCEM.PDF

- Place one finger on each of these bony landmarks and draw an imaginary line between them.
- Using your index fingers divide this line into thirds.
- At the junction of the lateral 1/3 and medial 2/3 make a mark. Your insertion point will be 1cm distal/caudal to this mark

COMPLICATIONS
- Intravascular injection
- Local anaesthetic toxicity
- Temporary or permanent nerve damage
- Infection
- Block failure
- Injury secondary to numbness/weakness of
- Allergy to any of the preparations used

10. BIER'S BLOCK
- According to the 2014 RCEM[268] Best practice guideline on intravenous regional anaesthesia (IRVA or Bier's block):
  o 0.5% or 1% prilocaine without preservative
  o No preparation with adrenaline
  o **Prilocaine 3mg/Kg**
  o If 0.5% prilocaine unavailable, use half volume of 1% plain prilocaine and the same volume of normal saline (eg instead of 40ml 0.5% plain prilocaine, use 20 ml 1% plain prilocaine and dilute with 20ml normal saline)
  o Bupivacaine should NOT be used

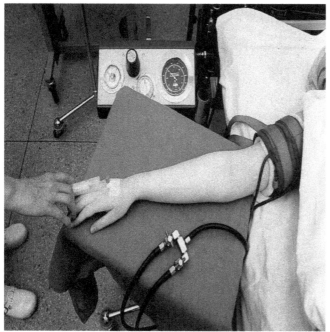

Image Source: Wikipaedia.org

CONTRAINDICATIONS
- o Allergy to local anaesthetic
- o Uncooperative or confused patient
- o Morbid obesity (cuff unreliable of obese arms)
- o Peripheral vascular disease,
- o Raynaud's phenomenon
- o Severe hypertension,
- o Scleroderma,
- o Epilepsy
- o Sickle cell disease or trait,
- o Methaemoglobinaemia
- o Procedures needed in both arms
- o Infection in the affected limb
- o Lymphoedema

PROCEDURE[269]:
- o Ensure patient is on a **cardiac monitor,**
- o Ensure that **two doctors** are present throughout the procedure (one of which should have adequate airway management training).
- o **Elevate the injured arm** for three minutes to exsanguinate the limb
- o Apply and inflate the **double-cuff tourniquet** and inflate to 100mmHg above the systolic BP or to 300mmHg (whichever is greater)
- o **Check for the absence of radial pulse,** Inject the **0.5%/1% plain prilocaine**
- o Warn the patient about the cold/hot sensation and mottled appearance of the arm
- o Check for anaesthesia, may have touch but not pain, after five minutes
- o If anaesthesia inadequate, flush cannulae with 10-15 ml normal saline
- o Remove the cannula, Lower arm on to a pillow and check tourniquet not leaking
- o Perform the reduction of the fracture and obtain check x-ray,
- o Watch for signs of toxicity.
- o The cuff must be inflated for a minimum of **20 minutes and a maximum of 45 minutes.**
- o If satisfied with the post reduction position of fracture, deflate the cuff observing the patient and monitor.
- o Observe the patient and limb closely for signs of delayed toxicity until fully recovered.
- o Check limb circulation prior to discharge.
- o Arrange patient follow up and analgesia as appropriate.

---

[268] *Intravenous Regional Anaesthesia for Distal Forearm Fractures (Bier's Block)-RCEM March 2014.pdf*

[269] *Intravenous Regional Anaesthesia for Distal Forearm Fractures (Bier's Block)-RCEM March 2014.pdf*

Section VI. Practical Procedures

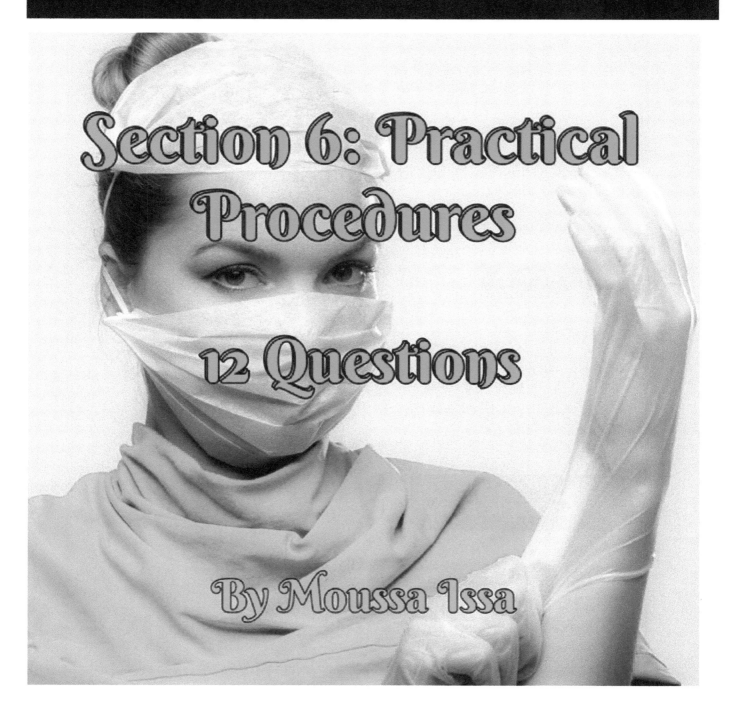

Section 6: Practical Procedures

12 Questions

By Moussa Issa

Ebook for only £3/month!

Get our Reading App for your Android smartphone or tablet to start enjoying the Moussa Issa eBookstore discovery and digital reading experience.

Download our APP on your Smart device Now.

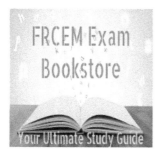

FRCEM Exam eBookstore

FRCEM Exam Bookstore   Books & Reference

PEGI 3

Offers in-app purchases
This app is compatible with all of your devices.

Installed

A static eBook with little interactivity cannot draw your attention any more. Thus it is essential to engage readers with interactive reading experience.
Moussa Issa eBookstore proves to be on top of the interactive eBook game, enabling readers to watch integrated videos related to the subject directly on the page.
The additional flipping effect makes the eBook fully interactive and dynamic.

Customize your experience with multiple font and page styles and social sharing tools.

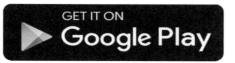
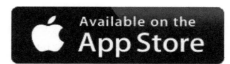

Distributed by Moussa Issa Bookstore Ltd
Website: www.moussaissabooks.com
Email: info@moussaissabooks.com
eBook subscription: www.moussaissabooks.com/read-ebook-online

1. Arterial Cannulation

INDICATIONS

- Continuous monitoring of blood pressure in acute illness or major surgery
- Serial sampling of arterial blood during resuscitation
- Inability to use non-invasive blood pressure monitoring (e.g., burns, morbid obesity)
- Continuous infusion of vasoactive inotropes (e.g., phentolamine for reversal of local anaesthesia)
- Angiography
- Embolization

CONTRAINDICATIONS

- **Absolute**
  o Circulatory compromise in the extremity
  o Third-degree burns of the extremity
  o Raynaud's syndrome
  o Thromboangiitis obliterans (Buerger's disease)
- **Relative**
  o Recent surgery in the extremity
  o Local skin infection
  o Abnormal coagulation
  o Insufficient collateral circulation
  o First- or second-degree burns of the extremity
  o Arteriosclerosis

COMPLICATIONS

- Hemorrhage
- Hematoma (at puncture site)
- Infection (at insertion site or systemic)
- Thrombosis
- Arteriovenous fistula
- Pseudoaneurysm formation
- Exsanguination (secondary to dislodgement of catheter)
- Cerebrovascular accident (CVA; secondary to air embolism)

LANDMARKS

- The radial artery lies between the brachioradialis tendons and flexor carpi radialis tendons, approximately 1-2 cm from the wrist, medial to the bony head of the distal radius.
- The initial puncture site should be as distal as possible, but at least 1 cm proximal to the styloid process, to avoid puncture of the retinaculum flexorum and the small superficial branch of the radial artery.
- Ultrasound guidance may be utilized to assist in identifying the artery and also to visualize cannulation of the vessel[270].

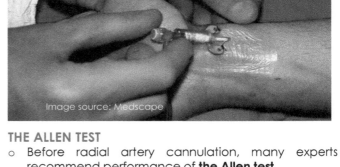

Image source: Medscape

THE ALLEN TEST

o Before radial artery cannulation, many experts recommend performance of **the Allen test.**
o This procedure evaluates for adequate collateral circulation to the hand via the ulnar artery.
o Elevate the hand and ask the patient to make a fist for 30 seconds while applying simultaneous pressure to the ulnar and the radial arteries to occlude them.
o Instruct patient to repeatedly clench the fist tightly to exsanguinate the hand while occlusion of the arteries is maintained.
o Without releasing digital pressure on arteries, instruct patient to extend fingers and observe palmar surface to confirm blanching of skin.
o Release pressure on ulnar artery only and observe palmar surface for reperfusion.
  ▪ If reperfusion of the hand does not occur within 5–10s, ulnar arterial blood flow may be compromised and radial artery cannulation should not be attempted.
  ▪ If reperfusion is brisk, repeat the test releasing pressure on radial artery only and observing palmar surface for reperfusion.
  ▪ If the return of rubor takes longer than 5–10 s, radial artery puncture should not be performed.

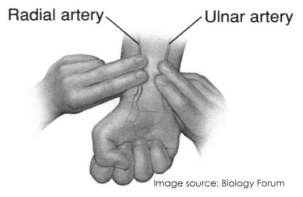

Radial artery   Ulnar artery

Image source: Biology Forum

---

[270] *Corcos T. Distal radial access for coronary angiography and percutaneous coronary intervention: A state-of-the-art review. Catheter Cardiovasc Interv. 2019 Mar 01;93(4):639-644.*

2. Peripheral Venous Cannulation

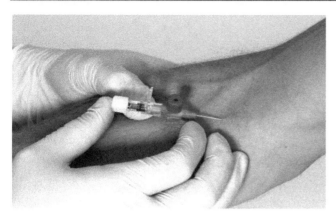

INDICATIONS

o Administration of intravenous medicines.
o Transfusions of blood or blood components.
o Maintenance or correction of hydration levels if unable to tolerate oral fluids.
o Potential venous access.

CONTRAINDICATIONS

o Extremities that have massive edema,
o Burns or injury
o The presence of infection as suggested by inflammation, phlebitis, cellulitis.
o The presence of injury or damage (e.g. fracture, Stroke, oedema, lymphadenopathy).
o Veins which are mobile or tortuous, or sited near a bony prominence.
o If intravenous therapy is predicted to be long-term.
o Continuous infusions or therapies which are vesicant or have a pH of 9.

COMPLICATIONS

o Thrombophlebitis
o Leakage

PERIPHERAL IV SITES

o The preferred site in the emergency department is the **veins of the forearm**, followed by the **median cubital vein** that crosses the antecubital fossa.
o In trauma patients, it is common to go directly to the **median cubital vein** as the first choice because it will accommodate a large bore IV and it is generally easy to catheterize.

o In circumstances where the veins of the upper extremities are inaccessible, the veins of **the dorsum of the foot** or **the saphenous vein** of the lower leg can be used. In circumstances in which no peripheral IV access is possible a central IV can be started.
o In general, the upper limb is the preferred site for placing an intravenous cannula. This is because of the increased incidence of thrombophlebitis and thrombosis with lower limb infusions[271], as well as the need to often immobilise the patient if a drip is sited in the lower limb. The non-dominant upper limb is preferred as an initial option.

1. VENOUS CUTDOWN

• The establishment of venous access is essential to the treatment and resuscitation of both the medically and traumatically ill patient.
• Adequate venous access allows the delivery of fluids, blood products, medications, and repeated blood draws[272].

INDICATIONS

o Saphenous vein cutdown is indication for the purpose of **eme**
o **rgency venous access** when attempts to gain access via peripheral or percutaneous routes have failed.
o Burns, Shock, Asystole or PEA, Sclerosed veins of IVDU.

CONTRAINDICATIONS

o Alternative option exists for venous access
o Coagulopathy or bleeding diathesis
o Vein thrombosis
o Overlying cellulitis
o Major trauma at the proposed site
o Injury proximal to the proposed site

COMPLICATIONS

---

271 Clutton-Brock TH (1984) How to set up a drip and keep it going. Br J Hosp Med 32:162–167

272 Ker K, Tansley G, Beecher D, Perner A, Shakur H, Harris T, Roberts I. Comparison of routes for achieving parenteral access with a focus on the management of patients with Ebola virus disease. Cochrane Database Syst Rev. 2015 Feb 26;(2):CD011386.

o Failed cannulation
o Creation of a false passageway in the vessel wall
o Hemorrhage
o Air embolus
o Venous thrombosis
o Infection
o Nerve / Artery/ Vein transection
o Damage of surrounding structures

LANDMARK

o Locate the **great saphenous vein 1 cm anterior and 1 cm superior to the medial malleolus**

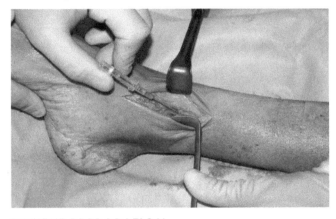

PATIENT PREPARATION

o Local anaesthesia is used (1% lidocaine with or without epinephrine).
o The patient is placed in a supine position with the foot externally rotated.
o A tourniquet can be placed above the ankle but is not necessary.

2. INTRAOSSEOUS CANNULATION

INDICATIONS

o Urgent venous access is required after **3 failed attempts** at venous cannulation
o **Difficulty in establishing venous access**, as in the following settings: Burns, Obesity, Edema, Seizures
o **Condition necessitating rapid high-volume fluid infusion**, such as the following: Hypovolemic shock, Burns
o **Afford access to the systemic venous circulation**, as with the following: Cardiopulmonary arrest, Burns, Blood draws, Local anaesthesia and Medication infusion.

LANDMARKS

• If possible, avoid areas of burns or of skin infection
  o **Proximal tibia**: Anteromedial surface, 2-3 cm below the tibial tuberosity
  o **Distal tibia**: Proximal to the medial malleolus
  o **Distal femur**: Midline, 2-3 cm above the external condyle

o Sternum, Deltoid, Iliac crest

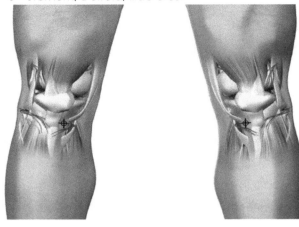

CONTRAINDICATIONS

o Proximal ipsilateral fracture
o Ipsilateral vascular injury
o Osteogenesis imperfecta
o Osteoporosis
o In a general manner, IO access should not be used in severe genetic or acquired bone diseases, imperfect osteogenesis, osteoporosis and osteomyelitis[273].

COMPLICATIONS

o Failure to enter the bone marrow, with extravasation or subperiosteal infusion
o Through and through penetration of the bone
o Osteomyelitis (rare in short term use)
o Growth plate injury
o Local infection,
o Skin necrosis,
o Pain
o Compartment syndrome,
o Fat and bone microemboli have all been reported (rare)

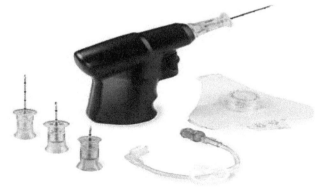

273 Cotte J, Prunet B, d'Aranda E, Asencio Y, Kaiser E. A compartment syndrome secondary to intraosseous infusion. Ann Fr Anesth Reanim. 2011;30(1):90–1. doi: 10.1016/j.annfar.2010.05.038.

3. Central Venous Cannulation

INTRODUCTION

- A central venous line (CVL) is a large-bore central venous catheter that is placed using a sterile technique (unless an urgent clinical scenario prevents sterile technique placement) in certain clinical scenarios[274].

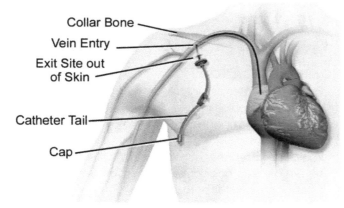

Collar Bone
Vein Entry
Exit Site out of Skin
Catheter Tail
Cap

Image source: Wikipaedia.org

ANATOMY

- In emergency medical practice, there are three possible sites for CVL placement in the adult patient.
- Each has advantages and disadvantages.
- The placement sites include the internal jugular vein, femoral vein, and subclavian vein.
- The right internal jugular vein and left subclavian vein are the most direct paths to the right atrium via the superior vena cava. The femoral veins are compressible sites and as such may be more appropriate for coagulopathic patients.
- The subclavian vein approach is at higher risk for pneumothorax than the internal jugular vein approach. Ultrasound guidance can be very helpful in all approaches and is the recommended approach. However, when ultrasound guidance is not feasible for various reasons, such as the emergency nature of a procedure, lack of equipment, or a patient's anatomy in a situation where there is limited room for the ultrasound transducer in the subclavian approach while manipulating the needle, CVLs may be placed using anatomical landmarks without ultrasound.

INDICATIONS

- There are many different indications for placing a CVL, but in emergency medicine, the most common indications include:
  - Fluid resuscitation (including blood products)
  - Drug infusions that could otherwise cause phlebitis or sclerosis (e.g., vasopressors and hyperosmolar solutions)
  - Central venous pressure monitoring, pulmonary artery catheter introduction
  - Emergency venous access (due to difficult peripheral intravenous access)
  - Transvenous pacing wire placement

CONTRAINDICATIONS

- Contraindications include: distorted local anatomy (such as for trauma), infection overlying the insertion site, or thrombus within the intended vein.
- Relative contraindications include coagulopathy, hemorrhage from target vessel, suspected proximal vascular injury, or combative patients.

EQUIPMENT

- Most central line kits include:
  - Syringe and needle for local anesthetic
  - Small vial of 1% lidocaine
  - Syringe and introducer needle
  - Scalpel
  - Guidewire
  - Tissue dilator
  - Sterile dressing
  - Suture and needle
  - Central line catheter (of which there are several types, including triple-lumen, dual-lumen, and large bore single-lumen)

- In addition, the operator will require a sterile gown, cap, sterile gloves, sterile gauze, sterile saline, face mask, and a sterile cleansing solution such as chlorhexidine.
- The operator should ensure that ultrasound, sterile ultrasound gel, and a sterile ultrasound probe are part of the setup as well.

PREPARATION

- Place the patient in the appropriate position for the site selected, then prepare the site in a sterile fashion using the sterile solution, sterile gauze, and sterile drapes.

---

[274] *Derderian SC, Good R, Vuille-Dit-Bille RN, Carpenter T, Bensard DD. Central venous lines in critically ill children: Thrombosis but not infection is site dependent. J. Pediatr. Surg. 2019 Sep;54(9):1740-1743.*

- For the internal jugular and subclavian approach, place the patient in reverse Trendelenburg with the head turned to the opposite side of the site.
- For the femoral vein, place the patient in the supine position with the inguinal area exposed; this usually means the target leg should be bent at the knee with the lateral aspect resting on the stretcher or bed. It is recommended to place the patient on cardiopulmonary monitoring for the duration of the procedure.

TECHNIQUE

The steps are as follows:

1. Infiltrate the skin with 1% lidocaine for local anesthesia around the site of the needle insertion.
2. Use the bedside ultrasound to identify the target vein.
3. If using landmarks for the subclavian vein CVL, the needle should be inserted approximately 1 cm inferior to the junction of the middle and medial third of the clavicle. If using landmarks for the femoral line CVL, the needle insertion site should be located approximately 1 cm to 3 cm below the inguinal ligament and 0.5 cm to 1 cm medial to where the femoral artery is pulsated.
4. Insert the introducer needle with negative pressure until venous blood is aspirated. For the subclavian CVL, insert the needle at an angle as close to parallel to the skin as possible until contact is made with the clavicle, then advanced the needle under and along the inferior aspect of the clavicle. Next, direct the tip of the needle towards the suprasternal notch until venous blood is aspirated. Whenever possible, the introducer needle should be advanced under ultrasound guidance to ensure the tip does not enter the incorrect vessel or puncture through the distal edge of the vein.
5. Once venous blood is aspirated, stop advancing the needle. Carefully remove the syringe and thread the guidewire through the introducer needle hub.
6. While still holding the guidewire in place, remove the introducer needle hub.
7. If possible, use the ultrasound to confirm the guidewire is in the target vessel in two different views.
8. Next, use the scalpel tip to make a small stab in the skin against the wire just large enough to accommodate the dilator (and eventually, the central venous catheter). Insert the dilator with a twisting motion.
9. Advance the CVL over the guidewire. Make sure the distal lumen of the central line is uncapped to facilitate passage of the guidewire.

10. Once the CVL is in place, remove the guidewire. Next, flush and aspirate all ports with the sterile saline.
11. Secure the CVL in place with the suture and place a sterile dressing over the site.

COMPLICATIONS

- Potential complications should be explained to the patient if possible while obtaining informed consent.
- Complications include:
  o Pain at cannulation site,
  o Local hematoma,
  o Infection (both at the site as well as bacteremia),
  o Misplacement into another vessel (possibly causing arterial puncture or cannulation),
  o Vessel laceration or dissection,
  o Air embolism,
  o Thrombosis, and
  o Pneumothorax requiring a possible chest tube[275].

CLINICAL SIGNIFICANCE

- Clinical pearls for consideration:
  o A chest X-ray should be performed immediately for the internal jugular and subclavian lines to ensure proper placement and absence of an iatrogenic pneumothorax.
  o Be sure you are withdrawing venous blood before dilation and cannulation of the vessel.
  o If internal jugular CVL attempt is unsuccessful, move to the ipsilateral subclavian vein.
  o Never attempt the opposite side without a chest X-ray or ultrasound first to avoid bilateral pneumothoraces.
  o Never let go of the guidewire as it may migrate distally into the vessel.
  o Never force the wire on insertion because it may cause damage to the vessel or surrounding structures.
  o Forcing the wire could also cause it to kink making removal difficult or impossible.
  o Always place your finger over the open hub of the needle to prevent an air embolism.
  o Always confirm placement with ultrasound, looking for reverberation artifact of the needle and/or tenting of the vessel wall.
  o Needles cannot be visualized on ultrasound. Wires can be visualized so the operator can confirm at that step as well.
  o A venous blood gas can be aspirated off a femoral line to ensure it is not arterial.

---

[275] Pare JR, Pollock SE, Liu JH, Leo MM, Nelson KP. Central venous catheter placement after ultrasound guided peripheral IV placement for difficult vascular access patients. Am J Emerg Med. 2019 Feb;37(2):317-320.

4. Arterial Blood Gas Sampling

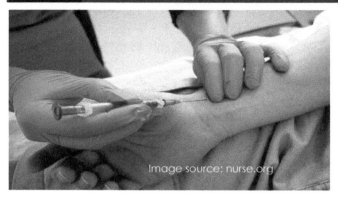
Image source: nurse.org

INDICATIONS FOR ABG SAMPLING
o To interpret oxygenation levels
o To assess for potential respiratory derangements
o To assess for potential metabolic derangements
o To monitor acid-base status
o To assess carboxyhaemoglobin in CO poisoning
o To assess lactate
o To gain preliminary results for electrolytes and Haemoglobin
o Can be conducted as a one-off sample or repeated sampling to determine response to interventions

CONTRAINDICATIONS TO ABG SAMPLING
o **Absolute:**
   ▪ Absent pulse
   ▪ Thromboangiitis obliterans (Buerger disease)
   ▪ Full-thickness burns over the cannulation site
   ▪ Inadequate circulation to the extremity
   ▪ Raynaud syndrome

o **Relative:**
   ▪ Anticoagulation
   ▪ Coagulopathy
   ▪ Atherosclerosis
   ▪ Inadequate collateral flow
   ▪ Infection at the cannulation site
   ▪ Partial-thickness burn at the cannulation site
   ▪ Previous surgery in the area
   ▪ Synthetic vascular graft

EQUIPMENT REQUIRED FOR ABG SAMPLING
o Gloves,
o Sharps bin,
o Cleaning swab
o Gauze,
o Tape,
o ABG syringe

PROCEDURE FOR ABG SAMPLING
o Consent the patient verbally after explaining the procedure
o Set up a tray with a sharps bin
o Expel excess heparin from ABG syringe
o Palpate for radial pulse
o Transfix artery between forefinger and middle finger
o Insert ABG syringe into palpated artery
o Depending on the syringe it may self-fill or you may need to withdraw the plunger carefully.
o Remove needle and syringe after sample gained (only 1-2ml required)
o Arterial blood samples should be obtained in strict anaerobic conditions and should be placed on ice and held at 0° C until analysis. Any air bubbles introduced during the sampling procedure will lead to overestimation of arterial oxygen tension (PaO_2) and underestimation of arterial carbon dioxide tension ($PaCO_2$) [276].

POST PROCEDURE CARE
o Apply pressure to area with gauze and tape.
o Advise patient to continue giving pressure for 5-10 minutes
o Take sample to the analyser as soon as possible
o Ensure the result is labelled with the patient's details and documented in the notes
o Ensure inspired oxygen concentration is clearly documented

IN THE EVENT OF FAILURE
• Call for senior help

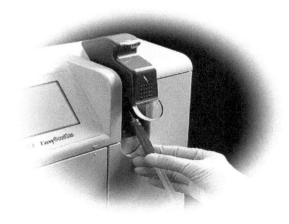

---

[276] Gilbert HC, Vender JS. Arterial blood gas monitoring. Crit Care Clin. 1995 Jan. 11 (1):233-48.

5. Lumbar Puncture

INDICATIONS

- **Diagnostic**
  - Evaluation for the possibility of a central nervous system (CNS) infection: Viral, Bacterial, and Fungal Meningitis and Encephalitis
  - Evaluation for inflammatory processes: Multiple Sclerosis, Guillain-Barré syndrome
  - Evaluation for spontaneous subarachnoid hemorrhage (SAH)
  - Suspicion of CNS diseases: oncological and metabolic processes
- **Therapeutic**
  - Therapeutic reduction of cerebrospinal fluid (CSF) pressure
  - Procedures requiring lower body analgesia or anesthesia
  - Intrathecal antibiotic administration for some types of meningitis
  - Chemotherapy and methotrexate for some forms of leukemia and lymphomas

CONTRAINDICATIONS

- Presences of increased intracranial pressure (ICP), regardless of cause, can increase risk of cerebral or cerebellar brainstem herniation at the level of the foramen magnum.
- Use of anticoagulants (e.g., warfarin, enoxaparin, etc) due to increased risk of developing an epidural hematoma.
- Evidence of cellulitis or abscess over the area where LP would be performed due to risk of introducing infection into the subarachnoid space.
- Significant degenerative joint disease or prior back surgeries where hardware maybe in place (*Note*: many of these patients may require an LP under fluoroscopy)

COMPLICATIONS

The following are in order of most concerning to the least:

- Herniation of the brainstem
- Accidental puncture of the aorta or vena cava leading to retroperitoneal hematoma
- Accidental puncture of the spinal cord from being in wrong location
- Infection being introduced into the subarachnoid space
- Pain over the LP site
- Headache from CSF leak

  - Can worsen with sitting up or standing, and if lasting longer than 1-2 days may require a blood patch in the area of the LP puncture site
- Lumbar puncture should be performed only after a neurologic examination but should never delay potentially life-saving interventions, such as the administration of antibiotics and steroids to patients with suspected bacterial meningitis[277].

PROCEDURE

- **Positioning**
  - Determined by practitioner preference or patient capability.
  - Options: **lateral recumbent position, upright sitting position**.
  - **Lateral recumbent position** is preferred to obtain accurate opening pressure and to reduce the risk of postpuncture headache.
  - Both positions require the patient to arch the lower back toward the practitioner in order to open up the intervertebral spaces (obtain the "fetal position" or arch "like a cat").
  - Shoulders and hips should remain aligned during process.

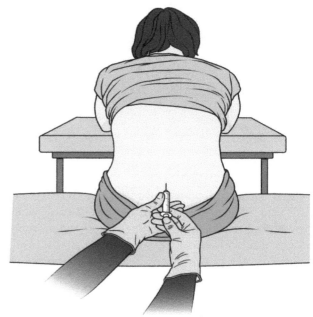

Image source: Macmillan.org

[277] de Gans J, van de Beek D, European Dexamethasone in Adulthood Bacterial Meningitis Study Investigators. Dexamethasone in adults with bacterial meningitis. N Engl J Med. 2002 Nov 14. 347(20):1549-56.

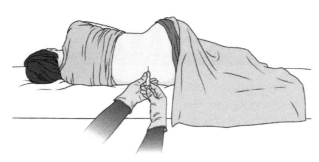

Image source: Macmillan.org

- **LANDMARKS**
  - Determined by palpation.
  - Draw a visual line between the superior aspects of the iliac crests that intersects the midline at the L4 interspace.
  - The L3–4 and L4–5 spaces are preferred because these points are below the termination of the spinal cord.
  - Palpate the posterosuperior iliac crests with the midpoint of a visual line that connects the two crests representing the L4 spinous process.
  - Palpate the space between the L3–4 or the L4–5 spinous processes and mark where the needle will be placed.

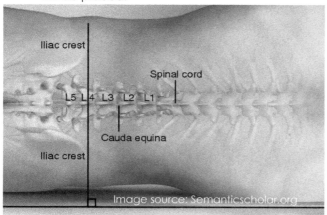

Image source: Semanticscholar.org

BEFORE THE PROCEDURE

- Verify that no contraindications exist. This may include doing a CT head to rule out active bleeding, midline shift, space-occupying lesions or signs of brain swelling.
- Obtain informed consent with appropriate documentation
- Do a baseline neurologic exam with special notation on the strength, sensation and ability to move extremities
- Wash hands, open the lumbar puncture tray without compromising sterility and consider any extra supplies (i.e., spinal needles or extra tubes)

DURING THE PROCEDURE

- Position the patient either in lateral decubitus / fetal position, or sitting upright leaning forward over a small table,
- Locate the L3/L4 space by locating the superior iliac crests and placing your thumbs midline to the spine. Palpate above and below to determine the widest space and attempt to mark location with the nail of your thumb or create a small indentation with an object like pen or needle cap,
- Aseptically clean the skin using chlorhexidine skin prep. Put on sterile gloves, facemask, and protective gear per institutional policy.
- Draw up and inject 10 mL of 1% or 2% lidocaine (preservative free; without epinephrine) to the area
- Insert the spinal needle directed at a slight cephalad angle (imagine aiming towards the umbilicus) and with the bevel of the needle oriented to the longitudinal fibers in attempt to separate the fibers instead of cutting them
- The entry into the subarachnoid space is commonly described as feeling a "pop" sensation, the needle insert (obturator) is then removed and CSF should begin to drip out.
- Attach the sterile manometer to the end of the spinal needle to measure the opening pressure
  - Normal opening pressures: **< 20 cm H2O**
  - Measuring opening pressure is very important for evaluation for cryptococcal meningitis or pseudotumor cerebri
  - If blockage of CSF flow to the spinal subarachnoid space is suspected, the clinician may perform a Queckenstedt-Stookey test
- Empty the manometer into CSF tube #1 and about 10 drops of CSF into tubes #2 - 4
- Measure the closing pressure (if indicated)
- Reinsert the needle insert (obturator) and withdraw the spinal needle and immediately apply pressure and an adhesive bandage over the insertion site

AFTER THE PROCEDURE

- There is no evidence that it has any effect on the development of post-LP headache.
- There is no harm in having the patient lie flat if they desire to do so.
- Immediately label the CSF tubes have the tubes hand carried/delivered to the lab for analysis
- If meningitis is suspected, initiate empiric antibiotics with or without steroids based on the clinical scenario. Repeat neurologic assessment to evaluate for any changes post-LP.
- Document the procedure, number of attempts, opening and closing pressure (if applicable), total amount of CSF drained.

6. Pleural & Pericardial Tap
I. THORACENTESIS

- Thoracentesis is a procedure that is performed to remove fluid from the thoracic cavity for both diagnostic and/or therapeutic purposes[278].

BEDSIDE ULTRASONOGRAPHY

- Before the procedure, **bedside ultrasonography** can be used to determine the presence and size of pleural effusions and to look for loculations.
- During the procedure, **bedside ultrasonography** can be used in real time to facilitate anaesthesia and then guide needle placement.

INDICATIONS

- **Therapeutic thoracentesis** is performed to relieve dyspnea, hypoxia, or otherwise compromised respiratory function due to a large pleural effusion.

- **Diagnostic thoracentesis** is performed to aid in the diagnosis and workup of:
  - Pleural effusions of unknown cause
  - Unilateral pleural effusions
  - Pleural effusions originally determined to be due to heart failure but persisting after 3 days of diuresis

CONTRAINDICATIONS

- **Absolute**
  - None
- **Relative:**
  - Coagulopathy,
  - Thrombocytopenia.
  - Small or loculated pleural effusion. These will increase the risk of missing the effusion and causing lung injury.
  - Positive-pressure ventilation.
  - Skin infection over the needle insertion site.

PERIPROCEDURAL CARE

- **Informed Consent:** should be obtained from the patient or parent if minor.
- Provide a focused set of risks and complications.
- Discuss how these risks can be avoided or prevented (e.g., proper positioning, ensuring that the patient remains as still as possible during the procedure, adequate analgesia).

PATIENT PREPARATION

- Patient preparation includes **adequate anaesthesia** and **proper positioning.**

ANESTHESIA

- In addition to **local anaesthesia, mild sedation** may also be considered.
- **IV Midazolam or Lorazepam.**
- The skin, subcutaneous tissue, rib periosteum, intercostal muscle, and parietal pleura should all be well infiltrated with local anaesthetic.

POSITIONING

- Thoracentesis is done in either a supine or sitting position depending on patient comfort, underlying condition, and the clinical indication[279].
- **Patients who are alert and cooperative** are most comfortable in a **seated position,** leaning slightly forward and resting the head on the arms or hands or on a pillow, which is placed on an adjustable bedside table. This position facilitates access to the posterior axillary space, which is the most dependent part of the thorax.
- **Unstable patients** and those who are unable to sit up **may be supine** for the procedure.

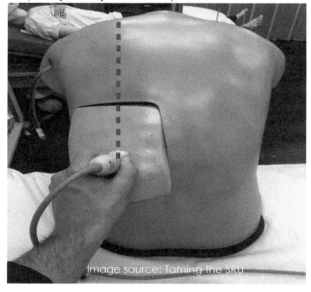

Image source: Taming the SRU

[278] Leo F, Makowska M. [Thoracentesis - Step by Step]. Dtsch. Med. Wochenschr. 2018 Aug;143(16):1186-1192.

[279] Alzghoul B, Innabi A, Subramany S, Boye B, Chatterjee K, Koppurapu VS, Bartter T, Meena NK. Optimizing the Approach to Patients With Pleural Effusion and Radiologic Findings Suspect for Cancer. J Bronchology Interv Pulmonol. 2019 Apr;26(2):114-118.

LANDMARK

- Traditionally, this is **between the 7th and 9th rib spaces** and between the **posterior axillary line and the midline.**

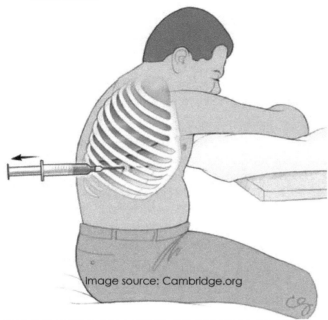

Image source: Cambridge.org

DIAGNOSTIC ANALYSIS OF PLEURAL FLUID

The following laboratory tests should be requested:

- **pH level**
- **Gram stain, Culture, Cell count and Differential**
- **Glucose level, protein levels,** and **lactic acid dehydrogenase** (LDH) level
- **Cytology**
- **Creatinine level** if Urinothorax is suspected
- **Amylase** level if oesophageal perforation or pancreatitis is suspected
- **Triglyceride levels** if chylothorax is suspected (e.g., after coronary artery bypass graft [CABG], especially if the inferior mesenteric artery [IMA] was used; milky appearance is not sensitive

COMPLICATIONS

- Pneumothorax
- Re-expansion pulmonary edema
- Hemothorax, hematoma
- Intra-abdominal organ injury
- Air embolism, Empyema
- Damage to the intercostals or internal mammary vessels, Diaphragmatic injury,
- Cough, Pain
- Risk of Catheter fragment left in the pleural space.

CONSIDERATIONS

- If available, the use of bedside ultrasound is highly recommended because ultrasound guidance has been shown to substantially reduce the risk of pneumothorax.

- Before the procedure, the height, width, and depth of the effusion can be appreciated by scanning the chest and viewing the effusion through the intercostal spaces.
- The use of ultrasound aids in selecting the needle insertion site by:
  - Visualizing the distance, the needle must pass to reach the parietal pleura
  - Confirming the thickness of the effusion in the site selected is at least a minimum of 1.5 cm
  - Providing the clinician with a view of the effusion and surrounding structures through the complete respiratory cycle
- With these items in mind, the needle insertion site can be selected with confidence and marked before beginning the procedure.
- In addition, the use of bedside ultrasound in real time will allow the clinician to visualize the needle as it passes toward and enters the pleural space. This use requires sterile probe covers.

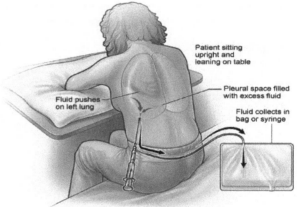

Patient sitting upright and leaning on table

Pleural space filled with excess fluid

Fluid pushes on left lung

Fluid collects in bag or syringe

Image source: Wikipaedia

- **Re-expansion pulmonary edema** is a rare but feared complication of thoracentesis.
- The cause is not fully understood. Historically it was thought that re-expansion pulmonary edema was caused by removing too large a volume of fluid from the pleural space (>1–1.5 L).
- Another theory is that re-expansion pulmonary edema is caused when great negative intrapleural pressures (<20 cmH2O) are generated during the procedure. The low incidence of this complication has yielded inconclusive evidence.
- In light of this, it is prudent to continue to limit the volume of pleural fluid removed to no more than 1–1.5 L.
- **Pleural manometry** is not widely available for use in the emergency department, but should also be considered if available to maintain intrapleural pressures from reaching more negative values.

II. PERICARDIOCENTESIS

INDICATIONS

- **Therapeutic:** Treatment of hemodynamic compromise from cardiac tamponade
- **Diagnostic:** To diagnose the cause or presence of a pericardial effusion

CONTRAINDICATIONS

- **Absolute**
  o Aortic dissection
  o Need for immediate surgery for trauma patients
- **Relative**
  o Coagulopathy
  o Anticoagulant therapy
  o Thrombocytopenia

- If the pericardiocentesis is unsuccessful, a bedside thoracotomy can be performed to allow for pericardiotomy and drainage of pericardial tamponade[280].

MATERIALS AND MEDICATIONS

- Antiseptic (e.g., Chloraprep)
- 1 % lidocaine
- 25-gauge needle, 5/8-in. long
- 18-gauge catheter-type needle, 1½-nch long
- Syringes (10, 20, and 60 mL)
- Ultrasound (US) machine and cardiac/phased array probe
- Sterile US probe cover
- Cardiac monitor

PROCEDURE

- Identify the point of maximal effusion with US. Evaluate for hypoechoic or anechoic (dark) effusion around the heart, between the pericardial sac and the myocardium.
- A patient with hemodynamic compromise from a pericardial effusion or tamponade will have right ventricular collapse, septal bulging, and dilation of the inferior vena cava.
- Diastolic collapse of the right ventricular free wall can be absent in elevated right ventricular pressure and right ventricular hypertrophy or in right ventricular infarction.
- Measure the distance from the skin surface to the effusion border to assess the expected needle depth.

- Choose the needle trajectory based on the point of maximal effusion in the path with the fewest intervening structures.
- The most commonly used approaches are left parasternal, apical, and subxiphoid. For complex loculated posterior pericardial effusions, optional techniques such as transatrial and transbronchial may be performed by specialists.
- These types of loculated effusions can occur in autoimmune diseases, infective pericarditis, after cardiac surgery, and after radiotherapy.
- **Sterile preparation:** prepare the skin of the entire lower xiphoid and epigastric area with antiseptic. Prepare the US transducer with a sterile sleeve.
- **Local anaesthetic:** if the patient is awake, anesthetize the skin and planned route of the needle.
- **Pericardial needle insertion:** depends on approach used.

1. SUBXIPHOID APPROACH

- The US transducer is placed just inferior to the xiphoid process and left costal margin.
- Insert the needle between the xiphoid process and the left costal margin at a 30–45° angle to the skin.
- Aim for the left shoulder.

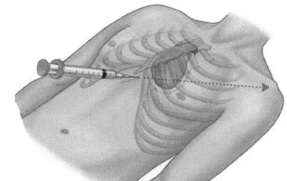

Image source: Heartbeatkenya

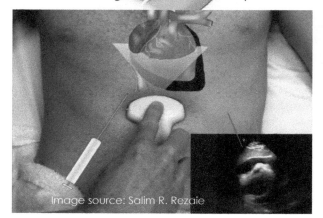

Image source: Salim R. Rezaie

---

[280] Honasoge AP, Dubbs SB. *Rapid Fire: Pericardial Effusion and Tamponade. Emerg. Med. Clin. North Am. 2018 Aug;36(3):557-565.*

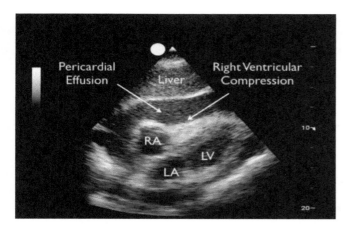

2. APICAL APPROACH

- The US transducer is placed at the patient's point of maximal impulse and aimed at the patient's **right shoulder for a four-chamber view of the heart.**
- Insert the needle in the fifth intercostal space 1 cm lateral to and below the apical beat, within the area of cardiac dullness.

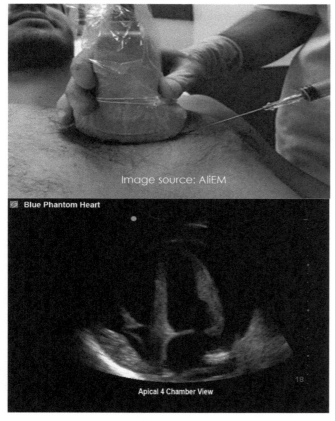

3. PARASTERNAL LONG-AXIS APPROACH

- The US transducer is placed obliquely on the left sterna border between the fourth and fifth ribs with the transducer, **indicator aimed at the right shoulder.**
- Insert the needle perpendicular to the skin in the fifth intercostal space medial to the border of cardiac dullness.

- Visualize and feel a giving way as the needle penetrates the pericardium. Removal of fluid confirms successful entry. Remove fluid with the goal of restoring hemodynamic stability.
- Aspiration of fluid should result in improvement in blood pressure and cardiac output.
- Remove the catheter and apply a dressing.
- **Optional:** Place a pigtail catheter using the Seldinger technique for continued drainage.

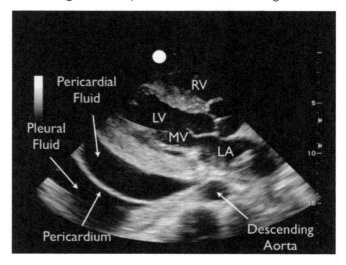

COMPLICATIONS

- Pericardiocentesis, when done in the hands of experienced physicians, has good outcomes but complication rates still occur in about 5-40% of cases. Most complications present early and need immediate attention. The use of ultrasound or fluoroscopy is highly recommended to lower the risk of complications[281].
- Any vital structure within reach of the pericardial needle has the potential for injury:
  - Pneumothorax;
  - Hemothorax;
  - Coronary vessel laceration;
  - Hemopericardium;
  - Heart chamber lacerations;
  - Intercostal vessel injury;
  - Dysrhythmias;
  - Ventricular tachycardia;
  - Puncture of the liver, diaphragm, or gastrointestinal tract;
  - Bacteremia;
  - Purulent pericarditis;
  - Air embolisms;
  - Pleuropericardial fistulas.

---

[281] Lekhakul A, Assawakawintip C, Fenstad ER, Pislaru SV, Thaden JJ, Sinak LJ, Kane GC. Safety and Outcome of Percutaneous Drainage of Pericardial Effusions in Patients with Cancer. Am. J. Cardiol. 2018 Sep 15;122(6):1091-1094.

7. Intercostal Drain-Open
I. NEEDLE THORACOSTOMY

INDICATIONS

- Needle decompression thoracostomy is a procedure used in the emergent treatment of a tension pneumothorax.
- Tension pneumothorax is a clinical diagnosis.
- Decompression treatment should not be delayed in order to obtain radiographic confirmation.
- The following scenarios illustrate some of the clinical signs that *may* be present in such patients:
- ***Awake patient* with suspected or confirmed tension pneumothorax**
  - o Chest pain
  - o Respiratory distress
  - o Decreased breath sounds with hyperresonance and/or subcutaneous emphysema
  - o Trachea deviated away from the side of the pneumothorax
  - o Tachycardia
  - o Falling pulse oximetry (SpO2)
  - o Shock

- ***Ventilated patient* with suspected or confirmed pneumothorax (often insidious)**
  - o Increased resistance to ventilation
  - o Hypotension
  - o Elevated central venous pressure
  - o Tachycardia
  - o Decreased breath sounds with hyperresonance and/or subcutaneous emphysema
  - o Trachea deviated away from the side of the pneumothorax
  - o Falling SpO2
  - o Shock

- **Injured patient (especially with penetrating chest trauma) with suspected or confirmed tension pneumothorax**
  - o In arrest
  - o Unexplained hypotension
  - o Apnea
  - o Decreased breath sounds with hyperresonance and/or subcutaneous emphysema

ABSOLUTE INDICATIONS

- Patient in acute respiratory distress with rapid decompensation secondary to suspected or confirmed tension pneumothorax

- Injured patient in extremis with apnea, unexplained hypotension, or arrest
- Tube thoracostomy (TT) is the gold standard treatment for tension pneumothorax[282].
- Needle thoracotomy (NT) has been originally suggested as an immediate and simple temporary method for chest decompression, serving as a bridge to TT. When successful, it can be a life-saving intervention, relieving the elevated intrapleural pressure[283].
- NT was never designed to be a definitive treatment for pneumothorax.

CONTRAINDICATIONS

- None

MATERIALS

- Large-bore needle/angiocatheter (min of 16 gauge)
- 10-mL syringe (optional)
- One-way valve (optional)
- Betadine (povidone-iodine) swab/chlorhexidine scrub
- Tape

PROCEDURE

- Expose the anterior chest at the level of the second intercostals space on the affected side.
- Alternatively, expose the chest wall at the level of the anterior axillary line in the fourth or fifth intercostal space on the affected side.
- Cleanse the area with a Betadine swab or chlorhexidine scrub.
- Using a gloved hand, locate the second intercostal space at the midclavicular line.
  - The first rib is normally not felt.
  - The second rib is felt just below the clavicle.
  - The second intercostal space is the area between the second and the third ribs.

---

[282] *Garchitorena Ramirez MA, Delos Santos NC Doble F, et al. Comparative study between manual aspiration and closed tube thoracostomy in the management of pneumothorax secondary to trauma: a prospective randomized control trial done in a tertiary hospital specialized in trauma. J Am Coll Surg 2012; 215: S100–1.*

[283] *Dominguez KM, Ekeh AP, Tchorz KM, et al. Is routine tube thoracostomy necessary after prehospital needle decompression for tension pneumothorax? Am J Surg2013; 205:329–32; discussion 332.*

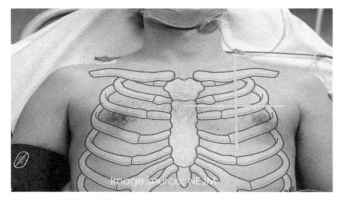

Image source: NEJM

- **Note:** Alternatively, **this procedure may also be performed on the midaxillary line in the fourth intercostal space of the affected side**. The same general steps listed later are employed in this approach and care is taken to avoid the neurovascular bundles inferior to the fourth rib.
- Insert the needle/angiocatheter perpendicular to the chest wall into the second intercostal space just above the superior edge of the third rib to avoid the intercostal neurovascular bundle.

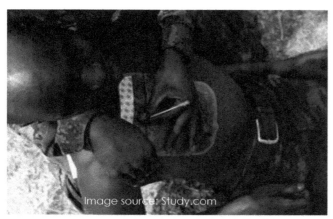

Image source: Study.com

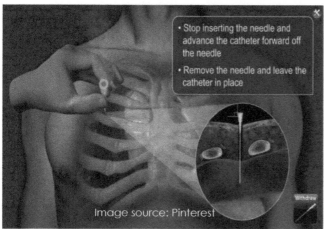

- Stop inserting the needle and advance the catheter forward off the needle
- Remove the needle and leave the catheter in place

Withdraw

Image source: Pinterest

- o This step may be done with or without a syringe attached.
- o Local anesthesia is usually unnecessary but may be used if the patient is not in extremis.

- Carefully walk the needle over the third rib and advance until the pleural space is entered.
- o Entry into the pleural space is accompanied by a **"popping"** sound or a sensation of **"giving way."**
- If you are able to withdraw air with the syringe or hear a **"hiss"** of air escaping through the angiocatheter during expiration and inspiration, then placement is considered successful.
- After removing the needle, secure the angiocatheter in place with tape.

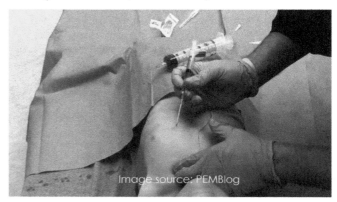

Image source: PEMBlog

- **Caution:** Do not reinsert needle into the angiocatheter owing to the danger of sheering the angiocatheter.
- Assess the patient and evaluate the effectiveness of the procedure.
- o The patient should exhibit immediate and obvious improvement in respiratory status including improved lung sounds and vital signs.
- o The procedure may be repeated if the patient is not improving.
- o Excess pleural air may be aspirated through the angiocatheter with a syringe.
- **Obtain a chest radiograph to confirm success.**
- o Repeat in 6 h.
- Because needle decompression is only a temporizing measure, **tube thoracostomy** must be performed for definitive management of the pneumothorax.

COMPLICATIONS
- Failure to resolve the tension pneumothorax.
- Obese or muscular patients may require a longer needle and catheter to reach the pleural space or, alternatively, may require proceeding immediately to tube thoracostomy.
- Iatrogenic pneumothorax.
- Laceration of intercostal artery or nerve.
- Rapid re-expansion may result in the development of pulmonary edema.
- Infection.

II. CHEST TUBE THORACOSTOMY

- Tube thoracostomy is the most commonly performed surgical procedure in thoracic surgery.
- It is defined as insertion of a tube (chest tube) into the pleural cavity to drain air, blood, bile, pus, chyle or other fluids[284].

INDICATIONS
- Spontaneous pneumothorax
- Tension pneumothorax (or suspected)
- Iatrogenic pneumothorax
- Penetrating chest injuries
- Hemopneumothorax in acute trauma
- Patient in extremis with evidence of thoracic trauma
- Empyema/Chylothorax/hemothorax/
- Post-thoracic surgery
- Bronchopleural fistula

CONTRAINDICATIONS
- **Absolute:** Emergent thoracotomy
- **Relative**
  - Coagulopathy
  - Pulmonary bullae
  - Pulmonary, pleural, or thoracic adhesions
  - Loculated pleural effusion or empyema
  - Skin infection over the chest tube insertion site

COMPLICATIONS
- Improper placement for pneumothorax
- Tube dislodgment
- Pain, Bleeding, Infection,
- Damage to local structures,
- Empyema (TT introduces bacteria into the pleural space)
- Retained pneumothorax (may require second TT)
- Re-expansion pulmonary edema
- Subcutaneous emphysema

PRE-PROCEDURE
- **Written consent:** should be gained for Pain, failure of procedure, bleeding, infection, damage to surrounding structures and pneumothorax if the procedure is for an effusion.
- **Aseptic technique:** All drains should be inserted with full aseptic precautions (washed hands, gloves, gown, antiseptic preparation for the insertion site and adequate sterile field) in order to avoid wound site infection or secondary empyema.

- **Patient position:** The most commonly used position is with the patient lying at 45° with their arm raised behind the head to expose the axillary area or in a forward lean position. The procedure may also be performed with the patient lying on their side with the affected side uppermost.
- **Premedication/local anaesthetic**

LANDMARKS
- **The 5th intercostal space anterior to the mid-axillary line** for most situations.
- This area is commonly known as the **"safe triangle"**.
- Any other placement should be discussed with a senior clinician (apical pneumothorax), placement of a chest tube in the **2nd intercostal space** should be considered. A specific position may also be required for a loculated effusion.

TRIANGLE OF SAFETY (SAFE TRIANGLE)

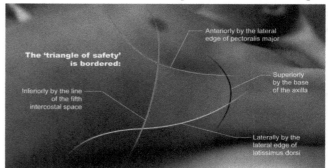

The 'triangle of safety' is bordered:

Anteriorly by the lateral edge of pectoralis major

Superiorly by the base of the axilla

Inferiorly by the line of the fifth intercostal space

Laterally by the lateral edge of latissimus dorsi

- The triangle of safety is an anatomical region in the **axilla** that forms a guide as to the safe position for intercostal catheter (ICC) placement.
- The 'safe triangle' is an anatomical area which is bounded by the lateral border of the pectoralis major anteriorly, the lateral border of the latissimus dorsi laterally, the line of the 5th intercostal space inferiorly and the base of the axilla superiorly[285].

POST INSERTION
- CXR
- Watch for complications:
  - **Not draining:** check for kinking
  - **Organ injury** (lung, liver, spleen, heart, vessel): careful insertion
  - **Blood loss:** careful observation
  - **Surgical emphysema:** small hole and good suturing
  - **Infection:** sterile technique

---

[284] Systematic approach to pneumothorax, haemothorax, pneumomediastinum and subcutaneous emphysema. Mattox KL, Allen MK Injury. 1986 Sep; 17(5):309-12.

[285] Havelock T., et al. "Pleural procedures and thoracic ultrasound: British Thoracic Society pleural disease guideline 2010". Thorax 65.2 (2010): ii61-eii76.

8. Chest Drain - Seldinger

INDICATIONS OF SELDINGER TECHNIQUES

o Angiography,
o Insertion of chest drains and central venous catheters,
o Insertion of PEG tubes using the push technique,
o Insertion of the leads for an artificial pacemaker or implantable cardioverter-defibrillator, and
o Numerous other interventional medical procedures.

COMPLICATIONS

o Hemorrhage: Puncture of the intercostal artery.
o Organ perforation
o Infection : non-aseptic technique.
o Inadequate "stay" suture allowing the chest tube to fall out.
o Tube blockage
o Pneumothorax if the procedure is for an effusion.

PROCEDURE

- **Consent the patient** for pain, failure of procedure, bleeding, infection, damage to surrounding structures and pneumothorax if the procedure is for an effusion.
- **Small-bore Seldinger chest drain insertion**
  o Ensure full aseptic conditions are maintained at all times; Perform surgical hand wash, don apron and sterile gloves.
  o Open pack keeping contents sterile, take additional equipment from assistant in a sterile fashion. Clean the skin using Antiseptic skin preparation such as Chlorhexidine. Apply sterile drape and Make a small incision (3-5 mm) in the skin where the drain is to be inserted
  o Using the needle and syringe in the pack gently insert (avoiding excess force) towards the upper border of the chosen rib aspirating continuously until air in the syringe confirms the position of the needle in the pleural cavity
- **Best Practice Statement**
  o Air or fluid must be aspirated before wire is inserted (stop and get help or arrange USS guidance if you cannot achieve this).
  o Both the needle and dilator should be inserted without force
- **Rationale:** Confirm correct position and minimise risk of damage to underlying structures
  o Hold the needle steady and remove the syringe.
  o Feed the wire gently through the needle into the pleural cavity

o Remove the needle leaving the guide-wire in place, make sure that the wire does not shear.
o Feed the first dilator down over the wire and into the pleural cavity. Repeat the process for the second dilator if present.
o Remove the dilator leaving the wire in place. Estimate the depth of insertion on the scale on the drain from the apex to the skin. Feed the 12F chest drain over the wire until it is in the pleural cavity to desired depth. Remove the wire making sure that the chest drain stays in position **DO NOT LET GO OF THE DRAIN NOW.**
o Attach the end of the drain onto the underwater seal system and make sure that the chest drain bottle is placed below the patient. Check that the water in the chest drain is bubbling or swinging, if in doubt ask the patient to cough gently. An adhesive dry dressing such as MEPORE is normally all that is required to secure the drain to the skin
o Remove the drape and Dispose of all waste and sharps appropriately

- Ultrasound guidance has been shown to detect fluid more accurately than by chest radiography, to decrease the incidence of failed aspirations and the incidence of complications, and to be significantly better than clinical examination in choosing a site for safe aspiration or drain insertion[286].

POST-PROCEDURE

o Place drain on free drainage but monitor closely
o **Analgesia**
o **Post procedure CXR**
o **Document procedure clearly** and document length of drain inserted
o **Respiratory review** and advise on onward management

IN THE EVENT OF FAILURE

o Stop procedure and Seek senior help
o Re-review imaging and patient with a senior colleague to ensure presence of fluid
o Consider further imaging or chest drain insertion in radiology.

---

[286] Diacon AH, Brutsche MH, Soler M. Accuracy of pleural puncture sites. A prospective comparison of clinical examination with ultrasound. Chest 2003;**123**:436–41.

9. Ascitic Tap-Paracentesis

- **Abdominal paracentesis** is a simple bedside or clinic procedure in which a needle is inserted into the peritoneal cavity and ascitic fluid is removed[287].
- **Diagnostic paracentesis** refers to the removal of a small quantity of fluid for testing.
- **Therapeutic paracentesis** refers to the removal of five liters or more of fluid to reduce intra-abdominal pressure and relieve the associated dyspnea, abdominal pain, and early satiety[288].

- **Causes of transudative ascites include the following:**
  - Heart failure
  - Hepatic cirrhosis
  - Alcoholic hepatitis
  - Fulminant hepatic failure
  - Portal vein thrombosis

- **Causes of exudative ascites include the following:**
  - Peritoneal carcinomatosis
  - Inflammation of the pancreas or biliary system
  - Nephrotic syndrome
  - Peritonitis
  - Ischemic or obstructed bowel

INDICATIONS
- **Diagnostic tap** is used for the following:
  - New-onset ascites - Fluid evaluation helps to determine aetiology, differentiate transudate versus exudate, detect the presence of cancerous cells, or address other considerations.
  - Suspected spontaneous or secondary bacterial peritonitis
- **Therapeutic tap** is used for the following:
  - Respiratory compromise secondary to ascites
  - Abdominal pain or pressure secondary to ascites (including abdominal compartment syndrome)

CONTRAINDICATIONS
- An acute abdomen that requires surgery
- Severe thrombocytopenia
- Coagulopathy
- Pregnancy

- Distended urinary bladder

---

287 Runyon BA. Ascites and spontaneous bacterial peritonitis. In: Sleisenger and Fordtran's Gastrointestinal and Liver Diseases, 8th edition, Feldman M, Friedman L, Brandt LJ (Eds), Elsevier, 2010. p.1517.

288 Runyon BA, AASLD Practice Guidelines Committee. Management of adult patients with ascites due to cirrhosis: an update. Hepatology 2009; 49:2087.

- Abdominal wall cellulitis
- Distended bowel
- Intra-abdominal adhesions

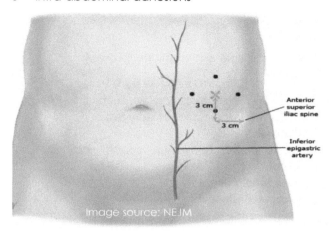

Image source: NEJM

COMPLICATIONS
- Persistent leakage from the needle insertion site
- Abdominal wall hematoma
- Bowel perforation
- Introduction of infection
- Hypotension (after a large-volume paracentesis)
- Dilutional hyponatremia
- Hepatorenal syndrome
- Bleeding
- Postparacentesis circulatory dysfunction

PRE-PROCEDURE
- **Consent patient and explain procedure:** Consent for infection, bleeding, pain, failure, damage to surrounding structures (especially bowel perforation – rare), leakage
- **Positioning:** Lie patient flat and examine clinically to confirm ascites. **Ultrasound** area for insertion
- **Define landmarks: Aim for 1/3 to ½ of the way between the anterior superior iliac spine and the umbilicus** avoiding vessels and scars.

PROCEDURE FOR ASCITIC TAP
- Position the patient supine in the bed with their head resting on a pillow.
- Select an appropriate point on the abdominal wall in the right or left lower quadrant, lateral to the rectus sheath.
- If a suitable site cannot be found with palpation and percussion consider using ultrasound to mark a spot.
- Clean the site and surrounding area with 2% Chlorhexidine and apply a sterile drape.

- Anaesthetise the skin with Lidocaine using the orange needle.
- Anaesthetise deeper tissues using the green needle, aspirating as you insert the needle to ensure you are not in a vessel before infiltrating with lidocaine.
- Use a maximum of 10mls of Lidocaine.
- Take a clean green needle and 20ml syringe and insert through the skin advancing and aspirating until fluid is withdrawn
- Aspirate 20ml,
- Remove needle and apply sterile dressing

TECHNICAL CONSIDERATIONS

- Depending on the clinical situation, fluid may be sent for the following laboratory tests:
  o **Gram stain**
  o **Cell count** (elevated counts may suggest infection)
  o **Bacterial culture**
  o **Total protein level**
  o **Triglyceride levels** (elevated in chylous ascites)
  o **Bilirubin level** (may be elevated in bowel perforation)
  o **Glucose level**
  o **Albumin level,** used in conjunction with serum albumin levels obtained the same day (used to calculate SAAG; see the Ascites Albumin Gradient calculator)
  o **Amylase level** (elevation = pancreatic source)
  o **Lactate dehydrogenase (LDH) level**
  o Cytology

SERUM-ASCITES ALBUMIN GRADIENT (SAAG)

o The serum-ascites albumin gradient (SAAG) can be used to identify the cause of the ascites.
o It is calculated by subtracting the albumin concentration in the Ascites from the albumin concentration in the serum.

SAAG = serum albumin – ascites albumin

o **A high gradient (>1.1 g/dL)** suggests portal hypertension.
o Such conditions may include the following:
  ▪ Cirrhosis, Fulminant hepatic failure
  ▪ Veno-occlusive disease
  ▪ Hepatic vein obstruction (i.e., Budd-Chiari syndrome)
  ▪ Congestive heart failure
  ▪ Nephrotic syndrome
  ▪ Protein-losing enteropathy
  ▪ Malnutrition, Myxedema, Ovarian tumors
  ▪ Pancreatic ascites, Biliary ascites, Malignancy
  ▪ Trauma, Portal hypertension

o **A low gradient (SAAG < 1.1 g/dL)** indicates nonportal hypertension and suggests a peritoneal cause of ascites. Such conditions may include the following:
  ▪ Primary peritoneal mesothelioma
  ▪ Secondary peritoneal carcinomatosis
  ▪ Tuberculous peritonitis
  ▪ Fungal and parasitic infections (eg, Candida, Histoplasma, Cryptococcus, Schistosoma mansoni, Strongyloides, Entamoeba histolytica)
  ▪ Sarcoidosis

PEARLS AND PITFALLS

o The preferred site of entry is in the midline of the abdomen, below the umbilicus.
o **Postparacentesis circulatory dysfunction (PPCD)** occurs secondary to hypovolemia after large-volume paracentesis (>4 L) in cirrhotic patients.
o It is associated with worsening hyponatremia, renal dysfunction, shorter time to ascites recurrence, and increased mortality.
o Prevention of PPCD has been demonstrated with the administration of **6–8 g of albumin per liter** of Ascites removed.
o Polymorphonuclear lymphocyte **(PMN) count greater than 250/mm³** is diagnostic of **spontaneous bacterial peritonitis.**

SPONTANEOUS BACTERIAL PERITONITIS

- Infection of ascitic fluid without intra-abdominal infection usually occurs in patients with chronic liver disease due to translocation of enteric bacteria. Common pathogens include:
  o Escherichia coli,
  o Klebsiella pneumoniae,
  o Enterococcal species, and
  o Streptococcus pneumoniae.
- Patients with renal failure who use abdominal peritoneal dialysis are also at increased risk, as are children with nephrosis or systemic lupus erythematosus.
- Anaerobic bacteria are not associated with spontaneous bacterial peritonitis (SBP).
- An ascitic fluid polymorphonuclear leukocyte (PMN) count > 250/µL (neutrocytic ascites), with the percentage of PMNs in the fluid usually greater than 50%, is presumptive evidence of SBP.
- Patients whose ascitic fluid meets these criteria should be treated empirically, regardless of symptoms.
- Secondary bacterial peritonitis is defined as infected ascitic fluid associated with an intra-abdominal infection.

10. Airway Protection
I. BAG-VALVE-MASK VENTILATION

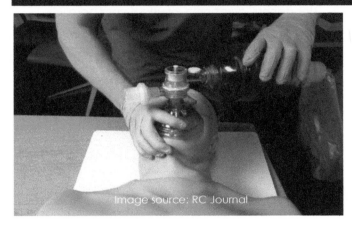

Image source: RC Journal

INDICATIONS
- Hypoxia
- Hypoventilation/apnea
- Rescue maneuver if failed intubation

CONTRAINDICATIONS
- **Absolute**
  o Inability to ventilate due to lack of seal (thick beard, deforming facial trauma)
  o Inability to ventilate secondary to complete upper airway obstruction
  o Active, adequate spontaneous ventilation
- **Relative**
  o Full stomach (aspiration risk)
  o After induction and paralysis during rapid sequence intubation (aspiration risk)

MATERIALS
- Bag valve mask (BVM) with reservoir
- Oxygen connector tubing
- Nasal pharyngeal airway/oral pharyngeal airway
- Lubricant jelly

PROCEDURE
- Position patient in "sniffing" position.
- Open the airway with chin-lift/head-tilt or jaw thrust maneuvers.
- Place airway adjuncts to maintain airway patency.
  o Use oral airway in unconscious patients.
  o Use nasal airway in semiresponsive patients.
- Attach oxygen tubing to high-flow oxygen (15 L/min).
- Place appropriately sized mask on patient's face covering the nose and mouth.

- **For one-handed technique,** use nondominant hand to make a **"C"** with index finger and thumb on top of the mask and form an **"E"** with the rest of the fingers using them to pull up on the mandible (**E–C technique**).
- Use the dominant hand to provide bag ventilations.
- **For two-handed,** two-person technique (preferred), make two semicircles with index fingers and thumbs of both hands-on top of the mask and use the rest of the fingers to pull up on the mandible.

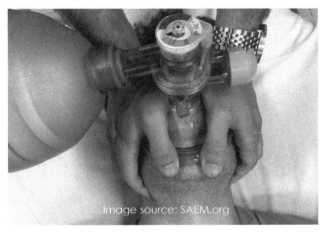

Image source: SAEM.org

- Consider the **Sellick maneuver (cricoid pressure)**[289] to compress the oesophagus against the cervical vertebrae, preventing gastric insufflation.
- Ventilate patient providing reduced tidal volume breaths (500 mL) at a rate of 10–12 breaths per minute.
- Give each breath gently over 1–1.5 s to avoid high peak pressures, avoiding gastric insufflation.
- Prepare for definitive airway as dictated by the clinical scenario.

COMPLICATIONS
- Stomach inflation may lead **to vomiting and aspiration**.
- Increased positive thoracic pressure may cause **decreased preload, worsening cardiac output, and/or hypotension**.
- **Hypoventilation** (inadequate O2 tidal volume, airway patency, or mask seal).

---

[289] *Sellick BA. Cricoid pressure to control regurgitation of stomach contents during induction of anaesthesia. Lancet 1961;2:404–6*

II. CRICOTHYROIDOTOMY

- Up to seven intubation attempts in 1000 end up in a **"can't intubate/can't ventilate"** situation in the emergency department.
- These are considered failed airways that may require a surgical airway to maintain ventilation and oxygenation.

INDICATIONS

- The emergency cricothyrotomy is the final step in the emergency airway management algorithm, becoming necessary when you find yourself in a **CICO scenario**. (Cannot Intubate, Cannot Oxygenate is also sometimes referred to as "Cannot Intubate, Cannot Ventilate")[290].
- Failure to recognize and intervene in a CICO scenario can rapidly lead to brain hypoxia and patient death. A percutaneous airway must be established immediately in a CICO scenario[291].
- The emergency cricothyrotomy is indicated in any CICO scenario. Some situations in which a physician may encounter CICO include[292]:
  - Oral or maxillofacial trauma
  - Cervical spine trauma
  - Profuse oral hemorrhage
  - Copious emesis
  - Anatomic abnormalities that prevent endotracheal intubation

CONTRAINDICATIONS

- Airway protection achievable using a less invasive strategy
- Tracheal transection
- The presence of laryngeal pathology[293] (e.g., tumor, fracture)
- Paediatric patients younger than 8 years
- Other relative contraindications to performing a cricothyroidotomy are:
  - Coagulopathy,
  - Massive neck swelling or Hematoma in the neck;
  - Distortion of the anatomy.
  - Unfamiliarity with the technique

---

290 Paix BR, Griggs WM. Emergency surgical cricothyroidotomy: 24 successful cases leading to a simple 'scalpel-finger-tube' method. Emerg Med Australas. 2012 Feb;24(1):23-30.

291 Hamaekers AE, Henderson JJ. Equipment and strategies for emergency tracheal access in the adult patient. Anaesthesia. 2011 Dec;66 Suppl 2:65-80.

292 Schroeder AA. Cricothyroidotomy: when, why, and why not? Am J Otolaryngol. 2000 May-Jun;21(3):195-201.

293 Kress TD, Balasubramaniam S. Cricothyroidotomy. Ann Emerg Med. 1982 Apr;11(4):197-201.

COMPLICATIONS

- Bleeding
- ETT misplacement (false passage, through the thyrohyoid membrane, unintentional tracheostomy)
- Hoarseness, dysphonia, or vocal cord paralysis
- Subglottic or laryngeal stenosis
- Damage to thyroid cartilage, cricoid cartilage, or tracheal rings
- Perforated esophagus
- Infection
- Aspiration

EQUIPMENT

- Yankauer suction
- Scalpel (preferably #20 blade)
- Gum elastic bougie
- Cuffed tracheostomy tube 6.0
- 10 cc syringe
- Securement device
- Ventilator and tubing

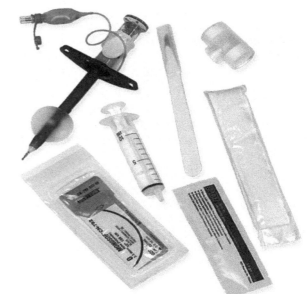

Image source: Medshop.Com

PROCEDURE

- Apply topical antiseptic.
- Remove the 15-mm ETT ventilator connector from the ETT end.
- Place copious Surgilube on the bougie and railroad over the end of the bougie.
- Palpate the thyroid notch, cricothyroid membrane, and hyoid bone for orientation.
- Stabilize the thyroid between the thumb and the middle finger of the nondominant hand.

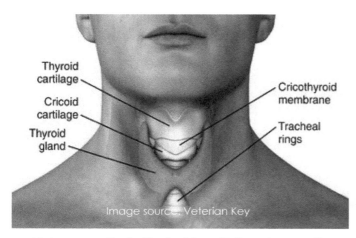

Image source: Veterian Key

- o Make a vertical skin incision (2–3 cm) over the cricothyroid membrane.
- o Palpate with the index finger to verify the cricothyroid membrane location.
- o Use stabilization of the thyroid and palpation to maintain orientation of the anatomy.

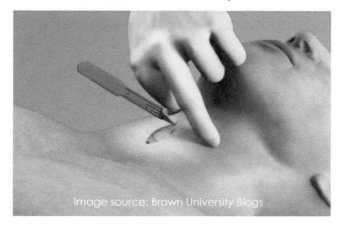

Image source: Brown University Blogs

- o Make a 1.5-cm horizontal incision through the lower half of the membrane.
- o Insert a tracheal hook into the incision, then rotate such that hook faces superiorly.
- o Withdraw at a 45° angle in a cephalad direction, applying gentle traction to the thyroid cartilage.

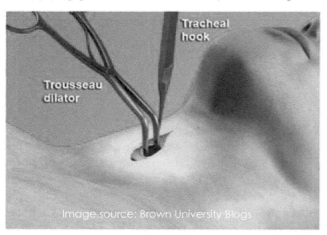

Image source: Brown University Blogs

- o Place the Trousseau dilator into the incision transversely and open the membrane incision vertically.
- o Insert a cuffed ETT (5.0–6.0) or TT (6.5–7.0) into the incision between the prongs of the dilator in the horizontal access.
- o Rotate both the dilator and the ETT toward the head of the patient and then direct the tube downward into the trachea while removing the dilator.

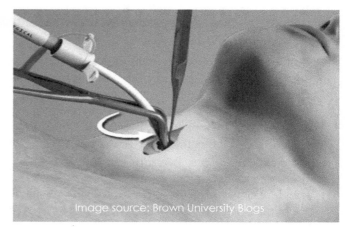

Image source: Brown University Blogs

- o Inflate the ETT cuff and ventilate the patient.
- o Verify the position of the ETT via auscultation, EtCO 2, and chest x-ray.
- o Once placement of the tube has been verified, the tracheal hook can be removed.
- o Secure the ETT.

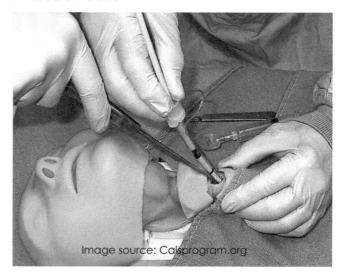

Image source: Calsprogram.org

11. Defibrillation & Cardioversion

I. UNSYNCHRONIZED CARDIOVERSION

INTRODUCTION[294]

- **Defibrillation** is the therapeutic use of electricity to depolarize the myocardium so coordinated contractions can occur. The term *defibrillation* is usually applied to an attempt to terminate a nonperfusing rhythm (e.g., ventricular fibrillation or pulseless ventricular tachycardia)
- **Cardioversion** is the application of electricity to terminate a still perfusing rhythm (e.g., ventricular tachycardia with a pulse, supraventricular tachycardias including atrial arrhythmias) to allow a normal sinus rhythm to restart.
- By this definition, cardioversion is a less urgent procedure compared to defibrillation, although the patient requiring cardioversion may be hypotensive or hemodynamically unstable, rather than in cardiac arrest.

⤷ *Unsynchronized cardioversion or defibrillation is the delivery of a high - energy shock as soon as the button is pushed on defibrillator. This means it can be delivered anywhere in the cardiac cycle. By contrast, synchronized cardioversion delivers a low-energy shock at the peak of the R wave in the cardiac (QRS) cycle.*

INDICATIONS

- Ventricular fibrillation (VF)
- Pulseless ventricular tachycardia (VT)
- Cardiac arrest due to or resulting from VF

CONTRAINDICATIONS

- **Absolute**
  - Conscious patient
  - Presence of a pulse
  - Pulseless electrical activity (PEA)
  - Asystole
  - Multifocal atrial tachycardia
  - Defibrillation without knowing the rhythm

  - A second Defibrillation before 2 min (or five cycles) of CPR,
  - Advanced Directive, Physician Order for Life-Sustaining Treatment (POLST) indicating no cardiopulmonary resuscitation (CPR) or do not resuscitate (DNR)
- **Relative**
  - Potential electrical catastrophe (explosive environment [i.e., operating rooms])
  - Dysrhythmias due to enhanced automaticity such as in digitalis toxicity and catecholamine-induced arrhythmia (because mechanism of tachycardia remains after the shock)
- **Factors that are not contraindications**
  - Pregnancy.
  - Chest trauma.
  - Automatic implantable cardiac defibrillators
  - The patient is on a wet or moist surface.
  - Piercings on the chest.

MATERIALS AND MEDICATIONS

- Electrocardiogram (ECG) monitor/defibrillator.
- Self-adhesive Defibrillation pads or Defibrillation paddles (paddles may be more successful than self-adhesive pads, but they have more complications and pose more danger to operators).
- Conductive gel for Defibrillation paddles (not ultra sound gel).
- ECG electrodes.
- Supplemental oxygen.
- Intubation equipment as needed

COMPLICATIONS

- **Skin burns** (most common and likely due to improper technique).
- **Injury to cardiac tissue** (myocardial necrosis secondary to burn): ST segment elevation that lasts longer than 2 min usually indicates myocardial injury unrelated to the shock.
- **Abnormal heart rhythms** (usually benign like atrial, ventricular, and junctional premature beats).

---

[294] *Tintinalli's Emergency Medicine: A Comprehensive Study Guide, 8e,* **Chapter 23: Defibrillation and Cardioversion by** *Marcus E. H. Ong; Swee Han Lim; Anantharaman Venkataraman*

Synchronised cardioversion[295]

- If the patient is conscious, carry out cardioversion under sedation or general anaesthesia.
- Ensure that the defibrillator is set to synchronised mode.
  - For a broad-complex tachycardia or atrial fibrillation, start with 120–150 J and increase in increments if this fails.
  - Atrial flutter and regular narrow-complex tachycardia will often be terminated by lower energies: start with 70–120 J.

	BROAD COMPLEX TACHYCARDIA	NARROW COMPLEX TACHYCARDIA
IRREGULAR	o AF with a BBB o Pre-excited AF o Torsade's de pointes	o Atrial Fibrillation o Atrial flutter with variable block o Multifocal Atrial Tachycardia
REGULAR	o VT o SVT with BBB o Sinus tachycardia with BBB o Atrial flutter with BBB	o Sinus tachycardia o Atrial Flutter o Re-entrant SVT

PROCEDURE

- Defibrillation should be promptly performed in conjunction with or before administration of induction or sedative agents to facilitate intubation.
- Assess the ABCs (airway, breathing, circulation).
- Open the airway with a head tilt/chin lift (or jaw thrust in a suspected traumatic patient). If the patient is apnoeic, provide breaths with a bag-valve-mask (BVM) and observe chest rise.
- Check for pulses. If absent, start CPR.
- CPR should be initiated before any shock while getting all equipment ready for at least 2 min to provide adequate circulation to the brain and heart. Wipe off the patient's chest if moist or wet.
- Remove transdermal patches, jewellery, and piercings if possible.
- Attach ECG electrodes to the patient.
- The self-adhesive Defibrillation pads or Defibrillation paddles can be used as ECG electrodes to access the rhythm.
- **Paddles:** With conductive gel applied to the metal surface, place one paddle on the patient's right chest, just below the clavicle, near the sternal border.

---

[295]https://www.resus.org.uk/resuscitation-guidelines/peri-arrest-arrhythmias/

- The other should be on the left chest, midaxillary line above the fifth or sixth intercostal space.
- The long axis of the paddles should be perpendicular to the ribs to allow for better transduction of current through the chest.

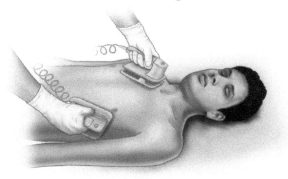

- **Pads:** Same placement as paddles except that pads can be placed in any orientation as long as they are in full contact with the chest.
- If a lot of breast tissue is present, push the tissue to one side or lift it away and place the paddles or pads underneath.
- An error in pad or paddle placement can distort the rhythm into looking like a rhythm that does not require defibrillation.
- Place the ECG monitor/defibrillator into a mode to acquire a rhythm from the pads or paddles.
- Stop CPR and assess the rhythm and pulse for no longer than 10 s.
- If VF or pulseless VT is observed, then switch the defibrillator to charge mode. Charge to **200 J.**
- Continue CPR while the defibrillator is being charged.
- When the defibrillator indicates that it is charged, clearly order that everyone stop touching the patient and observe that there is no physical contact before defibrillating the patient.
- If using the paddles, apply extra force to the chest through the paddles to deflate the lungs to allow for better defibrillation. The operator should observe a muscle twitch during defibrillation.
- Restart CPR for 2 min or five cycles.
- Another operator may charge (but not fire) the defibrillator while CPR is being performed to expedite the time between pulse/rhythm check and the initiation of a shock.
- After 2 min or five cycles of CPR, assess the rhythm and pulse and repeat steps above and give appropriate Advanced Cardiac Life Support (ACLS) medications.
- If successful return of spontaneous circulation (ROSC) occurs, initiate the hypothermia protocol per hospital guidelines.

II. SYNCHRONIZED ELECTRICAL CARDIOVERSION

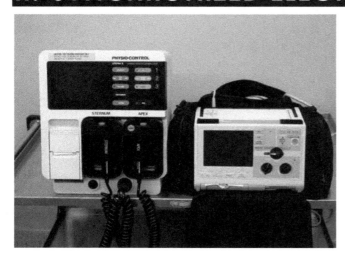

- Tachycardia is defined as >100 beats per minute

INDICATIONS
- Non-sinus-rhythm tachycardias with a pulse including:
  - Atrial fibrillation
  - Atrial flutter
  - Monomorphic ventricular tachycardia (VT)
  - Refractory or unstable supraventricular tachycardia (SVT)
- Unstable signs and symptoms including acute coronary syndrome, decreased level of consciousness, chest pain, dyspnea, pulmonary edema, and hypotension

CONTRAINDICATIONS
- **Absolute**
  - Ventricular fibrillation and pulseless or polymorphic (irregular) VT require unsynchronized electrical cardioversion (defibrillation), not synchronized cardioversion.
  - Known atrial thrombus.
  - Sinus tachycardia.

- **Relative**
  - Digitalis toxicity-related tachycardia
  - Atrial fibrillation of greater than 48 h duration without anticoagulation
  - Multifocal atrial tachycardia
  - Electrolyte abnormalities
  - Left atrial diameter greater than 4.5 cm
  - Patients with low probability of maintaining sinus rhythm and readily return to atrial fibrillation
  - Patients with sick sinus syndrome or sinoatrial blockage who will require a pacemaker for maintenance of stable rhythm

MATERIALS AND MEDICATIONS
- Airway management equipment (laryngoscopes, endotracheal tubes)
- Cardiac monitoring, pulse oximetry, end-tidal CO_2 monitoring
- Cardioverter/defibrillator
- Sedation and analgesic medications

PROCEDURE
- Obtain a 12-lead ECG and intravenous (IV) access.
- If possible, correct underlying electrolyte abnormalities that may cause or contribute to the patient's arrhythmia.
- Discuss risks, benefits, and alternatives (including pharmacological cardioversion) with the patient and obtain consent.
- Prepare airway equipment and Advanced Cardiac Life Support (ACLS) code drugs.
- Consider IV sedation (e.g., propofol, midazolam).
- Provide IV analgesia (e.g., fentanyl, morphine).
- Place defibrillator adhesive pads (8- to 12-cm diameter in adults) or paddles on the patient. Paediatric-sized pads/paddles should be used if the patient is less than 10 kg.
- The first paddle/pad is placed to **the right of the sternum** at the second/third intercostal space.
- The second paddle/pad can be placed in one of two equally efficacious positions:
  - **Anterolateral position**—left fourth/fifth intercostals space in the midaxillary line.
  - **Anteroposterior position**—between the spine and the edge of the left scapula.

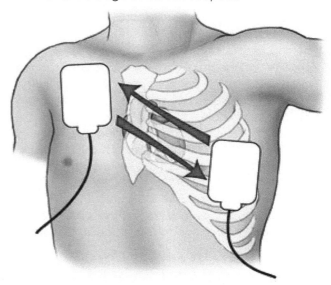

Anterolateral pad placement – Source: Nurse Key

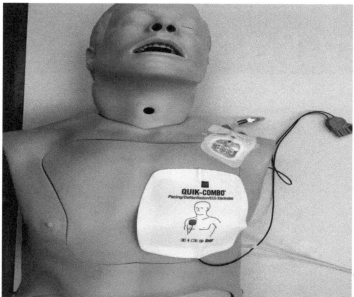

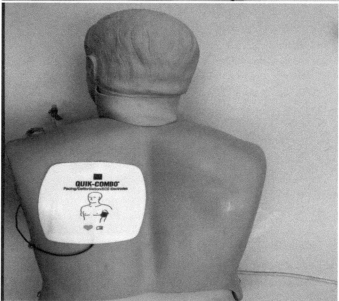

Anteroposterior pad placement – Source: SAEM

- Turn the defibrillator/cardioverter into synchronized mode—marker above R-waves will be present.
- Select the energy level to be delivered based on the underlying rhythm.

  - ↓ **Regular VT (with pulses)—Adults**: 100 J (monophasic or biphasic), 200 J for subsequent shocks
  - ↓ **Atrial fibrillation**—120–200 J (biphasic), 200 J (monophasic), 360 J for subsequent shocks
  - ↓ **Atrial flutter and paroxysmal SVT**—50–100 J (biphasic), 100 J for subsequent shocks
  - ↓ **Paediatric dosage** (regular and pulsed VT or SVT)—0.5–1 J/kg, up to 2 J/kg for subsequent shocks.

- Announce that you are going to deliver the shock on the count of three, and ensure that everyone is clear of the patient.
- Deliver the shock by pressing button marked "SHOCK."
- If using paddles, apply firm pressure and keep paddles in place until shock is delivered.
- Reassess the patient's pulse and cardiac rhythm.
- Repeat with escalating energy in a stepwise fashion if cardioversion is unsuccessful.

COMPLICATIONS

- **Superficial burns** if there is inadequate gel.
- **Induced arrhythmias** (bradycardia in patients with previous inferior myocardial infarction, atrioventricular block, VT, ventricular fibrillation, asystole).
- Improperly synched cardioversion may rarely induce **ventricular fibrillation**.
  - o Ectopy of the atria or ventricle in first 30 min after cardioversion
  - o Atrial clot embolization in patients without adequate anticoagulation
- Apnea, hypoxia, hypercarbia, or hypotension may occur from sedation/analgesia.
- Medical professionals who incidentally touch the patient during shock delivery may be shocked or burned.
- Rarely, fire has occurred as a consequence of poor pad placement and a hyperoxygenated environment

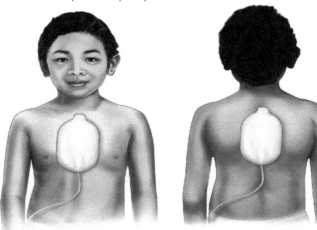

Paediatric pad placement - Source: Link.springer.com

12. Temporary Pacemakers

INTRODUCTION

- There are two types of artificial pacemaker: Temporary and Permanent.
  - **Permanent (epicardial) pacemakers** are implanted by means of a surgical procedure and are used to treat permanent conduction problems.
  - **Temporary pacemakers** are used in emergency situations for transient conduction disturbances or prophylactically for anticipated dysrhythmias.
    - Temporary pacemakers may be **invasive** (transvenous) or **non-invasive** (transthoracic).
    - Temporary non-invasive pacemakers are typically available to clinicians as part of a cardiac resuscitation system, complete with defibrillation, cardioversion and monitoring capabilities.

USES

- Life-threatening or unstable bradyarrhythmia[296]

DESCRIPTION

3 types of pacing equipment:

1. Semi-rigid, bipolar pacing lead (under II guidance)
2. Paceport PA catheter
3. Balloon flotation leads (ECG or pressure guided)

METHOD OF INSERTION AND/OR USE

(1) Flotation Catheter

Can be inserted by ECG guidance as follows:

- Connect pacing wire to pacing box (black to negative, red to positive)
- Set to demand
- Check box and batteries are OK
- Turn rate to 30 bpm greater than intrinsic rate
- Set output to 4mA
- Insert wire to 15-20cm
- Inflate balloon
- Advance observing ECG for changes in ECG morphology and capture of pacing rate (if using II direct wire to RV apex)
- Approximate depth 35-40cm
- Once pacing captured deflate balloon and decrease mA to find threshold and double.
- Get patient to cough to check that wire doesn't dislodge.
- Tape wire securely so it doesn't move

(2) Semi-rigid wire

- Insert under II guidance until leads up against right ventricular wall
- Connect to control box
- Set output and sense to minimum and to an appropriate rate
- Gradually increase output until capture takes place (ideal capture @ 2mA)

(3) Paceport on PA

- Insert PAC
- Attach pressure transducer to RV port to ensure in RV
- Attach adaptor to TV port and insert probe to the reference mark
- Attach ECG monitoring and advance until ST elevation indicates contact with epicardium
- Secure and connect side port to a saline flush
- Commence pacing

COMPLICATIONS

- arrhythmia
- microshock
- CVL insertion complications
- myocardial perforation
- infection

TEMPORARY PACEMAKER TROUBLESHOOTING [297]

OVERVIEW

Problems with pacing:

- Output failure
- Failure to capture

Problems with sensing:

- Oversensing
- Undersensing

Pacemaker syndromes:

- Cross-talk
- Pacemaker syndrome
- Pacemaker-mediated tachycardia
- Sensor-induced tachycardia
- Runaway pacemaker
- Lead displacement dysrhythmia
- Twiddler's syndrome

---

[296] *Life In Th fast Lane: Temporary Transvenous Cardiac Pacing, by Dr Chris Nickson, last update April 23, 2019*

[297] *Life In Th fast Lane: Temporary Pacemaker Troubleshooting, by Dr Chris Nickson, last update March 25, 2019*

GENERAL MANAGEMENT[298]

- **Review rhythm strip and 12 lead ECG**
- **Check integrity of circuit** (start at patient -> pacing box): lead placement, polarity, integrity, tightly connected to correct port of pacing box (atrial/ventricular), battery, settings
- **Check mode**
- **Check rate**
- **Check capture threshold** (find threshold and double it for safety)
- **Check sensitivity** (normal = 2-5mV) – changes with position
- **Fixes:** change patient position, reverse bipolar pacing leads, convert to unipolar pacing, replace pacing equipment, return to OT for reinsertion of epicardial wires
- **Back up plan in emergency:** transcutaneous or tranvenous pacing, atropine, adrenaline, isoprenaline, ephedrine, electrolyte correction

FAILURE TO PACE DUE TO OUTPUT FAILURE

- No electrical output at the pacing wire tips (pacing spikes absent on ECG)
- **Causes:**
  - Lead malfunction,
  - Unstable connection,
  - Insufficient power,
  - Cross-talk inhibition,
  - Oversensing (see below),
  - Apparent failure to pace
- **Approach:**
  - Check power, battery and connections
  - Increase output to maximum (20mA atrial and 25mA ventricular)
  - Switch to an asynchronous mode to prevent oversensing (AOO, VOO)
  - Connect the pacemaker directly to the pacing lead (occasionally the connecting wires may be faulty)
  - Prepare for transcutaneous pacing
  - Prepare for cpr and chronotropic drugs

FAILURE TO CAPTURE

- Visible pacing spikes are seen on ECG but no electrical capture on ECG or cardiac contraction seen in arterial line or SpO2 waveform
- Usually due to some specific mechanical problem (wires no longer connected to heart, wires not tightly connected to cable, cable not connected to correct port, output setting to low)

- **Other causes:**
  - Fibrosis at wire-myocardium interface,
  - MI,
  - Electrolyte imbalance,
  - Post-defibrillation,
  - Drugs (Flecanide, Sotalol, Betablockers, Lignocaine, Verapamil)
- **Approach:**
  - Correct exacerbating causes
  - Tight and confirm all external connections
  - Increase output if possible
  - Bipolar leads may be tried in reverse positions or can try convert to unipolar pacing
  - In bipolar leads, the negative electrodes develop fibrosis first -> use other electrode and plug into negative terminal and insert return electrode in the subcutaneous tissue (create unipolar circuit)
  - May need temporary transvenous wire

FAILURE TO SENSE

- Produces atrial pacing when not appropriate
- Due to specific setting of sensitivity (including AOO mode)
  - Same mechanisms as failure to capture and pace
  - Decrease absolute value of sensitivity (making it easier to inhibit)

OVERSENSING

- Oversensing occurs when electrical signal are inappropriately recognised as native cardiac activity and pacing is inhibited
- Produces inappropriate/excessive inhibition of atrial pacing -> confuses pacemaker into thinking that there has been a return to spontaneous atrial activity
- These inappropriate signals may be large P or T waves, skeletal muscle activity or lead contact problems
- Abnormal signals may not be evident on ECG
- Reduced pacemaker output / output failure may be seen on ECG monitoring if the patient contracts their rectus or pectoral muscles (due to oversensing of muscle activity)
- Usually due to settings on the pacemaker
  - Increase absolute value of sensitivity (making it harder to inhibit)
  - In DDD external electrical impulses can also be misinterpreted as atrial activity causing pacemaker mediated tachycardia
  - Increase sensitivity threshold or switch to an asynchronous mode (AOO, VOO).

---

[298] *Life In Th fast Lane: Temporary Pacemaker Troubleshooting, by Dr Chris Nickson, last update March 25, 2019*

CROSS TALK

- In dual chamber pacing it is possible that the atrial pacemaker spike will be sensed by the ventricular wire and is misinterpreted as a ventricular depolarisation - Inhibits ventricular pacemaker output (ventricular standstill)
- The opposite can happen as well
  - Reduce sensitivity in atrial or ventricular channel
  - Reduce mA delivered to the ventricular or pacing wire

PACEMAKER MEDIATED TACHYCARDIA[299]

- Also known as endless-loop tachycardia or pacemaker circus movement tachycardia
- VDD or DDD pacing problem
- Can switch to VVI or DVI (but may lose AV synchrony)
- **Mechanisms:**
  (1) atrial sensing of a ventricular spike
  - Interpreted as an endogenous atrial depolarisation
  - Another ventricular impulse- Use an atrial blanking period (now preset into box)
  (2) retrograde conduction between ventricle and atrium through AV node or accessory pathway
  - Retrograde p waves being sensed as native atrial activity with subsequent ventricular pacing
  - Paced ventricular complex results in further retrograde conduction with retrograde p wave generation
  - 'Endless' loop of periodicity
  - Re-entry tachycardia
    - Adjustable post ventricular (pacing spike) atrial refractory period (PVARP) or slowing AV conduction e.g. adenosine or activation of magnet mode.
- Results in a paced tachycardia with the maximum rate limited by the pacemaker programming
- Newer pacemakers contain programmed algorithms designed to terminate PMT. May result in rate-related ischaemia in the presence of IHD

PACEMAKER SYNDROME

- Caused by improper timing of atrial and ventricular contractions resulting in AV dyssynchrony and loss of atrial "kick"
- Variety of clinical symptoms including fatigue, dizziness, palpations, pre-syncope
- Associated decrease in systolic blood pressure > 20 mmHg during change from native rhythm to paced rhythm

TWIDDLER'S SYNDROME

- Patient manipulation of the pulse generator (accidentally or deliberately)
- The pacemaker rotates on its long axis, resulting in dislodgement of pacing leads
- Can result in diaphragmatic or brachial plexus pacing (e.g. arm twitching) depending on extent of lead migration

LEAD DISPLACEMENT DYSRHYTHMIA

- A dislodged pacing wire may float around inside the right ventricle intermittently "tickling" the myocardium and causing ventricular ectopics or runs of VT alternating with failure of capture.
- If the paced QRS morphology changes from a LBBB pattern (indicating RV placement) to a RBBB pattern (indicating LV placement), this suggests that the electrode has eroded through the interventricular septum. A chest x-ray will usually help to confirm the diagnosis.

RUNAWAY PACEMAKER[300]

- This potentially life-threatening malfunction of older-generation pacemakers is related to low battery voltage (e.g. overdue pacemaker replacement)
- The pacemaker delivers paroxysms of pacing spikes at 2000 bpm, which may provoke ventricular fibrillation
- Paradoxically, there may be failure to capture — causing bradycardia — because the pacing spikes are very low in amplitude (due to the depleted battery voltage) and because at very high rates the ventricle may become refractory to stimulation
- Application of a magnet can be life saving but definitive treatment requires replacement of the pacemaker

SENSOR INDUCED TACHYCARDIA

- Modern pacemakers are programmed to allow increased heart rates in response to physiological stimuli such as exercise, tachypnoea, hypercapnia or acidaemia
- Sensors may "misfire" in the presence of distracting stimuli such as vibrations, loud noises, fever, limb movement, hyperventilation or electrocautery (e.g. during surgery). This misfiring leads to pacing at an inappropriately fast rate
- The ventricular rate cannot exceed the pacemaker's upper rate limit (usually 160-180 bpm)
- These will also usually terminate with application of a magnet

---

[299] *Life In Th fast Lane: Temporary Pacemaker Troubleshooting, by Dr Chris Nickson, last update March 25, 2019*

[300] *Life In Th fast Lane: Temporary Pacemaker Troubleshooting, by Dr Chris Nickson, last update March 25, 2019*

13. Large Joint Examination
I. KNEE CLINICAL EXAMINATION

- **Inspection:**
  - Observe both knees together. Note any asymmetry of the joint or quadriceps muscles.
  - Ask patient to lie supine. Whenever possible, ensure patient can lie comfortably with head back, legs straight, and toes up

- **Assess temperature** by placing back of hand to shin then ipsilateral knee, repeated for both legs.
  - Commonly, the knee will feel cooler than the shin.
  - If knee feels warmer than shin, suspect inflammation.
  - Try the "crossover test" with one hand on one knee and one on the other knee. Decide if there's a temperature difference. Next, cross the hands to test the opposite knee. If there's a temperature difference, it will be exagerated by this maneuver.

- **Assess for fluid**
  - Method 1: Gently press just medial of the patella, then move the hand in an ascending motion. Then press firmly on the lateral aspect of the knee.
    - Commonly, no fluid will be appreciated.
    - A medial aspect that 'bulges' out after lateral pressure (positive "bulge sign") is consistent with a moderate amount of fluid.
    - A medial aspect that does not bulge but tensely reflects lateral pressure is consistent with a large amount of fluid.
  - Method 2: Assess for fluid by placing one hand superior to the patella and with slight downward pressure milk the suprapatellar pouch which emptys into the knee joint. Next use the other hand to push to push on the patella. If there is an effusion, the patellar will bounce off the underlying bone (patella tap test).
    - A palpated or audible tap indicates a "ballotable" knee and is consistent with at least a moderate amount of fluid.

- **Assess for tendon pathology** by firmly palpating the superior pole of the patella and then the inferior to assess patellar femoral syndrome.
  - Tenderness at the *superior* insertion is consistent with quadriceps tendon pathology.
  - Tenderness at the *inferior* insertion is consistent with patellar tendonitis, "Jumpers knee."
    - In the patient with direct patellar trauma & isolated patellar tenderness, an x-ray is indicated to evaluate for fracture.

- **Assess for cartilage pathology**
  - Apley's grind test (patellar cartilage tear): By placing palm on patella and applying firm pressure while manipulating the patella in the sagittal plane. Crepitus is significant only when accompanied by tenderness, in which case it is consistent with patellar cartilage pathology.
  - McMurray test (meniscus cartilage tear):
    - Lateral meniscus tear: With patient supine, fully flex the knee, place forefingers on lateral side of joint line, then with applying valgus stress and internal rotation of leg, extend the knee looking for <u>both</u> pop/click and pain
    - Medial meniscus tear: With patient supine, fully flex the knee, place forefingers on medial side of joint line, then with applying varus stress and external rotation of leg, extend the knee looking for <u>both</u> pop/click and pain[301].

- **Assess for laxity**
  - While supine, ask patent to flex knee and set foot on examination table. Sit on the foot to immobilize it and grasp the head of the tibia with both hands and pull anteriorly.
    - Movement greater than 1cm (positive anterior drawer sign) is consistent with an anterior cruciate ligament (ACL) tear.
    - Do not attempt to elicit an anterior drawer sign with legs hanging; the extra degree of freedom will confound any findings.
    - Lachman test: flex the knee only 20-30 degrees (rather than 90 degrees in anterior drawer sign), then attempt to pull tibia anterior relative to the femur. If positive, a deficient ACL will demonstrate increase movement forward. This test is thought to be more sensitive than the anterior drawer sign.
  - Attempt to hyperextend knee by placing one hand superior to the patella and the other posterior to the heel. More than 2-3cm (i.e. able to place one or two fingers beneath the heel when leg is extended and flat) is abnormal.
  - With both hands, flex and extend the knee. Repeat while introducing medial and lateral rotation. Determine if any "locking" or "catching" is present. With leg straight, apply valgus stress and varus stress to text deviation greater than a few centimeters.

---

[301] *Introduction to the Knee Exam by Mark Genovese. Available at* https://stanfordmedicine25.stanford.edu/the25/knee.html

1. PATELLOFEMORAL ASSESSMENT

o An evaluation for effusion should be conducted with the patient supine and the injured knee in extension. **The suprapatellar pouch** should be milked to determine whether an **effusion** is present.

o Patellofemoral tracking is assessed by observing the patella for smooth motion while the patient contracts the quadriceps muscle. The presence of crepitus should be noted during palpation of the patella.

A. PATELLAR APPREHENSION TEST

o With fingers placed at the medial aspect of the patella, the physician attempts to sublux the patella laterally. If this manoeuvre reproduces the patient's pain or a giving-way sensation, **patellar subluxation** is the likely cause of the patient's symptoms.

o Both the superior and inferior patellar facets should be palpated, with the patella subluxed first medially and then laterally.

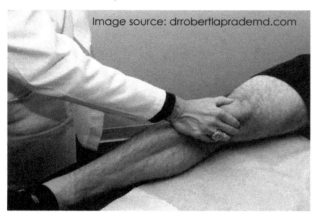

Image source: drrobertlaprademd.com

2. ANTERIOR CRUCIATE LIGAMENT

A. ANTERIOR DRAWER

o **Description**
  ▪ The Anterior Drawer test examines for **any tearing or laxity of the ACL ligament.**

o **Manoeuvre**
  ▪ Have the patient lying on their back with their knee bent as close to 90° as possible, with the foot resting on the table.
  ▪ Place both hands behind tibia and pull the tibia forward, using a force between 15-20 lbs.
  ▪ The test can also be performed with the foot externally rotated (turned out) to 15°.

o **Positive Findings**
  ▪ **Increased anterior movement of the tibia** on the injured side compared to the non-injured side is considered to be a positive test.
  ▪ Up to 3 mm of forward movement of the tibia is considered normal.

▪ The Grading: **Grade 1 = 5 mm, Grade 2 = 5 to 10 mm, Grade 3 > 10 mm.**

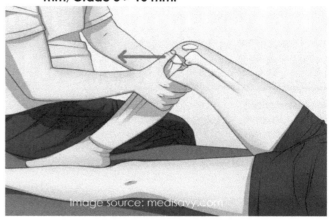

Image source: medisavy.com

B. THE LACHMAN TEST

o It is another means of assessing the integrity of the anterior cruciate ligament.

o The test is performed with the patient in a supine position and the injured knee flexed to 30 degrees.

o The physician stabilizes the distal femur with one hand, grasps the proximal tibia in the other hand, and then attempts to sublux the tibia anteriorly.

o **Lack of a clear end point** indicates a positive Lachman test.

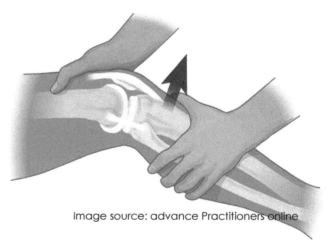

Image source: advance Practitioners online

3. POSTERIOR CRUCIATE LIGAMENT

A. POSTERIOR DRAWER

o **Description:**
  ▪ The posterior drawer test is used to **examine the Posterior Cruciate Ligament (PCL).**

o **Manoeuvre**
  ▪ Have the patient lying on their back with their knee bent as close to 90° as possible with their foot resting on the table.
  ▪ Place both hands behind the tibia, and push backwards on the proximal shin/tibia looking for instability backwards. Use a force between 15-20 lbs.

o **Positive Findings**
  ▪ Upon application of a posterior force to the upper shin, an increase in backwards motion in comparison to the other side is indicative of a positive test.

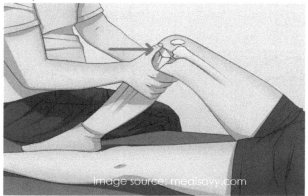
Image source: medisavy.com

4. MEDIAL & LATERAL COLLATERAL LIGAMENTS

A. VALGUS STRESS TEST
o **Description**
  ▪ The valgus stress test **checks for medial joint laxity**, which usually represents an injury to the **medial collateral ligament (MCL)**.
o **Manoeuvre**
  ▪ Have patient lie on their back. Position one hand at the joint line on the outer part of the knee. Have the other hand fixed on the ankle of the affected side.
  ▪ Flex the knee between 20° and 30° and apply a **medial or valgus** force to the knee.
  ▪ In order to test the MCL, as well as the posterior medial capsule, the test can be repeated at 0° with the knee in full extension.

o **Positive Findings**
  ▪ A positive test demonstrates **increased medial joint laxity** compared to the unaffected side.
  ▪ Grading system: **Grade 1= 5mm, Grade 2= 5 to 10mm, Grade 3= >10 mm.**

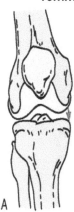
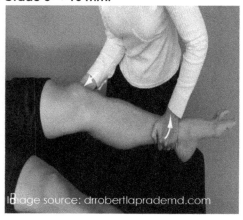
Image source: drrobertlaprademd.com

B. VARUS STRESS TEST
o **Description**
  ▪ The varus stress test checks for joint laxity on the outside of the knee, which usually represents an injury to the **lateral collateral ligament (LCL).**
o **Manoeuvre**
  ▪ With the patient lying on their back, position one hand at the joint line on the outer part of the knee.
  ▪ Fix the other hand on the ankle of the affected side.
  ▪ Flex the knee between 20° and 30° and apply a **lateral or varus** force to the knee.
  ▪ This can be done either by reaching over the top of the knee, or by approaching the patient from the inside aspect of the knee with the leg off to the side.
  ▪ The test can also be repeated at 0° with the knee in full extension.

o **Positive Findings**
  ▪ A positive test demonstrates **increased lateral joint laxity** compared to the unaffected side.
  ▪ Grading system: **Grade 1= 5mm, Grade 2= 5 to 10mm, Grade 3= >10 mm.**

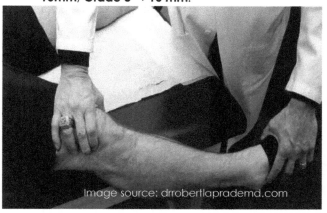
Image source: drrobertlaprademd.com

5. MENISCI

A. MCMURRAY'S TEST
o **Description**
  ▪ This test checks for **meniscal tears** and other internal derangement in the knee.
o **Manoeuvre**
  ▪ With the patient supine, and their hip and knee bent to 90°, grasp the heel in one hand.
  ▪ Place the other hand over the knee, with the thumb and fingers on the joint line.
  ▪ Gently rotate the tibia with the heel internally rotated with a mild valgus force (for the lateral compartment) and externally rotated with a mild varus force (for the medial compartment).

- o **Positive Findings**
  - ▪ **Painful clicking along the joint line**, or **any pain over the joint line** that reproduces the patient's symptoms is considered to be a positive test.

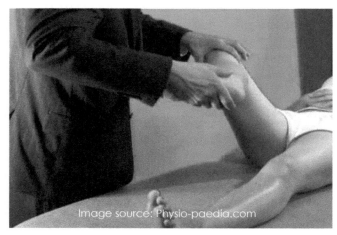

Image source: Physio-paedia.com

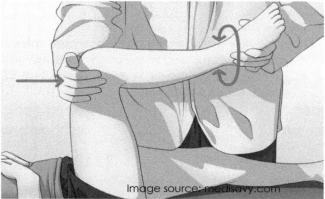

Image source: medisavy.com

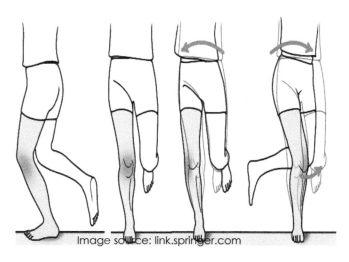

Image source: link.springer.com

- o **Positive Findings**
  - ▪ The twisting movement will reproduce pain of a meniscal injury.
  - ▪ The pain is typically localized to joint line, and patients typically have more pain with the knee bent at 20° rather than 5°.

B. THESSALY'S TEST
- o **Description**
  - ▪ This functionally tests **meniscus tears in the standing position**.
  - ▪ Since bending and twisting movements while weight bearing often reproduce pain from meniscus tears, this test recreates the exacerbating movements.
- o **Manoeuvre**
  - ▪ Have the patient stand on one foot with the foot flat on the floor.
  - ▪ Hold the patient's hand for support and have them initially bend on the standing knee to 5° of flexion.
  - ▪ Ask the patient to twist at the knee, making sure they are internally and externally rotating at the knee rather than at the pelvis or back.
  - ▪ Check for any reproduction of pain symptoms.
  - ▪ Next, have the patient bend the knee deeper to 20°degrees and again actively twists on knee.

II. SHOULDER PHYSICAL EXAMINATION

EXAMINATION

o Inquire about the patient's hand dominance, as well as their occupation and recreational activities. Establish their chief complaint: pain, instability, weakness, or loss of range of motion.

o Establish an approximate

o timeline for when the injury occurred and what event or mechanism, if any, lead to the injury or onset of symptoms.

o For patients who report a dislocation, it should be asked what position the arm was in at the time of the dislocation, and what the frequency of dislocations or subluxations were. Establish what type of activities of daily living the patient can and cannot perform. Such activities include simple everyday tasks like getting dressed, lifting an object overhead, sleeping on the shoulder, brushing your teeth, combing your hair, putting on shoes, and carrying or lifting objects like groceries.

PALPATION

o Bony structures to palpate should include: the sternoclavicular joint, the clavicle, the acromioclaviular joint, the coracoid process, the borders of the scapula, and the greater and lesser tuberosities of the humerus.

o Soft tissue landmarks should include: the subacromial bursae, the supraclavicular fossa, the long head of the biceps tendon, the trapezius, and other associated muscles and tendons.

RANGE OF MOTION

o **Active range of motion** performed by the patient is typically assessed first, and can be affected by both pain and motor function. The patient can be either seated or standing during the assessment, and movements to be tested should include forward flexion, extension, internal/external rotation, and abduction/adduction.

o **Passive range of motion** is performed by the clinician with the patient seated or supine in the same planes previously stated. This is used to isolate motion for an accurate evaluation of soft tissue.
  - Normal flexion: 0° to 170-180°
  - Normal extension is said to be 60°.
  - Normal internal rotation is said to be 90°
  - Normal external rotation is around 60-70°.
  - Normal adduction is typically 30°
  - Normal Abduction motion can range from 0° - 180°

o An example of limited passive range of motion can be seen in cases of frozen shoulder.

1. FROZEN SHOULDER: EXTERNAL ROTATION

o To improve range of motion, special exercises such as Codman's Pendulum can be performed to help relax the muscles around the shoulder, reduce pain, and increase motion.

A. CODMAN'S PENDULUM

o Have the patient standing in a relaxed position, and tell them to swing their weak arm in a circular motion while keeping their shoulder nice and relaxed.

o Be sure they swing their arm in both the clockwise and counter clockwise directions.

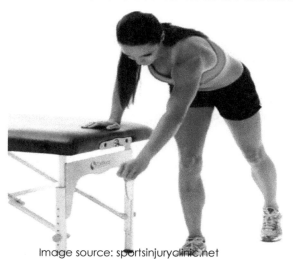

Image source: sportsinjuryclinic.net

2. ROTATOR CUFF STRENGTH TESTING:

+ *Supraspinatus:* abduction >>> Empty can test
+ *Subscapularis:* internal rotation >>> Lift-off test
+ *Infraspinatus and Teres minor:* external rotation >>> External rotation test

A. EMPTY CAN TEST

o **Description:** The empty can test is used to evaluate the strength and integrity of the **supraspinatus muscle and tendon**.

o **Manoeuvre:**
  - Have the patient stand with their shoulder abducted to 90° and horizontally adducted forward 30° with the thumbs pointing down towards the floor, as if they are pouring out a can.
  - Ask the patient to maintain this position.
  - Proceed to apply downward resistance to the patient's forearm.

- A variation of this test can be done at 30° abduction instead of 90°, where the supraspinatus should function in relative isolation.
  - o **Positive findings:** Decreased strength or pain on resisted testing.

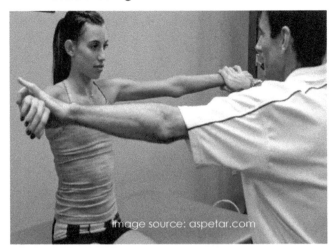

Image source: aspetar.com

B. EXTERNAL ROTATION

- o **Description:** The external rotation test examines the **strength of the infraspinatus and teres minor.**
- o **Manoeuvre:**
  - With the patient's arms at their side, externally rotated 45° and elbow flexed to 90°, the examiner applies an internal rotation moment to assess the strength of the external rotators.
- o **Positive Findings:** Decreased strength or pain on resisted testing. Significant weakness of the infraspinatus may be indicative of **suprascapular nerve palsy,** where the infraspinatus become denervated.
- o This can be due to trauma, ganglion cyst or illness.

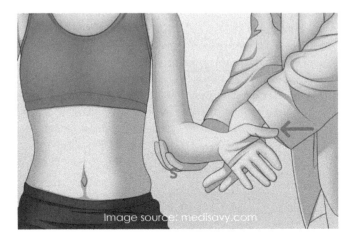

Image source: medisavy.com

C. LIFT-OFF TEST

- o **Description: The lift off test** evaluates the muscular strength of the **subscapularis.**
- o **Manoeuvre:** With the patient seated or standing, have them internally rotate their arm behind their back.
- o Then ask the patient to lift the back of their hand off their lower back.
- o If they are unable to complete this task, apply resistance to the palm to assess the strength of the subscapularis.
- o **Positive findings:** Inability to lift the dorsum of hand off the back.

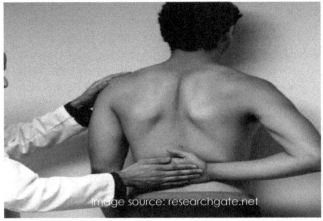

Image source: researchgate.net

3.   IMPINGEMENT/ROTATOR   CUFF SPECIAL TESTS:

A. NEER'S IMPINGEMENT

- o **Description:** The Neer impingement test assesses the presence of impingement of the rotator cuff, **primarily the supraspinatus,** as it passes under the subacromial arch during forward flexion.
- o **Manoeuvre:** Stabilize the scapula with one hand while applying passive forced flexion of the arm.
- o **Positive findings:** Pain in the anterior shoulder or reproduction of the patient's symptoms.

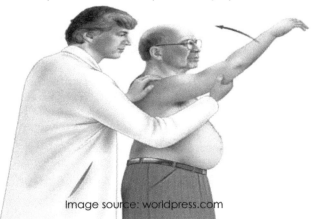

Image source: worldpress.com

B. HAWKIN'S KENNEDY IMPINGEMENT TEST

- o **Description:** The Hawkin's test is used to evaluate **impingement of rotator cuff and subacromial bursa.**
- o **Manoeuvre:** The patient is seated or standing and with their arm forward flexed to 90°and their elbow bent to 90°. Stabilize the top of the shoulder while internally rotating the arm at the forearm.
- o **Positive Findings:** Pain in the anterior shoulder or reproduction of the patient's symptoms with the test.

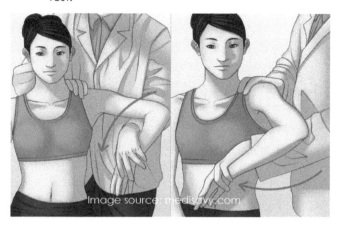

Image source: medisavy.com

4. INSTABILITY SPECIAL TESTS

A. LOAD AND SHIFT TEST

- o **Description:** The Load and Shift test **examines integrity of shoulder stability in the anterior and posterior directions.**
- o **Manoeuvre:** Have the patient seated or supine with their arm relaxed and resting at their side.
- o Grasp the head of the humerus with thumb and fingers and apply an anterior and posterior glide from the resting position.
- o **Positive Findings:** Excessive gliding of the humeral head is considered to be a positive test.

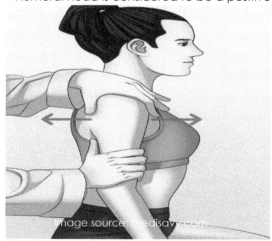

Image source: medisavy.com

B. APPREHENSION- RELOCATION TEST

- o **Description:**
  - **The apprehension test**, described by Row and Zarin, **tests for anterior instability of the shoulder.**
  - **The relocation test**, described by Jobe, is used in conjunction with the apprehension test to **distinguish between anterior instability and primary impingement of the shoulder.**
- o **Manoeuvre:**
  - To perform the apprehension test, have the **patient supine**, with their arm abducted and elbow flexed to 90°.
  - **Gently externally rotate the arm.**
  - Once the patient becomes apprehensive or complains of pain, proceed with the relocation and surprise test by applying a posterior force to the humeral head.
- o **Positive Findings:**
  - **For the apprehension test,** the patient may complain of pain or be apprehensive that their arm may dislocate as it is externally rotated.
  - **The relocation test** is positive if the symptoms of apprehension reduce, or if the clinician is able to externally rotate the shoulder further without any increase in pain or apprehension.
  - If the symptoms persist following the posterior directed force, the pain is associated with primary impingement and not anterior shoulder instability.

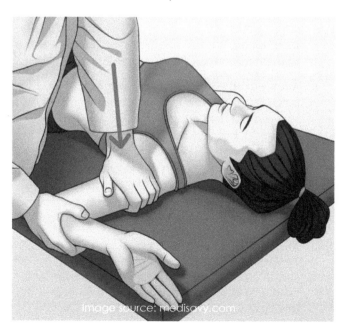

Image source: medisavy.com

C. SULCUS SIGN

- **Description:** The sulcus sign tests for **inferior instability caused by laxity of the inferior glenohumeral ligament complex.**

- **Manoeuvre:** Have the patient seated with their arm resting at their side. Grasp the patient's upper arm and apply a distal force to it.

- **Positive Findings:** Increased inferior movement of the humeral head or the visible development of a sulcus at the glenohumeral joint are positive findings.

- A positive test can often suggest that the patient has multidirectional instability, especially if there are other signs of join instability.

- The pain associated with labral tears is described as being deep in the shoulder.

- Pain situated over the acromioclavicular joint is associated with acromioclavicular joint pathology such as **osteoarthritis or a shoulder separation,** rather than labral pathology.

- Pain in the AC joint is usually equal with the palm down or the palm up.

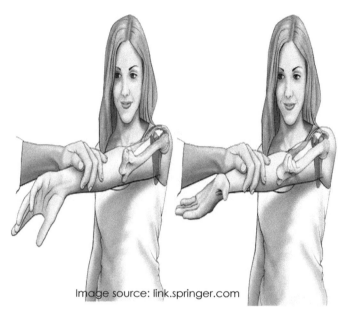

Image source: link.springer.com

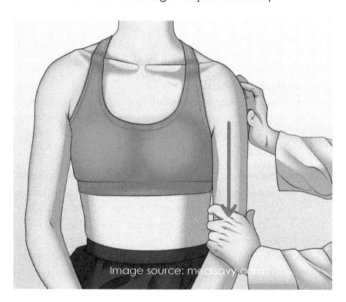

Image source: medisavy.com

5. LABRAL SPECIAL TESTS

A. O'BRIEN'S TEST

- **Description:** This test examines **the integrity of the glenoid labrum and the acromioclavicular joint.**

- **Manoeuvre:** With the patient seated or standing, instruct the patient to raise their arm into 90° of forward flexion with their elbow extended, and then adduct their arm 10-15°.

- Have the patient internally rotate their arm and point their thumb down to the ground.

- Apply a downward force to the arm.

- Then instruct the patient to externally rotate their arm and point their thumb towards the ceiling. Again, apply a downward force.

- **Positive Findings:** Positive findings for labral pathology occur when the first test reproduces pain, while the second test decreases or eliminates pain.

III. ANKLE PHYSICAL EXAMINATION

EXAMINATION

o Assessment of gait pattern, standing posture, and shoe wear pattern.

o Any obvious gross deformity, malalignment, or atrophy should also be observed and noted.

- **PALPATION**
  o Bony structures to palpate: shaft of tibia and fibula, traveling down the borders of both the medial and lateral malleoli. Palpation of the neck and dome of the talus should also be performed. This can be done by inverting and everting the foot, and palpating just anterior to the medial and lateral malleoli.

  o Soft tissue palpation should include all the ligamentous structures: the anterior talofibular ligament, the posterior talofibular ligament, the calcaneofibular ligament, the deltoid ligament complex, and the anterior tibiofibular syndesmosis.

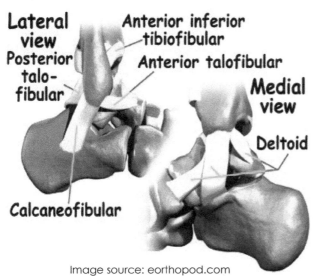

Image source: eorthopod.com

  o Palpation of the muscle tendons: The peroneus longus and brevis tendon can be palpated as **it passes posterior to the lateral malleolus and courses below the distal pole towards the base of the fifth metatarsal.**

  o On the medial aspect of the ankle, palpation of the posterior tibialis, flexor digitorum longus, and flexor hallucis longus can be done. These three tendons pass posterior to the medial malleolus.

  o Finally, along the anterior aspect of the ankle, the body and tendon of the tibialis anterior, extensor hallucis longus, and extensor digitorum longus can be palpated.

- **RANGE OF MOTION**
  o There are **four main motions** that occur at the ankle joint: **dorsiflexion, plantar flexion, inversion, and eversion**.

  o Range of motion **should always be compared bilaterally** and any deficits should be noted.

  o Limitation of motion may be a result of pain, swelling, or scar tissue from a chronic injury.

  o Finally, resistive range of motion should be tested to assess for any muscular weaknesses or injuries.

1. TALAR TILT TEST

o **Description:** The Talar Tilt Test is a ligamentous stress test that examines **the integrity of the lateral ankle ligaments**, particularly the **calcaneofibular ligament.**

o **Manoeuvre:** Have the patient in the seated position, with their knee bent and foot in a neutral or slightly dorsiflexed position. Stabilize the distal tibia with one hand while applying an **inversion force to the foot.**

o **Positive Findings:** Positive findings include any pain in the ankle or increased joint laxity. Depending on the positioning of the ankle, pain may be experienced over either the calcaneofibular ligament or the anterior talofibular ligament.

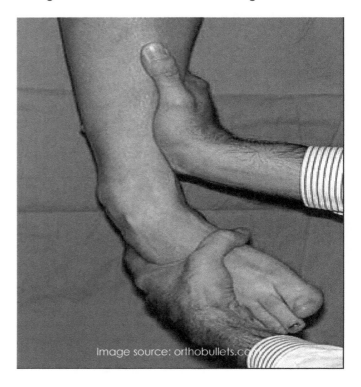

Image source: orthobullets.com

2. ANTERIOR DRAWER

o **Description:** The anterior drawer test is used to examine the **integrity of the anterior talofibular ligament**, which is frequently injured during an **inversion ankle sprain**.

o **Manoeuvre:** Have the patient seated with their knee bent and their ankle in a neutral position at 0° or 90° to the leg. Stabilize the distal tibia with one hand, while grasping the heel with the other hand. Apply an anterior force to the heel. This test should be performed bilaterally to compare for differences in anterior translation.

o **Positive Findings:** Pain or increased joint laxity in the injured ankle **indicates disruption of the anterior talofibular ligament.** A dimple may also be visually seen by the clinician while performing this test.

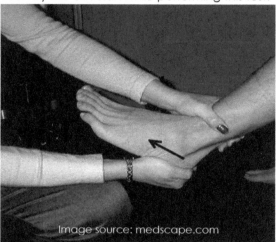

Image source: medscape.com

3. EXTERNAL ROTATION OR KLEIGER'S TEST

o **Description:** The test is used to help **identify syndesmotic injuries.**

o **Manoeuvre:** Have the patient seated with their knee bent on the exam table. Stabilize the distal tibia while externally rotating the foot. External rotation of the talus applies pressure to the lateral malleolus, causing a widening of the tibiofibular joint.

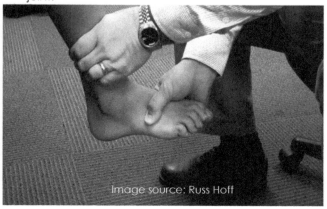

Image source: Russ Hoff

o **Positive findings:** Increased external rotation of the foot when compared bilaterally, or any pain in the anterolateral ankle joint is considered to be a positive finding.

4. THOMPSON'S TEST

o **Description:** This test is utilized to evaluate the **integrity of the heel cord.**

o **Manoeuvre:** Have the patient lying prone on a table with their foot extended off the edge. Squeeze the calf muscle at position slightly distal to the place of widest girth. Examine the movement at the foot.

o **Positive Findings:** A positive test occurs when **the calf is squeezed and no plantar movement occurs at the foot.** This indicates **Achilles tendon rupture.**

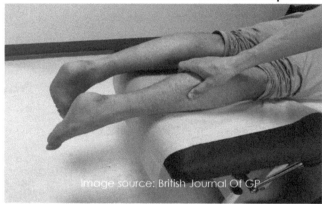

Image source: British Journal Of GP

5. COMPRESSION TEST

o **Description:** This test examines **the integrity of the distal tibiofibular joint**. It can also **assess for fractures of the tibia and fibula.**

o **Manoeuvre:** Have the patient sitting supine with their foot on the table. Grasp the mid-calf and squeeze the tibia and fibula together. Gradually move distally towards the ankle while continuing to apply the same amount of pressure.

o **Positive findings:** Any pain in the lower leg may be indicative of a fracture or syndesmotic sprain.

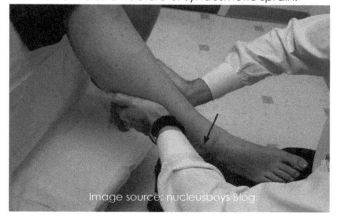

Image source: nucleusboys Blog

14. Reduction of Dislocation/ Fracture

I. SHOULDER DISLOCATION REDUCTION TECHNIQUES

INDICATIONS
- Subjective history of new-onset dislocation or recurrent dislocations combined with clinical assessment consistent with shoulder dislocation.

ANTERIOR DISLOCATIONS (96 %)
- Typical mechanism of injury being indirect, with combination of abduction, extension, and external rotation. Rarely, the etiology is a direct blow to the posterior shoulder.
- Prominent acromion with a palpable drop off below the acromion and subclavicular region fullness is consistent with anterior shoulder dislocation.

POSTERIOR DISLOCATIONS (4 %)
- Mechanism of injury is indirect with a combination of internal rotation, adduction, and flexion.
- Precipitating events include seizure, electrical shock, and falls.
- More subtle presentation.
- Patient will maintain arm locked in internal rotation and adduction; he or she cannot externally rotate.
- Shoulder is flattened anteriorly and rounded posteriorly.
- Ultrasound can be used to prevent missed or delayed diagnosis

INFERIOR DISLOCATIONS (LUXATION ERECTA)
- Arm will be held flexed in overhead position.
- Radiographs reveal shoulder dislocation.
- Ultrasound can be used to identify the nature of the dislocation (anterior or posterior) and can be determined by the position of the humeral head relative to the transducer and glenoid.
- Although at this point, it should not replace radiographs owing to missed fractures.
- Advantages may include less radiation (decreased need for postreduction x-rays) and re-sedation if reduction is not complete.

CONTRAINDICATIONS
- **Associated fracture:** warrants orthopedic evaluation.
- **Associated neurovascular deficit:** May attempt reduction once but avoid multiple attempts.

MATERIALS AND MEDICATIONS
- 1 % lidocaine, with syringe and needle and povidoneiodine prep if administering local anesthesia
- Moderate sedation medications if administering moderate sedation
- Bed sheet for traction-countertraction method
- Dangling weight for Stimson maneuver

PROCEDURE
- **Physical examination**
  - Compare affected with unaffected shoulder.
  - Perform a complete neurovascular examination: test axillary, radial, ulnar, and median nerves for sensory deficit and motor function.
- **Radiographs**
  - Always obtain before attempting reduction for assessment of possible fracture and type and position of dislocation.
  - Obtain three views: **anteroposterior, scapular Y, and axillary lateral views.**
  - Anterior dislocations: humeral head appears anterior to the glenoid fossa on lateral or Y views.
  - Posterior dislocations: on anteroposterior view (vacant glenoid sign, 6-mm sign, lightbulb sign; on lateral or Y view: humeral head appears posterior to glenoid fossa).
- **Pain management and sedation**
  - Decide whether to use intra-articular lidocaine versus procedural sedation and analgesia.
  - For intra-articular lidocaine
    - Use 10–20 mL of 1 % lidocaine.
    - Attach a 1.5-in., 20-gauge needle.
    - Prepare the shoulder with povidone-iodine.
    - Insert the needle lateral to the acromion process and 2 cm inferiorly into the sulcus.
    - After withdrawing to ensure that the needle is not in a vessel, inject 10–20 mL lidocaine into the joint.

- **Reduction techniques:** it is important for the emergency department physician to be familiar with several different techniques.
  The following techniques are presented:

1. STIMSON MANEUVER

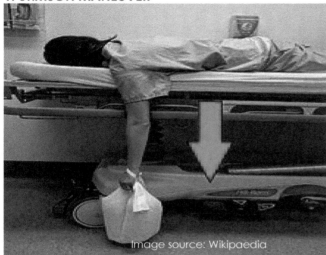

Image source: Wikipaedia

- Patient is placed prone with 2.5–5 kg of weight hanging from the wrist.
- Reduction may be facilitated by traction and external rotation of the arm.
- A success rate of 96 % has been reported using the combined prone position, hanging weights, intravenous drug therapy, and scapular manipulation.
- **Advantage:**
  - Can be performed by one person only.
- **Disadvantages:**
  - Requires time to gather materials;
  - The danger involved in the patient falling off the stretcher,
  - Requiring staff to monitor the patient.

2. SCAPULAR MANIPULATION TECHNIQUE

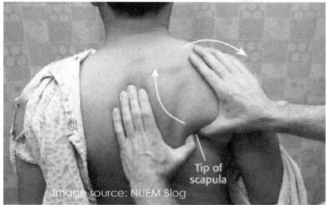

Tip of scapula

Image source: NUEM Blog

- Place the patient in the prone position with the affected arm hanging downward.
- Apply traction down on the arm.

- Locate the inferior tip of the scapula. Simultaneously push the inferior tip of the scapula medially toward the spine and use the other hand push the superior scapula laterally.
- **Advantages:**
  - High success rate, greater than 90 %;
  - Very safe to perform.
- **Disadvantages:**
  - It requires the patient to assume the prone position;
  - May require another person to perform traction.

3. EXTERNAL ROTATION METHOD

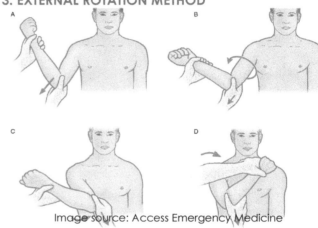

Image source: Access Emergency Medicine

- Place the patient in the supine position with the affected arm adducted directly next to the patient's side with the elbow flexed to 90°.
- The operator uses one hand to direct downward traction on the affected arm while maintaining it next to the patient's side.
- The operator uses the other hand to hold the patient's wrist and guide the arm into slow external rotation.
- Reduction usually takes place between 70° and 110° of external rotation.
- **Advantages:**
  - Requires no strength by operator;
  - Well tolerated by patients.
- **Disadvantage:**
  - Patient may have persistent dislocation during procedure,
  - Requiring operator to make adjustments.

4. MILCH TECHNIQUE

- Technique looks as though one is reaching up to grab an apple from a tree.
- Abduct the injured arm up to the overhead position. Once in the overhead position, apply gentle vertical traction with external rotation.
- An adjustment may need to be made if the reduction does not occur easily; push the humeral head upward into the glenoid fossa.

- **Advantages:**
  - o Lack of complications;
  - o Patient tolerance
- **Disadvantage:**
  - o Variable success rate reported: 70–90 %

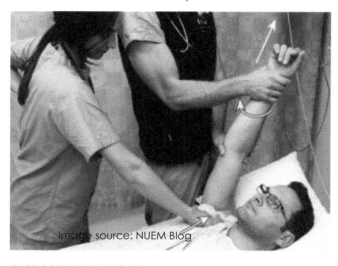

Image source: NUEM Blog

5. SPASO TECHNIQUE

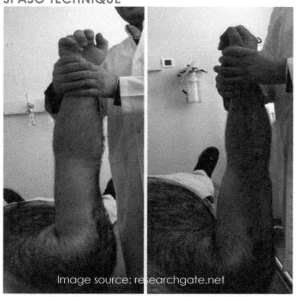

Image source: researchgate.net

- o Place the patient in the supine position.
- o Operator grasps the affected arm at the wrist and lifts the straight arm directly upward while applying longitudinal traction.
- o Apply external rotation.
- **Advantages:**
  - o Single operator,
  - o High level of success
- **Disadvantage:**
  - o May require more time to allow the shoulder muscles to relax
  - o

6. HIPPOCRATES METHOD or TRACTION-COUNTERTRACTION TECHNIQUE

- o With the patient is sitting up, have an assistant wrap a sheet around the upper chest and under the axilla of the affected shoulder.
- o Have the assistant wrap the sheet behind her or his back. Now have the patient lay supine.
- o Wrap another sheet around the flexed elbow of the affected arm and behind the operator's back.
- o Both the operator and the assistant lean back, applying gentle traction.
- **Advantage:**
  - o Many older physicians are familiar with this method and, therefore, have a high degree of success.
- **Disadvantages:**
  - o Requires two people;
  - o May cause skin tears on elderly patients.

7. POSTERIOR SHOULDER DISLOCATION REDUCTION

- o Give adequate premedication.
- o Place the patient supine and apply lateral traction on the proximal humerus.
- o Have an assistant apply anterior pressure to the posteriorly located humeral head.
- **Advantage:**
  - o Logical methods for reduction
- **Disadvantages:**
  - o Require sufficient premedication because often posterior dislocations present late;
  - o May require open reduction

POSTREDUCTION

- Obtain postreduction x-rays.
- There is some literature on using ultrasound to confirm adequate reduction, which allows repetitive assessments throughout procedure, as well as reduce radiation
- Do a postreduction neurovascular examination.
- Sling and swath or shoulder immobilizer for 2–3 weeks.
- Orthopedic follow-up in 1 week.

COMPLICATIONS

- **Fractures**
- Adhesive capsulitis, or **frozen shoulder**; especially a concern in the elderly with prolonged immobilization in sling
- **Brachial plexus injury**, especially of the axillary nerve
- **Vascular laceration**, most commonly of the axillary artery
- **Rotator cuff tears**

II. ELBOW DISLOCATION REDUCTION

INDICATIONS

- Any dislocation of the elbow joint.
- Direction of the dislocation (i.e., anterior, posterior, lateral and divergent radius, and ulnar dislocations) is determined by the position of the ulna relative to the joint space.

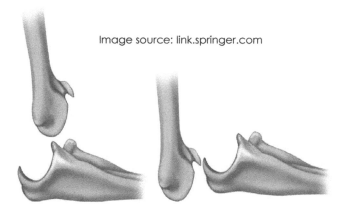

Image source: link.springer.com

CONTRAINDICATIONS

- **Relative**
  - Compound fracture dislocation

MATERIALS AND MEDICATIONS

- Parenteral sedation and analgesia medications
- Local anaesthetic for local and intra-articular anesthesia
- Splinting material
- Stockinette
- Padding
- Elastic bandage
- Tape
- Sling

PROCEDURE FOR POSTERIOR DISLOCATIONS

- Obtain a true lateral and anteroposterior radiographs of the affected elbow.
- Ensure adequate sedation and analgesia.
- Consider intra-articular analgesia.
- Check the neurovascular status of affected extremity.
- Follow a selected method for reduction as detailed later.
- Following successful reduction gently flex the elbow to ensure full range of motion.
- Place a long-arm posterior splint with the elbow in at least 90° flexion and secure the arm in a regular sling.
- Check neurovascular status.
- Obtain a postreduction radiograph of the elbow.

METHOD A

- Position the patient on a stretcher in the supine position.
- Apply steady traction at the supinated distal forearm keeping the elbow slightly flexed, while an assistant applies countertraction to the midhumerus with both hands.

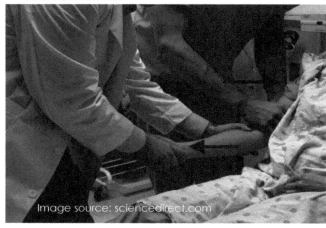

Image source: sciencedirect.com

METHOD B

- Position the patient on a stretcher in the supine position.
- Extend the affected extremity over the edge of the stretcher.
- Apply traction to the supinated forearm slightly flexed at the elbow, while an assistant holds the distal humerus with both hands and uses thumbs to apply pressure to the olecranon as if pushing it away from the humerus.

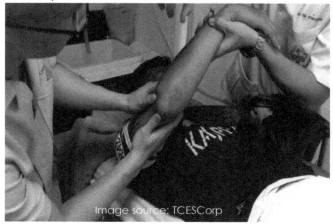

Image source: TCESCorp

METHOD C

- Position the patient on a stretcher in the prone position.
- Hang the affected extremity over the side of the stretcher toward the floor.

o Apply downward traction to the pronated distal forearm and with the other hand just above the patient's antecubital fossa lift the humerus toward you.

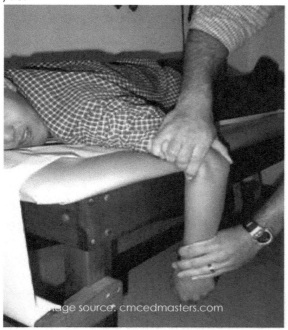

Image source: cmcedmasters.com

PROCEDURE FOR ANTERIOR DISLOCATIONS

o Follow pre- and postprocedure steps as documented for the posterior dislocation.
o Position the patient on a stretcher in the supine position.
o With one hand, apply traction to the supinated distal forearm with the elbow extended, while an assistant applies countertraction with both hands around the distal humerus.
o With the other hand apply downward and backward pressure over the proximal forearm just below the antecubital fossa.

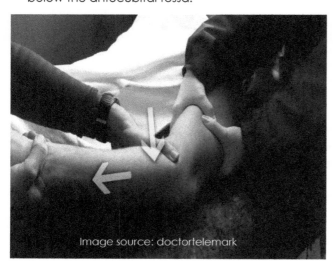

Image source: doctortelemark

PULLED ELBOW
PROCEDURE FOR RADIAL HEAD SUBLUXATIONS (PULLED ELBOW)

▪ This procedure can normally be performed without any sedation or parenteral analgesia.
▪ Position the patient, most commonly a child aged 1–3 years, facing forward on the caretaker's lap.
▪ Hold the flexed elbow of the affected extremity placing your thumb firmly over the radial head.
▪ With the other hand, take the child's hand and wrist, and in one continuous movement, hyperpronate and flex the Forearm.
▪ Another method is to supinate and flex the forearm instead of hyperpronating it.
▪ Leave the room, encourage the caretaker to engage the child with distracting activities and reexamine the child in 10–20 min, at which stage, if reduction was successful, the child should be using the extremity normally again.
▪ No postreduction radiograph or immobilization is required.

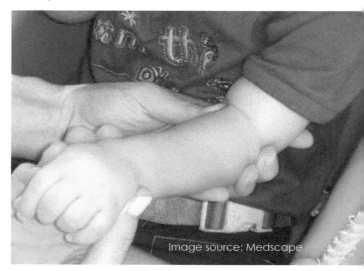

Image source: Medscape

COMPLICATIONS

• Concomitant fractures
• Vascular injury, most commonly to the brachial artery
• Median nerve injury/entrapment
• Recurrent dislocation—rare

III. DISTAL INTERPHALANGEAL JOINT REDUCTION

- Distal interphalangeal (DIP) joint dislocation is rare.
- It occurs when an axial force is applied to the distal phalanx

INDICATIONS

- DIP joint reduction is performed to alleviate functional and anatomical derangements resulting from DIP joint dislocation, commonly dorsal, from axial compression.

CONTRAINDICATIONS

- **Absolute**
  - o Absence of radiographic confirmation (anteroposterior, true lateral, and oblique) of simple DIP joint dislocation, especially in pediatric cases
- **Relative**
  - o Open joint dislocation, associated fracture, or entrapped volar plate
  - o Digital neurovascular compromise

Finger Dislocation

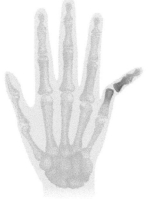
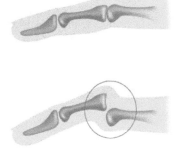

Image source: g4physio.co.uk

PROCEDURE

- o Place the patient in the seated position with the arms at rest on a bedside table or supported by an assistant.
- o Pronate the patient's hand, remove rings if present, and rest on a flat surface.
- o Insert a 25-gauge needle at the dorsolateral aspect of the base of the finger to form a wheal to reduce patient discomfort.

- o Advance the needle and direct anteriorly toward the phalangeal base.
- o Inject 0.5–1 mL of local anaesthetic as the needle is withdrawn 1–2 mm from the point of bone contact.
- o Inject an additional 1 mL of local anaesthetic continuously as the needle is withdrawn.
- o The injection should never render the tissue tense nor be circumferential.
- o Hyperextend the DIP joint while applying longitudinal traction, followed by immediate joint flexion at the base of the distal phalanx.
- o Place finger(s) in an aluminium digital dorsal splint in slight flexion for 2 weeks.
- o Postreduction radiograph is recommended for confirmation.

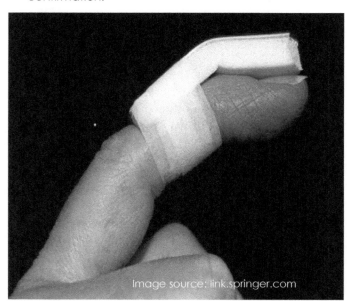
Image source: link.springer.com

Padded aluminium splint applied to block the DIP joint in flexion but allow further flexion, which encourages active flexion of that joint when the PIP joint flexes

COMPLICATIONS

- Irreducible dislocations
- Stiffness
- Recurrent dislocation
- Extensor lag in joints with residual subluxation
- Associated with dorsal joint prominences, swan-neck/ boutonnière deformity, and degenerative arthritis

IV. HIP DISLOCATION REDUCTION

INDICATIONS

- Displacement of the femoral head in relation to the acetabulum without concomitant femoral neck, head, or acetabulum fractures:
  - **Posterior hip dislocations** make up 80–90 % of cases.
  - **Anterior hip dislocations** make up 10–15 % of cases.
    - These are classified into obturator, pubic, iliac, central, or inferior types.
    - Central dislocations are associated with comminuted acetabulum fractures, and inferior dislocations are a rare occurrence normally occurring in children younger than 7 years of age.
  - **Prosthetic hip dislocations**

CONTRAINDICATIONS

- **Absolute**
  - Femoral neck fracture: attempted reduction may increase the displacement of the fracture and increase the probability of avascular necrosis.

- **Relative**
  - Fractures in other parts of the affected lower extremity: these may limit the pressure that can be applied necessary for traction during reduction.

MATERIALS AND MEDICATIONS

- Parenteral sedation and analgesia medications
- Sheet or belt to fi x the pelvis to the stretcher
- Knee immobilizer
- Abduction pillow

PROCEDURE

- Check the neurovascular status of the affected extremity.
- Obtain anteroposterior (AP) views of the pelvis and lateral views of the hip.
- Ensure adequate parenteral sedation and analgesia.
- Decide upon a technique, as detailed later, and position the patient accordingly.
- Once the hip has been successfully reduced, test the joint for stability by moving it gently thought its range of motion.
- Place a knee immobilizer and an abduction pillow between the knees.

- Check the neurovascular status.
- Obtain repeat AP films of the pelvis.

1. STIMSON MANEUVER

- Place the patient prone on the stretcher with the affected extremity hanging over the edge and the hip flexed to 90°.
- Flex the knee and the foot to 90°.
- Apply downward pressure to the area just distal to the popliteal fossa with a hand or knee while using the opposite hand to internally and externally rotate the hip at the ankle.
- Have an assistant simultaneously manipulate the displaced femoral head into position with both hands, applying downward pressure over the affected buttock.

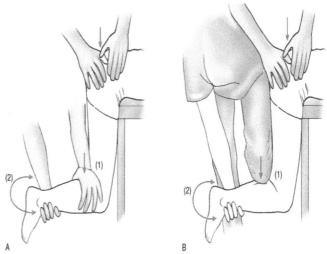

Stimson maneuver with hand and Knee
Image source: accessemergencymedicine.mhmedical.com

2. ALLIS MANEUVER

- Position the patient supine on the stretcher.
- The operator should stand on the stretcher to achieve maximum leverage or have the patient on a backboard on the ground. Have an assistant apply downward pressure to both iliac crests.
- Apply constant, gentle upward traction in line with the deformity while maneuvering the hip to 90° flexion and through internal and external rotation.
- Have a second assistant provide lateral traction to the midthigh.
- Once the femoral head has cleared the outer lip of the acetabulum, continue traction while keeping the hip in external rotation and gently abducting and extending the hip.

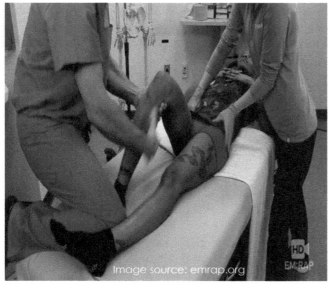
Allis technique

3. WHISTLER TECHNIQUE

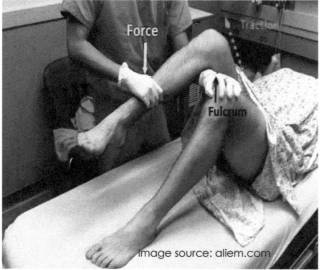
Whistler technique

o Position the patient supine on the stretcher with the knee and hip flexed to 45°. Have an assistant stabilize the pelvis with downward pressure on both iliac crests.

o Stand on the side of the affected extremity and place one arm under the knee, resting the hand on the flexed knee of the unaffected extremity.

o Secure the ankle of the affected extremity with the other hand and elevate the shoulder of the opposite arm, providing upward traction at the distal thigh and a strong fulcrum to reduce the dislocation.

o Internal and external rotation can be achieved with the opposite hand at the ipsilateral ankle.

4. CAPTAIN MORGAN TECHNIQUE

o Position the patient supine on the stretcher with the knee and hip flexed to 90°.

o Stabilize and fix the pelvis with a sheet tied securely over the pelvis and under the stretcher.

o Standing on the side of the affected extremity, the operator's foot should be resting perpendicular on the stretcher with the knee placed under the patient's knee.

o With the opposite hand, apply downward pressure to the ankle and provide a sustained upward force to the patient's thigh by elevation of the knee through plantar flexion of the toes and upward pressure of the other hand placed behind the patient's knee.

o Internal and external rotation can be applied simultaneously if necessary, by gently twisting the ankle.

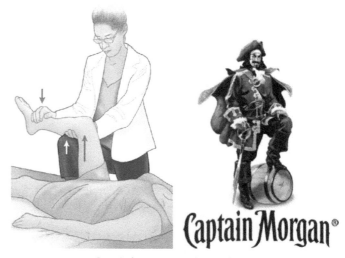
Captain Morgan technique
Image source: accessemergencymedicine.mhmedical.com

COMPLICATIONS

• Sciatic nerve injury
• Avascular necrosis of the femoral head due to delay in adequate reduction
• Inability to perform reduction due to occult fractures and fracture fragments, incarceration of the joint capsule, or associated tendons
• Unstable or irreducible dislocations
• Traumatic arthritis and joint instability

V. KNEE DISLOCATION REDUCTION

INDICATIONS
- Dislocation of the knee/fibular head/patella

CONTRAINDICATIONS
- **Absolute**
  - None
- **Relative**
  - Immediate availability of orthopedic consultation

MATERIALS AND MEDICATIONS
- Parenteral sedation and analgesia medications
- Knee immobilizer or splinting materials

1. KNEE (FEMUR/TIBIA) DISLOCATION REDUCTION
- Assess **neurovascular function.**
- Pre-treat the patient with sedation or analgesia as appropriate. Position the patient supine with the affected leg fully extended.
- Instruct an assistant to stand near the patient's hip and, facing the patient's affected knee, grasp the distal femur firmly with both hands to fix it in place.
- Stand near the patient's foot and, facing the patient's affected knee, grasp the distal tibia and apply straight traction in a distal direction.
- Longitudinal traction-countertraction alone, as described previously, will usually reduce the dislocation. If reduction does not occur, proceed with the following steps.
- While applying straight traction in a distal direction to the tibia with the dominant hand, with the nondominant hand:

❖ **Anterior dislocation:** push the proximal tibia in a posterior direction.

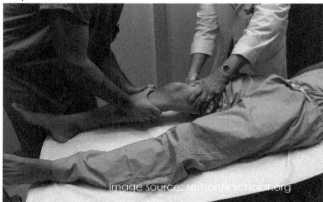

Anterior dislocation of the knee: the proximal tibia is pushed in a posterior direction. The *arrows* indicate the direction in which force should be applied by the operator during reduction of dislocation

❖ **Posterior dislocation:** lift the proximal tibia in an anterior direction.

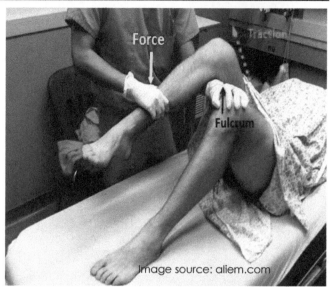

Posterior dislocation of the knee: the proximal tibia is pushed in an anterior direction. The *arrows* indicate the direction in which force should be applied by the operator during reduction of dislocation

❖ **Lateral dislocation:** push the proximal tibia in a medial direction.

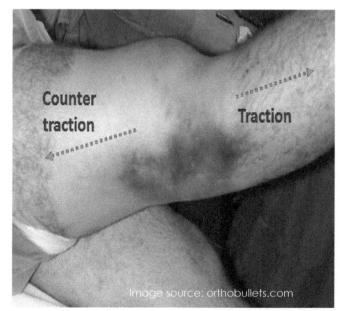

Lateral dislocation of the knee: the proximal tibia is pushed in a medial direction. The *arrows* indicate the direction in which force should be applied by the operator during reduction of dislocation.

❖ **Medial dislocation:** push the proximal tibia in a lateral direction.

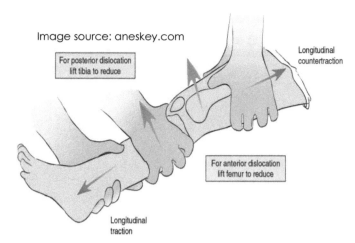

Image source: aneskey.com

For posterior dislocation lift tibia to reduce

Longitudinal countertraction

For anterior dislocation lift femur to reduce

Longitudinal traction

❖ **Rotary dislocation:** rotate the proximal tibia into proper linear alignment with the femoral condyles.

• Reduction may be facilitated by the use of two assistants rather than just one.

• The second assistant grasps the distal tibia and applies straight traction in a distal direction, freeing the operator to manipulate the proximal tibia as described previously using both hands.

• After reduction, **reassess neurovascular function** and, if available, obtain **angiography.**

• **Immobilize the knee in 15° of flexion** in a knee immobilizer or long-leg posterior splint.

COMPLICATIONS

• Distal ischemia (even requiring amputation)
• Degenerative arthritis
• Joint instability due to ligamentous injury

PEARLS AND PITFALLS

o Dislocations of the knee are described in terms of the tibia's position in relation to the femur.

o All knee dislocations require orthopedic evaluation at the earliest possible opportunity.

o Owing to the frequency of associated popliteal artery and peroneal nerve injury, a neurovascular examination should be performed before and after any attempts at reduction or manipulation of the knee.

o Dislocations of the knee should be reduced as soon as possible, particularly if distal neurovascular compromise exists.

o Operative ligamentous repair is often required approximately 2 weeks postreduction (once acute swelling has resolved) to achieve the maximum functional recovery.

o If the knee hyperextends more than 30° when the horizontal leg is lifted by the foot, the knee is considered severely unstable.

o This is likely due to a previous dislocation, and thus, the knee should be evaluated for the neurovascular complications of dislocation.

o Because the joint capsule is commonly disrupted during knee dislocation, synovial fluid may diffuse into the surrounding tissue, such that an effusion is not always present.

o A posterolateral dislocation may be irreducible because the medial femoral condyle traps the medial capsule within the joint.

2. FIBULAR HEAD DISLOCATION REDUCTION

o Assess **neurovascular function.**

o Pre-treat the patient with sedation or analgesia as appropriate. Position the patient supine.

o Flex the knee to 90° to relax the biceps femoris tendon.

o Instruct an assistant to stand near the patient's hip and, facing the patient's affected knee, grasp the distal femur firmly with both hands to fix it in place.

o Stand near the patient's foot and, facing the patient's affected knee, grasp the distal tibia and apply straight traction in a distal direction with the dominant hand and with the nondominant hand.

❖ **Anterior dislocation:** push the fibular head in a posterior direction.

❖ **Posterior dislocation:** push the fibular head in an anterior direction

• Reduction may be facilitated by the use of two assistants rather than just one.

• If a second assistant is available, instruct the second assistant to stand near the patient's foot and, facing the patient's affected knee, grasp the distal tibia and apply straight traction in a distal direction.

• This enables the operator to grasp and move the proximal fibula as described previously using both hands.

• Reduction is often signified by a palpable and audible click as the fibula snaps back into position.

• After reduction, **reassess neurovascular function** and, if available, obtain **angiography.**

• After reduction, patients should receive orthopaedic referral, avoid weight-bearing for the first 2 weeks, and then gradually increase weight-bearing over the next 6 weeks.

• Typically, **immobilization is not required** following reduction of an isolated fibular head dislocation

COMPLICATIONS

• Peroneal nerve injury
• Fibular head instability/subluxation
• Degenerative arthritis

PEARLS AND PITFALLS

o Fibular head dislocations are usually anterolateral, but these do not result in neurovascular compromise.

o A knee joint effusion is usually not seen in a fibular head dislocation because the tibiofibular ligaments are contained within a separate synovium.

o **Anterior dislocations** typically result from a fall on the flexed, adducted leg, often combined with ankle inversion.

o Flexion of the knee relaxes the fibular collateral ligament, reducing the stability of the tibiofibular joint.

o **Superior dislocation** is accompanied by interosseus membrane damage and proximal displacement of the lateral malleolus.

o **Posterior fibular head dislocations** usually result from direct trauma to the flexed knee and may be accompanied by **peroneal nerve injury.**

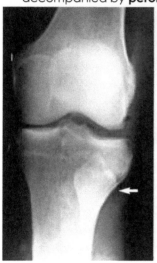 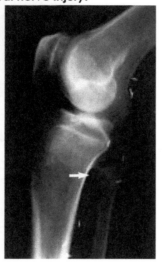

3. LATERAL PATELLAR DISLOCATION REDUCTION

o pre-treat the patient with sedation or analgesia as appropriate.

o Stand at the side of the affected knee and, facing the knee, grasp the distal tibia and slowly extend the knee with one hand, and with the other hand simultaneously apply gentle pressure to the patella in a medial direction.

• The lateral edge of the patella may be lifted slightly to facilitate its travel over the femoral condyle during reduction.

• After reduction, the knee should be immobilized in full extension in a knee immobilizer or long-leg posterior splint, and the patient should receive orthopedic referral, avoid weight-bearing for the first 2 weeks, and then gradually increase weight-bearing over the next 6 weeks.

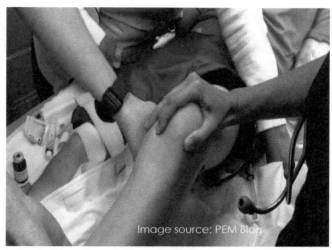

Image source: PEM Blog

Lateral dislocation of the patella: the patella is pushed in a medial direction. The *arrow* indicates the direction in which force should be applied by the operator during reduction of dislocation.

COMPLICATIONS

• Failure of reduction
• Degenerative arthritis
• Recurrent dislocation/subluxation

PEARLS AND PITFALLS

o Patellar dislocation occurs most frequently among adolescents.

o Patellar dislocation typically occurs in the setting of external rotation combined with a strong valgus force and quadriceps contraction.

o Patellar dislocations are described in terms of the patellar relationship to the normal knee joint.

o **The most common patellar dislocations are lateral.**

o If a spontaneous reduction has occurred, a knee effusion and tenderness along the medial aspect of the patella are likely to be present on examination, and the patellar apprehension test will be positive.

o To perform the patellar apprehension test, flex the knee to 30° and push the patella laterally. If the patient senses an impending redislocation, the test is considered positive.

o Isolated lateral patellar dislocations do not usually require hospitalization, but orthopedic follow-up is recommended owing to the likelihood of persistent instability.

o Intracondylar and superior dislocations require surgical reduction.

o Patients with an isolated patellar dislocation typically present with the knee in 20–30° of flexion and the patella displaced laterally.

o Dislocations tend to be recurrent, particularly in patients with patellofemoral anatomical abnormalities.

VI. ANKLE DISLOCATION REDUCTION

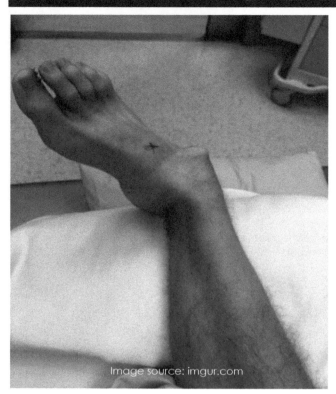

Image source: imgur.com

INDICATIONS

- Dislocation of the ankle joint.
- This is defined by the articulation of the talus with the mortise that is formed by the distal tibia and fibula.
- Dislocations can be posterior, anterior, superior, or lateral and are classified by the **position of the talus in relation to the tibial mortise.**

CONTRAINDICATIONS

- **Relative**
  - Open dislocations where there is no evidence of acute neurovascular compromise are better managed definitively in the operating room to avoid further contamination.

MATERIALS AND MEDICATIONS

- Parenteral sedation and analgesia medications
- Local anaesthetic for local and intra-articular anesthesia
- Splinting material
- Stockinette
- Padding
- Elastic bandage
- Tape
- Sheet

PROCEDURE

- **Check the neurovascular status** of the affected foot and ankle.
- If there is no evidence of critical neurovascular compromise, **obtain a lateral and an anteroposterior radiograph** of the affected ankle.
- Ensure adequate parenteral sedation and analgesia to maximize success and limit pain and suffering.
- Position the patient on a stretcher with the knee flexed at 90° over a folded pillow or rolled-up sheet or with the lower leg and knee hanging over the edge of the stretcher.

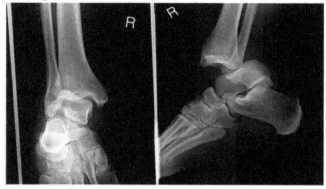

1 POSTERIOR DISLOCATIONS

- Hold the heel in one hand and pull with longitudinal traction.
- With the other hand, hold the top of the foot and gently plantarflex it downward, while an assistant provides countertraction at the back of the midcalf.

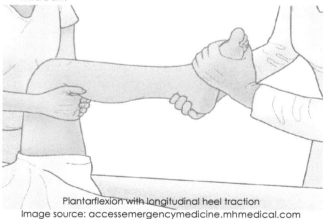

Plantarflexion with longitudinal heel traction
Image source: accessemergencymedicine.mhmedical.com

- Continue longitudinal traction at the heel and countertraction at the calf.
- Dorsiflex the foot while another assistant applies downward pressure to the distal anterior leg.

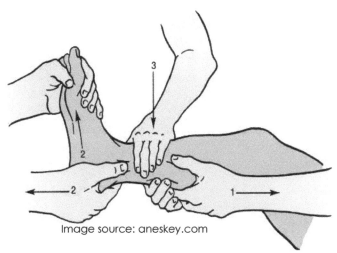

Image source: aneskey.com

Dorsiflexion with longitudinal heel traction

o Examine foot for restoration of normal anatomy and for any new lacerations or defects to the skin.
o **Recheck neurovascular integrity.**
o Place the leg in a sugar-tong splint with the foot at 90°.
o **Recheck neurovascular integrity.**

2 ANTERIOR DISLOCATIONS
o Hold the heel in one hand and pull with longitudinal traction.
o With the other hand, hold the top of the foot and dorsiflex, while an assistant provides countertraction at the back of the midcalf.

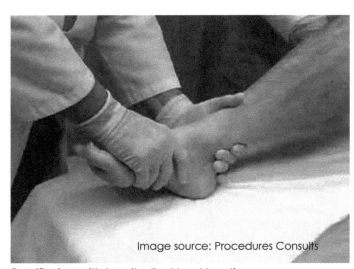

Image source: Procedures Consults

Dorsiflexion with longitudinal heel traction

o Continue longitudinal traction at the heel and countertraction at the calf.
o Keeping the foot at 90° to the leg, hold the foot firmly and push the foot downward toward the floor while another assistant applies upward pressure to the distal posterior leg.

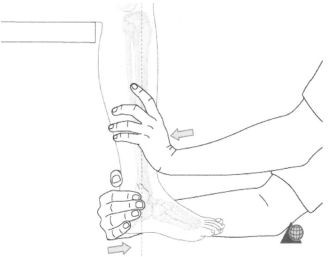

Downward movement of foot (toward the floor) with longitudinal heel traction
Image source: aofoundation.org

o Examine the foot for restoration of normal anatomy and for any new lacerations or defects to the skin.
o **Recheck neurovascular integrity.**
o Place the leg in a sugar-tong splint with the foot at 90°.
o **Recheck neurovascular integrity.**

COMPLICATIONS
• Compound fractures
• Neurovascular injury
• Skin and soft tissue damage
• Compartment syndrome

PEARLS AND PITFALLS
• **PEARLS**
  o The ankle rarely dislocates without associated fractures.

• **PITFALLS**
  o Ankle dislocation is an orthopedic emergency, and reduction should not be delayed by imaging if there is evidence of neurovascular impairment.
  o Complications that are exacerbated by delay in management include concomitant fractures, gross deformity of the ankle, severe stretching and tenting of the skin with resultant skin blisters, skin necrosis, and possible conversion to a compound fracture.
  o Be sure to check the radiograph carefully for commonly associated fractures notably of the malleoli.

15. Joint Aspiration
I. ARTHROCENTESIS

I. KNEE & SHOULDER JOINTS ASPIRATION

INDICATIONS

- Diagnosis of septic joint
- Diagnosis of traumatic effusion
- Diagnosis of inflammatory effusion
- Diagnosis of crystal-induced arthritis
- Therapeutic relief of pain from effusion

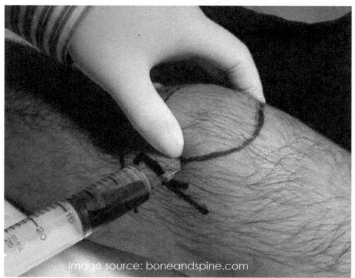

Knee arthrocentesis

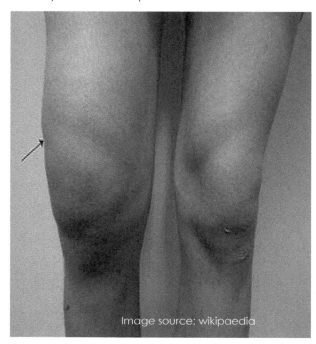

Image source: wikipaedia

CONTRAINDICATIONS

- Severe coagulopathy
- Skin infection over the needle insertion site
- Joint prosthesis
- Patients with Bacteremia or sepsis (except to diagnose a septic joint)

PROCEDURE

o Informed consent may be required.

o Position the patient appropriately. The joint should be placed in slight flexion.

o Palpate the joint and identify anatomical landmarks.

❖ **For knee arthrocentesis**, the needle should be inserted at the midpoint of either the medial or the lateral side of the patella.

❖ **For acromioclavicular (AC) joint arthrocentesis**, the needle should be inserted at the superior surface of the AC joint.

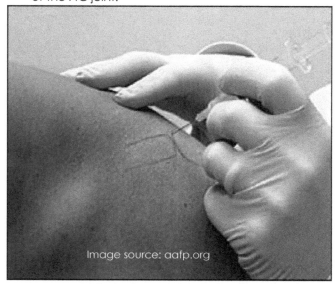

Acromioclavicular joint arthrocentesis

❖ **For glenohumeral joint arthrocentesis**, there are two approaches:

1. In the anterior approach, the needle is inserted into the groove lateral to the coracoid process.

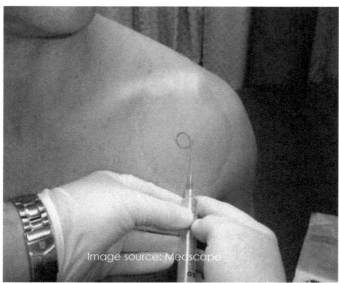

Glenohumeral joint arthrocentesis: anterior approach

2. In the posterior approach (preferred), the needle is inserted below the posterior border of the acromion process and lateral to the border of the scapula.

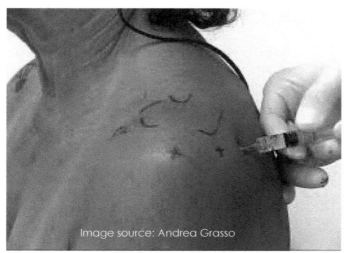

Glenohumeral joint arthrocentesis: posterior approach

o Prepare the skin and drape in a sterile fashion.
o Using lidocaine (drawn up in 5-mL syringe), anesthetize the skin with the 25-gauge needle.
o Secure the 18- to 22-gauge needle on the 5- to 50-Ml syringe (depending on the size of the joint) and insert it into the skin.

o Advance the needle slowly into the joint space while aspirating until joint fluid can easily be withdrawn
o While inserting the needle into the joint space, avoid scraping the needle against the bone.
o If fluid cannot be aspirated easily, the catheter can be repositioned further in the joint space or turned by 45° sequentially as needed.
o Once the joint fluid is aspirated, pull out the needle and hold pressure with gauze. Bleeding should be minimal.
o Place a band-aid or other dressing over the site.
o Send the synovial fluid to the laboratory.
o Generally, laboratory analyses may include:
  ▪ **Crystals,**
  ▪ **Protein,**
  ▪ **Glucose,**
  ▪ **Cell count and differential,**
  ▪ **Culture and sensitivity, and gram stain.**

COMPLICATIONS
• Introduction of infection
• Bleeding
• Dry tap

PEARLS AND PITFALLS
• The preferred site of entry is over the extensor surface of the joint. This will reduce the risk of damage to tendons, ligaments, and blood vessels.
• When assessing synovial fluid, **the Rule of Twos** may be used to differentiate among normal, inflammatory, and septic fluid.
  o **Normal synovial fluid** has less than 200 white blood cells (WBCs)/mm³.
  o **Noninflammatory synovial fluid** has 200–2000 WBCs/mm³.
  o **Inflammatory synovial fluid** has greater than 2000 WBCs/mm³ (but <50,000 WBCs/mm³).
  o **Septic synovial fluid** has greater than 75,000 WBCs/mm³. Only septic synovial fluid will have a positive Gram stain and culture.

16. Mechanical Ventilator
I. NON-INVASIVE VENTILATION (NIV)

- Include machines used to ventilate and oxygenate patients without the need to perform the invasive procedure of intubation. These machines can only be used on a spontaneously breathing patient.
- The two most common forms of NIV are:
  o **CPAP**
  o **BiPAP**

I. CPAP

o This is **C**ontinuous **P**ositive **A**irway **P**ressure.
o It's a pressure exhale applied during the respiratory cycle that helps keep air passages open so that the next breath comes in easier. Since it keeps the airways patent, it assures **adequate oxygenation** and is often prescribed to increase oxygenation

Indications	Hypoxemia due to:
	o CCF, CPO, Pneumonia, asthma, COPD,
	o Near drowning
	o Obstructive Sleep Apnea
Cautions "CARS"	o **C**ardiogenic shock o **A**gitated patient o **R**ight ventricular failure o **S**evere obstructive airways disease
Contraindications	o Immediate endotracheal intubation indicated o Respiratory arrest or inadequate spontaneous ventilation o Worsening life-threatening hypoxia o Unconscious patient unable to protect own airway
How to deliver NIV	o Correctly fitting mask o Supplemental O$_2$ o Commence PEEP at 5-7.5 cm H$_2$O and increase to 10cm as tolerated o Continue for 30min/hr until reduction in dyspnoea and saturations are maintained off NIV
Complications "DAW - HIPS"	o **D**ry mouth o **A**spiration o **W**orsening right ventricular failure o **H**ypercapnoea, o **I**ntolerance due to anxiety, o **P**neumothorax o **S**kin/Eye discomfort,

II. BiPAP

- This is an acronym for **Bi**-level (or **Bi**phasic) **P**ositive **A**irway **P**ressure.
- It provides a combination of both **IPAP** and **EPAP**.
- **Indications of NIV:**
  o **Hypercapnic respiratory failure during an acute exacerbation of COPD with:**
    - Arterial pH <7.35.
    - Arterial PaCO$_2$ >6kPa (if acute onset).
    - Tachypnoea >25 breaths/min

A. IPAP

o This is **I**nspiratory **P**ositive **A**irway **P**ressure.
o It is a pressure during inspiration that assists a patient obtain an adequate **tidal volume.**
o Because it provides assistance with inhalation, it therefore **decreases the work of breathing required** to get air in.
o Because it assures **adequate ventilation**, it is often prescribed to **blow off carbon dioxide (CO2).**

B. EPAP

o This is **E**xpiratory **P**ositive **A**irway **P**ressure.
o It is the same thing as CPAP.
o EPAP is simply used here so you know you're talking about CPAP on a BiPAP machine.
o EPAP is used to **improve oxygenation.**

INCLUSION CRITERIA FOR NIV
o Primary diagnosis of COPD exacerbation
o Able to protect airway
o Conscious and cooperative
o Patient's wishes considered
o Potential for recovery of quality of life that will be acceptable to the patient
o NIV can be considered in the unconscious if within a critical care setting or intubation is inappropriate

EXCLUSION CRITERIA FOR NIV ARE:
o Life threatening hypoxaemia
o Intubation and ventilation is possible and would be in patient's best interests
o Inability to protect the airway
o Confusion
o Agitation
o Undrained pneumothorax

o Fixed upper airway obstruction
o Facial burns/trauma
o Recent facial or upper airway surgery
o Vomiting
o Copious respiratory secretions

o Bowel obstruction
o Upper gastrointestinal surgery
o Severe co-morbidity
o Patient moribund

II. INVASIVE MECHANICAL VENTILATION

INDICATIONS FOR INVASIVE MECHANICAL VENTILATION:

o A decision to intubate and proceed with mechanical ventilation should normally be made **within 4 hours of starting NIV**, as improvements should usually be apparent during this time.
o Patients with COPD should be considered for ITU treatment when necessary, especially if they are more unwell i.e. **pH < 7.26**.
o The Global Initiative for Chronic Obstructive Lung Disease 2013 guideline states the following may be **indications for invasive mechanical ventilation**:
  ▪ NIV failure
  ▪ Inability to tolerate NIV
  ▪ Respiratory or cardiac arrest
  ▪ Respiratory pauses with loss of consciousness or gasping for air
  ▪ Reduced consciousness or uncontrolled agitation
  ▪ Massive aspiration
  ▪ Persistent inability to remove respiratory secretion
  ▪ Heart rate <50 with loss of alertness
  ▪ Haemodynamic instability unresponsive to fluid and vasopressors
  ▪ Life threatening hypoxaemia

COMPLICATIONS OF MECHANICAL VENTILATION

- **Complications of intubation**
  o Upper airway and nasal trauma,
  o Tooth avulsion,
  o Oral-pharyngeal laceration,
  o Laceration or hematoma of the vocal cords,
  o Tracheal laceration,
  o Perforation,
  o Hypoxemia,
  o Intubation of the oesophagus.

  o Inadvertent intubation of the right mainstem bronchus
  o Aspiration: rates are 8–19% in intubations performed in adults without anaesthesia.
  o Sinusitis, tracheal necrosis or stenosis, glottic edema,
  o Ventilator-associated Pneumonia may occur with prolonged use of endotracheal tubes.

- **Ventilator-induced lung injury (VILI)**
  o Barotrauma
  o Volutrauma

SETTING UP NIV

- Consultant/Senior Decision maker to commence NIV.
- Set EPAP at 4 – 5 cm H_2O and IPAP at 10 cm H_2O.
- Set back-up breathing frequency to 8 – 10 breaths/minute.
- Select appropriate size mask (full face in preference to nasal) to fit patient.
- Explain procedure to patient.
- Hold mask in place to allow patient to familiarize themselves.
- Attach pulse oximeter.
- Commence NIV, holding mask in place initially.
- Secure mask in place with straps/headgear to prevent leaks – do not attach too tightly!
- Reassess patient after a few minutes.
- Check for leaks and refit mask if necessary.
- Add O_2 to maintain SpO_2 >85%.
- Instruct patient how to remove the mask and summon help.
- Increase IPAP gradually up to about 12 - 15 cmH$_2$O over 1 hr.
- Clinical assessment and, if appropriate, check ABG at 1 hour.
- If procedure fails, institute alternative management plan

III. MODES OF MECHANICAL VENTILATION

1. VOLUME-LIMITED VENTILATION

- Volume-limited ventilation (**also called volume-controlled or volume-cycled ventilation**) requires the clinician to set the peak flow rate, flow pattern, tidal volume, respiratory rate, positive end-expiratory pressure (applied PEEP, also known as extrinsic PEEP), and fraction of inspired oxygen (FiO_2). Inspiration ends once the inspiratory time set has elapsed.
- Volume-limited ventilation can be delivered via several modes, including:
  - Controlled Mechanical Ventilation (CMV),
  - Assist Control (AC),
  - Intermittent Mandatory Ventilation (IMV),
  - Synchronized intermittent mandatory ventilation (SIMV)

1. Controlled Mechanical Ventilation (CMV)

- During CMV, the minute ventilation is determined entirely by the set respiratory rate and tidal volume. The patient does not initiate additional minute ventilation above that set on the ventilator.
- This may be due to pharmacologic paralysis, heavy sedation, coma, or lack of incentive to increase the minute ventilation because the set minute ventilation meets or exceeds physiologic need. CMV does not require any patient work.

2. Assist Control (AC)

- During AC, the clinician determines the minimal minute ventilation by setting the respiratory rate and tidal volume. The patient can increase the minute ventilation by triggering additional breaths. Each patient-initiated breath receives the set tidal volume from the ventilator.
- Consider the following example. If the clinician sets the respiratory rate to 20 breaths per minute and the tidal volume to 500 mL, the lowest possible minute ventilation is 10 L per minute (20 breaths per minute times 500 mL per breath).
- If the patient triggers an additional 5 breaths beyond the preset 20 breaths, the ventilator will deliver 500 mL for each additional breath and the minute ventilation will be 12.5 L per minute (25 breaths per minute times 500 mL per breath).
- Pressure regulated volume control (PRVC) is similar to AC. The main difference is that the ventilator is able to autoregulate the inspiratory time and flow so that the tidal volume generates a smaller rise in the plateau airway pressure.

3. Intermittent Mandatory Ventilation (IMV)

- IMV is similar to AC in two ways: the clinician determines the minimal minute ventilation (by setting the respiratory rate and tidal volume) and the patient is able to increase the minute ventilation. However, IMV differs from AC in the way that the minute ventilation is increased. Specifically, patients increase the minute ventilation by spontaneous breathing, rather than patient-initiated ventilator breaths.
- Consider the following example. If the clinician sets the respiratory rate to 10 breaths per minute and the tidal volume to 500 mL per breath, the lowest possible minute ventilation is 5 L per minute (10 breaths per minute times 500 mL per breath). If the patient initiates an additional 5 breaths beyond the preset 10 breaths, the tidal volume for each additional breath will be whatever size the patient is able to generate and the minute ventilation will be some amount greater than 5 L per minute.
- The precise minute ventilation depends on the size of the tidal volume for each spontaneous breath.

4. Synchronized intermittent mandatory ventilation (SIMV)

- SIMV is a variation of IMV, in which the ventilator breaths are synchronized with patient inspiratory effort. SIMV (or IMV) can be used to titrate the level of ventilatory support over a wide range. This is an advantage unique to these modes. Ventilatory support can range from full support (set respiratory rate is high enough that the patient does not overbreathe) to no ventilatory support (set respiratory rate is zero).
- The level of support may need to be modified if hemodynamic consequences of positive pressure ventilation develop. In one study, cardiac output, mean blood pressure, pulmonary capillary wedge pressure, and oxygen consumption were all better when the level of support provided by SIMV was less.

COMPARISONS

- SIMV and AC are the most frequently used forms of volume-limited mechanical ventilation.
- Possible advantages of SIMV compared to AC include better patient-ventilator synchrony, better preservation of respiratory muscle function, lower mean airway pressures, and greater control over the level of support. In addition, auto-PEEP may be less likely with SIMV.

- In contrast, AC may be better suited for critically ill patients who require a constant tidal volume or full or near-maximal ventilatory support than 50 percent

2. PRESSURE-LIMITED VENTILATION

- Pressure-limited ventilation (also called pressure-cycled ventilation) requires the clinician to set the inspiratory pressure level, inspiratory to expiratory (I:E) ratio, respiratory rate, positive end-expiratory pressure (applied PEEP), and fraction of inspired oxygen (FiO_2). Inspiration ends after delivery of the set inspiratory pressure.
- The tidal volume is variable during pressure-limited ventilation. It is related to inspiratory pressure level, compliance, airway resistance, and tubing resistance. Specifically, tidal volumes will be larger when the set inspiratory pressure level is high or there is good compliance, little airway resistance, or little resistance from the ventilator tubing.
- In contrast, the peak airway pressure is constant during pressure-limited ventilation. It is equal to the sum of the set inspiratory pressure level and the applied PEEP. As an example, a patient with a set inspiratory pressure level of 20 cm H_2O and an applied PEEP of 10 cm H_2O will have a peak airway pressure of 30 cm H_2O.
- Pressure-limited ventilation can be delivered using the same modes of ventilation that deliver volume-limited ventilation:
  o During pressure-limited controlled mechanical ventilation (CMV; also called pressure control ventilation), the minute ventilation is determined entirely by the set respiratory rate and inspiratory pressure level. The patient does not initiate additional minute ventilation above that set on the ventilator.
  o During pressure-limited assist control (AC), the set respiratory rate and inspiratory pressure level determine the minimum minute ventilation. The patient is able to increase the minute ventilation by triggering additional ventilator-assisted, pressure-limited breaths.
  o During pressure-limited intermittent mandatory ventilation (IMV) or synchronized intermittent mandatory ventilation (SIMV), the set respiratory rate and inspiratory pressure level determine the minimum minute ventilation. The patient is able to increase the minute ventilation by initiating spontaneous breaths.

3. PRESSURE SUPPORT VENTILATION

- Pressure support ventilation (PSV) is a flow-limited mode of ventilation that delivers inspiratory pressure until the inspiratory flow decreases to a predetermined percentage of its peak value. This is usually 25 percent.
- For PSV, the clinician sets the pressure support level (inspiratory pressure level), applied PEEP, and FiO_2.
- The patient must trigger each breath because there is no set respiratory rate. The tidal volume, respiratory rate, and minute ventilation are dependent on multiple factors, including the ventilator settings and patient-related variables (e.g., compliance, sedation). In general, a high-pressure support level results in large tidal volumes and a low respiratory rate. The work of breathing is inversely proportional to the pressure support level, provided that inspiratory flow is sufficient to meet patient demand. In other words, increasing the level of pressure support decreases the work of breathing. The work of breathing is also inversely proportional to the inspiratory flow rate.

DISADVANTAGES

- PSV is poorly suited to provide full or near-full ventilatory support. The following characteristics of PSV are disadvantages in that setting:
  o Each breath must be initiated by the patient. Central apnea may occur if the respiratory drive is depressed due to sedatives, critical illness, or hypocapnia due to excessive ventilation.
  o An adequate minute ventilation cannot be guaranteed because tidal volume and respiratory rate are variable.
  o Ventilator asynchrony can occur when PSV is employed for full ventilatory support, potentially prolonging the duration of mechanical ventilation.
  o PSV is associated with poorer sleep than AC. Specifically, there is greater sleep fragmentation, less stage 1 and 2 non-rapid eye movement (NREM) sleep, more wakefulness during the first part of the night, and less stage 3 and 4 NREM sleep during the second part of the night.
  o Relatively high levels of pressure support (e.g., >20 cm H_2O) are required during full ventilatory support to prevent alveolar collapse (which can lead to cyclic atelectasis and ventilator-associated lung injury) and to attain a stable breathing pattern. Such high levels of pressure support are not as comfortable as moderate levels (e.g., 10 to 15 cm H_2O)

III. MANAGING INITIAL MECHANICAL VENTILATION IN THE ED

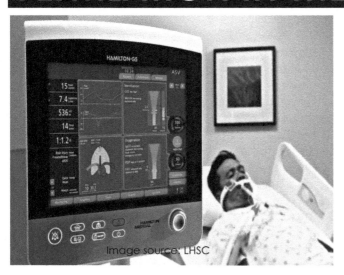

Image source: LHSC

INTRODUCTION

- The ventilator lectures given to most fledgling emergency physicians are often so complex and abstruse that many simply resign themselves to mute dependence on the respiratory therapist's settings.
- This piece represents a hopeful departure from this complexity. Understanding 2 simple ventilator strategies, lung protective and obstructive, will give a good foundation and management base for the first few hours of an emergency department (ED) patient's care.

LUNG PROTECTIVE STRATEGY

- The lung protective strategy focuses on low-tidal volume ventilation to reduce ventilator-associated lung injury such as barotrauma and volutrauma.
- It is appropriate for patients already demonstrating signs of acute lung injury and may also be used for any intubated patient to prevent disease state progression into acute lung injury.
- **This strategy should be chosen for any patient intubated in the ED who does not have obstructive disease** (asthma or chronic obstructive pulmonary disease).

Mode

- **Volume-assist control Mode** has numerous advantages for critically ill ED patients, including **availability** on all ventilators.
- The mode also **prevents patient fatigue** by offering full respiratory support.

- In my ED, the theoretical benefits of other modes (primarily a perception of increased patient comfort) are outweighed by the safety and ease of volume-assist control. Once the mode is selected, only 5 other settings must be chosen:

1. Tidal Volume

- Is for Alveolar Protection
- Set the initial tidal volume to **8 mL/kg.**
- This initial setting is appropriate for all intubated ED patients.
- The weight used is the patient's predicted body weight (based on patient's height) rather than actual body weight.
- This lower volume takes into account decreased functional lung volume (i.e., "baby lung"), caused by derecruited or shunted alveoli, in a patient with acute lung injury.
- In a critically ill patient without current acute lung injury, these small tidal volumes may minimize lung injury.
- The tidal volume may need to be further decreased as discussed below. This setting should not be changed to achieve $PaCO_2$ goals (with the exception of patients with severe metabolic acidosis).

2. Inspiratory Flow Rate

- Is for Patient Comfort
- When we breathe, we inspire a large amount of gas at the beginning of the breath that tapers to a small amount toward the end. This is called a **decelerating flow pattern**.
- Although some newer ventilators allow this flow pattern while in the volume-assist control mode, most ED ventilators do not. Instead, they deliver a fixed inspiratory flow rate.
- Erring on the side of excess flow toward the end of the breath is more comfortable than inadequate flow at the beginning of the breath.
- An initial setting of **60 L/minute** usually leads to adequate flow for patient comfort.
- If a patient looks like he or she is trying to inhale more gas at the beginning of an inspiration, this setting can be titrated up.
- Lack of attention to this setting may lead to an increased sedation or analgesia need but is unlikely to affect patient outcome.

3. Respiratory Rate

- Is for Titrating Ventilation
- The goal PaCO2 should be chosen according to the patient's illness and acid-base status. Once this value is determined, the only setting that should be used to achieve this goal is the respiratory rate.
- Respiratory rates as high as **30 to 40 breaths/min** are acceptable to achieve PaCO2 goals.
- **An initial rate of 15 to 16 breaths/min** should allow normocapnia in most patients.
- After 20 to 30 minutes, **venous or arterial blood should be drawn f**or blood gas testing to allow further titration.
- End tidal CO2 can be used as a spur to increase the respiratory rate if the ETCO2 value is greater than the PaCO2 goal; however, a low ETCO2 level should not trigger a decreasing of the respiratory rate. Physiologic shunt, decreased cardiac output, and dead space may lead to ETCO2 values that significantly underestimate the PaCO2 (remember this rule: all we can say is the PaCO2 is at least as high as the ETCO2). If PaCO2 goals cannot be achieved with even rapid respiratory rates, one should consider permissive hypercapnia.

4. PEEP and FiO2 Are for Titrating Oxygenation

- When faced with a low SpO2, one may think it seems intuitive to increase the FiO2.
- Unfortunately, this strategy has only a short-lived effect. Once the FiO2 reaches greater than 50%, any continuing hypoxemia is due to physiologic shunt. The solution to this shunt is to increase mean airway pressure through Positive End Expiratory Pressure (PEEP). The ARDSnet strategy guides clinicians to increase FiO2 and PEEP in tandem to allow alveolar recruitment.
- Immediately after intubation, **decrease the FiO2 to 30% to 40%** and **assign the patient a PEEP of 5 cm H2O.** Using the chart in Table below, rapidly titrate to PEEP-FiO2 combinations that result in an SpO2 of 88% to 95%.

FiO2 and PEEP scale from ARDSnet ARMA trial.

A. Lower PEEP:FiO₂ Combination													
FiO₂	0.3	0.4	0.4	0.5	0.5	0.6	0.7	0.7	0.7	0.8	0.9	0.9	0.9	1.0
PEEP	5	5	8	8	10	10	10	12	14	14	14	16	18	18-24

B. Higher PEEP:FiO₂ Combination												
FiO₂	0.3	0.3	0.4	0.4	0.5	0.5	0.5	0.6	0.7	0.8	0.8	0.9	1.0
PEEP	12	14	14	16	16	18	20	20	20	20	22	22	22-24

- Allowing patients to achieve a saturation of 100% exposes them to excess pressure and hyperoxia.
- Often, the initial PEEP and FiO2 settings used to achieve saturation goals will need to be titrated downward; eventually, progressive alveolar recruitment will result in a saturation of 100%.

- At this point, PEEP- FiO2 combinations should be decreased according to Table above.
- Downward titration should proceed at a slower pace than upward titration to avoid losing the hard-won alveolar recruitment.

5. Checking for Alveolar Safety

- Immediately after intubation, and subsequently every 30 to 60 minutes, a plateau pressure should be checked. Whereas the peak pressure on a ventilator represents a combination of alveolar pressure and large airway and ventilator equipment resistance, the plateau pressure approximates the pressure on and in the alveoli. By pressing the inspiratory hold button on the ventilator at the end of a breath, the plateau pressure can be measured.
- It is crucial that the patient be adequately sedated in order not to resist this breath hold. If the plateau pressure is greater than or equal to 30 cm H2O, there is the potential for alveolar injury.
- The solution to this issue is **to decrease the tidal volume by 1 mL/kg until a plateau pressure of less than 30 cm H2O is achieved.**
- **Tidal volumes as low as 4 mL/kg** are acceptable, although rarely necessary in the ED.
- In such cases, you will likely need to increase the respiratory rate to maintain PaCO2 goals.
- If you have reached the limit of respiratory rate titration, the patient should be allowed to maintain permissive hypercapnia. In patients who are already demonstrating established severe acute lung injury (PaO2/FiO2 <200 mm Hg), rapid titration of the tidal volume to 6 mL/kg should occur even if the plateau pressures are acceptable.

OBSTRUCTIVE STRATEGY

- Usually, the only patients who require diversion from the lung protective strategy outlined above are the **asthmatic and chronic obstructive pulmonary disease patients experiencing bronchospasm.**
- These obstructed patients will experience air trapping and barotrauma because they are unable to fully exhale when exposed to the rapid respiratory rates of the lung protective strategy.
- **The best ventilatory strategy in the obstructive patient is to avoid intubation altogether.**
- These patients often respond to aggressive pharmacologic and noninvasive ventilatory strategies.
- If forced to intubate because of worsening mental status, be aware that the ventilator will often make the pulmonary situation worse rather than better.

- The obstructive patient receiving ventilator treatment requires **deep sedation during the first few hours of care**.
- Paralysis is often unnecessary if deep sedation and analgesia are provided. If paralysis is used, the treatment should be short-lived. Intubation and mechanical ventilation should not represent the end of the pharmacologic treatment of bronchospasm, but rather an opportunity to maximize these medication regimens.
- **The primary goal** of the ventilator strategy for obstructive patients is to allow time to exhale. All settings are aligned to the aim of allowing a full exhalation after each ventilator breath.

Mode
- Just as in the lung injury strategy, I select the volume assist control mode. In my practice, any putative benefits of other modes have no applicability to the early stages of the postintubation period and are outweighed by the safety and familiarity of volume-assist control.

Tidal Volume
- Use the same initial **8 mL/kg** predicted body weight as for the lung injury strategy. This setting should not need to be titrated.

Flow
- Some texts recommend increasing the inspiratory flow rate to decrease the time required for inhalation, in turn allowing a longer period for the subsequent exhalation.
- This will serve only to increase the peak pressure, causing unnecessary alarms without producing any clinically meaningful change in the expiration time.
- **A setting of 60 to 80 L/minute** is more than enough flow for these patients.

Respiratory Rate
- Allows Time to Exhale This is the primary titratable setting to safely manage the intubated patient with obstructive lung disease. Decreasing the respiratory rate allows more time for expiration.
- These patients will inevitably become hypercapnic when the respiratory rate is set properly.
- This hypercapnia should be permitted. **A starting rate of 8 to 10** should be used and then titrated as discussed below.

PEEP and FiO2
- In isolated obstructive disease, patients receiving even a modicum of supplemental FiO2 should not experience difficulty achieving adequate levels of oxygen saturation. **An FiO2 of 40%** should allow an SpO2 greater than 88%.

- Higher FiO2 levels may be used when necessary.
- There are no compelling data to suggest any benefit in the application of PEEP within the first few hours postintubation. Inappropriately high PEEP can be deleterious. As such, a PEEP of 0 is my recommendation when managing patients in the ED. Some resuscitationists' preferences may dictate setting low levels of PEEP (≤5), but again there is no definitive evidence to support this practice.

Peak Pressure Alarm
- Peak pressures represent resistance in an obstructive patient's large airways as a result of bronchospasm. Often, high peak pressures will be necessary to ventilate past this obstruction.
- These elevated pressures are not transmitted to the alveoli and thus convey no harm to the lung parenchyma. If the peak pressure alarm of the ventilator is set too low, the ventilator may terminate the breath prematurely, and the patient will receive little or no alveolar ventilation.
- To prevent this, **increase the peak pressure alarm setting until the full breath of 8 mL/kg** is allowed to be delivered. In obstructed patients, the peak pressure may be quite high, but the plateau pressure should remain well below the 30 cm H2O (as long as the patient is being allowed to fully exhale), ensuring the safety of this strategy.

Summary table for the 2 ventilator strategies.

	Lung Protective Strategy	Obstructive Strategy
Mode	Volume assist control	Volume assist control
Tidal volume	Start at 8 mL/kg PBW; adjust for plateau pressure goal	8 mL/kg PBW
Inspiratory flow rate	Start at 60 L/min; adjust for comfort	60–80 L/min
Respiratory rate	Start at 16 breaths/min; adjust for PaCO2 goal	Start at 10 breaths/min; adjust to allow full expiration
PEEP	Start at 5 cm H2O; adjust according to table	0 cm H2O (some may treat pt with PEEP 5 cm H2O)
FiO2	Start at 40%; adjust according to table	Start at 40%; adjust for SpO2 88%
Check for safety	Measure plateau pressure. If <30 cm H2O decrease tidal volume by 1 mL/kg	Measure plateau pressure or observe flow time graph. If plateau pressure ≥30 cm H2O or flow/time graph shows incomplete expiration, decrease respiratory rate

17. End-Tidal Capnography

INTRODUCTION

- End-tidal capnography (end-tidal CO_2, $PETCO_2$, $ETCO_2$) refers to the graphical measurement of carbon dioxide partial pressure (mm Hg) during expiration.
- The American Society of Anesthesiologists (ASA) endorses end-tidal capnography as a standard of care for general anaesthesia, moderate sedation, and deep sedation.
- Accordingly, other specialities, including critical care and emergency medicine, are more frequently implementing end-tidal capnography monitoring.

MONITORING AN INTUBATED PATIENT

- Immediately following intubation, the following checks should be performed.
- These checks should also be performed when taking over an intubated patient, such as following an out of hospital intubation:
- Attach a pulse oximeter (if not already in place).
- Connect a capnometer if available.
- Auscultate the patient in both axillae and over the stomach.
- Pulse oximetry assesses patient oxygenation, not ventilation.
- In the event of a misplaced (i.e. oesophageal) endotracheal tube, the saturations may only drop slowly, not immediately.
- Thus, pulse oximetry has limited use as a rapid check of correct intubation.
- Capnometers respond rapidly to falls in expired CO_2 and immediately indicate the absence of expired CO_2.
- Hence capnometry is the gold standard monitor for correct intubation: **lack of expired CO2 suggests oesophageal intubation.**
- When monitoring a ventilated patient, **a sudden drop in expired CO2 to zero** indicates an **equipment problem** such as a disconnection in the breathing system, extubation or ventilator failure.
- A more **gradual fall in expired CO2** suggests a **patient problem** such as a drop in cardiac output due to cardiac arrest, inadequate external cardiac compressions or pulmonary embolism.
- As the lungs are still ventilated, expired CO_2 falls more slowly as CO_2 is washed out of the lungs over several breaths.

1. CAPNOGRAPHY WAVEFORM INTERPRETATION

- Capnography waveform interpretation can be used for diagnosis and ventilator-trouble shooting.
- The CO2 waveform can be analysed for 5 characteristics: **Height/ Frequency/ Rhythm / Baseline / Shape**

NORMAL CAPNOGRAM PHASES

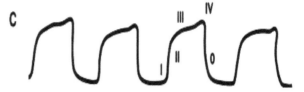

4 PHASES:

- **Phase I (inspiratory baseline):** beginning of exhalation, CO2 level is ZERO.
- **Phase II (expiratory upstroke):** alveolar gas begins to mix with the dead space gas and the CO2 rises rapidly.
- **Phase III (alveolar plateau):** elimination of CO2 from the alveoli; usually.
- **An additional phase IV** (terminal upstroke before phase 0) may be seen in pregnancy
- **Phase 0 (inspiratory downstroke):** the beginning of the next inspiration

CLINICAL USES OF CAPNOGRAPHY

- Monitoring Ventilation: Hyperventilation and Hypoventilation.
- Confirming, Maintaining, and Assisting Intubation
- Measuring Cardiac Output during CPR
- Monitoring Sedated Patients
- Ventilating Head Injured Patients
- Perfusion Warning Sign

LIMITS OF CAPNOMETRY

- There may be little or no CO2 output in low or zero cardiac output states. Capnometry may not detect endobronchial intubation. Endobronchial intubation may be suspected by asymmetrical chest movement following intubation, and should be detected by auscultation.
- Ventilation of a patient with an uncuffed endotracheal tube that is significantly too small may result in a large leak with expiration around the tube rather than through it, especially if PEEP is used. As no expired gases are flowing through the breathing system, the capnometer may give a misleadingly low or even zero reading.
- Auscultation should be performed over both axillae, as in small patient's breath sounds may transmit from one side of the chest to the other.
- Auscultation is also performed over the stomach, as the sound of air entry into the stomach may be misinterpreted as lung air entry unless the stomach is auscultated as well for comparison.

2. CAUSES OF ABNORMAL ETCO2

FLAT ETCO2 TRACE

- Ventilator disconnection
- Airway misplaced – extubation, oesophageal intubation
- Capnograph not connected to circuit
- Respiratory/Cardiac arrest
- Apnoea test in "brain death" dead patient
- Capnography obstruction

INCREASED ETCO2

CO2 Production

- Fever
- Sodium bicarbonate
- Tourniquet release
- Venous CO2 embolism
- Overfeeding

Pulmonary perfusion

- Increased cardiac output
- Increased blood pressure

Alveolar ventilation

- Hypoventilation
- Bronchial intubation
- Partial airway obstruction
- Rebreathing

Apparatus malfunctioning

- Exhausted CO2 absorber
- Inadequate fresh gas flows
- Leaks in ventilator tubing
- Ventilator malfunctioning

DECREASED ETCO2

CO2 production

- Hypothermia

Pulmonary perfusion

- Reduced cardiac output
- Hypotension
- Hypovolemia
- Pulmonary embolism
- Cardiac arrest

Alveolar ventilation

- Hyperventilation
- Apnea
- Total airway obstruction
- Extubation

Apparatus malfunctioning

- Circuit disconnection (note low airway pressures)
- Leaks in sampling tube
- Ventilator malfunctioning

SUDDEN DROP IN ETCO2 TO ZERO "DOPES"	SUDDEN INCREASE IN ETCO2
- **D**isplacement/ **D**isconnection - **O**bstruction/ **P**neumothorax - **E**quipment failure, - Breath **S**tacking	- ROSC during cardiac arrest - Correction of ET tube obstruction

SUDDEN CHANGE IN BASELINE (NOT TO ZERO)	ELEVATED INSPIRATORY BASELINE
- Calibration error - CO2 absorber saturated: check capnograph with room air - Water drops in analyser or condensation in airway adapter	- CO2 rebreathing (soda lime exhaustion) - Contamination of CO2 monitor (sudden elevation of baseline and top line) - Inspiratory valve malfunction (elevation of the baseline, prolongation of downstroke, prolongation of phase III)

3. COMMON CAPNOGRAM PATTERNS

- Pattern recognition of common changes in the capnogram can be useful in coming to a rapid diagnosis during mechanical ventilation (see patterns above):

1. Normal

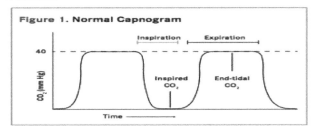

Figure 1. Normal Capnogram

2. Flat line: DARC (+DOPES)

- o **D**isconnection
- o **A**pnoea
- o **R**espiratory arrest
- o **C**ardiac arrest

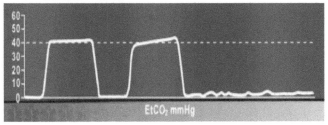

3. Up-sloping plateau phase (increased alpha-angle):

- o Ventilation-perfusion mismatch
- o Lower airway obstruction: bronchospasm, asthma, COPD
- o Partial airway obstruction: pathological, secretions, tube kinking.

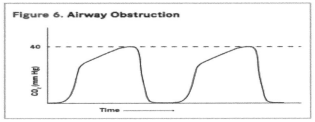

Figure 6. Airway Obstruction

4. High plateau and end-tidal CO2:

- o Hypoventilation
- o Increased CO_2 production (metabolic), e.g. malignant hyperpyrexia.

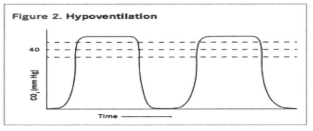

Figure 2. Hypoventilation

5. Low plateau and end-tidal CO2:

- o Hyperventilation.

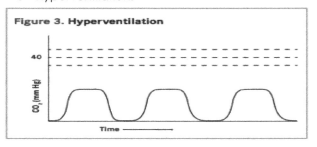

Figure 3. Hyperventilation

6. Progressively rising plateau and baseline:

- o Re-breathing within an anaesthetic breathing system.

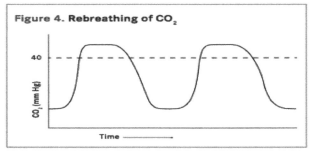

Figure 4. Rebreathing of CO_2

7. Oscillations in down slope of tracing:

- o Cardiac oscillations.

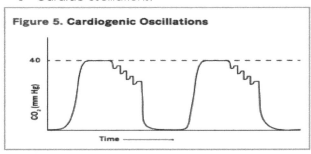

Figure 5. Cardiogenic Oscillations

8. Notched plateau phase:

- o This capnopgraphy waveform demonstrates the "curare cleft" in the alveolar plateau.
- o This is caused by the patient making spontaneous respiratory effort during mechanical ventilation due to neuromuscular blockade wearing off.

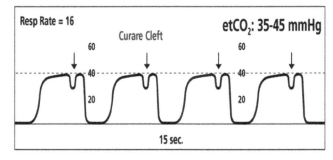

Resp Rate = 16   Curare Cleft   etCO2: 35-45 mmHg

15 sec.

RELATIONSHIP BETWEEN END-TIDAL AND ARTERIAL CO2

- EtCO2 reflects PaCO2 but is usually lower than PaCO2 by 0.3–0.6kPa in health. An increase in the difference between EtCO2 and PaCO2 develops in the presence of ventilation-perfusion mismatch, due to an increase in physiological dead space.
- Arterial – end-tidal PCO2 (a-ET PCO2) difference is therefore a good measure of dead space ventilation, except when the phase III plateau is steeply up-sloping, which can result in a zero or negative a-ET PCO2 difference.
- Reduced cardiac output, poor pulmonary perfusion, and pulmonary embolism are common situations that result in an increased a-ET PCO2.
- These conditions will cause an underestimation of PaCO2 from EtCO2.

COLORIMETRIC CO2 DETECTORS

- Colorimetric detectors are small disposable devices that can be attached directly to an endotracheal tube to confirm the presence of CO2 in respiratory gas.
- They comprise a pH sensitive chemical that changes colour as gas containing CO2 in the range of 2–5% CO2 passes over it but will remain unchanged if lower than this.

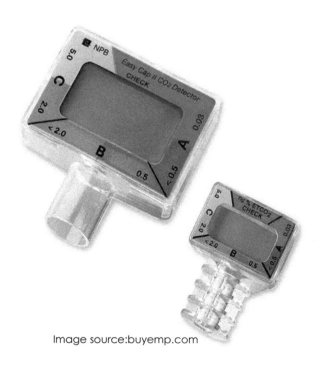

Image source:buyemp.com

- It is therefore a useful aid to help confirm correct placement of an endotracheal tube when formal capnography is unavailable.

4. HOW TO ANALYZE THE WAVEFORM?

- Use an algorithm or systematic process for analysis.
- This can be divided into several steps:
  - Look for presence of exhaled CO2 (Is a waveform present?)
  - Inspiratory baseline (Is there rebreathing?)
  - Expiratory upstroke (What is the shape i.e. steep, sloping, or prolonged?)
  - Expiratory/alveolar plateau (Is it sloping, steep, or prolonged?)
  - Inspiratory downstroke (Is it sloping, steep, or prolonged)
  - Ensure you evaluate the height, frequency, rhythm, baseline, and shape.

  With these thoughts in mind, let's discuss some clinical scenarios.

CLINICAL CASES...
Case 1:

- Before you can reassess your other two patients, you receive an EMS radio call. They were called to the scene of a patient in PEA, and they have started compressions and will be at your doorstep in 3 minutes.
- The patient arrives, with the crew doing high quality CPR.
- The patient continues with no pulse, leads and ETCO2 are connected, one amp of epinephrine is given, and US shows a heart rate of 40 bpm.
- Your waveform capnography shows 10 mm Hg, and the person completing CPR is tiring. As the team leader, you ask another team member to take over.

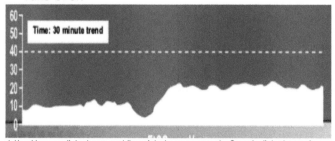

http://www.slideshare.net/larryide/capnography?next_slideshow=1

- *This waveform with a dip shows the time to transition to a different provider, with improved perfusion with the new provider doing compressions, as the CO2 has increased indicating better tissue perfusion.*
- After another minute of CPR, the ETCO2 jumps to 40.
- **A sudden increase in ETCO2 is seen in ROSC during arrest or correction of an ETT obstruction.**

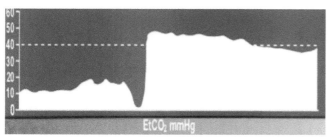

http://www.slideshare.net/larryide/capnography?next_slideshow=1

- You now have return of pulses and are preparing to intubate the patient.
- Unfortunately, the resident completing it is not confident in his view and is unsure of tube placement. Your waveform shows the following:

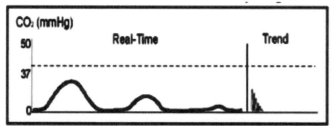

Fig 6.20.4. *This waveform shows a **tapering of the ETCO2**, suggestive of oesophageal intubation.*

- You ask the resident to remove the ETT. He obtains an improved view with videoscope and passes the ETT without difficulty. The waveform looks normal, and the patient is now stable.

Case 2:
- Finally, you have time to go reassess your COPD patient.
- Just as you enter the resuscitation bay, he has a **desaturation to 88% while on FiO2 of 100%**, and your waveform is flat.

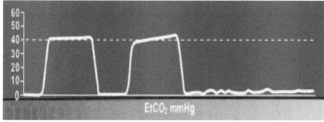

http://www.slideshare.net/larryide/capnography?next_slideshow=1

- You are now pretty tired of these flat waveforms, and you immediately curb your sphincter response while running to the bedside.
- Your mind quickly goes through the **DOPES mnemonic** (**D**isplacement/**D**isconnection, **O**bstruction, **P**neumothorax, **E**quipment failure, Breath **S**tacking) and you see that while moving the patient, **the ETT became disconnected from the circuit**. You reconnect, with increase in saturation and good waveform.

WHAT ARE OTHER CAUSES OF A SUDDEN FLAT ETCO2 TRACING?
- Extubation,
- Ventilator disconnection
- Capnography not connected to circuit,
- Obstruction of capnography,
- Oesophageal intubation.
- Cardiorespiratory arrest,
- Apnea test in brain dead patient,

Case 3:
- After caring for an ankle sprain and beginning the workup of a patient with chest pain, you again reassess the patient with COPD. You notice a steadily increasing EtCO2 baseline in your COPD patient. The waveform looks like this...

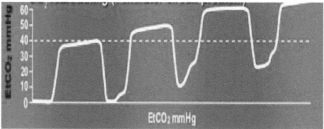

http://www.slideshare.net/larryide/capnography?next_slideshow=1

- The waveform reflects **an elevation of baseline**, as well as the **plateau**, indicating **incomplete exhalation. The CO2 is not being appropriately removed.**
- **This is often due to:**
  o Insufficient expiratory time,
  o Inadequate inspiratory flow, or
  o Faulty expiratory valve.
- **Rebreathing** can also appear with the following waveform **with baseline elevation**, which is due **to inadequate exchange of CO2.**

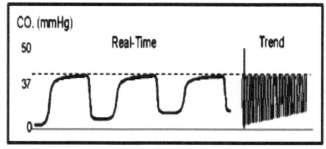

http://www.paramedicine.com/pmc/End_Tidal_CO2.html.

INCREASED ETCO2 CAN BE DUE TO FOUR COMPONENTS:
  o **Increased CO2 production** (fever, NaHCO3 administration, tourniquet release, and overfeeding syndrome).

- o **Pulmonary perfusion increase** (increased cardiac output, increased blood pressure).
- o **Alveolar ventilation decrease** (hypoventilation, bronchial intubation, partial airway obstruction, rebreathing).
- o **Equipment malfunction** (exhausted CO2 absorber, inadequate fresh gas flow, ventilator tubing leak, ventilator malfunction).

- • **Once you slow down his respiratory rate and increase the flow rate**, his saturations and **waveform improve**.
- • Suddenly, the alarm alerts you to high pressures in the circuit, and his waveform shows:

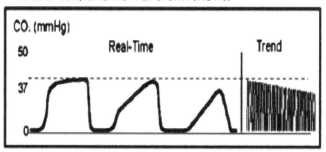

http://www.paramedicine.com/pmc/End_Tidal_CO2.html

- • *This waveform is due to **obstruction of the ETT**, either through **ETT kink, foreign body in airway, bronchospasm, or mucous plug**.*

- • You see high peak pressures and suction the tube, while ordering an in-line duoneb.
- • Five minutes later the **patient again improves**.

Case 4:

- • After all this excitement, you prepare for **the sedation of the 8-year-old male** with forearm fracture requiring reduction. The sedation and reduction go smoothly with ketamine. He is starting to wake from his dissociative state, and you see this:

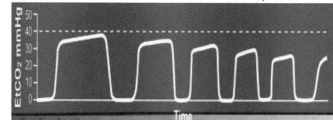

http://www.slideshare.net/larryide/capnography?next_slideshow=1

- • *This waveform demonstrates **hyperventilation**.*
- • ***Notice the baseline is unchanged.** This waveform **shows steadily decreasing plateau, reflecting tachypnoea**, increase in tidal volume, decreased metabolic rate, or fall in body temperature.*

A DECREASING ETCO2 HAS SEVERAL ETIOLOGIES:

- o **Decreased CO2 production** (hypothermia)
- o **Pulmonary perfusion decrease** (reduced cardiac output, hypotension, pulmonary embolism, cardiac arrest)
- o **Alveolar ventilation increase** (hyperventilation, apnea, total airway obstruction, extubation)
- o **Apparatus malfunction** (circuit disconnection, leak in sampling, ventilator malfunction)

WHAT IF HIS RESPIRATORY RATE HAD STARTED TO DECREASE?

- • **The alveolar plateau will begin to steadily increase**, which is due to decrease in respiratory rate, decreased tidal volume, increased metabolic rate, and hyperthermia.
- • Notice the baseline is still close to 0, so CO2 is appropriately exchanged.

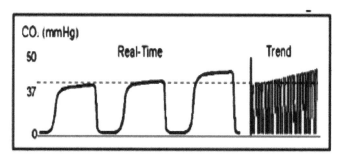

http://www.paramedicine.com/pmc/End_Tidal_CO2.html

- • Just before you send the COPD patient to the ICU, the nurse grabs you, as the waveform has now changed.

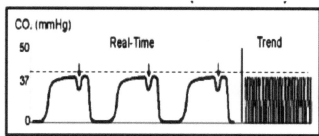

http://www.paramedicine.com/pmc/End_Tidal_CO2.html

- • *This small dip in the alveolar plateau is known as a **"curare cleft."***
- • This waveform appears when the **paralytic begins to subside and the patient tries to breathe during partial paralysis.**
- • **You increase the analgesic drip**, and the patient is transferred to the ICU.

18. Tracheostomy Tube Displaced

I. ADULT TRACHEOSTOMY TUBE DISPLACED

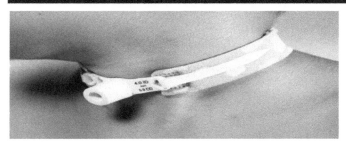

What is your first step once you confirm that the tracheostomy tube is displaced?

- Call for help
- Give/switch 100% oxygen
- Check capnography (ETCO2): if not on, put it on
- Call for difficult airway trolley
- Look if the chest is moving or not?

What will you do if the patient is breathing normally and the ETCO2 trace is normal?

Suggests tracheostomy displacement unlikely
- Consider other causes for deterioration (pneumothorax, bronchospasm)
- Assess breathing and circulation, follow ALS algorithm if necessary

What will you do if the patient is not breathing normally and the ETCO2 trace is not normal?

- Suggests a problem with tracheostomy:
  - Is tracheostomy blocked? – pass suction catheter via tracheostomy, ensure inner tube removed
  - Has cuff herniated over end of tracheostomy? – deflate and reinflate cuff

What will you do if the patien is deteriorating?

- Deflate tracheostomy cuff and remove tracheostomy
- Cover tracheostomy with sterile gauze and occlusive dressing
- Ventilate with 100% O2 using bag and facemask with Guedel airway and two hands on mask
- Consider LMA/I-gel/ Proseal LMA
- Intubate if you have the skills
- When senior help arrives consider:
  - GEB guided insertion of tracheostomy (extreme care if tracheostomy tract <7 days old)
  - RSI and oral reintubation.

II. CHILD TRACHEOSTOMY TUBE DISPLACED

What will be your first Resuscitation steps In the event of finding an unresponsive tracheostomised child?

- Attempt to arouse the child while calling for help
- Attempt to suction the airway

What if there is difficulty suctioning or the tracheostomy tube is blocked?

- Change the tracheostomy tube immediately and attempt suctioning again

What If this fails?

- Consider inserting a smaller size tracheostomy tube

What If this fails?

- A tracheal suction tube is passed down the lumen of the smaller tube and an attempt is made to guide the tracheostomy tube over the suction tube

What If this fails?

- If still unsuccessful, a flexible endoscope with a tube first threaded over it may be used by experienced staff to insert the tracheostomy tube under direct vision
- Concurrently with the above steps, any other possible means of ventilating the child are employed i.e. bag & mask, endotracheal tube intubation etc.; the possibility of doing this depends on the underlying pathology
- Only experienced personnel should use tracheostomy dilators or an artery clip to dilate the tracheal stoma if it has started to close down
- Check whether the child is breathing after reinserting the tracheostomy tube; a self-inflating bag ventilation device may be required to provide rescue breaths.

19. Tracheal Tube Displaced

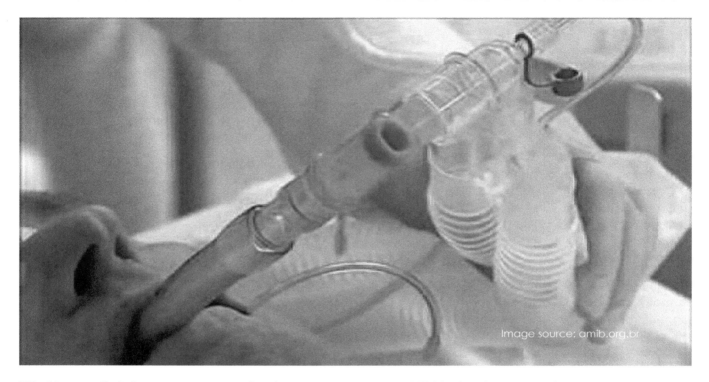

Image source: amib.org.br

What is your first step once you confirm that the endotracheal tube is displaced?

- Give 100% oxygen
- Check capnography (ETCO2): if not on, put it on
- Call for difficult airway trolley
- Look if the chest is moving or not?

What if the patient is breathing normally and the ETCO2 trace is normal. What will you do?

- Suggests problem with tracheal tube unlikely
- Consider other causes for deterioration (pneumothorax, bronchospasm)
- Assess breathing and circulation, follow ALS algorithm if necessary

What if the patient is not breathing normally and the ETCO2 trace is not normal. What will you do?

- Suggests a problem with tracheal tube (TT):
  - o Check TT markings at teeth- has TT been pushed in or partially fallen out?
  - o Is TT blocked? – pass suction catheter
  - o Is patient biting on TT? - give ATRACURIUM 50mg IV
  - o Has cuff herniated over end of TT? - deflate and reinflate cuff

What will you do if the patient is deteriorating?

- Remove tracheal tube and call for senior anaesthetist
- Ventilate with 100% O2 using bag/mask with Guedel airway + two hands on mask
- Consider LMA/I-gel/ Proseal LMA
- Oral tracheal intubation if you have the skills

What if the patient is not deteriorating?

- 100% Oxygen and await senior anaesthetist
- Paralyse
- Consider passing bronchoscope via TT ± railroading TT into place
- If no doubt, laryngoscopy and re-intubation

20. Fluid Challenge

I. ALGORITHMS FOR IV FLUID THERAPY IN ADULTS

Adapted from NICE CG174

ALGORITHM 1: ASSESSMENT

Using an **ABCDE approach, assess whether the patient is hypovolaemic and needs fluid resuscitation**
Assess volume status taking into account clinical examination, trends and context. Indicators that a patient may need fluid resuscitation include: systolic BP <100mmHg, HR>90bpm, capillary refill >2sec or peripheries cold to touch, RR>20bpm, NEWS≥5, 45°passive leg raising suggests fluid responsiveness.

YES

NO

ALGORITHM 2: FLUID RESUSCITATION

Assess the patient's likely fluid and electrolyte needs:
- History: previous limited intake, thirst, abnormal losses, comorbidities
- Clinical Examination: Pulse, BP, capillary refill, JVP, Oedema (peripheral/pulmonary), postural hypotension

Initiate treatment:
- Identify cause of deficit and respond
- Give a fluid bolus of 500ml of crystalloid (containing sodium in the range of 130-154 mmol/l) over 15 minutes

Can the patient meet their fluid and/or electrolyte needs orally or enterally?

YES

Ensure nutrition and Fluid needs are met:
Also see support in adults
(NICE CG 32)

NO

Reassess the patient using the ABCDE approach:
Does the patient still need fluid resuscitation?
Seek expert help if unsure

Does the patient have complex fluid or electrolyte replacement or abnormal distribution issues?
Look for existing deficits or excesses, ongoing abnormal losses, abnormal distribution or other complex issues

YES

ALGORITHM 4: REPLACEMENT AND REDISTRIBUTION

YES

NO

Does the patient have signs of shock?

NO

ALGORITHM 3: ROUTINE MAINTENANCE

YES

NO

Give maintenance IV Fluids:
Normal daily fluid and electrolyte requirements:
- 25-30ml/kg/day water
- 1 mmol/kg/day Sodium, Potassium, Chloride
- 50-100g/day Glucose (e.g. Glucose 5% contains 5g/100ml)

>2000ml given?

YES

Seek expert help

NO

Give a further fluid bolus of 250-500ml of crystalloid

Reassess and monitor the patient:
- Stop IV Fluids when no longer needed
- Nasogastric Fluids or enteral feeding are preferable when maintenance needs are more than 3 days.

ALGORITHM 4: REPLACEMENT AND REDISTRIBUTION

Existing fluid or electrolyte deficits or excesses.

Check for:
- Dehydration
- Fluid overload
- Hyperkalaemia/Hypokalaemia

Ongoing abnormal fluid or electrolyte losses
Check ongoing losses and estimate amounts.

Check for:
- Vomiting and NG tube loss
- Biliary drainage loss
- High/low volume ileal stoma loss
- Diarrhoea/ excess colostomy loss
- Ongoing blood loss. e.g. melaena
- Sweating/ fever/ dehydration

Redistribution and other complex issues
Check for:
- Gross oedema
- Severe sepsis
- Hypernatraemia/ hyponatraemia
- Renal, liver and/or cardiac impairment
- Post-operative fluid retention and redistribution
- Malnourished and refeeding issues

Seek expert help if necessary

Prescribe by adding to or substracting from routine maintenance, adjusting for all other sources of fluid and electrolytes (oral, enteral and drug prescriptions)

Monitor and reassess fluid and biochemical status by clinical and laboratory monitoring

Adapted from NICE CG174 [302].

---

[302] *Intravenous fluid therapy in adults in hospital – NICE **Clinical guideline [CG174]** Published date: December 2013 Last updated: May 2017*

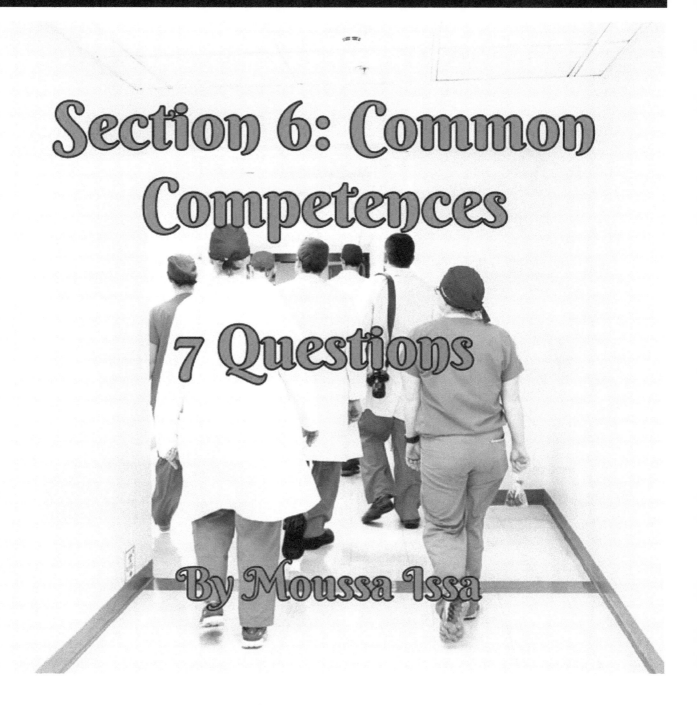

Section VII. Common Competences

Section 6: Common Competences

7 Questions

By Moussa Issa

Ebook for only £3/month!

Get our Reading App for your Android smartphone or tablet to start enjoying the Moussa Issa eBookstore discovery and digital reading experience.

Download our APP on your Smart device Now.

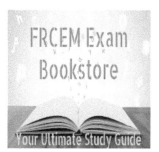

FRCEM Exam eBookstore

FRCEM Exam Bookstore   Books & Reference

PEGI 3

Offers in-app purchases

ⓘ This app is compatible with all of your devices.

Installed

A static eBook with little interactivity cannot draw your attention any more. Thus it is essential to engage readers with interactive reading experience.

Moussa Issa eBookstore proves to be on top of the interactive eBook game, enabling readers to watch integrated videos related to the subject directly on the page.

The additional flipping effect makes the eBook fully interactive and dynamic.

Customize your experience with multiple font and page styles and social sharing tools.

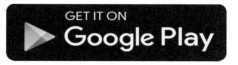

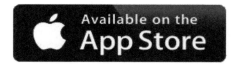

Distributed by Moussa Issa Bookstore Ltd

Website: www.moussaissabooks.com

Email: info@moussaissabooks.com

eBook subscription: www.moussaissabooks.com/read-ebook-online

1. Health Promotion & Public Health

I. STANDARD INFECTION CONTROL PRECAUTIONS

1. HAND HYGIENE

- Hand hygiene is a term used to describe processes that render the hands of health care workers safe (having reduced the number of micro-organisms present that are acquired through activities that involve touching patients, equipment or the environment in the workplace)[303].
- Hand Hygiene is a simple and very effective method of helping to prevent the spread of healthcare associated infection.
- Healthcare associated infections can have significant consequences for the resident leading to increased morbidity and mortality, extended bed stay, extra treatment and psychological stress.
- People, who are either ill and/or in residential care, have an increased risk of acquiring an infection. Minor infections for some people, may be very serious for others. Hand Hygiene is the single most important method of controlling infection.

WHO NEEDS TO CARRY OUT HAND HYGIENE?

- Most care activities involve the use of our hands.
- All disciplines of staff have responsibility to their residents, clients and to themselves to carry out effective hand hygiene. Hands are the principal route by which cross infection occurs.

WHY?

- Hands normally have a 'resident' population of microorganisms. These are:
  o Deep seated
  o Difficult to remove
  o Part of the body's natural defence mechanism
- They can be associated with infection following surgery, invasive procedures or in immunocompromised residents.

- Other microorganisms are picked up during every day activities and these are termed 'transient' microorganisms. These are:
  o Superficial and easily transferred to and from the hands
  o An important source of infection
  o Easily removed with good hand hygiene
- Many infections are caused by transient microorganisms.
- Effective hand hygiene will remove these transient microorganisms before they are transferred to:
  o surfaces
  o other residents or
  o susceptible sites on the same resident

WHAT TO USE FOR HAND HYGIENE?

- Good technique covering all surfaces is more important than the product used or the length of time taken.
- Good quality liquid soap and water is effective for social hand hygiene.
- Paper towels must be available for hand drying.

ALCOHOL HAND RUBS

- Alcohol hand rubs are recommended and are preferable in the healthcare setting for social and antiseptic hand hygiene. When using an Alcohol hand rub the preparation should be:
  o Dispensed as per manufacturers instructions.
  o Rubbed into all areas of the hands using the six step technique.
  o Rubbed in until hands are dry.
  o Used only on visibly clean hands. Exceptions to using Alcohol Hand Rubs
  o Alcohol hand rubs should not be used on visibly soiled hands.
  o Alcohol hand rubs should not be used after caring for residents with diarrhoeal illnesses including Clostridium difficile.

---

[303] *Essential Practice for Infection Prevention and Control Guidance for nursing staff.pdf*

My "5 Moments for Hand Hygiene" [304]

1. Moment 1- Before Touching the patient/resident

- o **When:** Clean the hands before touching the person you are delivering care to
- o **Why:** To protect the perons recieveing care from harmful micro-organisms carried on the HCWs hands
- o **Examples**
  - Helping someone to get washed or dressed
  - Prior to changing incontinence wear
  - Taking pulse, blood pressure, examination of skin, abdominal palpation

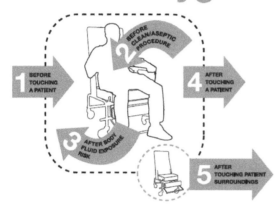

Your 5 Moments for Hand Hygiene

2. Moment 2 -Before a Clean/Aseptic Procedure

- o **When:** clean the hands immediately before performing an aseptic or clean procedure
- o **Why:** to protect against micro-organisms from entering the persons body
- o **Examples**
  - Oral care, giving eye drops, suctioning
  - Skin lesion care, wound dressing, giving an injection
  - Urinary catheter insertion and catheter care
  - Accessing /commencing a tube feeding system
  - Preparation of medication, or doing a dressing
  - Taking specimen samples including blood and urine

3. Moment 3 - After Body Fluid Exposure Risk

- o **When:** clean the hands immediately after an exposure risk to body fluids (and after glove removal)
- o **Why:** to protect the HCW and the healthcare environment from harmful micro-organisms
- o **Examples**
  - Clearing up urine, faeces, vomit, handling waste (soiled dressings, tissues, incontinence pads),
  - Cleaning of contaminated and visibly soiled material from equipment or the environment (bathroom, commodes)
  - Taking blood, urine or faecal samples, emptying urinary catheters

4. Moment 4 - After Touching the Client/Resident

- o **When:** clean the hands after directly touching the person you are when you have completed the care you are providing
- o **Why:** to protect the HCW and the healthcare environment from harmful micro-organisms
- o **Examples**
  - Helping someone to get washed, get dressed,
  - Taking pulse, blood pressure.
  - After completing an examination on someone

5. Moment 5 - After Touching the Patient/ Residents Surroundings

- o **When:** Clean the hands after touching any object or furniture or personal items belonging to the person you are caring for which includes their home , even if the person has not been touched
- o **Why:** to protect the HCW and the healthcare environment from harmful micro-organisms Examples
- o **Examples**
  - Touching personal items
  - Leaving someones home after providing care

GOOD PRACTICE WHEN CARRYING OUT HAND HYGIENE[305]

- Keep nails short, clean and cut smoothly
- Do not wear false or gel nails
- Remove all nail polish
- Restrict jewellery to a flat ring/wedding band
- Move ring to wash and dry underneath
- Remove wrist jewellery
- Shirts should have short sleeves or turned up sleeves

CARING FOR YOUR HANDS

- Care for your hands by using a moisturiser
- Do not wear gloves unnecessarily
- Any rashes, dermatitis or glove usage problems should be referred to the Occupational Health Department for advice and follow up

THINK.....

- What have you just done?
- What are you about to do?
- What type of hand hygiene procedure is needed?

---

[304] *WHO Guidelines on Hand Hygiene in Health Care*

[305] *Infection Prevention and Control Hand Hygiene for Staff.pdf - HSE 2014*

2. PERSONAL PROTECTIVE EQUIPMENT

- Personal protective equipment (PPE) includes items such as gloves, aprons, masks, goggles or visors.
- PPE is used to protect health care workers from harm, in this case from risks of infection.
- PPE such as gloves may also be required for contact with hazardous chemicals and some pharmaceuticals, for example, disinfectants or cytotoxic drugs.

DISPOSABLE GLOVES

- Gloves are not a substitute for hand hygiene and should be used when appropriate.
- Overuse of gloves is an increasing concern.
- Wearing gloves only when required is important, as the incorrect use of gloves can lead to several problems including:
  - Undermining local hand hygiene initiatives
  - Risk of skin problems such as contact dermatitis or exacerbation of skin problems on hands.
- As one element of PPE, gloves act as a control measure to reduce identified risks to health care workers including nursing staff.
- Where exposure cannot be avoided, as is the case with a number of health care related activities, personal protective equipment, including gloves should be used. Gloves should only be used if a risk assessment identifies them as necessary.
- Typically the use of gloves is justified when the wearer is at risk of exposure to blood/bodily fluids, non-intact skin or mucous membranes.
- In such circumstances the risk is exposure to blood bourne viruses (BBV) which can be referred to as a biological risk. Health care workers also need to protect themselves from chemical risks such as cytotoxic drugs and chemicals, in these cases gloves should also be worn.
- Gloves should be worn whenever contact with blood and body fluids, mucous membranes or non-intact skin is a risk, but should not be considered a substitute for hand hygiene. Hand hygiene must always be performed following the removal of gloves.
- Gloves should be put on immediately before the task is to be performed, then removed and discarded in the relevant waste stream as soon as that procedure is completed.
- Gloves should never be worn 'just in case' as part of routine nursing care. The choice of glove should be made following a risk assessment of the task about to be undertaken, the suitability of the gloves (including fit, comfort and dexterity) and any risks to the patient or to the health care worker.

- Glove good practise points[306]:
  - Gloves are not an alternative to hand hygiene
  - Gloves should only be worn if a risk assessment identifies the need
  - Gloves are not required for routine bed making or feeding patients

DISPOSABLE PLASTIC APRONS

- Disposable plastic aprons provide a physical barrier between clothing/skin and prevent contamination and wetting of clothing/uniforms during bathing/washing or equipment cleaning.
- Aprons should be worn whenever there is a risk of contamination of uniforms or clothing with blood and body fluids and when a patient has a known or suspected infection.
- As with gloves, aprons should be changed as soon as the intended individual task is completed.
- Aprons should not be worn routinely during shifts as part of normal activity but should be reserved for when required.

GOWNS

- Impervious (i.e. waterproof) gowns should be used when there is a risk of extensive contamination of blood or body fluids or when local policy dictates their use in certain settings.
- For example, maternity or A&E settings, or when there are high risk respiratory infections or infections caused by some multi-resistant bacteria[307].

MASKS

- Masks may be necessary if a suspected or confirmed infection may be spread by an airborne route – for example, multi-drugresistant tuberculosis or other high risk infections transmitted via the respiratory route.
- You should ensure that masks are always fitted correctly, are handled as little as possible, and changed at required time intervals, as recommended by manufacturer, between patients or operations. Masks should offer reliable, effective protection when used correctly.

VISORS OR GOGGLES

- Visors or goggles can be utilised to protect the eye membranes. Some visors can offer full face protection.
- The choice of visors or goggles will depend on task/procedure to be undertaken, a risk assessment of likely exposure, local policy and availability.

---

[306] *Essential Practice for Infection Prevention and Control Guidance for nursing staff.pdf p13-14*

[307] *Essential Practice for Infection Prevention and Control Guidance for nursing staff.pdf p13-15*

3. SAFE HANDLING & DISPOSAL OF SHARPS

- Sharps include needles, scalpels, stitch cutters, glass ampoules, bone fragments and any sharp instrument[308].
- The main hazards of a sharps injury are blood borne viruses such as hepatitis B, hepatitis C and HIV.
- It is not uncommon for staff to be injured by the unsafe or poor practice of others; for example, cleaners who sustain injuries as a result of sharps being placed in waste bins. Sharps injuries are preventable and learning following incidents should be put in place to avoid repeat accidents.
- Between 2004 and 2014, there were just under 5,000 significant occupational exposure incidents reported to the Public Health England[309].
- Significant exposures are percutaneous or mucocutanenous where the source patient is hepatitis B, hepatitis C or HIV positive.
- To reduce the risk of injury and exposure to blood borne viruses, it is vital that sharps are used safely and disposed of carefully, following your workplace's agreed policies on use of sharps.
- Education and guidance should be available through your employer on how to manage sharps safely.
- Some procedures have a higher than average risk of causing injury. These include surgery, intra-vascular cannulation, venepuncture and injection.
- Devices involved in these high-risk procedures include:
  o IV cannulae
  o Needles and syringes
  o Winged steel needles (known as butterfly needles)
  o Phlebotomy needles (used in vacuum devices).
- To reduce the use of needles and syringes, the use of 'safety engineered devices' to support staff undertaking cannulation, phlebotomy and so on should be supported by employing organisations.
- Safety engineered devices have a built in feature to reduce the risk of a sharps injury before, during and after use.
- Devices can be passive or active.
- For example, passive devices have an automatic safety mechanism that is activated after use, such as when a cannula is withdrawn from a patient's vein.
- An active device needs to be manually activated by the member of staff.

---

[308] *Essential Practice for Infection Prevention and Control Guidance for nursing staff.pdf p.16*

[309] *PHE, 2014*

4. USE OF INDWELLING DEVICES

- Indwelling devices are common in health care and when used appropriately provide valuable assistance to providing patient care and positive patient outcomes. However, the use of indwelling devices is not without risk and the development of infection occurs by their very nature as they bypass the body's natural defence mechanisms such as skin and mucous membranes.
- Common invasive devices (for example, urinary catheters, IV cannula or central venous catheters) are frequently responsible for HCAIs such as urinary tract, insertion site infections or bloodstream infections.

PREVENTION OF INTRAVASCULAR LINE ASSOCIATED INFECTIONS

- The use of peripheral or central vascular devices is a common cause of infection which can lead to life threatening blood stream infections (bacteraemia). The types of organisms implicated in these infections vary but frequently involve members of the staphylococcus family such as Staphylococcus aureus, meticillin-resistant staphylococcus aureus (MRSA), or coagulase negative staphylococci (CNS) in neonates.
- These may enter the device insertion site as a result of contamination from the skin during insertion of the device or as a result of contamination on staff hands during manipulation of the device.
- Peripheral intravascular cannulas represent the most common invasive device used and these may be temporary (for a few hours) or longer term provided they are clinically indicated and there are no complications identified.
- Prevention of infection is complex, and good practice is required at all stages of care whilst these devices are in situ. This includes, but is not limited to, insertion and ongoing management.

INSERTION

- Appropriate and thorough disinfection of the skin is crucial prior to insertion of any intravascular device – such as a central, peripheral, peripherally inserted central catheter (PICC) or femoral line.
- The proper use of an appropriate skin disinfectant product will reduce the number of viable micro-organisms present at the site of insertion, reducing the risk of contamination at the insertion site at the time of introduction. The use of 2% chlorhexidine in 70% isopropyl alcohol is recommended for skin disinfection unless a known sensitivity is present[310].

---

[310] *Loveday et al., 2014*

5. MANAGING ACCIDENTAL EXPOSURE TO BLOOD-BORNE VIRUSES

- Blood borne infections are most frequently associated with those caused by hepatitis B, hepatitis C and HIV which may be found in blood and other body fluids such as amniotic fluid, synovial fluid, vaginal fluid, semen, and breast milk.
- They are not associated with excretions such as saliva, urine, vomit or faeces unless blood is present. Accidental exposure to blood and body fluids can occur by:
  o Percutaneous injury – for example, from used needles, instruments, bone fragments or significant bites that break the skin
  o Exposure of broken skin – for example, abrasions, cuts or eczema
  o Exposure of mucous membranes, including the eyes and the mouth.

MANAGING THE RISK OF HIV

- The risk of acquiring HIV infection following occupational exposure to HIV-infected blood is low[311]. A risk assessment needs to be made urgently by someone other than the exposed worker about the appropriateness of starting post exposure prophylaxis (PEP), ideally an appropriately trained doctor designated according to local arrangements for the provision of urgent post-exposure advice.
- Counselling should also be considered for the individual exposed. If a health care worker is exposed to blood, high risk blood and body fluids or tissue known or strongly suspected to be contaminated with HIV, the use of antiretroviral post exposure prophylaxis (PEP) is recommended.
- Ideally, this is given within an hour of exposure (the incident), hence the importance in undertaking first aid immediately, followed by prompt reporting of the incident. Staff should ensure they are familiar with their local policies and procedures should such an incident occur in order to ensure prompt treatment for themselves or co-workers if affected.
- Advice and follow-up care from your occupational health provider will also be essential.

MANAGING THE RISK OF HEPATITIS B AND C
HEPATITIS B (HBV)

- The risk of contracting HBV from a sharps injury in a health care setting is much higher than HIV because the virus is more infectious and has greater prevalence.

- All nurses and health care assistants should be vaccinated against hepatitis B. Those at risk of occupational exposure, particularly health care and laboratory workers, should have their antibody titres checked one to four months after the completion of a primary course of vaccine[312].
- Refer to local policies for information on monitoring of antibody titre levels and boosters following exposure incidents.

HEPATITIS C (HCV)

- There is currently no vaccine available that can prevent infection following exposure to the hepatitis C virus.
- Prevention is the key to avoiding exposure and subsequent infection, and staff should ensure they comply with local blood borne diseases policy, sharps safety and wear appropriate protective clothing, reporting any exposure incidents as these occur.

6. ANTIMICROBIAL RESISTANCE (AMR)

- It is estimated that 10 million lives a year could be lost as a result of AMR by 2050 if we do not tackle this problem[313].
- Antimicrobial resistance occurs when micro-organisms become resistant to the drugs used to treat them. Some micro-organisms, especially those found in the environment are naturally resistant to antibiotics.
- Other micro-organisms have adapted to survive and developed mechanisms and changes within their genetic structure to allow them to become resistant as a method of their survival.
- As a result of AMR infections are harder to treat; this can lead to longer stays in hospital, longer courses of antimicrobials and ultimately treatment failure.
- Antimicrobial agents include antibacterials/ antibiotics (for bacterial infections), antifungal agents (for fungal infections) and antivirals (for viral infections).
- Antimicrobial agents can be used either systemically (within the body) or topically (for example, creams) and can be used as a prophylaxis (as a preventative measure, for example, before surgery) or as treatment when infection is present. Regardless of the method of use, antimicrobial agents are unique in that they only have an effect on the micro-organism causing the infection and not the host (patient).

---

[311] PHE, 2014

[312] DH, 2014 The Green Book

[313] O'Neill, 2016

- Antimicrobials are important because they allow the treatment of simple and complex infections.
- If antimicrobials such as antibiotics stop working then common medical procedures such as surgical treatments could be a greater risk of infections developing and we could once again see patients dying of infections, as occurred in the pre-antibiotic era.
- In order to reduce AMR a number of initiatives are underway locally, nationally and globally. This includes a requirement in the updated Health and Social Care Act (DH, 2015) for antimicrobial stewardship programmes to be demonstrated when organisations in England are inspected by the Care Quality Commission (CQC).
- Information on the activities undertaken by Scotland, Wales and Northern Ireland can be found by following the web links for these countries in the Further Resources section.
- It is important to refer to your local guidelines and procedures or contact your infection control team if you have any queries. This section of the document will highlight the main interventions which have been identified nationally across the United Kingdom to control AMR.

RAISING PUBLIC AWARENESS OF AMR

- It is important that everybody knows what they can do as individuals to help stop AMR.
- European antibiotic awareness days and a global antibiotic awareness week have highlighted the importance of this.
- Information is available regionally to support health care workers provide self-help information for patients who present to medical facilities with a range of common illnesses eg, NHS Choices.
- Public Health England has launched a new campaign aimed at the general public on raising awareness of the need for appropriate use of antibiotics[314].
  1. Improve hygiene and prevent the spread of infection. This intervention really highlights the importance of infection prevention and public health actions. Hand hygiene is a key intervention that all staff should be able to achieve to prevent the spread of infection. Other important factors within this intervention will include the cleanliness of the health care environment and knowledge of staff to prevent the spread of infection.

2. Improve the surveillance of AMR in humans and animals and measure the amount of antimicrobials that are consumed. Efforts to understand drug resistance and consumption are underway nationally. England collect data on both of these interventions via data collected routinely from laboratories displayed on the PHE Fingertips portal (https://fingertips.phe.org.uk/profile/amr-local-indicators) and via CQUIN (England only) collection on antimicrobial usage. It is important to collect and use this data as a means to measure the effects of interventions.

3. Rapid diagnostics to detect individuals with infections more quickly and treat them appropriately need to be developed. Alongside ensuring people need antimicrobials receive them this will also help reassure the patients that they do not need antimicrobials for the symptoms with which they present.

4. Other measures include reducing antimicrobial usage across the world including in agriculture. A great deal of antimicrobials are used for animals so it is important that efforts are made to reduce this. Other interventions include encouraging more individuals into infectious disease and associated specialities and carrying out global research into antimicrobial development. Further information on the interventions mentioned above and AMR can be found at: https://amr-review.org

---

[314] https:// campaignresources.phe.gov.uk/resources/ campaigns/58-keep-antibiotics-working

II. LONG TERM CONDITIONS CARE

1. HEALTH VISITOR

o The Health Visiting Team **work with all families before or after the birth of a child.**

o Their role is to:

   ▪ Assess the health needs of families, offering support as required.

   ▪ Encourage and support families to make healthy lifestyle choices through health education and health promotion information.

   ▪ Provide information about the many services available to support families.

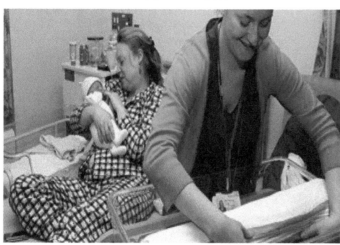

2. DISTRICT NURSES

o The District Nursing Team will provide high quality, safe and **effective nursing care to Adults who require care delivery in their own home.**

3. MIDWIFE

o Midwives are specialists in normal pregnancy and birth, and their role is to look after a pregnant woman and her baby throughout a phase of antenatal care, during labour **and birth, and for up to 28 days** after the baby has been born.

4. OCCUPATIONAL THERAPY

o Occupational Therapy provides practical support to people with physical and mental health disability, long term condition, or those experiencing the effects of ageing, to do the things they need or want to do.

o It enables people of all ages to carry out practical and purposeful activities.

o **This could be essential day to day tasks-**such as dressing, cooking, going shopping, to the things that make us who we are – our jobs, interests, hobbies and relationships.

o Occupational Therapy considers all our needs, for example physical, psychological, social and environmental, and helps to increase people's independence and satisfaction in all aspects of life.

5. PHYSIOTHERAPY

o The Physiotherapy service aims to provide the interventions needed to support people **to manage their Musculoskeletal conditions.**

o This will encompass assessment and treatment, management and advice of wider health issues, managing and supporting people to return to their work or meaningful activities.

6. COMMUNITY MENTAL HEALTH TEAM

o The service provides community focused **psychiatric assessment and treatment interventions for patients from 18 to 65 years of age.**

o Patients will have access to Nursing Staff, Occupational Therapists, Psychiatrists, Psychologists, Social Work, Area Crisis Service, Primary Care Mental Health Team and the voluntary sector.

7. COMMUNITY REHABILITATION TEAM

o The service provides multi-disciplinary **rehabilitation at home for adults with disabilities and older people.**

o The service provides Physiotherapy, Occupational Therapy, Nursing Services, Dietetic and Support Services to any adult (over 16years old) with a disability and older people in their own homes.

o Individuals will go through an assessment process to determine what type of rehabilitation package is necessary for their situation.

III. SCREENING PROGRAMMES

1. ABDOMINAL AORTIC ANEURYSM SCREENING PROGRAMME [315]

- o The NHS abdominal aortic aneurysm (AAA) screening programme is available for **all men aged 65 and over** in England.
- o The programme aims to reduce AAA related mortality among men aged 65 to 74.
- o **A simple ultrasound test** is performed to detect AAA.
- o The scan itself is quick, painless and non-invasive and the results are provided straight away.
- o A result letter is also sent to all patients' GPs.

2. BOWEL CANCER SCREENING PROGRAMME [316]

- o People eligible for screening receive an invitation letter explaining the programme, along with an information leaflet explaining **the benefits and risks of bowel cancer screening.**
- o About a week later, the programme should send a **faecal occult blood sampling kit.**
- o The kit includes simple instructions for:
  - Completing sampling at home.
  - Sending the samples to the laboratory
- o The sample is then processed and the results sent to the individual within 2 weeks.

- o **Colonoscopy**
  - Healthcare professionals should offer patients with an abnormal screening result a colonoscopy.
  - The **quality assurance guidelines for colonoscopy** explain how to complete the procedure.
  - If the procedure finds polyps, a wire loop passed down the colonoscope tube can remove them and these tissue samples must be tested for any abnormal cells that may be cancerous.

- o **Bowel scope screening**
  - The programme is also rolling out **bowel scope screening** to all men and women in **England aged 55.**

- Healthcare professionals should explain to people that this new test is not yet available everywhere across the country.
- The target is for all screening centres to be operational by December 2016.

3. BREAST SCREENING [317]

- o Eligible women, **aged 50 to 70**, receive an invitation letter explaining:
  - The programme
  - The benefits and risks of breast screening
- o Women do not always receive an invitation when they turn 50. They can expect their invitation within 3 years of their 50th birthday.
- o Women **cannot walk in and request breast screening unless they are over 70**, when they can request screening every 3 years.

- o **Age extension**
  - In some areas, women **aged 47 to 49 and 71 to 73** receive invitations for screening.
  - This is part of a study looking at whether to **extend the breast screening age range**.

- o **Higher risk women**
  - Women identified as having a **higher risk of breast cancer** should receive:
    - A formal assessment
    - The opportunity to discuss risk management options.

4. CERVICAL SCREENING [318]

- o NHS cervical screening programme is available to **women aged 25 to 64** in England.
- o All eligible women who are registered with a GP automatically receive an invitation by mail.
- o Women **aged 25 to 49** receive invitations **every 3 years.**
- o Women aged **50 to 64 receive invitations every 5 years.**
- o NHS Choices provides information for the public on the **cervical screening programme.**

- **SCREENING TESTS**
  - o Cervical screening is a method of preventing cancer by detecting and treating abnormalities of the cervix.

---

[315] https://www.gov.uk/topic/population-screening-programmes/abdominal-aortic-aneurysm

[316] https://www.gov.uk/topic/population-screening-programmes/bowel

---

[317] https://www.gov.uk/topic/population-screening-programmes/breast

[318] https://www.gov.uk/topic/population-screening-programmes/cervical

- o **Cervical cytology**
  - ▪ The programme uses liquid-based cytology (LBC) to collect samples of cells from the cervix.
  - ▪ The laboratory will examine these samples under the microscope to look for any abnormal changes in the cells.
- o **Human papillomavirus**
  - ▪ Human papillomavirus (HPV) is a common virus transmitted through sexual contact.
  - ▪ In most cases, a woman's immune system will clear the infection without the need for treatment.
  - ▪ HPV has over 100 subtypes, most of which do not cause significant disease in humans.
  - ▪ Known as high risk HPV (HR-HPV), some subtypes can cause cervical cancer.
  - ▪ In particular **HPV16 and HPV18.**

5. DIABETIC EYE SCREENING[319]

- o The eligible population for DES is all people **with type 1 and type 2 diabetes aged 12 or over.**
- o People already under the care of an ophthalmology specialist for the condition are not invited for screening.
- o The programme offers pregnant women with type 1 or type 2 diabetes additional tests because of the risk of developing retinopathy.
- o Screening gives people with diabetes and their primary diabetes care providers **information** about very early changes in their eyes.
- o Early warnings allow people to take preventative action to stop serious retinopathy developing.

PRINCIPE OF NOTIFICATION

- Registered medical practitioners (RMPs) have a statutory duty to notify the 'proper officer' at their **local council** or **local health protection team** (HPT) of suspected cases of certain infectious diseases.
- Complete a **notification form** immediately on diagnosis of a suspected notifiable disease.
- **Don't wait for laboratory confirmation** of a suspected infection or contamination before notification.
- Send the form to the proper officer **within 3 days**, or notify them verbally **within 24 hours** if the case is urgent, securely:
  - o By phone
  - o Letter

- o Encrypted email
- o Secure fax machine

- All proper officers must pass the entire notification to Public Health England (PHE) within 3 days of a case being notified, or within 24 hours for urgent cases.

LIST OF NOTIFIABLE DISEASES

- Diseases notifiable to local authority proper officers under the Health Protection **(Notification) Regulations 2010** [320]:
  - o Acute encephalitis
  - o Acute infectious hepatitis
  - o Acute meningitis
  - o Acute poliomyelitis
  - o Anthrax,
  - o Botulism
  - o Brucellosis,
  - o Cholera,
  - o Diphtheria
  - o Enteric fever (typhoid or paratyphoid fever)
  - o Food poisoning
  - o Haemolytic uraemic syndrome (HUS)
  - o Infectious bloody diarrhoea
  - o Invasive group A streptococcal disease
  - o Legionnaires' disease,
  - o Leprosy
  - o Malaria,
  - o Measles,
  - o Meningococcal septicaemia,
  - o Mumps
  - o Plague,
  - o Rabies,
  - o Rubella
  - o Severe Acute Respiratory Syndrome (SARS)
  - o Scarlet fever,
  - o Smallpox
  - o Tetanus
  - o Tuberculosis
  - o Typhus
  - o Viral haemorrhagic fever (VHF)
  - o Whooping cough
  - o Yellow fever

Report other diseases that may present significant risk to human health under the category 'other significant disease'.

---

[319] https://www.gov.uk/topic/population-screening-programmes/diabetic-eye

[320]https://www.gov.uk/guidance/notifiable-diseases-and-causative-organisms-how-to-report#list-of-notifiable-diseases

2. Ethics & Confidentiality

I. CONFIDENTIALITY & SHARING INFORMATION

THE PRINCIPLES OF CONFIDENTIALITY

- Confidentiality is central to the trust between doctors and patients and an essential part of good care.
- Without assurances about confidentiality, children and young people, as well as adults, may be reluctant to get medical attention or to give doctors the information they need to provide good care[321].
- Teenagers may be particularly concerned about keeping confidential information from their parents, schools, children's services, the police and other statutory agencies.
- Young people, parents and other adults receiving psychiatric care, and other vulnerable people might have similarly increased concerns about sharing confidential information.
- But sharing information appropriately is essential to providing safe, effective care, both for the individual and for the wider community.
- It is also at the heart of effective child protection.
- It is vital that all doctors have the confidence to act on their concerns about the possible abuse or neglect of a child or young person.
- Confidentiality is not an absolute duty.
- You can share confidential information about a person if any of the following apply[322]:
  - You must do so **by law**[323] **or in response to a court order**.
  - The person the information relates to has **given you their consent to share the information** (or a person with parental responsibility has given consent if the information is about a child who does not have the capacity to give consent).
  - It is justified in the **public interest** – for example, if the benefits to a child or young person that will arise from sharing the information outweigh both the public and the individual's interest in keeping the information confidential.

KEY POINTS

- **Tell an appropriate agency** promptly if you are concerned that a child or young person is at risk of, or is suffering, abuse or neglect.
- **Get advice** if you are concerned about the possibility of abuse or neglect, but do not believe that the child or young person is at risk of significant harm.
- **Ask for consent** to share information unless there is a compelling reason for not doing so.
- Information can be shared without consent if **it is justified in the public interest** or **required by law**.
- Do not delay disclosing information to obtain consent if that might put children or young people at risk of significant harm. Tell your patient what information has been shared, with whom and why, unless doing this would put the child, young person or anyone else at increased risk.
- Get advice if you are not sure what information to share, who to share it with or how best to manage any risk associated with sharing information.
- In England and Wales doctors are under a legal duty to report known cases of female genital mutilation in girls and young women aged under 18 to the police.

1. DISCLOSURES WITH CONSENT[324]

- Before disclosing any information to a third party **the patient's consent should be sought**.
- **Consent may be implied,** for example most patient understand that information about their health needs to be shared within the treating healthcare team.
- Implied consent is also acceptable for the purposes of clinical audit, provided patients have been made aware of this possibility by notices in the hospital and have not actively objected.
- **Express consent** is required if patient-identifiable information is to be disclosed for any other purpose, unless required by law or in the public interest.
- For the consent to disclose information to be valid, patients must be **competent to give consent and provided with information about the extent of the disclosure**.

---

[321] *Confidentiality and sharing information/ Ethical Guidance. London, General Medical Council*

[322] *General Medical Council (2017)* <u>Confidentiality: good practice in handling patient information</u> *London, General Medical Council.*

[323] *Multiagency practice guidelines: female genital mutilation and Mandatory reporting of female genital mutilation: procedural information*

[324] *Disclosing patients' personal information/ Ethical Guidance. London, General Medical Council*

- If a patient lacks capacity, demonstrated by the functional test of capacity advised in the Mental Capacity Act 2005, then disclosure of information **should be in the patient's best interest.**
- **If a patient, under the age of 16 years**, is able to understand the purpose and consequences of the disclosure (Gillick competent) they can give or withhold consent.
- **If the young person refuses disclosure** but this is necessary to protect the young person from serious harm (e.g. neglect or abuse) this is justifiable. The young person should be made aware of the disclosure and the reasons behind the disclosure.
- **If a young person is not competent to give consent,** someone with parental responsibility may consent to the disclosure on their behalf.
- **In a patient aged 16–17 who lacks capacity,** both the Mental Capacity Act 2005 and the Children Act 1989 can apply, depending on the circumstances.

2. DISCLOSING INFORMATION WITHOUT CONSENT

- If it is probable that a crime has been committed, the police will ask for more information.
- If the patient cannot give consent because, for example, they are unconscious, or refuses to disclose information or to allow you or your colleagues to do so, you can still disclose information if it is required by law or if you believe it is justified in the public interest.
- **Disclosures in the public interest may be justified when:**
  - Failure to disclose information may put the patient, or someone else, at risk of death or serious harm, or
  - Disclosure is likely to help in the prevention, detection or prosecution of a serious crime.
- If there is any doubt about whether disclosure without consent is justified, the decision should be made by, or with the agreement of, the consultant in charge, or the trust's Guardian.
- If practicable, you should seek the patient's consent to the disclosure, or tell them that a disclosure has been made unless, for example, that:
  - May put you or others at risk of serious harm, or
  - Would be likely to undermine the purpose of the disclosure, by prejudicing the prevention, detection or prosecution of a crime.
- You must document in the patient's record your reasons for disclosing information without consent and any steps you have taken to seek their consent, to inform them about the disclosure, or your reasons for not doing so.
- If there is no immediate public interest reason for disclosing personal information, no further information should be given to the police.
- The police may seek an order from a judge or a warrant for the disclosure of confidential documents. You should tell those responsible for the continuing care of the patient that further discussion with the patient is needed to ensure, for example, that they are fit to hold a firearms licence.

3. DISCLOSURES REQUIRED IN THE PUBLIC INTEREST

- It should be presumed that **clinical information should not normally be disclosed without the explicit, written consent of the patient**.
- Only information that is directly relevant to the case should be disclosed. In certain scenarios, releasing information to the police is in the public interest.
- The decision to release information should be made **by the Consultant in charge**, or his **deputy**.
- The Consultant in Charge should consider discussing this with another experienced colleague or the **Trust's Caldicott guardian**.
- Disclosure should be considered **where a serious crime has been committed.** 'Serious crime' has not been defined in law, but normally includes; rape, abuse of a child or vulnerable adult, terrorism, murder and injuries from guns and knives.
- Theft, burglary, fraud and damage to property are not generally regarded as serious crimes.
- In all cases the balance of breaching a patient's confidentiality and the possible harm caused by this should be weighed against the benefits of disclosing the information. The information should be anonymised if possible and the minimum, relevant information only should be disclosed.
- Patient consent should be sought if possible and the patient kept informed of any disclosures, unless this undermines the purpose of the disclosure.
- The ultimate decision about whether or not a disclosure was made in the public interest is determined by the courts. All decisions must be justified and clearly documented.
- A competent adult's wishes should generally be respected if they refuse to allow disclosure and no-one else will suffer. However, if the disclosure is to protect an incompetent patient from serious harm, there is an expectation that the relevant confidential information will be disclosed.
- If such information is not disclosed this will need to be justified.

4. REPORTING GUNSHOT & KNIFE WOUNDS[325]

- Disclosure of personal information about a patient without consent may be justified in the public interest **if failure to disclose may expose others to a risk of death or serious harm**.
- You should still seek the patient's consent to disclosure if practicable and consider any reasons given for refusal. Such a situation might arise, for example, when a disclosure would be likely to assist in the prevention, detection or prosecution of serious crime, especially crimes against the person.
- **When victims of violence refuse police assistance**, disclosure may still be justified if others remain at risk, for example, from someone who is prepared to use weapons, or from domestic violence when children or others may be at risk.

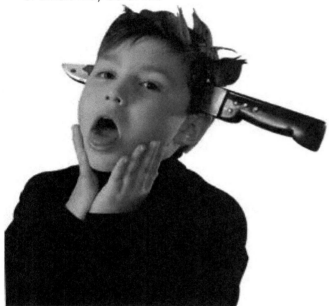

- If a patient's refusal to consent to disclosure leaves others exposed to a risk so serious that it outweighs the patient's and the public interest in maintaining confidentiality, or if it is not practicable or safe to seek the patient's consent, **you should disclose information promptly to an appropriate person or authority.**
- **You should inform** the patient before disclosing the information, if practicable and safe, even if you intend to disclose without their consent.
- The guidance in Confidentiality applies to all violent crime, but gunshot and knife wounds raise issues that warrant special consideration.
- That is not to suggest that information should not be disclosed to assist in the prevention, detection or prosecution of other serious crime.

A. GUIDANCE:

- **This guidance describes a two-stage process:**
  - **You should inform the police quickly** whenever a person arrives with a gunshot wound or an injury from an attack with a knife, blade or other sharp instrument.
  - This will enable the police to make an assessment of risk to the patient and others, and to gather statistical information about gun and knife crime in the area.
  - **You should make a professional judgement** about whether disclosure of personal information about a patient, including their identity, is justified in the public interest.
- The police are responsible for assessing the risk posed by a member of the public who is armed with, and has used, a gun or knife in a violent attack. They need to consider:
  - The risk of a further attack on the patient
  - The risk to staff, patients and visitors in the ED or hospital, and
  - The risk of another attack near to, or at, the site of the original incident.
- For this reason, the police should be informed whenever a person arrives at hospital with a gunshot wound. Even accidental shootings involving lawfully held guns raise serious issues for the police about, for example, **gun licensing.**
- The police should also be informed when a person arrives at a hospital with a wound from an attack with a knife, blade or other sharp instrument.
- The police should not usually be informed if a knife or blade injury is accidental, or a result of self-harm.
- If you are in doubt about the cause of the injury, you should if possible, consult an experienced colleague.
- Quick reporting at this stage may help prevent further incidents or harm to others.
- If you have responsibility for the patient, you should make sure that the police are contacted, but you can delegate this task to another member of staff.
- Personal information, such as the patient's name and address, should not usually be disclosed in the initial contact with the police.
- The police will respond even if the patient's identity is not disclosed.
- The police need to be informed quickly in order to respond to the risk to patients, staff and the public.
- They also need statistical information about the number of gunshot and knife injuries, and when and where they occur, to inform their own and their crime reduction partners' operational and strategic priorities.

---

[325] *Confidentiality: reporting gunshot and knife wounds/ **Ethical Guidance. London, General Medical Council***

B. MAKING THE CARE OF THE PATIENT YOUR FIRST CONCERN

- When the police arrive, **you should not allow them access to the patient** if this will delay or hamper treatment or compromise the patient's recovery.
- If the patient's treatment and condition allow them to speak to the police, you or another member of the healthcare team should **ask the patient whether they are willing to do so**.
- If they are not, you should explain what the consequences, if any, might be.
- You, the rest of the healthcare team, and the police must abide by the patient's decision.

C. CHILDREN AND YOUNG PEOPLE

- Any child or young person under 18 arriving with a gunshot wound or a wound from an attack with a knife, blade or other sharp instrument **will raise obvious child protection concerns.**
- You must inform an appropriate person or authority promptly of any such incident.
- Knife or blade injuries from domestic or occupational accidents might also raise serious concerns about **the safety of children and young people**.
- You should consider the advice on child protection in **0-18 years**: guidance for all doctors whenever you are concerned that a child may be the victim of abuse or neglect.
- You must be able to justify a decision not to share a concern that children or young people are at risk of abuse, neglect or other serious harm, having taken advice from a named or designated doctor for child protection or an experienced colleague, or a defence or professional body.

5. PROVIDING A WITNESS STATEMENT FOR THE POLICE [326]

- **SCOPE**
  - This document guides clinicians (Doctors and Emergency Nurse Practitioners) in how to prepare witness statement to use as evidence.
  - This document should standardise the content of a witness statement and defines emergency, urgent and standard statements.

- **THE STATEMENT**
  - Clinicians working in emergency departments have an important societal role in assisting the police.
  - A witness statement should be provided promptly after a request by the police.

- A witness statement is usually related to a patient attending the Emergency Department with injuries due to an alleged assault.
- The statement should only be issued after the patient has provided written consent or a request is issued by a judicial authority.
- The main purpose of a statement is to provide an evidence of facts that will be used in court.
- The statement is a way of providing evidence in court that is as valid as if the evidence was presented in person.
- It is for this reason that a declaration attesting to the truth of the statement is signed.
- Any dishonesty in a signed statement amounts to perjury and may lead to prosecution.
- The statement is a method of communicating medical information to a lay person and so medical terms should be explained in a way that is easy to understand with medical terms explained. It must be noted that an omission could be as improper as an invalid piece of information that is included.
- The police can request personal (not clinical) details regarding attendances to the Emergency Department **if the request is made in writing on Form 826C and** relates to a serious, arrestable crime (Police and Evidence Act 1984) or the Road Traffic Act 1988.
- The form must be signed by an Inspector or above.

A. EMERGENCY STATEMENTS

- There are uncommon occasions when the police request an emergency statement.
- A witness statement concerning a serious crime of violence, injury or death is required by a police officer at the first available opportunity.
- This statement will directly affect the ability of the police to investigate a serious offence or decision to be able to arrest, detain or charge a suspect within the limited time available under the law where appropriate.
- These statements will normally be confined to a description of the injury/injuries and a brief account of the nature of the treatment.
- **They should be obtained from the most senior doctor involved in the patient's initial care** and will be handed to the police without delay.
- In these circumstances the police will normally make the request due to either the serious nature of the case or because of time and legal constraints relating to a person in custody or whose detention is imminent.

---

[326] *Acting as a witness in legal proceedings/ **Ethical Guidance. London, General Medical Council***

o Where such a request is made, it will be on **the authority of an officer not below the rank of Inspector**, whose name will be provided to the Emergency Department being requested to provide the statement.

o These statements should be regarded as provisional and returned to the police as promptly as possible, **within 12 hours of a request.**

B. URGENT STATEMENTS

o This is a witness statement required to meet a deadline required for a prosecution, breach of which could seriously prejudice the continuation of the proceedings which will usually contain information which details a key element of an offence being charged or prosecuted.

o This should be provided **within 72 hours of a request**.

o Where the request for an urgent statement is made by the police it will be made on the authority of **The Criminal Justice case manager or the officer in charge of the case**.

o Where the request is made later in proceedings by The Crown Prosecution Service, it will be made by a named lawyer who has responsibility for and is actively reviewing the case.

C. STANDARD STATEMENTS

o These are all other cases where a witness statement is required from hospital medical staff, production of which will normally be not later than **two weeks from the receipt** of the request by the hospital liaison officer.

o The request for such statements will be made by the police via **The Criminal Justice Case Manager or an identified Police Liaison Officer.**

- **CONSTRUCTING THE STATEMENT**
  o The contents of the statement are based on the patient's records and other documents related to his or her attendance.
  o Medical history and history of other conditions or illnesses should not be a routine part of the statement unless relevant to the episode of attendance. The statement is better typed and a copy stored in a secure computer.
  o Hand written statements should be clear, legible, and in black ink.
  o A copy should be kept for future reference.

- **GIVING OPINION**
  o A witness statement is a professional statement of facts only. Opinion is given by experts only and this should be based on extensive experience, knowledge, and research.
  o Opinion should be justified and substantiated.

6. DOCTORS GIVING EVIDENCE IN COURT / WITNESS CARE [327]

o The Crown Prosecution Service will make every reasonable effort **to avoid calling a member of the hospital medical staff as a witness** to give oral testimony at the court.

o This will be done, wherever possible, by serving the evidence on the defence and seeking to agree it, or by identifying any issues in contention for further consideration.

o The service of the original medical notes exhibited to a statement, where this can be agreed and arranged will often avoid having to call a member of the medical staff as a witness.

o Where the original medical records or copies thereof are appended to statements the patient's address and telephone number and any information related to third parties (e.g. identity and addresses of next of kin, relatives or employers) should be removed or suitably obscured in any copy served on or shown to the defence.

o Prompt responses from medical staff for further information when required may also assist in avoiding the calling of such staff to give evidence.

- **When called to testify:**
  o The first duty of all witnesses is to the court.
  o Give evidence that is impartial, honest and not misleading.
  o Only give testimony and express opinions about issues that are within your professional competence.
  o Work within the timescales set by the court.

7. REPORTING CONCERNS TO THE DVLA[328]

o Confidential medical care is recognised in law as being in the public interest. However, there can also be a public interest in disclosing information: **to protect individuals or society from risks of serious harm,** such as serious communicable diseases or serious crime; or **to enable medical research, education** or other secondary uses of information that will benefit society over time.

o Personal information may, therefore, be disclosed in the public interest, without patients' consent, and in exceptional cases where patients have withheld consent, if the benefits to an individual or to society of **the disclosure outweigh both the public and the patient's interest in keeping the information confidential.**

---

[327] *General Medical Council (2013) Good medical practice London, GMC.*

[328] *Confidentiality: patients' fitness to drive and reporting concerns to the DVLA or DVA/ Ethical Guidance. General Medical Council*

o You must weigh the harms that are likely to arise from non-disclosure of information against the possible harm, both to the patient and to the overall trust between doctors and patients, arising from the release of that information.

o Disclosure of personal information about a patient without consent may be justified in the public interest if failure to disclose may expose others to a risk of death or serious harm.

o You should still seek the patient's consent to disclosure if practicable and consider any reasons given for refusal.

o The **Driver and Vehicle Licensing Agency** (DVLA) and **Driver and Vehicle Agency** (DVA) are legally responsible for deciding if a person is medically unfit to drive.

o This means they need to know if a driving licence holder has a condition or is undergoing treatment that may now, or in the future, affect their safety as a driver.

o You should seek the advice of an experienced colleague or the DVLA or DVA's medical adviser if you are not sure whether a patient may be unfit to drive.

o You should keep under review any decision that they are fit, particularly if the patient's condition or treatments change.

o The DVLA's publication Assessing fitness to drive – a guide for medical professionals includes information about a variety of disorders and conditions that can impair a patient's fitness to drive (See Major Presentations, Chapter 6 / TLoC).

o **The driver is legally responsible for informing the DVLA or DVA** about such a condition or treatment. However, if a patient has such a condition, you should explain to the patient:

  ▪ That the condition may affect their ability to drive (if the patient is incapable of understanding this advice, for example, because of dementia, you should inform the DVLA or DVA immediately), and

  ▪ That they have a legal duty to inform the DVLA or DVA about the condition.

o If a patient refuses to accept the diagnosis, or the effect of the condition on their ability to drive, you can suggest that they seek a second opinion, and help arrange for them to do so. You should advise the patient not to drive in the meantime.

o If a patient continues to drive when they may not be fit to do so, **you should make every reasonable effort to persuade them to stop.** As long as the patient agrees, you may discuss your concerns with their relatives, friends or carers.

o If you do not manage to persuade the patient to stop driving, or you discover that they are continuing to drive against your advice, **you should contact the DVLA or DVA immediately and disclose any relevant medical information**, in confidence, to the medical adviser.

o Before contacting the DVLA or DVA you should try to inform the patient of your decision to disclose personal information.

o You should then also inform the patient in writing once you have done so.

8. DISCLOSURES AFTER A PATIENT'S DEATH[329]

• The duty of confidentiality to a patient remains after their death. There are certain circumstances where disclosure may be justified.

• For example, responding to a complaint, including those made by bereaved relatives.

• The Access to Health Records Act 1990 allows relevant information to be disclosed to the 'personal representative' of the deceased (usually the executor of the will, or an administrator if there is no will) or anyone who may have a claim arising from the patient's death (e.g. a life insurance claim).

• If the patient requested that specific information remained confidential their views should be respected, subject to those disclosures required by law or justified in the public interest.

9. CALDICOTT GUARDIAN[330]

• In 1997 the Caldicott Report (named after the author **Dame Fiona Caldicott**) was produced, which identified weaknesses in the way parts of the NHS handled confidential patient data.

• The report made several recommendations, one of which was the appointment of a **Caldicott Guardian, a senior member of staff** with a responsibility to ensure patient data is kept secure.

• Each NHS organization has to appoint a Caldicott Guardian to fulfil this role. The six key principles of the Caldicott report are:

  o Justify the purpose(s) for using the confidential information.

  o Only use it when absolutely necessary.

  o Use the minimum that is required.

  o Access should be on a strict need-to-know basis.

  o Everyone must understand his or her responsibilities.

  o Understand and comply with the law.

---

[329] *Managing and protecting personal information / **Ethical Guidance. General Medical Council***

[330] *Storing and disposing of recordings / **Ethical Guidance. General Medical Council***

10. GDPR AND DATA PROTECTION ACT 2018

- **The General Data Protection Regulation (GDPR)** and the Data Protection Act 2018 (DPA) aim to strike a balance between the privacy rights of individuals and the ability of organisations to use personal information to conduct their business[331].
- The Data Protection Act defines UK law on the processing of data on identifiable, living people.
- It gives every living person, or their representative, the right to apply for access to their health records.

DATA PROTECTION OFFICER (DPO)

- The GDPR introduces the concept of a Data Protection Officer (DPO). The DPO's functions are set out in Art. 39 of the GDPR.
- These require the DPO to be involved on a day-to-day basis in data protection compliance and facilitating compliance through the implementation of tools such as data protection impact assessments, oversight of processing activities and additional subject rights processes.

DATA SUBJECT RIGHTS

- A data subject has certain rights conferred under the GDPR including:
  o Request access to his or her personal data
  o The right to be informed
  o The right to rectification
  o The right to erasure
  o The right to restrict processing
  o The right to data portability
  o The right to object
  o Rights in relation to automated decision making and profiling
- There are eight key principles that must be complied with when processing personal data:
  o Personal data should be processed fairly and lawfully.
  o Data should only be obtained for specified purposes and should not be further processed in a manner incompatible with these purposes.
  o Personal data should be adequate, relevant and not excessive in relation to the purposes for which they were collected.
  o Personal data should be accurate and where necessary kept up to date.
  o Personal data should not be kept longer than is needed for its intended purpose.
  o Personal data should be processed in accordance with the rights of the individual which the information concerns.

  o Appropriate measures should be taken against unauthorized or unlawful processing or destruction of personal data.
  o Personal data should not be transferred outside the European Economic Area.
- Applications for access to health records by the patient, or their representative, must be made **in writing or electronically to the Records Manager at the hospital, with the patient's signature.**
- A fee may be charged for the release of the information. Requests should be dealt with promptly, **within 21 days and no later than 40 days** after the request has been made.
- Access may be denied, or limited, where the information might cause serious harm to the physical or mental health, or condition of the patient, or any other person, or where giving access would disclose information relating to or provided by a third person who had not consented to the disclosure.

11. FREEDOM OF INFORMATION ACT 2000

- The Freedom of Information Act deals with access to official information and **gives individuals or organisations the right to request information from any public authority**[332].

- **Part I of the Act**
  o Anyone can make a request for information to any public authority providing it is **in writing, states the name and address of the enquirer,** and **describes the information requested.**
  o The authority has the duty to confirm or deny whether it holds the information, and if it does so, to supply it **within 20 working days from receipt of request**.
  o Authorities are not obliged to provide information where they cannot find it without assistance.

- **Part II of the Act**
  o Sets out exemptions where the right of access to information is not allowed or restricted.
  o These relate to issues such as national security, law enforcement, commercial interests, and data protection.

- Requests from someone about their personal information are dealt with under the **Data Protection Act (See Above).**

---

[331] *Data Protection Policy, **General Medical Council, 2018***

[332] *How to access information about what we do/**Ethical Guidance. General Medical Council***

II. CONSENT

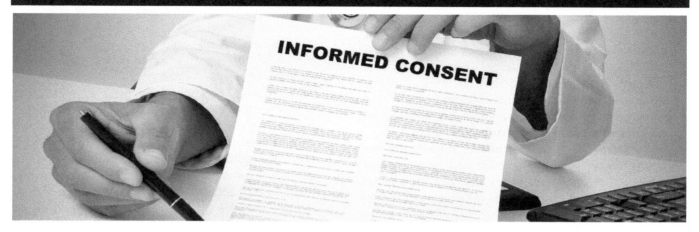

- **INTRODUCTION**
  - Consent is required for every examination, treatment, or intervention performed on a patient. **Consent may be explicit or implied**.
  - **Explicit consent** is when a patient actively agrees, either verbally or in writing.
  - **Implied consent** is signalled by the behaviour of an informed patient; for example, putting their arm out for a blood test.
  - There are exceptions where consent is not required, such as emergency treatment and where the law prescribes otherwise (e.g. mental health law).
  - There are only a few situations where written consent is legally required (e.g. the storage and use of gametes and embryos).
  - **Verbal consent is otherwise as valid as written consent**.
  - Consent forms do not prove valid consent they just provide some evidence that consent was obtained. Discussion with a patient regarding **consent should be documented in the notes** and state the purpose of the treatment, risks, benefits, and alternatives.

- **THE KEY PRINCIPLES FOR VALID CONSENT ARE:**
  - The patient must be competent.
  - The patient must be sufficiently informed to make a choice.
  - Consent must be given voluntarily.

- The GMC provides guidance on the type of information doctors should provide when gaining consent. This information includes:
  - The purpose of the investigation or treatment.
  - Details and uncertainties of the diagnosis. Options for treatment including the option not to treat.
  - Explanation of the likely benefits and probabilities of success for each option.
  - The risks such as known possible side effects, complications, and adverse outcomes, including where intervention or treatment may fail to improve a condition.
  - The name of the doctor with overall responsibility.
  - A reminder that the patient can change their mind.

- **WHO CAN GIVE CONSENT?**
  - The only person who can consent for a competent adult **is the patient themselves.**
  - **A young person of any age** can consent to treatment provided they are considered to be competent (**Gillick competent)** to make the decision.
  - **At the age of 16** there is a presumption that the patient is able to give valid consent.
  - However, **up to the age of 18 in England, Wales, and Northern Ireland, and age 16 in Scotland**, if the person is felt to lack capacity, a person with **parental responsibility** can give consent on behalf of the patient.
  - **A Lasting Power of Attorney** can consent on behalf of an adult patient once capacity is lost.

1. REFUSAL OF CONSENT

- Competent adult patients are entitled to refuse consent to treatment, even if doing so may result in permanent physical injury or death. The exception to this is where compulsory treatment is authorized by mental health legislation.
- Where the consequences of refusal are grave, it is important that the patient understands this.

- Doctors must respect a refusal of treatment if the patient is a competent adult, who is properly informed, and not being coerced.
- In England, Wales, and Northern Ireland, refusal of treatment by competent under-18s is not necessarily binding upon the doctors. The courts have ruled that patients under 18 have a right to consent to treatment, but not to refuse it if this would put their health in serious jeopardy.
- In such circumstances consent may be gained from an **adult with parental responsibility or a court**.
- **In Scotland**, it is likely that **neither parents nor the courts** are entitled to override a competent young patient's decision, although this has not been tested in the courts. Cases of refused consent are best discussed with senior medical staff, the hospital legal department, and/or medical defence societies.

2. CONSENT FOR EMERGENCY TREATMENT

- Consent should be sought for emergency treatment if the patient is competent.
- If consent cannot be obtained, medical treatment that is **in the patient's best interest**, and is immediately necessary to save life or avoid significant deterioration in the patient's health, should be provided.
- If the patient has appointed a **welfare attorney,** or there is a court-appointed deputy or guardian, this person, where practicable, must be consulted about treatment decisions.
- If the patient is **under 18 years old in England, Wales, and Northern Ireland**, or **under 16 in Scotland**, and unable to give consent due to lack of capacity or illness, **anyone with parental responsibility can provide consent.**
- If treatment is urgent and nobody with parental responsibility is available, treatment can proceed, without consent, **provided it is in the patient's best interest.**

3. REQUESTS FOR TREATMENT

- This case concerned a wide range of issues, most of which related to decision-making at the end of life.
- However, for the purposes of this guidance, the key point is the Court of Appeal's opinion that doctors are **under no legal or ethical obligation to agree to a patient's request** for treatment if they consider the treatment **is not in the patient's best interests.**

4. GILLICK COMPETENCE AND FRASER GUIDELINES

- Gillick competency and Fraser guidelines refer to a legal case which looked specifically at whether doctors should be able to give contraceptive advice or treatment to under 16-year-olds without parental consent.
- But since then, they have been more widely used to help assess whether a child has the maturity to make their own decisions and to understand the implications of those decisions.
- **The Fraser guidelines** refer to the guidelines set out by Lord Fraser in his judgment of the **Gillick** case in the House of Lords (1985), which apply specifically to contraceptive advice.
- Lord Fraser stated that a Doctor could proceed to give advice and treatment to a young person under the age of 16 if:
  o She had **sufficient maturity and intelligence** to understand the nature and implications of the proposed treatment,
  o She could **not be persuaded to tell her parents** or to allow her doctor to tell them,
  o She was **very likely to begin or continue having sexual intercourse** with or without contraceptive treatment,
  o Her **physical or mental health were likely to suffer** unless she received the advice or treatment,
  o The advice or treatment was in the **young person's best interests**.
- This case was specifically about contraceptive advice and treatment, but the case of Axon, R (on the application of) v Secretary of State for Health [2006] EWHC 37 (Admin) makes clear that the principles apply to decisions about treatment and care for sexually transmitted infections and abortion, too.
- As a result of this decision, a young person under 16 with capacity to make any relevant decision is often referred to as being **'Gillick competent'**.

Confidentiality source: GMC
http://www.gmc-uk.org/guidance/ethical_guidance

Consent and Capacity source: GMC
http://www.gmcuk.org/guidance/ethical_guidance/consent_guidance_common_law.asp

III. MENTAL CAPACITY

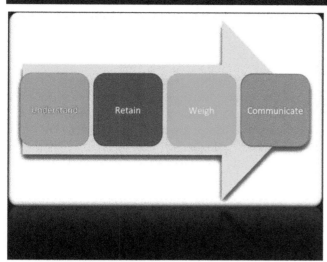

1. ASSESSING CAPACITY

- The Mental Capacity Act aims to protect people who lack capacity, and maximize their ability to make decisions. The Act came into full force in October 2007.
- The Act is underpinned by five statutory principles:
  - A person should be assumed to have capacity unless it is established that they lack capacity
  - A person should not be treated as lacking capacity unless all practical steps have been tried to enable capacity.
  - A person is allowed to make an unwise decision.
  - If a person lacks capacity then decisions should be made in their best interests.
  - Any decision made should be the least restrictive option.
- Patients should always be assumed to have capacity but if there is reason to believe a patient lacks capacity it should be assessed using the two-stage test:
  - Does the person have an impairment, or disturbance of the functioning, of their mind or brain?
  - Does the impairment or disturbance mean that the person is unable to make a specific decision when they need to?
- **A person lacks capacity** if they are unable to (any three will score a mark each): **"URUC"**
  - **U**nderstand the information relevant to the decision
  - **R**etain the information
  - **U**se or weigh the information
  - **C**ommunicate the decision (by any means)

2. ADVANCE DIRECTIVES AND CAPACITY

- **WHAT IS AN ADVANCE DECISION?**
  - An advanced decision (**'living will'**) allows an adult (over 18 years) with capacity to state how they wish to be treated if they suffer a loss of capacity.
  - Advanced decisions usually relate to the refusal of medical treatment but can be statements authorizing or requesting certain procedures or treatments. Advanced refusals of treatment are legally binding; however, advanced request or authorizations are not, but should be taken into account when assessing best interests. Valid and applicable advance decision to refuse treatment must be specific to the treatment in question.
  - It has the same force as a contemporaneous decision.
  - A Lasting Power of Attorney appointed before the advanced decision cannot overrule it, nor can the Court of Protection.
  - The refused treatments **must all be named in the advance decision**.
  - Patient may want to refuse a treatment in some situations, but not others. If this is the case, he/she needs to be clear about all the circumstances in which he/she wants to refuse this treatment. Patient can refuse a treatment that could potentially keep him/her alive (known as life-sustaining treatment). This includes treatments such as **ventilation and cardio- pulmonary resuscitation (CPR)**.
  - An advance decision is not the same as an **advance statement**.
  - Deciding to refuse a treatment is not the same as asking someone to end life or to help end your life; **Euthanasia and assisted suicide** are illegal under English law.

- **WHO MAKES AN ADVANCE DECISION?**
  - Patient makes the advance decision, as long as he/she has the mental capacity to make such decisions.
  - Patient may want to make an advance decision with the support of a clinician.
  - A decision to refuse life-sustaining treatment in the future needs to be:
    - Written down
    - Signed by the Patient
    - Signed by a witness

o If Patient wishes to refuse life-sustaining treatments in circumstances where he/she might die as a result, he/she needs to state this clearly in the advance decision.

- **IS AN ADVANCE DECISION LEGALLY BINDING?**
  o Yes, it is, as long as it:
    - Complies with the **Mental Capacity Act**
    - Is valid
    - Applies to the situation
  o If the advance decision is binding, it takes the place of decisions made in the patient's best interest by other people.
  o **AN ADVANCE DECISION MAY ONLY BE CONSIDERED VALID IF:**
    - The advanced decision must have been made by the patient when they were an adult (over 18), had capacity, and were properly informed.
    - The statement should specify precisely what treatment is to be refused and the circumstances in which the refusals should apply. The advanced decision will only apply once the patient lacks capacity to consent to or refuse treatment.
    - An advanced decision that relates to the refusal of life-sustaining treatments must be written, signed, and witnessed. The patient must acknowledge in the written decision that they intend to refuse treatment, even though this puts their life at risk.
  o **AN ADVANCED DECISION MAY BE INVALID IF:**
    - The decision was withdrawn while the person had capacity.
    - After the advance decision was made, a Lasting Power of Attorney was appointed and given express authority to make the treatment decisions covered by the advanced decision.
    - The person has done something that clearly goes against the advanced decision, which suggests they have changed their mind.

- If the possibility of an advanced decision is raised for a patient who currently lacks capacity, reasonable efforts must be made to find out the details of the decision. This may involve contacting the **patient's GP, looking at the hospital medical notes, and discussions with the patient's relatives**. If emergency treatment is required, this should not be delayed to look for an advanced decision **if there is no indication that one exists.**

- **If there is an indication that one exists**, the validity and applicability should be assessed and the decision adhered to, if valid.
- If the advanced decision is not valid or applicable, the treatment given **should be in the patient's best interest.**
- Advanced decisions can be overruled if the patient is being treated compulsorily under mental health legislation. However, a valid and applicable advanced refusal of treatment for conditions that are not covered by the compulsory powers of the legislation must be adhered to.

- **HOW DOES AN ADVANCE DECISION HELP?**
  o As long as it is valid and applies to the situation, an advance decision gives the health and social care team clinical and legal instructions about the patient's treatment choices.
  o An advance decision will only be used if, at some time in the future, the patient is not able to make his/her own decisions about the treatment.

- **DOES IT NEED TO BE SIGNED AND WITNESSED?**
  o **Yes, it does,** if choosed to refuse life-sustaining treatment – in which case, the advance decision must be written down, and both the patient and a witness must sign it.
  o Patient must also include a statement that the advance decision applies even if his/her life is at risk.

- **WHO SHOULD SEE IT?**
  o Patient has the final say on who sees it, but he/she should make sure that the family, carers, or health and social care professionals know about it, and know where to find it.
  o A copy can be kept in the medical records.

3. LASTING POWER OF ATTORNEY

- The Mental Capacity Act allows people over 18 years of age, who have capacity, to appoint a Lasting Power of Attorney (LPA).
- The person making the LPA is referred to as the **'Donor'.**
- A LPA can be appointed to make decisions on health and personal welfare, and/or property and financial affairs on behalf of the donor should they lose capacity in the future.
- The LPA is bound by the principles set out in the Mental Capacity Act and must make decisions in the donor's best interest.

- **A valid LPA requires** a signed certificate completed by an independent third party, which confirms that the donor understands the scope and purpose of the LPA and was not put under any pressure to make the LPA.
- The LPA must be registered with the Office of the Public Guardian. A personal welfare LPA can make healthcare decisions for the donor once they lack capacity and can consent on their behalf to treatment and social care decisions. There are specific situations when the LPA cannot consent to or refuse treatment:
  o When the donor has capacity to consent.
  o When the donor has made an advanced decision to refuse treatment (unless the LPA was appointed after the advanced decision and the donor gave permission to the LPA to refuse treatment).
  o When the decision relates to life-sustaining treatment and this has not been expressly authorised in the LPA.
  o When the donor is detained under the Mental Health Act.
- An LPA does not have the power to demand specific treatments if they are not felt to be necessary or appropriate. All LPAs are registered with the Office of the Public Guardian, who can confirm whether a patient has a LPA or not. If the medical team and LPA disagree on the best treatment for the patient, the case can be referred **to the Court of Protection**.
- Whilst a decision is reached the patient can be treated to prevent serious deterioration.

4. COURT OF PROTECTION
- The role of the Court of Protection is **to protect individuals who lack capacity** and **make difficult decisions about their care and welfare**.
- The Court of Protection can:
  o Determine whether an LPA is valid or not.
  o Give directions about using an LPA.
  o Remove an LPA.
  o Settle disputes over healthcare and treatment of a person lacking capacity.

5. INDEPENDENT MEDICAL CAPACITY ADVOCATES (IMCA)
- The role of an **IMCA** is to **support and represent a person who lacks capacity** in making a specific decision, who has no-one (other than paid carers) to support them.
- The IMCA:

  o Provides support for the person who lacks capacity.
  o Represents the person without capacity in discussions about proposed treatment.
  o Provides information to work out what is in a person's best interest.
  o Questions or challenges decisions that they believe are not in the best interests of the person lacking capacity.
  o Presents individuals' views and interests to the decision-maker.
- **The IMCA is not the decision-maker** and **cannot consent on behalf of the person** but the information and views expressed by the IMCA must be taken into account.
- An IMCA must be involved in decisions relating to providing, withholding, or stopping serious medical treatment. In an emergency situation, it is unlikely that there is time to instruct an IMCA so the patient should be treated according to best interest principles and any decisions clearly documented. If the IMCA disagrees with the proposed treatment and further discussion does not resolve this then the IMCA may use the formal complaints system to settle the case, or in more urgent cases, refer to the Court of Protection for a decision.

6. BEST INTERESTS
- The Mental Capacity Act states that any act done or decision made on behalf of a person who lacks capacity must be in their best interests.
- The Act sets out the factors that should be considered when deciding what is in a person's best interests:
  o Past and present wishes and feelings.
  o Beliefs and values that may have influenced the decision being made, if the person had capacity.
  o Other factors the patient would be likely to consider if they had capacity.
- In trying to assess the person's best interests you should:
  o Encourage the person who lacks capacity to participate in the decision. Avoid discrimination.
  o Try to identify all the issues most relevant to the person and to the decision being made.
  o If possible, defer the decision if the patient is likely to regain capacity.

Confidentiality source: GMC
http://www.gmc-uk.org/guidance/ethical_guidance
Consent and Capacity source: GMC
http://www.gmcuk.org/guidance/ethical_guidance/consent_guidance_common_law.asp

3. End of Lifecare in Elderly

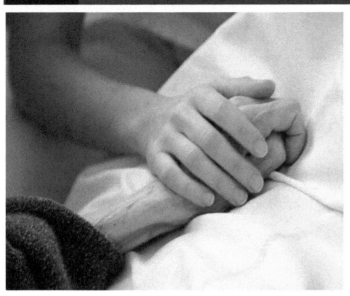

INTRODUCTION

- Dealing with patients who are near death or who have died is challenging. There may be difficult ethical decisions to make regarding resuscitation and inappropriate escalation of treatment and institution of palliative care. Many deaths in the Emergency Department are in tragic circumstances.
- After a death, the care given to the patient's family has a major influence on how they grieve.
- Achieving a dignified death for all patients who die in the ED should be a principal aim for ED clinicians, and can be a rewarding experience for all involved in caring for the patient and family.
- The National End of Life Care Strategy launched in 2008 aims to improve recognition of patients nearing death and to provide better palliative care in an appropriate setting.
- The number of people now dying at home has risen to 42.4%4, however between 56-78% of people wish to die at home.
- All ED doctors and nurses should receive regular training in all aspects of end of life care, communication, ethics, symptom control and caring for relatives.
- ED teams would benefit from fostering links with local palliative care services to help with training and improve services[333].

1. PATIENTS WHO ARE JUDGED TO BE DYING

MAKING END OF LIFE DECISIONS WITH PATIENTS – PRINCIPLES[334]

- We should start from a presumption of prolonging life and not hastening death. However, we should recognise that alleviating suffering is sometimes a more appropriate goal. In an emergency, the best treatment option gives most overall benefit and is least restrictive of the patient's future choices.
- Patients and their families should be involved with making decisions about their care wherever possible and appropriate.
- Patients who are vulnerable, have learning difficulties or cognitive impairment sometimes receive a poorer standard of end of life care.
- Staff should pay particular attention to how they communicate with these patients, and try to understand non-verbal cues if the patient is unable to talk. Emergency physicians should be familiar with assessing capacity and applying the principles of the Mental Capacity Act.

ADVANCE CARE PLANNING[335]

- The National End of Life Care Strategy encourages clinicians to make care plans for patients identified to be at the end of life (from whatever cause).
- Emergency Department staff may not be in a position to make those future plans, but can often identify patients coming to the end of their life.
- Patients may confide in us what care they do or do not want, and in particular where they want to be cared for. Patients should where possible be asked whether they have made any advanced care plans with their GP or specialist and whether these plans apply to the situation they are currently in.
- Access to documented end of life care plans varies around the country. Some departments have access to the patient's summary care record or electronic palliative care co-ordination systems (EPaCCS). It is recommended that EDs work with inpatient specialties and commissioners to be able to access these records. Any discussions we have with patients regarding future care, which could assist with end of life care planning, should be clearly documented and communicated to the patient's GP, care home and/or admitting team.

333 *End of Life Care for Adults in the Emergency Department, RCEM pdf - (March 2015)*

334 *End of Life Care for Adults in the Emergency Department, RCEM pdf - (March 2015)*

335 *End of Life Care for Adults in the Emergency Department, RCEM pdf - (March 2015)*

DISCHARGING END OF LIFE CARE PATIENTS HOME FROM THE ED[336]

- Discharging dying patients from the ED may be appropriate and is best practice if an appropriate care plan can be initiated and continued at home.
- A rapid discharge pathway is ideal where equipment, care and prescriptions can be accessed quickly.
- For example, if arranging patient transport is proving problematic, use of a private ambulance to facilitate transfer home may be appropriate.
- This may require access to medication to palliate symptoms, e.g. diamorphine, midazolam etc and in some cases syringe drivers which community nurses can use. In order for community nurses to administer the medication a community prescription form may be needed. The patient's regular medications should be reviewed before discharge in order to stop unnecessary medication taking.
- Copies of a discharge letter should be given to the family, care homes and the GP.
- The Emergency Department should be involved in the planning and organisation of services to enable patients to be discharged for care at home.

END OF LIFE CARE DISCUSSIONS IN ED[337]

- A senior named ED clinician should be involved with and responsible for every end of life care patient.
- This will usually be the ED Consultant but may be an ST4 or above out of hours, who should discuss such patients with their Consultant by phone as a minimum.
- When a patient is clearly dying, try to gauge the extent to which the patient and relatives want to be involved in treatment decisions.
- Involve the patient and their family as much as possible, in discussions about their care.
- Use the principles of breaking bad news outlined below.
- Remember that family have no legal right to make decisions on behalf of their relative unless they have an enduring right of attorney (for health decisions) and are registered with the office of the public guardian.
- However, where appropriate we should aim to involve family members in discussions, acknowledging their role and concerns.
- Family members are often able to tell us what their relative's wishes were in situations when the patient lacks capacity, helping a decision to be made in the patients **'best interests'.**

- If a patient who is dying has no capacity or means of expressing their opinions and has no family or friends to represent them, then an independent advocate should be sought.
- This may be a formal Independent Mental Capacity Advocate (IMCA) under the capacity act in England and Wales or more likely a chaplain or volunteer not directly involved in their care.
- In an emergency, the ED doctor is the most appropriate person to be able to take decisions in the patient's best interests.
- Document all discussions with patients and their family clearly in the patient's notes.
- Patients, as well as family, should be offered spiritual support from the hospital Chaplaincy or their own religious leader.
- Discuss the need for hydration and nutrition with the patient and their family.
- Usually intravenous (IV) hydration is not required but may occasionally make a patient more comfortable.

DO NOT ATTEMPT CARDIO-PULMONARY RESUSCITATION DECISIONS WITHIN THE ED[338]

- A DNACPR decision should be instituted if the patient wishes or a senior clinician, after appropriate consideration and discussion, feels that chest compression following a cardiac arrest would be futile or lead to unacceptable outcomes as a result of the patient's presenting condition or pre-existing co-morbidities.
- A DNACPR decision should always be discussed with the patient if they have capacity, unless it is felt that the discussion may cause physical or psychological harm, or unless the patient indicates that they do not want to be involved in treatment decisions.
- A concern that the discussion may cause distress alone is not sufficient grounds for not discussing the decision, 10. However, in some cases a discussion such as this will cause psychological harm particularly if the patient is very unwell, so a senior ED doctor should exercise careful judgement.
- DNACPR decisions should be discussed with a patient's family wherever possible. Discussions with patient and family should be clearly documented and if a decision is taken not to discuss a decision for DNACPR with a patient, the reasons should be clearly documented.
- A decision of DNACPR should be made by a senior doctor and in difficult circumstances should be shared with other senior colleagues.

---

336 *End of Life Care for Adults in the Emergency Department, RCEM pdf - (March 2015)*

337 *End of Life Care for Adults in the Emergency Department, RCEM pdf - (March 2015)*

338 *End of Life Care for Adults in the Emergency Department, RCEM pdf - (March 2015)*

- Advice from the trust legal team or medical defence organisation may be sought in very difficult circumstances. The final decision on whether a patient should receive CPR in the event of an arrest rests with the senior clinician. A patient cannot demand CPR if the treating clinician thinks the treatment is futile, however it is recommended that the patient is offered a second opinion.
- Some patients now come to hospital with a community DNACPR order. It is recommended that this is briefly reviewed to check that circumstances have not changed before converting this to a hospital DNACPR document. Some regions have multi-signatory, community-wide DNACPR orders which are valid for the emergency department. Patients nearing end of life should have a resuscitation decision made before leaving the ED.
- Resuscitation decisions made in the Emergency Department should be a trigger for the ED team to consider other aspects of care. Avoiding further escalation of treatment may be appropriate
- There is evidence that a DNACPR order can limit the care given to a patient. Therefore, it is important that a statement about what active care the patient is to have is also included, where appropriate. The Universal Form of Treatment Options (UFTO) is recommended as a tool to improve decision making and documentation.
- Uncommonly some patients with a DNACPR order may develop potentially reversible events such as a blocked tracheostomy tube, anaphylaxis or choking where resuscitation techniques would be appropriate while the reversible cause is treated.

ADVANCED DECISIONS REFUSING TREATMENT[339]

- If a patient has an advance directive an assessment should be made, by a clinician, of its applicability to the patient's current situation.
- **An advance directive is legally binding under the Mental Capacity Act (2005) in England and Wales if:**
  - The patient was over 18 and had capacity when it was made.
  - It is in writing, is signed and is witnessed.
  - It includes a statement 'even if life is at risk'.

- **An advance directive is not valid if:**
  - The patient was under undue influence at the time it was made.
  - The patient has since acted in a way that is inconsistent with its terms.
  - The patient has appointed a lasting power of attorney since the directive was made.

- An advanced directive in Scotland and Northern Ireland is not covered by statute but is likely to be binding under common law if the above criteria are met.
- In Scotland the patient can be 16 years or older.

COMMENCING PALLIATIVE CARE[340]

- Palliative care in hospitals has been identified as being variable in quality and lags behind hospice care and care at home.
- We should do our utmost to give good care.
- End of life patients should be made as comfortable as possible by requesting an air mattress or similar bed and turning the patient regularly if they are unable to do so themselves.
- End of life care should be tailored to the patient and their condition. The patient's current symptoms should be reviewed and adequate and appropriate medications prescribed for management of distressing symptom.
- Each intervention and likely side effects should be explained to the patient and family where possible.
- Use the minimum dose of medication to make the patient comfortable. Access palliative care support whenever necessary as these teams can provide valuable expertise and support.
- Decide on and document what hydration and nutrition are appropriate. Continue to offer regular drinks; or mouth care if the patient is unable to swallow. The patient's family may wish to participate in caring for their dying relative, if so, they should be helped by staff to do so.
- An end of life care checklist can be helpful in the ED as there are many facets to patient care. However, it should not be regarded as a prescription for care. All interventions and conversations should be documented.
- This may be in the ED notes or may be in specific end of life care documentation.

2. AFTER SUDDEN OR EXPECTED DEATH IN ED
2.1. BREAKING BAD NEWS[341]

- Breaking bad news should be carried out by the most experienced clinician available who knows the patient. The doctor should be sensitive of religious, cultural or other needs of the family.
- A good starting point is to find out what the family already know about the patient's current condition.
- Bad news should be communicated in a timely and sensitive way, avoiding **euphemisms and jargon.**

[339] *End of Life Care for Adults in the Emergency Department, RCEM pdf - (March 2015)*

[340] *End of Life Care for Adults in the Emergency Department, RCEM pdf - (March 2015)*

[341] *End of Life Care for Adults in the Emergency Department, RCEM pdf - (March 2015)*

- Listening is as important as talking when breaking bad news. A nurse should accompany the doctor when breaking bad news in order to support the family.

2.2. PROCEDURES NEAR AND AFTER DEATH [342]

- ED staff should refer all patients who are expected to die, and who are intubated and ventilated, to their local Specialist Nurse in Organ Donation (SNOD).
- Referral to the SNOD should be as early as possible as they can offer valuable support and guidance for the team and family. The SNOD will assess patient suitability for organ donation and approach the patient's next of kin for consent, if appropriate.
- Kidney donation from non-heart beating donors (now classified as 'donor after cardiac death') has been shown to have good outcomes even when the donor is elderly.
- Donors after brain death require brain stem death testing which is not usually carried out in the ED.
- Tissue (e.g. corneas and heart valves) can be retrieved up to 24 hrs after death. For tissue donation, referrals should be made via the National Referral Centre on: 0800 4320559.
- This service co-ordinates consent from family and tissue retrieval. The process of referral to the coroner varies between regions in the UK. Local policy should be followed.
- Hospitals should have guidelines on laying out the body. It is good practice to offer relatives the opportunity to take part in this taking into account religious and/or cultural practices.
- After a patient's death, departments should have an agreed process for informing the patient's GP and other professionals involved in the patient's care. This should occur within one working day.
- Departments could use an after-death checklist to ensure all tasks are completed. It is good practice to make arrangements for a doctor who can complete the death certificate and/or cremation form to be contactable the next working day by, for example, writing in the notes who can be contacted and how. This reduces delays for distressed families.

2.3. THE IDEAL ENVIRONMENT FOR THE PATIENT AND FAMILY [343]

- The Emergency Department can be a difficult place to care for the bereaved family, however every effort should be made to provide excellent care.

- All departments should have a relative's room to accommodate several family members that is close to the resuscitation room.
- The room should be private and ideally sound-proof.
- It should contain comfortable chairs and sofas, tissues and a telephone with direct dial access. Hot and cold drinks should be available. Access to outside space is valuable for patients and their families.
- A patient receiving palliative care should be cared for in a quiet room with space to accommodate family.
- Every patient and family should have access to a space that allows their cultural and spiritual needs to be met.
- A separate viewing room for family to see the body is valuable.
- Alternatively, the mortuary chapel of rest may be used.

2.4. CARE OF BEREAVED RELATIVES [344]

- A nurse should be assigned to care for and support the family both whilst the patient is being looked after in their last hours and after death.
- Clinicians may choose to book relatives as patients in order to extend the care they can give to them.
- Family should be offered spiritual support in the form of the hospital chaplain or other religious officers.
- Written information should be given to the family to guide them through obtaining a death certificate, coroner's processes and undertaker's arrangements.
- It is good practice to provide follow up for the relatives of a deceased patient. A letter of condolence to the family after the event is appreciated.
- Departments should consider giving the name and telephone number of a Consultant that relatives can contact at a later date.
- Providing the family with an appointment a few weeks after the death to discuss the events has been shown to help families with their grieving process.

2.5. STAFF SUPPORT [345]

- After every death or incident staff should be encouraged to talk together about the event.
- In many cases a formal debrief can be valuable.
- Further support should be available to staff through their supervisor or from occupational health.

---

[342] *End of Life Care for Adults in the Emergency Department, RCEM pdf - (March 2015)*

[343] *End of Life Care for Adults in the Emergency Department, RCEM pdf - (March 2015)*

[344] *End of Life Care for Adults in the Emergency Department, RCEM pdf - (March 2015)*

[345] *End of Life Care for Adults in the Emergency Department, RCEM pdf - (March 2015)*

4. Reporting Death to a Coroner

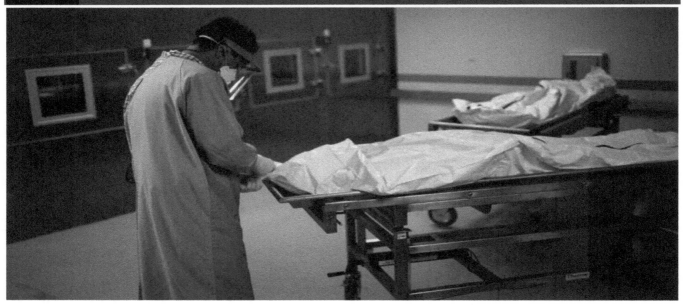

A Doctor may report the death to a coroner if the[346]:

- Cause of death is unknown
- Death was violent or unnatural
- Death was sudden and unexplained
- Person who died was not visited by a medical practitioner during their final illness
- Medical certificate is not available
- Person who died was not seen by the doctor who signed the medical certificate within 14 days before death or after they died
- Death occurred during an operation or before the person came out of anaesthetic
- Medical certificate suggests the death may have been caused by an industrial disease or industrial poisoning

The coroner may decide that the cause of death is clear. In this case:

1. The Doctor signs a medical certificate.
2. The family takes the medical certificate to the registrar.
3. The coroner issues a certificate to the registrar stating a post-mortem is not needed.

POST-MORTEMS

- The coroner may decide a post-mortem is needed to find out how the person died.
- This can be done either in a hospital or mortuary.

- One cannot object to a coroner's post-mortem - but if asked the coroner must tell (and the person's GP) when and where the examination will take place.

AFTER THE POST-MORTEM

- The coroner will release the body for a funeral once they have completed the post-mortem examinations and no further examinations are needed. If the body is released with no inquest, the coroner will send a form (**'Pink Form - form 100B'**) to the registrar stating the cause of death.
- The coroner will also send a **'Certificate of Coroner - form Cremation'** if the body is to be cremated.

- **If the coroner decides to hold an inquest**
- A coroner must hold an inquest if the cause of death is still unknown, or if the person:
  - Possibly died a violent or unnatural death
  - Died in prison or police custody
- One cannot register the death until after the inquest. The coroner is responsible for sending the relevant paperwork to the registrar.
- The death cannot be registered until after the inquest, but the coroner can give an interim death certificate to prove the person is dead.
- When the inquest is over the coroner will tell the registrar what to put in the register.

Article source: *https://www.gov.uk/after-a-death/when-a-death-is-reported-to-a-coroner*

---

[346] https://www.gov.uk/after-a-death/when-a-death-is-reported-to-a-coroner

INDEX

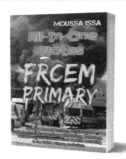
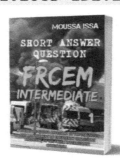
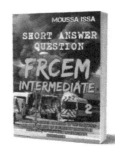
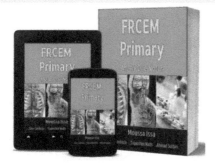
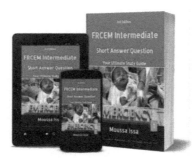
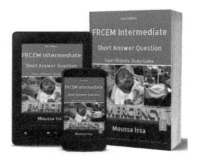
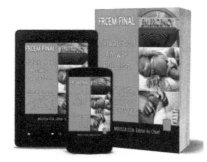
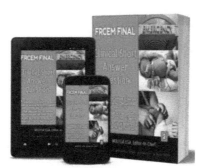
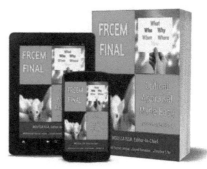
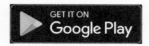
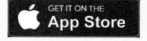

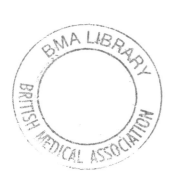
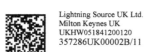

Lightning Source UK Ltd.
Milton Keynes UK
UKHW051841200120
357286UK00002B/11

9 781999 957582